Pig Health

Pig Health

JOHN CARR, BVSc, PhD, DPM, DiplECPHM, MRCVS

RCVS Recognised Specialist in Pig Medicine
James Cook University
Townsville, Australia

SHIH-PING CHEN, DVM, PhD

Principal Researcher
Agricultural Technology Research Institute
Taiwan

JOSEPH F. CONNOR, DVM, MS

Carthage Veterinary Service Ltd
Carthage
Illinois, USA

ROY KIRKWOOD, DVM, PhD, DiplECAR

Associate Professor Swine Production Medicine
University of Adelaide
Adelaide, Australia

JOAQUIM SEGALÉS, DVM, PhD, DiplECPHM, DiplECVP

European Specialist in Porcine Health Management
Researcher, Centre de Recerca en Sanitat Animal (IRTA)
Associate Professor, Veterinary School of the Universitat Autònoma de Barcelona
Barcelona, Spain

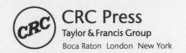

CRC Press
Taylor & Francis Group
Boca Raton London New York

CRC Press is an imprint of the
Taylor & Francis Group, an **informa** business

CRC Press
Taylor & Francis Group
6000 Broken Sound Parkway NW, Suite 300
Boca Raton, FL 33487-2742

First issued in paperback 2020

© 2018 by Taylor & Francis Group, LLC
CRC Press is an imprint of Taylor & Francis Group, an Informa business

No claim to original U.S. Government works

ISBN-13: 978-1-4987-0472-4 (hbk)
ISBN-13: 978-0-367-89340-8 (pbk)

Library of Congress Cataloging-in-Publication Data

Names: Carr, John, 1959- author. | Chen, Shih-Ping, author. | Connor, Joseph
F., author. | Kirkwood, R. N., author. |Segalés, Joaquim, author.
Title: Pig health / John Carr, Shih-Ping Chen, Joseph F. Connor, Roy
Kirkwood, Joaquim Segalés.
Description: Boca Raton : CRC Press, [2018]
Identifiers: LCCN 2017033138 (print) | LCCN 2017035547 (ebook) | ISBN
9781315157061 (eBook) | ISBN 9781498704724 (hardback : alk. paper)
Subjects: LCSH: Swine--Diseases. | MESH: Swine Diseases | Swine--physiology
Classification: LCC SF971 (ebook) | LCC SF971 .C27 2018 (print) | NLM SF 971
| DDC 636.4/0896--dc23
LC record available at https://lccn.loc.gov/2017033138

Visit the Taylor & Francis Web site at
http://www.taylorandfrancis.com

and the CRC Press Web site at
http://www.crcpress.com

CONTENTS

PREFACE

We introduce our book, *Pig Health*. The title was chosen specifically to reflect the fact that the veterinary profession needs to move away from disease management and towards health maintenance. Maintaining the health of our pigs is more difficult than just treating those few who become sick; it requires a holistic approach to veterinary care – a 360° veterinarian. We need to be promoting health rather than treating disease.

The pig represents many things to *Homo sapiens*. The importance of the pig to humans through the ages can be recognised by the Chinese word for home – a pig and a shelter: 家.

The pig provides over 40% of the meat protein eaten on this planet by people (**Figure A**). Therefore, nearly 3 billion people today and every day rely on the pig to provide them with food. It is vital that the veterinary profession continues to ensure that this vital meat protein source is healthy, nutritious, free from toxic residues and affordable. This book is directed towards the achievement of antibiotic-free farming for the majority of the pigs.

To children, the pig is a source of their future happiness through their piggy banks and the excellent films and cartoons introducing these fantastic animals to future generations of pig farmers and veterinarians. Pigs are also important as a companion animal. They are kept as loved pets by families in many parts of the world, and an increasing number are being used as sensory pets.

They can be ideal for children and adults with certain disabilities. The fact that the pig is relatively hairless makes them hypoallergenic. They do not jump and thus are less startling. That the pig and their companion can share identical feed makes them ideal.

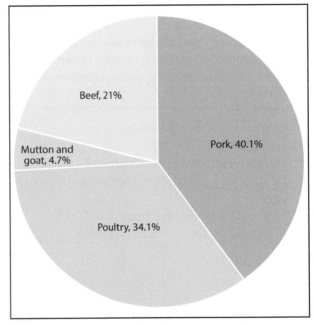

Fig. A **World meat and poultry consumption (adapted from U.S. Department of Agriculture data [2015]).**

Its sense of smell makes the pig a search animal, especially in the search for truffles. The pig is also a vital piece of the key for human medical research and potential xenotransplantation.

The fact that the pig is the most intelligent creature we farm creates its own unique opportunities for the pig veterinarian in managing the pig's mental health through toys and distractions. As the pig is a baseline artiodactyl (even-toed ungulates belonging to the Order Artiodactyla), understanding its biology can provide a great foundation for veterinarians dealing with animals of the Infraorder Ancodonta (hippos), Suborder Tylopoda (e.g. camels),

Order Cetacea (e.g. whales and dolphins) and the Suborder Ruminantia (e.g. giraffes).

Understanding the pig from a veterinary perspective provides students with the opportunity to appreciate:

- individual and population medicine;
- anatomy, physiology, pathology, microbiology and parasitology;
- animal husbandry;
- biosecurity;
- pharmacology and medicine management;
- economics and computer analysis systems;
- teaching, training, information transfer and web design;
- nutrition;
- genomics and metagenomics;
- transportation;
- slaughtering, meat processing and food health;
- farming on a global scale – hot and cold, wet and dry;
- entry into a global veterinary world, as illustrated by the authors' team work;

- and, most important, places the veterinarian right in the middle of the action as the spokesperson for the pig itself.

Animals are our passion; their health and welfare is our duty.
For:

> *I am fond of pigs.*
> *Dogs look up to us.*
> *Cats look down on us.*
> *Pigs treat us as equals!*
>
> Sir Winston Churchill
> *British politician (1874–1965)*

John Carr
Shih-Ping Chen
Joseph F. Connor
Roy Kirkwood
Joaquim Segalés

ACKNOWLEDGEMENTS

We are extremely grateful to our clients who allow us to treat and care for their pigs. Our clients and their pigs are the source of a great deal of practical knowledge which, combined with scientific questions, allowed for this book to be created.

We are also grateful to our friends and colleagues who have allowed us to use their photographs in this publication. Special thanks are offered to the members of the Swine and Wine group, Dr. Hyun-Sup Kim, Dr. Steve McCorist, Dr. Stan Done, Dr. Brad Thacker, Dr. Dachrit Nilubol and Dr. K.J. Yoon.

We also wish to thank all the members of the Taylor & Francis Editorial team and Peter Beynon in particular.

DEDICATION

We would like to dedicate this book to our parents.

Alan Stanley and Anne Carr

陳地火 and 陳蘇說

Glen Michael and Elizabeth Mary Connor

May and Arthur Cook

Jaume Segalés and Maria Coma

ACNV	automatically controlled natural ventilation	EU	European Union
AD	Aujeszky's disease	FA	fluorescent antibody (test)
ADG	average daily weight gain	FCR	feed conversion rate
ADV	Aujeszky's disease virus	FMD	foot-and-mouth disease
A/G	albumin/globulin (ratio)	FMDV	foot-and-mouth disease virus
AI	artificial insemination	FS	farrowing sows per batch
AIAO	all-in/all-out	FSH	follicle-stimulating hormone
ALP	alkaline phosphatase	GGT	gamma-glutamyl transferase
ALT	alanine aminotransferase	GnRH	gonadotropin-releasing hormone
APP	actinobacillus porcine pleuropneumonia	GPS	global positioning system
APPV	atypical porcine pestivirus	hCG	human chorionic gonadotropin
AR	atrophic rhinitis	H_2S	hydrogen sulphide
ASF	African swine fever	IgA	immunoglobulin A
ASFV	African swine fever virus	IgG	immunoglobulin G
AST	aspartate aminotransferase	IGF	insulin-like growth factor
AV	atrioventricular	IgM	immunoglobulin M
BF	breeding females per batch	IHC	immunohistochemistry
BVDV	bovine viral diarrhoea virus	IM	intramuscular
$CaCO_3$	calcium carbonate	ISH	in situ hybridisation
CFT	complement fixation test	IU	International unit
CK	creatine kinase	IV	intravenous
CNS	central nervous system	JE	Japanese encephalitis
CO	carbon monoxide	JEV	Japanese encephalitis virus
CO_2	carbon dioxide	kPa	kilopascal
COSHH	Control of Substances Hazardous to Health	LCT	lower critical temperature
		LDH	lactic acid dehydrogenase
CRI	constant rate infusion	LH	luteinising hormone
CSF	classical swine fever	MAC	*Mycobacteium avium* complex
CSFV	classical swine fever virus	MgO	magnesium oxide
CT	congenital tremor	MJ	millijoule
DIVA	differentiating infected from vaccinated animals	MLV	modified live vaccine
		MRP	maternal recognition of pregnancy
eCG	equine chorionic gonadotropin	MRSA	methicillin resistant *Staphylococcus aureus*
ECF	eosinophilic chemotactic cytokine		
EDTA	ethylenediamine tetra-acetic acid	NaCl	sodium chloride
ELISA	enzyme-linked immunosorbent assay	NAD	nicotinamide adenine dinucleotide
EP	enzootic (mycoplasma) pneumonia	NE	net energy
		NH_3	ammonia

NH$_4$	ammonium	PRRSV	porcine reproductive and respiratory syndrome virus
NIP	not in pig	PRV	pseudorabies virus
NSAID	non-steroidal anti-inflammatory drug	PSS	porcine stress syndrome
OCD	osteochondrosis dissecans	qPCR	quantitative polymerase chain reaction
OIE	World Organisation for Animal Health (Office International des Epizooties)	RH	relative humidity
		RT-PCR	reverse transcriptase polymerase chain reaction
ORF	open reading frame		
PAR	progressive atrophic rhinitis	SC	subcutaneous
PCMV	porcine cytomegalovirus	SD	standard deviation
PCR	polymerase chain reaction	SI	swine influenza
PCV2	porcine circovirus type 2	SIV	swine influenza virus
PCV2-RD	porcine circovirus type 2-reproductive disease	SMEDI	stillbirths, mummified, embryonic death and infertility
PCV2-SD	porcine circovirus type 2-systemic disease	SOP	standard operating procedure
		SVA	senecavirus A
PDNS	porcine dermatitis and nephropathy syndrome	SVD	swine vesicular disease
		TDS	total dissolved solids
PED	porcine epidemic diarrhoea	TGE	transmissible gastroenteritis
PEDV	porcine epidemic diarrhoea virus	TGEV	transmissible gastroenteritis virus
PEV	porcine teschovirus	TGF	transforming growth factor
PGF$_{2\alpha}$	prostaglandin F2 alpha	UCT	upper critical temperature
PHEV	porcine haemagglutinating encephalomyelitis virus	UK	United Kingdom
		USA	United States of America
PFTS	periweaning failure-to-thrive syndrome	UTJ	uterotubal junction
PG	prostaglandin	VE	vesicular exanthema
PIA	porcine intestinal adenomatosis	VEV	vesicular exanthema virus
PMWS	post-weaning multisystemic wasting syndrome	VS	vesicular stomatitis
		VSV	vesicular stomatitis virus
PO$_4$	phosphate	WB	numbers weaned per batch
ppm	parts per million	WSI	wean-to-service interval (WEI, wean-to estrus interval, in USA)
PPV	porcine parvovirus		
PR	pseudorabies		
PRCV	porcine respiratory coronavirus	ZnO	zinc oxide
PRDC	porcine respiratory disease complex	ZnSO$_4$	zinc sulphate
PRRS	porcine reproductive and respiratory syndrome		

eRESOURCES

You can access the resources (video clips and audio files) that are referenced in the text and listed in Appendix 3 (see page 479) via the companion website that accompanies the print and ebook editions of this book by using the following link:

https://www.crcpress.com/9781498704724

It will take you to a webpage where you can click on Downloads/Updates to access the resources themselves. The resources are indicated in the text by coloured icons: green for video VIDEO and blue for audio AUDIO.

The appendix not only lists the resources that can be found on the website but also gives clinical cases for you to review. The video cases will allow you to perform assessments of pig health and review normal pigs at various stages of production. The audio files are designed to strengthen your sense of hearing when making a clinical diagnosis.

CLINICAL EXAMINATION

'All groups are composed of individuals'

In order to carry out an examination of a pig it is important for the veterinarian to understand the normal behaviour, posture, vocalisation and alarm postures. Knowing the normal is necessary in order to be able to recognise the abnormal.

EXAMINATION OF THE PIG ALONE OR IN A GROUP

Introduction ▶ VIDEOS 1–5

In general practice, a detailed individual examination of a pig is rarely performed. It is, however, essential that you know the basics. All groups of pigs are made up of individuals and if you think that the problem is novel, a thorough examination from nose to tail is still required. To perform a clinical examination, it is important to follow a set procedure. Remember, more is missed from not looking than from not knowing. It will prove very useful to train with one or two colleagues. Verbally describing to each other what you are doing trains your mind in the required sequence.

Taking a history and making a start

It is essential to ask appropriate questions and then to wait and listen to answers given by the client. Watch the client's face to check for answers that may be difficult. Sometimes, if the client has missed something, they may not want to admit to making a mistake.

Talk to the client and consider the following line of enquiry (*Table 1.1*). History taking will continue after entering the building/room/pen and while examining the pigs as a group or as individuals.

- Prior to entry into the room (**Figures 1.1–1.3.**)
- Quietly enter the room. ▶ AUDIOS 1–6
- Listen. Quietly listen to the pigs for any change in normal pig noises. Of course, you need to know what are normal pig noises. This can only be achieved by spending time with pigs and observing them under normal non-stressed conditions. Recognising normal pig chatter

Table 1.1 **Outline of taking a history.**	
Number of pigs	Is the problem affecting a group or an individual only?
What has the client seen?	Is the pig eating, defecating, urinating, coughing, sneezing, lame or dying?
Severity of the problem?	How many are sick (morbidity) or dead (mortality)?
Location of the problem?	Which pens or age groups are affected?
When did the problem start?	Time, date, place?
How is the problem progressing?	Are more pigs getting sick within the group?
More than one problem?	How many different problems in same group?
Epidemiological consideration?	Has the problem spread to other groups?
Are there any other factors?	Factors that the client thinks are relevant to the situation?
What has the client done?	Action to alleviate the problem? What was the result of the action?

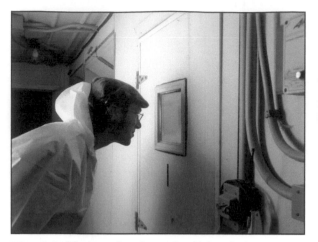

Fig. 1.1 Observe pigs through window before entering the room.

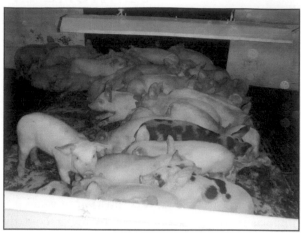

Fig. 1.2 Examine the pigs sleeping patterns and their defecation patterns.

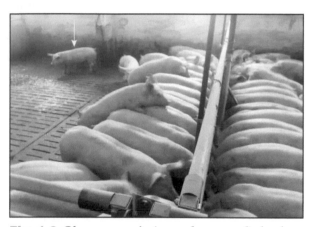

Fig. 1.3 Observe any pig (example arrowed) that has moved away from the group, especially during feeding.

is an important clinical process. In cases of *Actinobacillus pleuropneumoniae* infection or swine influenza there could be less noise. There could be more sneezing in cases of swine influenza or more coughing in cases of *Mycoplasma hyopneumoniae* infection.

- Smell. Is there a change in the smell of the room? A dead pig can be noticed first by the smell in the room. Diarrhoea, especially associated with classical swine fever, may have a particularly potent smell.
- Observe the animals. Type of animals affected with the clinical problem; are there any dead pigs in the pen? Note if the affected pigs are male, female or castrated animals.

EXAMINATION OF AN INDIVIDUAL PIG

Make contact both vocally and physically. Assess the body condition using a 1 to 5 scoring system (*Table 1.2*). In adult sows, using a backfat meter at the P2 measurement position may be useful.

Assess the weight of the pig and check that it is appropriate for its age. Commercial Large White/Landrace gilts are bred around 140 kg at 240 days of age. The sows will be approximately 200 to 250 kg depending on age. The boars will be approximately 300 to 400 kg depending on age.

Condition scoring can be easily taught on farms using a condition caliper, which allows a gradation of body condition (**Figure 1.5**). A change in an individual can then be assessed by using the caliper and photographing the results over time.

The expected growth rate of normal pigs is shown in **Figure 1.6**. Target growth rates of commercial pigs are shown in *Table 1.3*. The changes in shape of the pig as it grows should be noted. Boars will develop very large shoulders with very thick skin (**Figure 1.7**); this is normal.

The canines of pigs over 6 months of age will protrude beyond the mouth (**Figure 1.8**). In the male, these canines will continue to grow and the boar will spend many hours a day sharpening them into formidable weapons, which are dangerous. These tusks can grow back into the face and require removal using a Gigli wire to the gum level (**Figure 1.9**).

Table 1.2 **Scoring system (Figure 1.4).**

SCORE NUMBER	CONDITION	DESCRIPTION	SHAPE OF BODY
1	Emaciated	Hips and backbone visible (**1.4a**)	Bone structure apparent (ribs and backbone)
2	Thin	Hips and backbone noticeable and easily felt (**1.4b**)	Ribs and spine can be felt
2.5	Somewhat thin	Hips and backbone felt without palm pressure	Tube shaped but flat (slab) sides
3	Normal	Hips and backbone only felt with firm palm pressure (**1.4c**)	Tube shaped
3.5	Good condition	Hips and backbone only felt with difficulty	Tube shaped
4	Fat	Hips and backbone cannot be felt (**1.4d**)	Tending to bulge
5	Overfat	Hips and backbone heavily covered (**1.4e**)	Bulbous

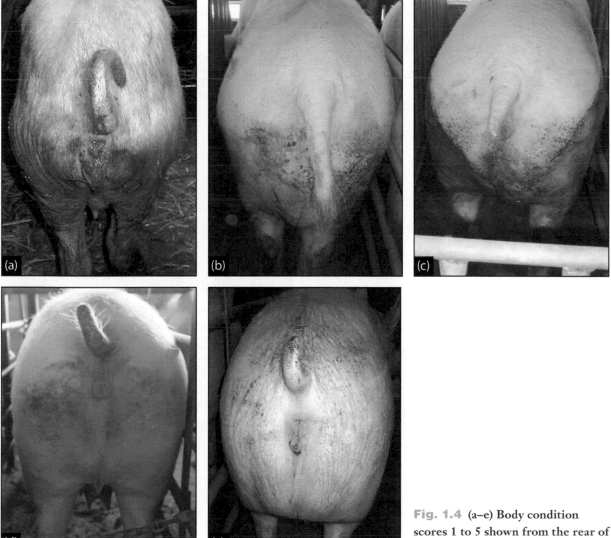

(a)   (b)   (c)

(d)   (e)

Fig. 1.4 (a–e) Body condition scores 1 to 5 shown from the rear of the pig. ▶ VIDEO 6

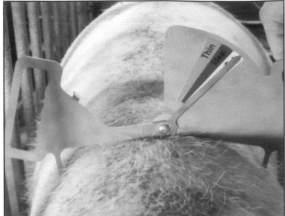

Fig. 1.5 Condition scoring of a sow using a caliper.

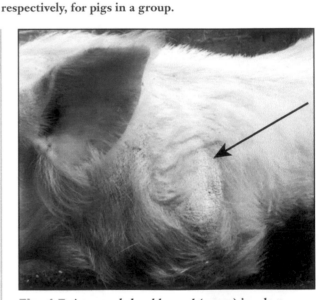

Fig. 1.6 Graph illustrating the expected growth curve of commercial pigs. The red and green lines represent the upper and lower expected rates of growth, respectively, for pigs in a group.

Table 1.3 **Age of the pig and target growth rate of commercial pigs.**			

AGE OF THE PIG		**DAILY LIVEWEIGHT**	
WEEKS	**DAYS**	**GAIN (g/day)**	**WEIGHT (kg)**
4	28	215	7.0
6	42	395	12.5
8	56	630	21.3
10	70	660	30.5
12	84	715	40.5
14	98	800	51.5
16	112	965	65.0
18	126	1,000	80.0
20	140	1,100	95.0
22	154	1,100	110.0

Fig. 1.7 A normal shoulder pad (arrow) in a boar older than 3 years of age.

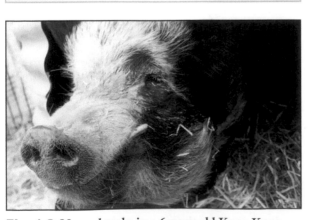

Fig. 1.8 Normal tusks in a 6-year-old Kune Kune.

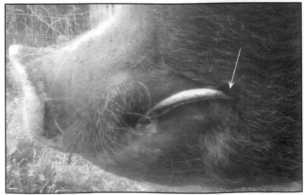

Fig. 1.9 Tusks may grow back into the face.

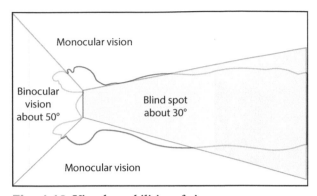

Fig. 1.10 Visual capabilities of pigs.

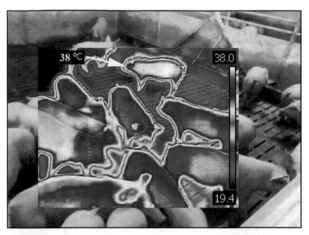

Fig. 1.11 Infrared technology makes identification of a pig with a higher temperature in a group possible. The pig arrowed is hotter (white) than the other pigs in the group (red) and warrants further investigation.

Pigs will generally try and face you as they are more vulnerable when approached from behind (**Figure 1.10**). The stockperson should stand about 60° behind the head, with the result that when moving forward the pig will move forward as well.

Check the breathing rate, which should be less than 20 breaths per minute for sows and boars. Above 40 the adult pig is heat stressed. Take the rectal temperature; normal is 39°C (**Figure 1.11**). (See *Table 1.4*.)

Examine the external genitalia while taking the rectal temperature. If possible, palpate the lumbar muscles, hind legs, abdomen and mammary area. Move your hands over the abdomen towards the chest. Some pigs may allow auscultation but this is generally unrewarding.

Pigs generally like to be scratched, particularly behind the ear and along the back. Check the head of the pig for any discharges from the nose, eyes and mouth. When handling the head be aware that the pig may try and bite.

Examination without physical restraint

Some pigs, notably young pigs, may allow the clinician to examine them without physical restraint. In addition, pet pigs with frequent human contact or selected breeding gilts may allow an examination sufficiently detailed to be rewarding.

Young pigs may be picked up and will generally settle, allowing visual examination (**Figure 1.12**). Ensure that the pig is held close to the body to avoid injury to the pig or handler.

With pet pigs, ask the owners to regularly handle their pigs, which will make examination easier.

Table 1.4 **Temperature, respiration and pulse rates.**

AGE/WEIGHT	RECTAL TEMPERATURE °C	°F	RESPIRATORY RATE (per minute)	PULSE RATE (per minute)
At birth	39.0	102.0	40–50	200–250
During suckling	39.2	102.5	30–40	80–110
At weaning	39.3	102.7	25–40	80–100
25–45 kg	39.0	102.5	30–40	80–90
45–90 kg	38.8	101.8	30–40	75–85
Pregnant sow	38.6	101.6	15–20	70–80
During farrowing	39.0– 40.0	102.0– 104.0	40–50	80–100
During lactation	39.1	102.5	20–30	70–80
Boar	38.6	101.5	15–20	70–80

Even training the pig to an anaesthesia mask may be extremely helpful in the event that the pig requires anaesthesia.

Examine the feet while standing. Grasp the pig's front legs firmly. The pig is likely to vocally object. Place the pig on its rear, holding its back with your knees. Palpation of the legs should start at the top and work down the leg to the feet. Note that pigs do not like having their feet examined (**Figure 1.13**).

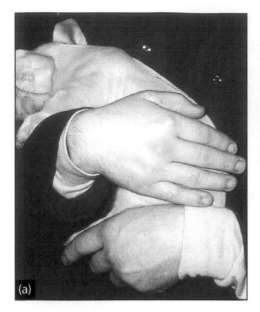

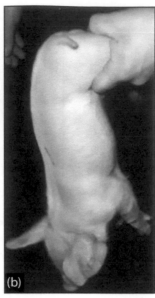

Fig. 1.12 (a) Holding a young pig close. (b) Holding a young pig by the hind leg.

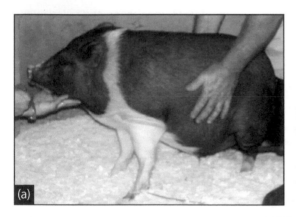

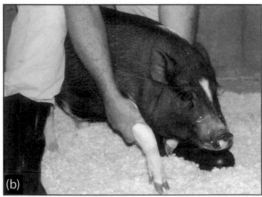

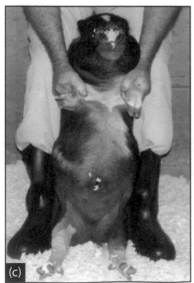

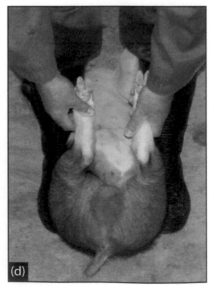

Fig. 1.13 Examination of the pig with restraint. (a) Make contact both vocally and physically. Approach the pig from behind. (b) Grasp both front legs by the elbow. (c) Raise the pig and place it on its behind, supporting its back with your legs. (d) Lower the pig between your legs and support its back with your feet.

Examination with physical restraint

Most pigs are not used to being handled. They become very vocal when caught and will not settle easily. Pigs will move as a herd or as individuals, so before moving a group of pigs think of escape routes they might take and then try to block them.

Pigs have a wide angle 330° vision, which allows them to see behind themselves without turning their heads. They are easily distracted by objects to the front and sides and sharp changes in floor texture and appearance. A shaft of sunlight is sufficient to affect pig movement. The behaviour and many clinical signs will be absent or changed in a physically restrained pig; breathing rate, heart rate and rectal temperature will all radically change in the restrained pig.

Pigs may be placed within a crate/stall or cart allowing the clinician to examine all surfaces of the pig without significant stress to clinician or pig (**Figures 1.14, 1.15**). Care needs to be taken to ensure your hands are not trapped between the pig and any metal work. Be aware that although they are in a cart, pigs are quite capable of jumping.

Collecting blood samples

Blood samples allow for analysis of the presence of pathogens in the blood, serology, biochemistry and haematological examination. Two methods of blood collection are described.

Piglets to 30 kg weaner weight

The blood sample is taken from the anterior vena cava (**Figures 1.16, 1.17**). The anterior vena

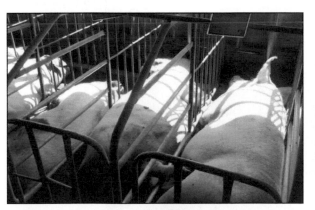

Fig. 1.14 Adult pigs restrained in a stall.

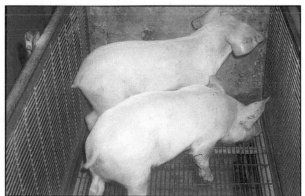

Fig. 1.15 Weaners restrained in a cart.

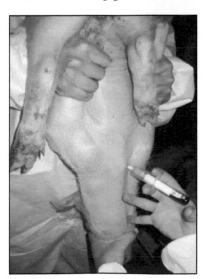

Fig. 1.16 Position to obtain a sample from the anterior vena cava of a weaned pig.

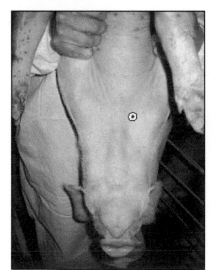

Fig. 1.17 Restraint to allow a blood sample to be obtained from a weaned pig, with a circle indicating the position for the blood collection.

cava is located on the left but needles are always inserted on the right to avoid damaging the left vagus nerve, which innervates the heart and diaphragm.

Grower/finishing and adult pigs

Grower, finisher and adult pigs may be bled from the jugular vein with a vacutainer and a 40 mm, 1.1 mm needle (**Figures 1.18, 1.19**). Keep the needle perpendicular to the skin and vertical. Do not move the needle laterally and medially when searching for the jugular vein as it will lacerate the neck, possibly causing a major haematoma.

Most problems occur because the needle is not in deep enough and the needle tip is bouncing off the jugular vein.

Wear ear protection when collecting samples from pigs as they are very vocal. The normal method of physical restraint is using a loop around the upper jaw behind the canines (**Figure 1.20**). The pig will normally pull back on the loop and stand still. Vocalisation is normal and the pig may act quite stressed, which can be alarming to the client. Mark the pig before releasing.

Once the snare is released the pig will stop vocalising and return to the rest of the group. As you

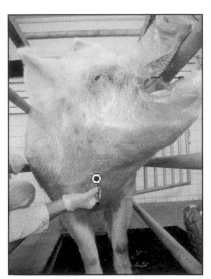

Fig. 1.18 Restaint of an older pig using a nose snare to raise the head. The circle indicates the required position of the needle.

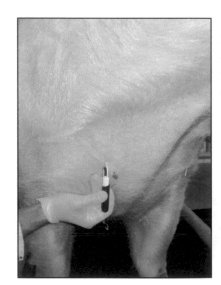

Fig. 1.19 Detail of blood collection from the jugular of an older pig.

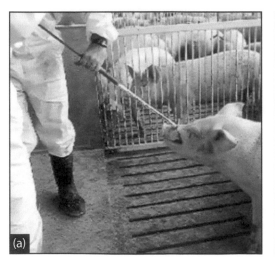

(a)

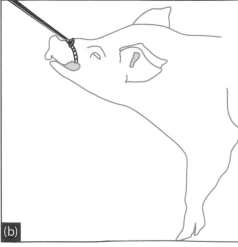

(b)

Fig. 1.20 (a) Restraint of an older pig using a nose snare. (b) Detail of the safe position of the nose snare behind the canines.

go to restrain the next pig, the one just restrained will often attempt to re-bite the snare and become recaptured.

Take special care with boars or lactating sows as they are armed with sharp canines and are quite capable of injuring people.

Chemical restraint

Some pigs are too difficult to handle, but examination is required and the veterinarian will need to sedate and even anaesthetise the pig to allow the examination to occur. It is important to realise that the behaviour and many clinical signs will be absent or changed in a chemically restrained pig.

There are a number of chemicals available but many are not licensed for pigs (*Tables 1.5, 1.6*). In addition, some sedative and anaesthetic drugs are not available in all countries. In some countries the product should not be used in a food producing animal. It is vital that the veterinarian decides how to use these products.

Changes that need to be recognised by members of the health team when examining a pig

The ability to clinically examine an individual pig and then a group of pigs is a learned process and improves with time and practice. Try to keep to the same systematic approach. Observe and note changes from normal. The following images illustrate some of the more obvious changes from normal that should be seen and recorded.

Clinical signs that are likely to be seen are shown in the following images (**Figures 1.21–1.105**). (See Clinical Quiz 1.1 on page 52.)

Table 1.5 Sedative medicines that may be useful in pigs.

Acepromazine	0.5 mg/kg IM	Good sedation, unreliable for surgery
Ketamine	15 mg/kg IM	Give acepromazine at least 10 minutes prior to ketamine
Diazepam	0.5–2 mg/kg IM	Sedation only
Ketamine	10–15 mg/kg IM	Good muscle relaxation
Xylazine	1–2 mg/kg IM	Moderate sedation at low doses, deep sedation at high doses
Ketamine	5–10 mg/kg IM	Good relaxation
	IV (for induction prior to inhalant anaesthesia)	Use ¼ to ½ dose for induction prior to inhalant anaesthesia
Azaperone	0.5 mg/kg	Mixing of pigs
	2–8 mg/kg	Sedation
	5–10 mg/kg	Knock-down

Table 1.6 Medicines that may be useful in achieving anaesthesia in a pig.

Xylazine	0.5–2.2 mg/kg IM	Anaesthesia with good analgesia and muscle relaxation. Intubation
Tiletamine/zolazepam (Telazol®)	3–6 mg/kg IM	possible. Apnoea may occur
Telazol®	4.4 mg/kg IM	Reconstitute powdered Telazol® with 250 mg xylazine (2.5 mL) and
Ketamine	2.2 mg/kg IM	250 mg ketamine (2.5 mL).
Xylazine	2.2 mg/kg IM	Dose at 1 mL/25–35 kg. Intubation possible, apnoea may occur. Duration: 45–90 minutes
Propofol	IV infusion Induction: 2–5 mg/kg CRI: 4–8 mg/kg/hr	Rapid onset, short duration, short, smooth recovery. Apnoea common, intubation recommended
Pentobarbital sodium (Euthatal®)	5–10 mL per 100 kg	Administer slowly. Note that underdosing results in excitability

Position of the pig in the pen
See **Figures 1.21–1.26**.

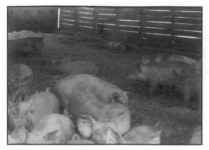

Fig. 1.21 Position away from other pigs.

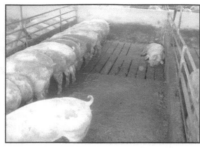

Fig. 1.22 Lying when others are standing and/or eating.

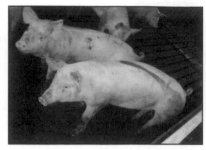

Fig. 1.23 Stockperson marks on back.

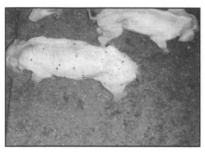

Fig. 1.24 Hairy pig. Note also the presence of flies on the skin.

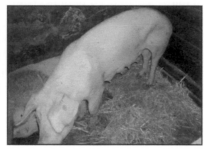

Fig. 1.25 Chronically affected pig. Note the loss of weight.

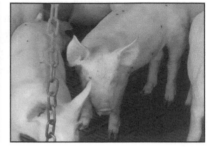

Fig. 1.26 Acutely affected pig. Note no loss of weight.

Skin changes
See **Figures 1.27–1.35**.

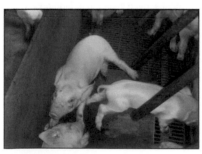

Fig. 1.27 Colour – paler than others in the group.

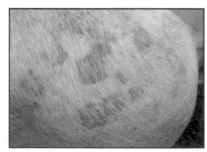

Fig. 1.28 Patchy skin necrosis.

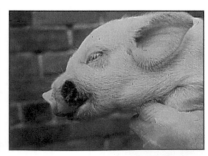

Fig. 1.29 Necrosis around the mouth.

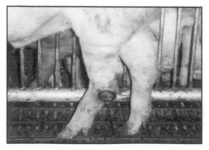

Fig. 1.30 Ulceration of the skin.

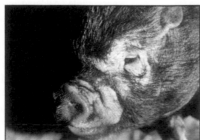

Fig. 1.31 Scaly skin.

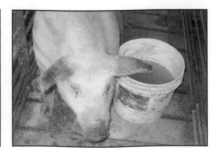

Fig. 1.32 Cyanosis of extremities.

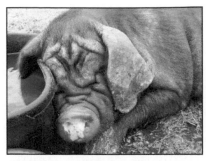

Fig. 1.33 Too much skin.

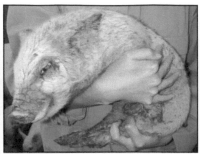

Fig. 1.34 Greasy skin.

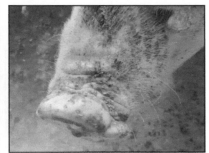

Fig. 1.35 Vesicles and blisters.

Presence of lumps

On the legs: See **Figures 1.36–1.38**.

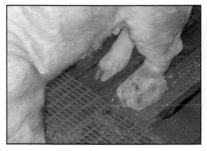

Fig. 1.36 Bush foot.

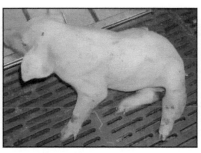

Fig. 1.37 Swollen joints.

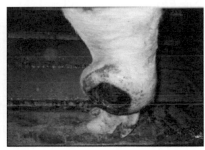

Fig. 1.38 Granuloma.

Elsewhere on the body: See **Figures 1.39–1.44**.

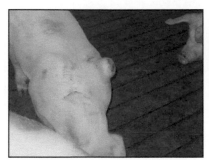

Fig. 1.39 Shoulder abscess.

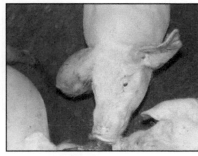

Fig. 1.40 Haematoma of the ear.

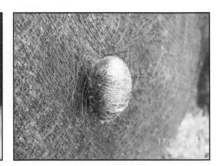

Fig. 1.41 Skin tumour.

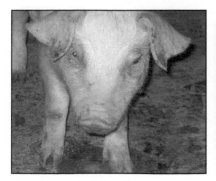

Fig. 1.42 Eyelid oedema.

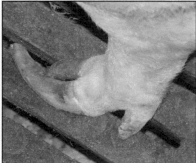

Fig. 1.43 Hoof overgrowth.

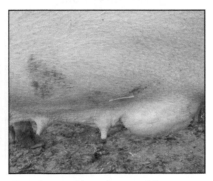

Fig. 1.44 Chronic mastitis.

Hernia
See **Figures 1.45–1.47**.

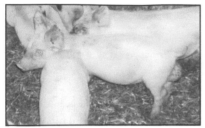

Fig. 1.45 Scrotal hernia.

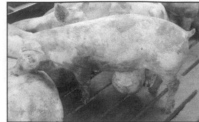

Fig. 1.46 Umbilical hernia.

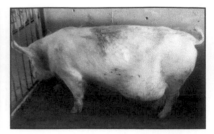

Fig. 1.47 Acquired hernia.

Configuration
See **Figures 1.48–1.53**.

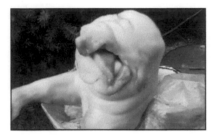

Fig. 1.48 Congenital defect.

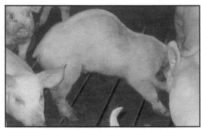

Fig. 1.49 Kinky back.

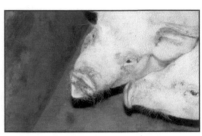

Fig. 1.50 Deviation in angle.

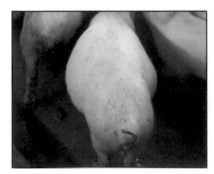

Fig. 1.51 Swollen abdomen.

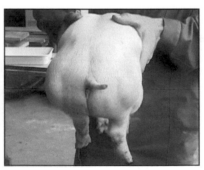

Fig. 1.52 Muscle changes.

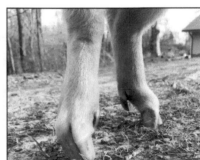

Fig. 1.53 Limb shape.

Evidence of vice
See **Figures 1.54–1.56**.

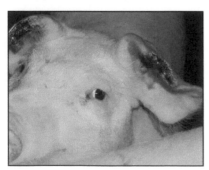

Fig. 1.54 Ear biting.

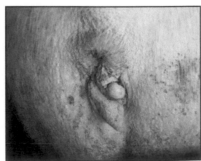

Fig. 1.55 Bitten vulva.

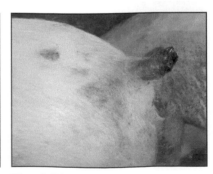

Fig. 1.56 Tail biting.

Prolapses

See **Figures 1.57–1.59**.

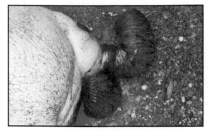

Fig. 1.57 Uterine prolapse.

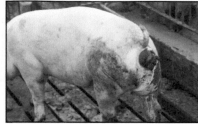

Fig. 1.58 Rectal or vaginal prolapse.

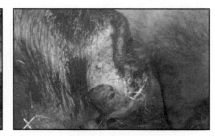

Fig. 1.59 Perineum prolapse.

Animal's breathing

See **Figures 1.60, 1.61**. Note the number of breaths per minute. A sow or boar breathes 20 times per minute. A rate of over 40 and visible is abnormal.

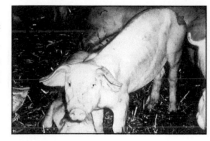

Fig. 1.60 Heave line.

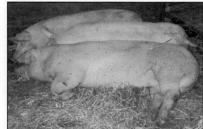

Fig. 1.61 Deep breathing.

Locomotor and behaviour changes

See **Figures 1.62–1.70**.

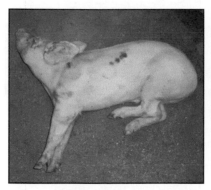

Fig. 1.62 Meningitis.

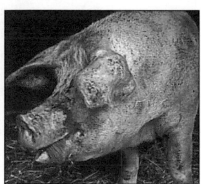

Fig. 1.63 Neurological deficit.

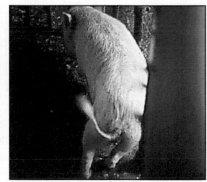

Fig. 1.64 Scratching.

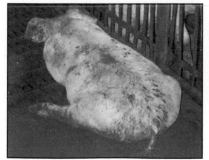

Fig. 1.65 Paraplegia.

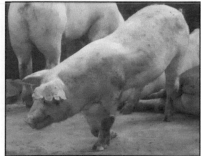

Fig. 1.66 Lame: high up the leg, leg held low.

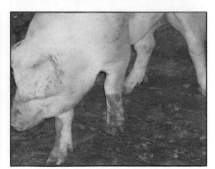

Fig. 1.67 Lame: low down in the leg, leg held high.

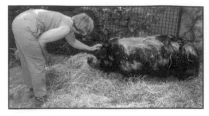

Fig. 1.68 Pig's behaviour to humans.

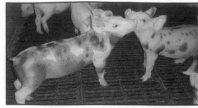

Fig. 1.69 Pig's behaviour to each other.

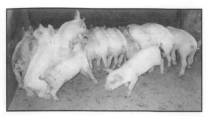

Fig. 1.70 Pig's grouping.

Presence of a discharge
See **Figures 1.71–1.76**.

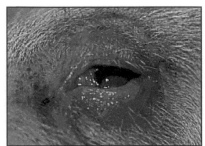

Fig. 1.71 Ocular.

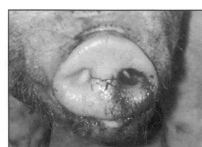

Fig. 1.72 Nasal.

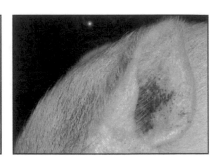

Fig. 1.73 Aural.

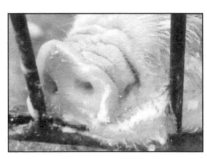

Fig. 1.74 Oral.

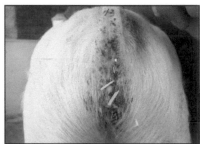

Fig. 1.75 Anal.

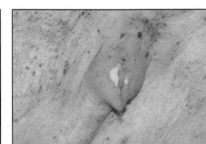

Fig. 1.76 Vulval.

Other observed changes associated directly with the pig
See **Figures 1.77–1.79**.

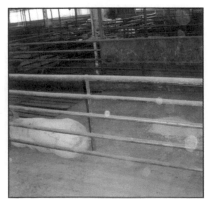

Fig. 1.77 Refusal of feed.

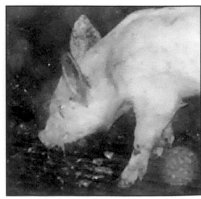

Fig. 1.78 Vomiting.

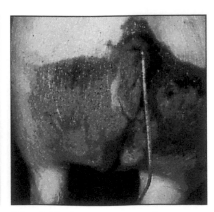

Fig. 1.79 Note any parasites.

Look around the pen and observe the faecal consistency
See **Figures 1.80–1.88**.

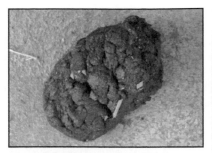

Fig. 1.80 Normal faeces.

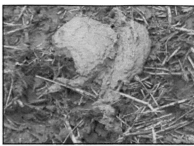

Fig. 1.81 Loose faeces.

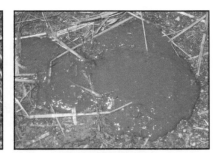

Fig. 1.82 Diarrhoea.

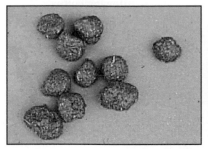

Fig. 1.83 Constipated.

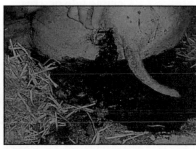

Fig. 1.84 Blood: melaena.

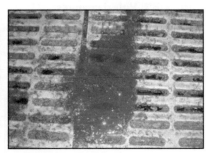

Fig. 1.85 Blood: red.

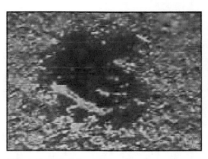

Fig. 1.86 Mucus in the faeces.

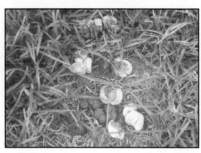

Fig. 1.87 Note the color of faeces: white shown, often yellow to green.

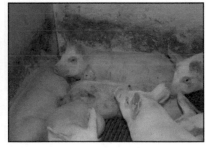

Fig. 1.88 Look also on the walls and surroundings for faecal staining.

Urinary tract
See **Figures 1.89–1.91**.

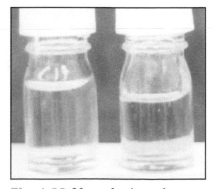

Fig. 1.89 Normal urine colours.

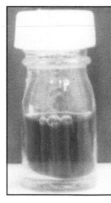

Fig. 1.90 Smokey urine.

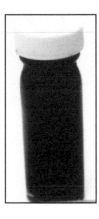

Fig. 1.91 Blood in the urine.

Note changes with the normal reproductive cycle
See **Figures 1.92–1.94**.

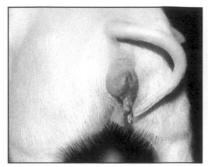

Fig. 1.92 Vulval changes.

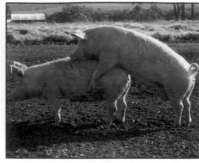

Fig. 1.93 Coming into oestrus.

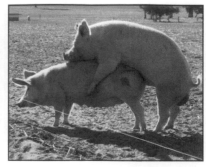

Fig. 1.94 Allowing coitus.

Abnormal reproductive signs
See **Figures 1.95–1.103**.

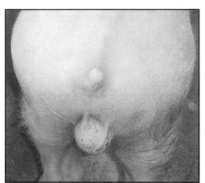

Fig. 1.95 Monorchid.

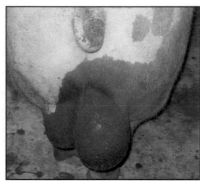

Fig. 1.96 Testicular atrophy.

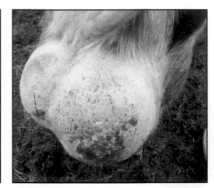

Fig. 1.97 Orchitis.

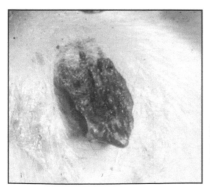

Fig. 1.98 Necrotic vulva.

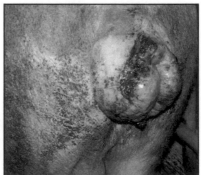

Fig. 1.99 Swollen vulva.

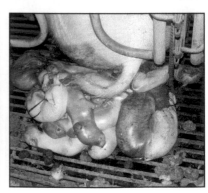

Fig. 1.100 Abortion.

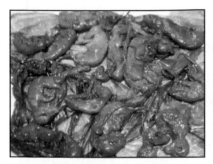

Fig. 1.101 Mummified piglets.

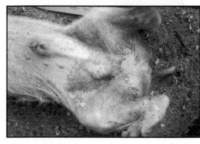

Fig. 1.102 Late mummified piglet.

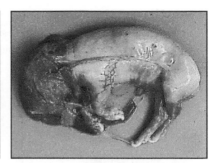

Fig. 1.103 Stillborn piglet.

Swollen lymph nodes
See **Figures 1.104, 1.105**.

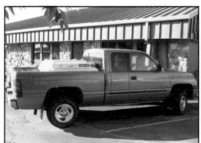

Fig. 1.104 Unilaterally swollen lymph node.

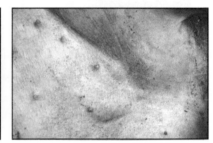

Fig. 1.105 Bilaterally enlarged lymph nodes.

CLINICAL EXAMINATION OF THE FARM

Pigs generally live in a population on a farm. It is important that the clinician is able to systematically examine the farm; this includes not only examination of the pigs but also their environment and the ability of the stockpersons looking after the pigs.

A systematic approach will take the veterinarian through a typical farrow-to-finish farm visit. Modifications to this approach may be required for multisite systems.

Getting to the farm
See **Figures 1.106–1.108**.

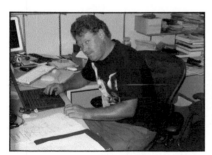

Fig. 1.106 Examine the farm records and arrange the visit. This may even be done at the last visit, but needs at least 2 weeks notice.

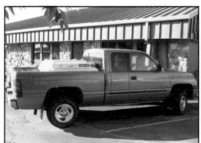

Fig. 1.107 Ensure your own biosecurity is adequate – truck clean. It is imperative that you are not a risk to the farm, real or perceived.

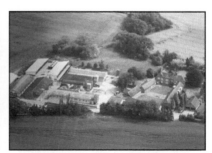

Fig. 1.108 Examine the surrounding area for local farms as you approach the farm, especially on the first visit. Drive around the farm's locality.

Locality of the farm

The locality of the farm will have a significant impact on the presence of potential diseases on the farm.

Entering the farm
See **Figures 1.109–1.114**.

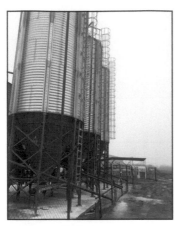

Fig. 1.109 Walk the outer perimeter, ensuring that it is secure. Note areas that can be improved (e.g. can feed trucks be kept out?).

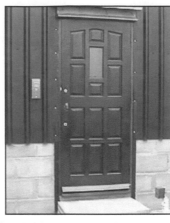

Fig. 1.110 Examine the entry facilities. Does the klaxon or horn work and attract attention? Are restriction notices clear?

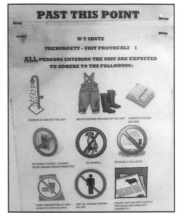

Fig. 1.111 Abide by farm biosecurity rules. Ensure that biosecurity notices are well posted.

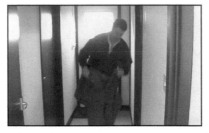

Fig. 1.112 As an absolute minimum, do not wear your own outer clothing, always wear farm clothing or disposable overalls.

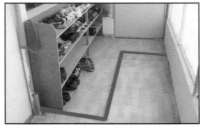

Fig. 1.113 In addition to farm outer clothing, boots or protective foot wear should be provided by the farm.

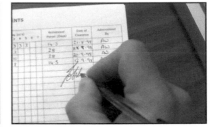

Fig. 1.114 Discuss farm targets and expectations in the farm office. Review pig flow, particularly all-in/all-out status. Sign the visitors book.

Medicine check
See **Figures 1.115–1.120**.

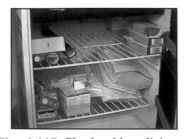

Fig. 1.115 Check cold medicine storage, including the max/min thermometer. The refrigerator must run at 2–8°C. Freezing vaccines will cause their inactivation.

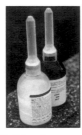

Fig. 1.116 Check warm medicine storage hygiene and medicine use. Many antibiotics have a maximum storage temperature of 25°C. This may be difficult in the summer.

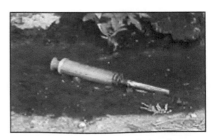

Fig. 1.117 Check needle, syringe and disposal systems. Medical products must be kept away from children at all times. Disposal through the regular rubbish is not acceptable.

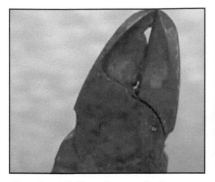

Fig. 1.118 Examine teeth clippers and other instruments used in processing. Ensure protocols are followed. Are the protocols necessary?

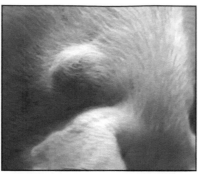

Fig. 1.119 Injection techniques. The photo shows a neck abscess/ granuloma due to poor injection technique.

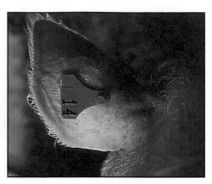

Fig. 1.120 Pig identification systems, including pre-slaughter. Look for evidence of poor pig identification, which can impair records.

Examination of the farm building

The farm should be examined progressively using the protocols described in the following figure captions. First, an overall check is required for each building (**Figures 1.121–1.126**).

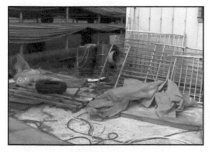

Fig. 1.121 Outside security. Rodent control is a vital part of disease control. Ensure there are no rodent access points. Do rodent boxes contain bait?

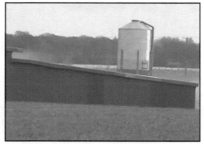

Fig. 1.122 Outside ventilation system. The inlets and outlets should be visually inspected from the outside. Bird nests and obstructions are common findings.

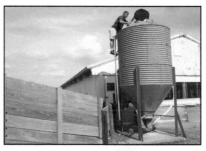

Fig. 1.123 Feed may be stored in a variety of places. Commonly, bulk feed is stored in a bin. Climb up to the top of the bin and examine the bin's hygiene and cleaning protocols.

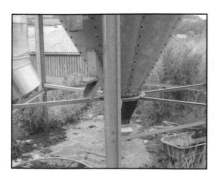

Fig. 1.124 Vermin control. Feed spills attract rodents, birds and flies.

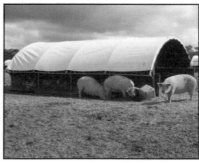

Fig. 1.125 Examine pigs without entering the building/room.

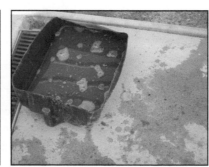

Fig. 1.126 Room biosecurity. Foot baths must be clean.

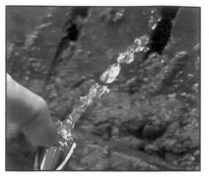

Fig. 1.127 Examine the water.

On entering the building, note the sleeping pattern of the undisturbed pigs. Next, quietly enter the room and observe any biosecurity arrangements. Review the basic environmental necessities. This requires the clinician to understand the basic husbandry requirements for water, food, floor and good air quality for each age group of pigs (**Figures 1.127–1.30**).

Although the clinical examination of pigs is covered in detail elsewhere, note that the level of investigation expected of the stock is the same as that required to investigate the environment (**Figures 1.131, 1.132**).

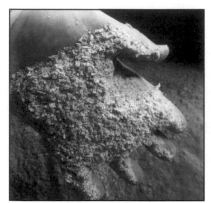

Fig. 1.128 Examine the feed.

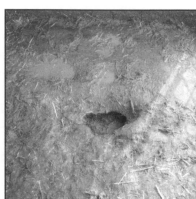

Fig. 1.129 Examine the floor.

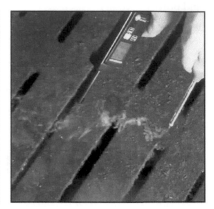

Fig. 1.130 Examine the air and ventilation system.

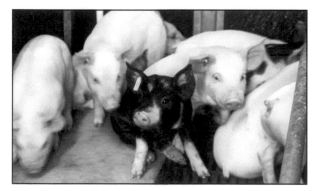

Fig. 1.131 Stock. Examine the pigs themselves.

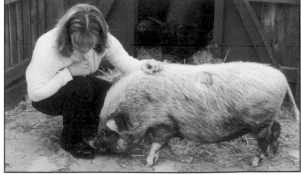

Fig. 1.132 Watch the interaction between stockpersons and the animals.

Farm walk

The farm walk requires a set protocol. The following is a suggested walk to minimise the spread of potential pathogens by following the pig flow from birth to finish. The aim should be to move from the clean part of the farm to the progressively 'dirty' part of the farm (**Figures 1.133–1.144**).

Prepare and send the report with any advice attachments within one working week.

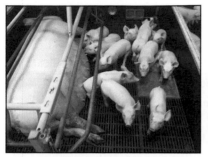

Fig. 1.133 Farrowing area.

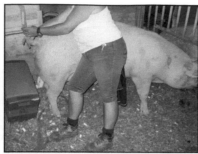

Fig. 1.134 Sow breeding area.

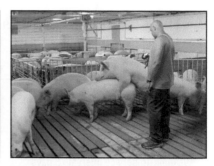

Fig. 1.135 Gilt breeding area.

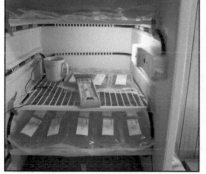

Fig. 1.136 Artificial insemination storage area.

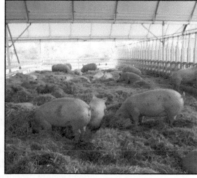

Fig. 1.137 Gestation area.

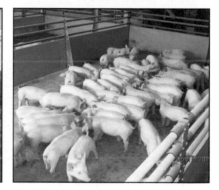

Fig. 1.138 Nursery.

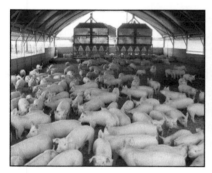

Fig. 1.139 Grow/finish area.

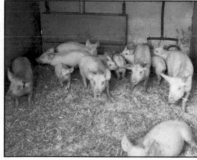

Fig. 1.140 Hospital pens/areas.

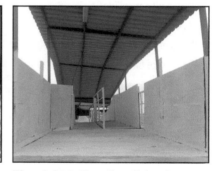

Fig. 1.141 Examine animal loading and entry points.

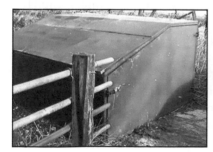

Fig. 1.142 Dead animal disposal.

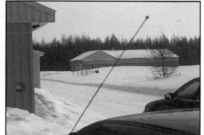

Fig. 1.143 Isolation area. To enter this may need change of clothing etc.

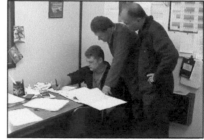

Fig. 1.144 Explain your findings to the farm health team.

Table 1.7 **Farm production expectations for a pig unit.**

	TARGET	INTERFERENCE
Reproduction		
Number of gilts available for service	6/100 sows	<5/100 sows
Age at first service	220 days	>250 or <200 days
Weaning-to-service interval	5 days	>7 days
Repeat matings; regular returns*	8	>9
Irregular returns (other times)	3	>4
Empty days per sow	12	>14
Abortions (%)	<1	>1.5
Sows NIP (%)	1	>2
Culled pregnant (%)	1	>2
Deaths pregnant (%)	1	>2
Farrowing rate (%)	87	<82
Vaginal discharge more than 7 days post service (%)	<1	>1.5
Sows culled per year (%)	38	>42
Sow parity at culling	6–7	>8
Sow deaths per year (%)	<5	>5
Number of boars no AI	5/100	<5 or >6 /100
Number of boars AI + natural	3/100	<3 or >4/100
Matings per week per boar	4	<2 or >6
Farrowing house performance		
Total born/sow	15	<13
Pigs born alive/sow	14	<12.5
Stillborn rate (%)	<7	>10
Piglets mummified (%)	<1.5	>2.5
Litter scatter (sows with <7 piglets) (%)	<10	>15
Pre-weaning losses (28 days)	10	>14
Piglets weaned per litter	12	<11
Litters per sow per year	2.35	<2.3
Piglets weaned per sow per year	28	<25

(*Continued*)

Table 1.7 (*Continued*) **Farm production expectations for a pig unit.**

	TARGET	INTERFERENCE
Feeding herd performance		
Finishing rate (7 to 110 kg) (%)	>96	<94
Pigs sold per sow per year	26	<22
Feed parameters		
Sow feed in tonnes per year	1.1	>1.2
Total tonnes farm feed per sow per year	8.5	<7 or >9.5
Food conversion 7–110 kg	2.2	>2.5
Daily gain 10–110 kg (g/day)	650	<600
Days to market 110 kg	160	>180
Dressing (%)	75%	<72%

* A regular return occurs between 18 and 24 days post breeding.
NIP, not in pig; AI, artificial insemination.
A 100 sow unit producing 25 pigs per sow per year sold at 90 kg dead weight produces enough pig meat to feed over 9,000 people per year if the consumption is 24.5 kg person/year.

FARM PRODUCTION

In order to understand normal, it is essential to have target expectations for production. There are two ways of looking at production; one is through the traditional method based around the sows, and the alternative is to look at numbers based around kg meat output. Each client may have different expectations and it is essential to understand your client's expectation of their pigs. Note that within a farm health team there may be fundamental differences. The owner may be primarily interested in financial returns based around kg meat output, whereas the manager may be primarily interested in output based on the sows on which the staff bonuses are paid. Production expectations for a pig farm are shown in *Table 1.7*. The interference point is where the farm team needs to discuss measures to investigate and correct any management issues on the farm.

POST-MORTEM EXAMINATION OF PIGS

Commercial pigs will go the slaughterhouse and this provides an ideal opportunity for the veterinarian to obtain information on the background levels of disease in both a specific batch and, through repeated examinations either by the slaughterhouse or government scheme, a degree of spacial and temporal analysis.

Post-mortem examination in the slaughterhouse

On the moving slaughter line, diseases are mainly reviewed by quick gross examination of organs (**Figures 1.145–1.156**). While crude, this will allow for an overview on a number of pigs to be obtained and a score on the health of the farm awarded. This must never be confused with a careful post-mortem examination. Identification of individual animals can never

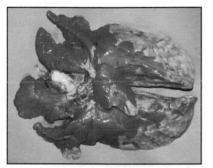

Fig. 1.145 Consolidation.

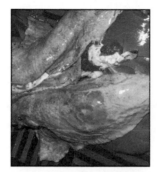

Fig. 1.146 Pleuropneumonia.

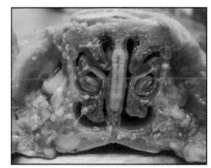

Fig. 1.147 Turbinate integrity.

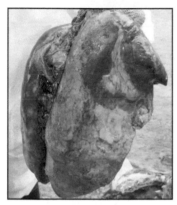

Fig. 1.148 Pleurisy.

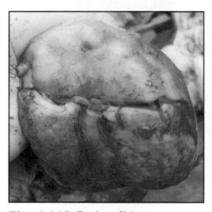

Fig. 1.149 Pericarditis.

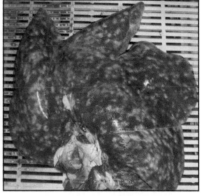

Fig. 1.150 White (milk) spot liver.

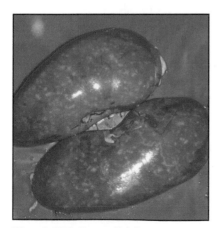

Fig. 1.151 Interstitial nephritis.

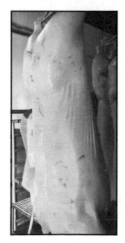

Fig. 1.152 Mange skin lesions.

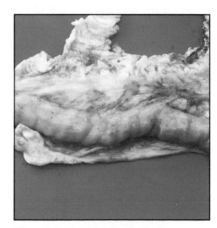

Fig. 1.153 Intestinal changes.

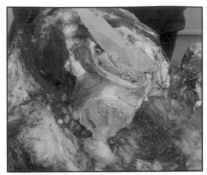

Fig. 1.154 Abscessation.

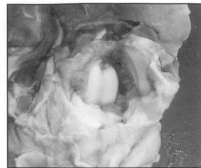

Fig. 1.155 Arthritic/bursal lesions.

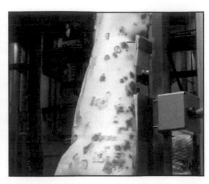

Fig. 1.156 Erysipelas/skin blemish.

be assumed. In the slaughterhouse tattoo marks may be poor and there may be a disconnect between the carcase and the offal on the line.

The major organs to be examined are the skin, lung, heart and liver. The skin should be examined as the pigs move to the eviseration area. Special investigations may be carried out on the intestinal tract and nasal cavity. The veterinarian should also carefully check the casualty and reserved line where abscessation, joint and other skin problems may be revealed.

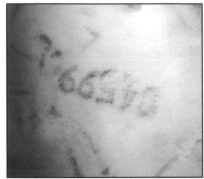

Fig. 1.157 Clarity of slap marking allowing meat traceability.

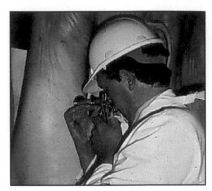

Fig. 1.158 Basic conformation, P2 backfat depth, etc.

In the slaughterhouse, the clinician is able to recognise disease conditions but not the causative pathogen. Further, the clarity of the slap marks (tattoos) and basic conformation can be assessed (**Figures 1.157, 1.158**).

Other issues

Changes in disease prevalence can be monitored over time; for example, for enzootic (mycoplasma) pneumonia score (**Figure 1.159**). This can allow for seasonal change in disease patterns to be recognised and thus impact on management changes or the choice of vaccine, for example.

Understanding the economic impact of pathogens may allow the clinician to place a value on preventive medicine programmes.

Post-mortem examination of the individual pig

Clinical examination of pigs on the farm may involve the post-mortem examination of any dead pigs found on the farm or following euthanasia of pigs exhibiting selected clinical signs.

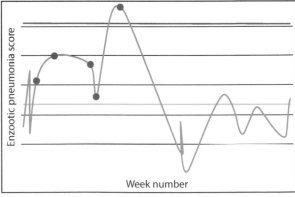

Fig. 1.159 The change in enzootic (mycoplasma) pneumonia score over time. The green line is the mean score over time. The red line is 3 SDs above the mean line. Using statistical process control measures, an assessment of the farm's health can be achieved. The red points indicate that at these times the farm was out of control: three points together above the mean and one point more than 3 SDs above the mean.

Euthanasia of pigs

There are a number of methods available to allow for safe, effective and humane euthanasia of

Table 1.8 **Euthanasia techniques available in different age groups/weight of pigs.**

	PIGLETS <3 WEEKS OLD BIRTH–6 kg	NURSERY PIG <10 WEEKS 6–30 kg	GROWING PIG 30–75 kg	FINISHING PIG 75 kg +	MATURE SOW OR BOAR
Blunt trauma	Yes	No	No	No	No
Gunshot	No	Yes	Yes	Yes	Yes
Captive bolt	No	Yes	Yes	Yes	Yes
Electrocution	Yes	Yes	Yes	Yes	Yes
Carbon dioxide	Yes	Yes	Not practical	Not practical	Not practical
For veterinarians only					
Anaesthetic overdose	Yes	Yes	Yes	Yes	Yes

pigs (*Table 1.8*). However, there may be local legal requirements; for example, exsanguination may be required after use of a captive bolt and pithing.

Blunt trauma: A sharp, firm blow with a heavy blunt instrument on the top of the head over the brain is an efficient way of humanely killing pigs less than 6 kg in weight (3 weeks of age) (**Figure 1.160**). It is essential that the blow is administered swiftly, firmly and with absolute determination. If there is any doubt whether the pig is dead, the blow should be repeated. If necessary, exsanguinate by severing the carotid artery.

Gunshot and penetrating captive bolt: Training in firearms is essential. The animal should be restrained by a rope or snare over the upper jaw held by an assistant. These methods stun or kill by concussive force and penetration into the brain (**Figures 1.161, 1.162**).

In larger animals (>75 kg) it is recommended that the carotid (neck) artery is severed once the pig is stunned. The captive bolt should be positioned against the forehead as shown (**Figures 1.162, 1.170**). A loose-bullet firearm must be held 10 cm from the skull (do not press against the forehead).

In old boars it may take more than one attempt to stun the pig.

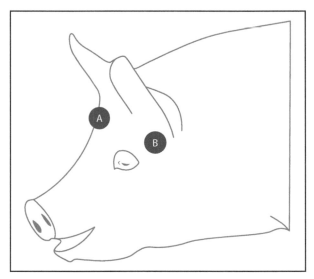

Fig. 1.161 Site of euthanasia using a live round. A indicates the recommended position for the temporal method – firearm only. Do not place the gun directly onto the skin – leave a 10 cm gap. B indicates the recommended position for the frontal method directed upwards at 20 degrees towards the brain. Sever the carotid artery after shooting where required.

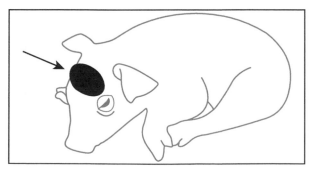

Fig. 1.160 Site of blunt trauma for euthanasia of piglets less than 6 kg.

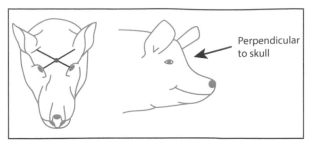

Fig. 1.162 Site of euthanasia using a captive bolt. Place the gun at the middle of a cross made from the back of the ear with the medial canthus of each eye. Keep the captive bolt against the skin and perpendicular to the skull. In pigs over 60 kg use a detonation cap in the captive bolt to drive the bolt at speed through the skull. Pith the pig after shooting and sever the carotid artery after stunning with a captive bolt gun.

Carbon dioxide: Carbon dioxide (CO_2) causes rapid onset of anaesthesia with subsequent death due to respiratory arrest. Since CO_2 is heavier than air, when constructing a container for swine euthanasia the outlet valve should be located at the top so that the container can be completely filled with CO_2 while air is allowed to escape. For small pigs, a garbage can, with the inlet and outlet valves installed in the lid, plus a plastic bin liner can be used. After checking for complete euthanasia the bag containing the pigs can be removed. CO_2 has a taste/smell that pigs might find distressing. Nitrous oxide is an alternative agent.

Electrocution: This is not common in Europe but is widely used in America and Asia. Electrocution induces death by insensibility of the brain followed by heart failure. Electrocution is a two-step procedure (**Figure 1.163**):

1 Pig rendered unconscious – place electrodes on opposite sides of the head so that the current travels through the brain.
2 Pig euthanasia – place electrodes so that the current is redirected through the heart of the unconscious pig.

Large market weight pigs require a minimum current of 1.25 amps at 300 v for 1 second.

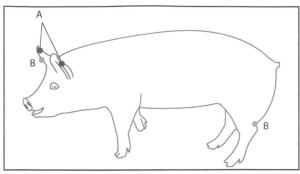

Fig. 1.163 Site of attachment of electrical cables to enable euthanasia through electrocution. A indicates the correct position for step 1 to render the pig unconscious. B indicates the correct position to induce heart fibrillation and death. Severe the carotid artery after stunning by electrocution.

Anaesthetic overdose: This is only for administration by a licensed veterinarian. Pentobarbitone may be administered intraperitoneally and allow the anaesthetic to sedate the animal, which may take 10 minutes. Safe euthanasia can then be achieved with intravenous pentobarbitone using intracardiac, intraportal or (careful) ear vein injection.

Euthanasia method must be noted on each post-mortem examination: Note the visual appearance of the euthanasia method; bullet-hole, captive bolt entry-hole, exsanguination and injection site. There will be barbiturate around the heart after an intracardiac injection for euthanasia, which may be mistaken for pericarditis.

Post-mortem procedure

The veterinarian should be prepared to carry out a systematic post-mortem examination and so must have all the equipment and sampling systems necessary before the examination starts. To enhance biosecurity, farms should have their own post-mortem equipment. The post-mortem examination should be carried out in a quiet, dedicated, easily cleaned area.

Post-mortem equipment

Personal hygiene is important. Disposable protective gloves should be worn. Hands must be washed

Fig. 1.164 (a) Personal hygiene. (b) Protective gloves.

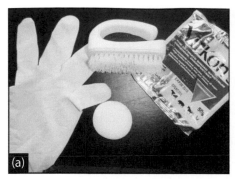

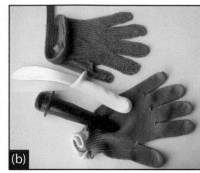

Fig. 1.165 Sawing implements.

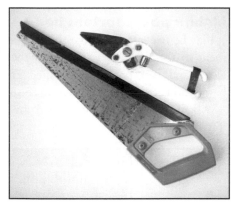

before and after the post-mortem examination (**Figure 1.164a**). All equipment, especially the knives, should be disinfected.

To gain access to major body cavities a sharp knife is required. If available, use protective gloves (i.e. chain mail or kevlar) for the non-knife hand (**Figure 1.164b**). To gain access to the chest, head and pelvis of sows, a saw and bone cutting tools may be necessary (**Figure 1.165**). Scissors are an important part of the post-mortem equipment, and are underutilised.

Animal, sample and farm identification

As in any investigation, having a secure chain of custody is essential. In this investigation the chain of custody is achieved by farm and building identification, individual animal ear tag and DNA sampling. The post-mortem findings may become part of a legal investigation.

Ensure cameras and video recorders are set for the correct date and time. Take a photograph of the pig's ear tag or notch. If the pig does not have any identification, place a tag in its ear or paint a number (pen/date) on the animal's side (**Figure 1.166a**). A waterproof camera or smart phone is very useful (**Figure 1.166b**).

The farm needs to be carefully identified by GPS and other map references. Obtain a map of the farm and identify each building. Google Earth may be a useful resource. An example of a farm under investigation is shown in **Figure 1.167**. Create a farm map to ensure all animal buildings are systematically examined (in this particular case there were 23 buildings). As each building is examined the age of the animals inside needs to be determined

Fig. 1.166 (a) Identifcation, note taking. (b) Recording camera, which is waterproof.

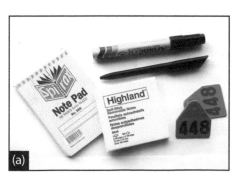

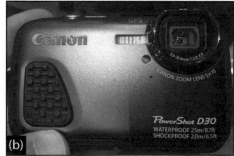

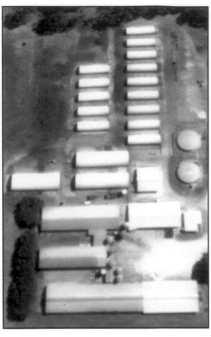

Fig. 1.167
Farm,
building
and pen
identification.

Sample collection and retrieval

A range of scissors, scalpels and forceps is required. A small tray to hold samples prior to processing can be very useful (**Figure 1.168a**).

Sample collection capabilities should include: blood tubes (clotted and unclotted blood); microscope slides for blood smears; litmus paper for pH examination; a syringe and needle for aspiration; a swab and liquid collection vessel (aerobic, anaerobic and virus collection); plastic bag for whole organ collection; a ruler scale (**Figures 1.168b, c**).

Mobile post-mortem box

It may be necessary to take the post-mortem equipment to the farm. It is vital that the equipment is clean and can be easily cleaned and disinfected before and after the examination (**Figure 1.169**).

All items should be placed in plastic bags. This also helps to keep it clean in the field.

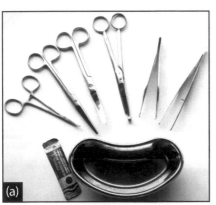

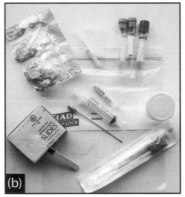

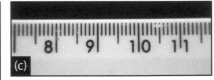

(c)

Fig. 1.168 (a–c) Requirements for sample collection.

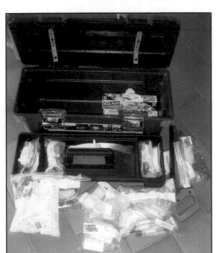

Fig. 1.169
The farm post-mortem kit, which is easy to clean and keep clean – biosecurity is king!

Post-mortem examination

Normally, the veterinarian will post-mortem an animal to determine its cause of death. For a population veterinarian, however, the actual cause of death is of interest but is not the primary reason for carrying out the post-mortem examination. The veterinarian's responsibility is to the living pigs not a dead pig. The post-mortem examination will collect information on what is not there. It will also determine which diseases/pathogens, present or absent, may affect the health of the herd. The fact that there is no evidence of foot and mouth disease is not only useful but a vital observation. Therefore, the examination must be complete and follow a systematic approach.

Only after the end of the examination should the veterinarian determine the importance of each finding in the cause of death. It is not possible in many cases for a cause to be determined on only gross examination. In many cases there will be several pathogenic processes found in the individual pig. The importance of each of these pathogenic processes needs to be determined before coming to a final diagnosis.

The following images (**Figures 1.170–1.230**) illustrate a systematic procedure for gross post-mortem examination of a pig. The procedure described assumes that the veterinarian is right handed. Highlighted are the diseases the clinician should be considering in each organ system.

(For details on anatomical structures, refer to the beginning of the chapter for each body system.)

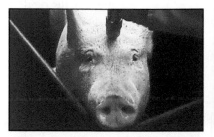

Fig. 1.170 It will be necessary to carefully euthanase the pig prior to the post-mortem examination.

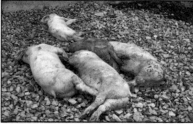

Fig. 1.171 Select an area where the post-mortem examination can take place where it is not too visible and biosecurity can be maintained. The area shown is not adequate.

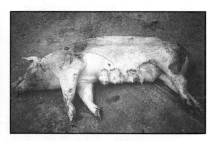

Fig. 1.172 Place the dead pig in lateral recumbency. Note the sex and body condition and estimate the weight. Note any cutaneous blood (swine fever) or jaw swelling (anthrax). Wash the pig if required.

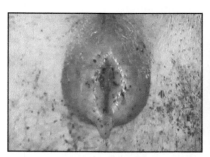

Fig. 1.173 Examine the anus and external genitalia for evidence of oestrus or discharges.

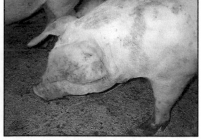

Fig. 1.174 Examine the external surface of the pig for evidence of fighting and septicaemia. Note any skin lesions (erysipelas) or body distortions (atrophic rhinitis).

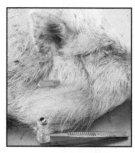

Fig. 1.175 Note the presence of wax in the ear. Take samples for mange.

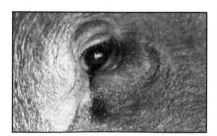

Fig. 1.176 Examine the eyes for evidence of dehydration and discharges (oedema disease).

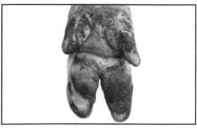

Fig. 1.177 Examine the legs and feet. Look for any indication of vesicles (foot and mouth disease, swine vesicular disease).

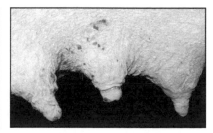

Fig. 1.178 Examine the mammary glands.

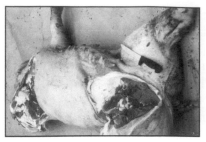

Fig. 1.179 Make deep incisions into the axilla on the left leg. Move to the left hind leg and cut into the groin area, exposing the femoral joint.

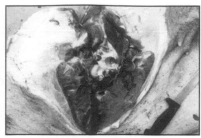

Fig. 1.180 Detail of the cut femoral joint. Note: In young animals the femoral head may separate along the epiphysis.

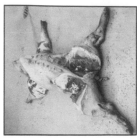

Fig. 1.181 Continue to the right hind leg and the right axilla. Lay the animal out as shown in dorsal recumbency. Note the inguinal lymph nodes (porcine circovirus type 2-systemic disease [PCV2-SD]).

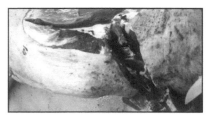

Fig. 1.182 Make a deep transverse cut into the neck immediately cranial to the manubrium.

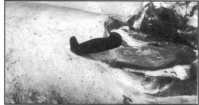

Fig. 1.183 Stand on the left. On the right hand chest make a cut along the line of the costochondral junction cartilages.

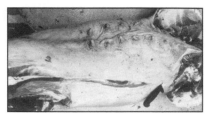

Fig. 1.184 Continue the cut under the skin towards the groin area. Place the sharp edge under the skin.

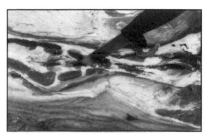

Fig. 1.185 Return to the chest then cut through the right costochondral junctions.

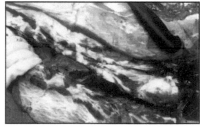

Fig. 1.186 Carefully part the opened chest so that the internal organs are not penetrated by the knife.

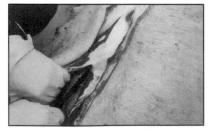

Fig. 1.187 Cut carefully into the peritoneal cavity. Do not puncture any of the abdominal organs.

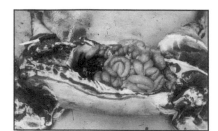

Fig. 1.188 Lay the ventral body wall over to the left side to reveal the visceral contents.

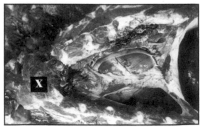

Fig. 1.189 Return to the chest and cut through the front ribs (x). Open up the chest by physical force, breaking the ribs. Consider how easy the ribs break.

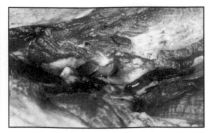

Fig. 1.190 Cut up the lateral side of the neck to the incisive part of the lower jaw.

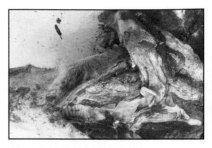

Fig. 1.191 Continue the dissection through the hyoid bones and release the tongue.

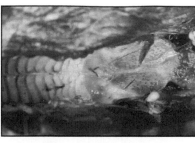

Fig. 1.192 Note the condition of the tonsils (Aujeszky's disease/pseudorabies).

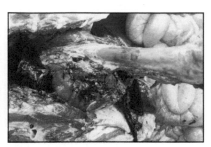

Fig. 1.193 Gripping the tongue, pull caudally and release from the carcase by cutting any dorsal attachments.

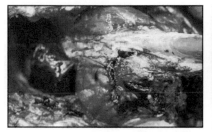

Fig. 1.194 Pull the contents of the chest caudally to the diaphragm.

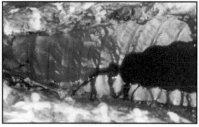

Fig. 1.195 Continue the cut until the lungs and heart are removed from the thoracic cavity. Note any pleural adhesions (*Actinobacillus pleuropneumoniae* infection).

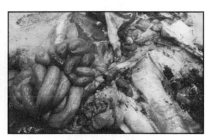

Fig. 1.196 Carefully cut through the diaphragm and dorsal attachments of the stomach and liver.

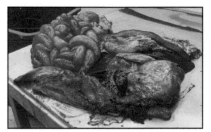

Fig. 1.197 Remove the viscera to a place for further investigation.

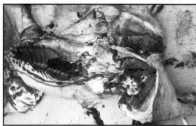

Fig. 1.198 Examine the pleura and peritoneal cavity for adhesions.

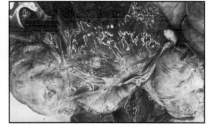

Fig. 1.199 Examine the distal oesophagus. If there is no evidence of pathology, separate the lung and heart from the stomach and liver.

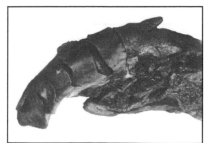

Fig. 1.200 Examine the tongue and mouth; check for vesicles (foot and mouth disease, swine vesicular disease).

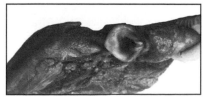

Fig. 1.201 Examine the throat.

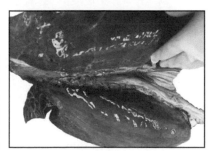

Fig. 1.202 Cut along the length of the oesophagus.

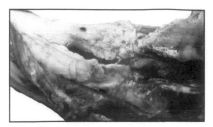

Fig. 1.203 Open up the trachea; note the tracheal rings are incomplete.

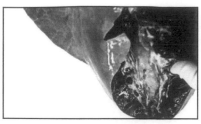

Fig. 1.204 Continue the cut down the bronchi to the end of the diaphragmatic lobe of the lung.

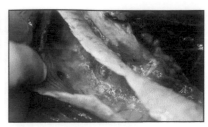

Fig. 1.205 Remember to open the tracheal bronchus into the right apical/cranial lobe.

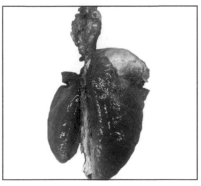

Fig. 1.206 Examine the lungs in detail. The particular diseases to note are enzootic (mycoplasma) pneumonia, pleuropneumonia, Glässer's disease and pneumonic abscessation.

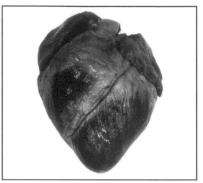

Fig. 1.207 Examine the pericardial surface for pericarditis (Glässer's). Examine the internal surfaces by opening the right atrium through the right atrioventricular valve. Open the right ventricle along the interventricular septum. Find the pulmonary artery and cut though the valve. Turn the heart over and repeat the same with the left side of the heart. Examine the heart valves (endocardiosis/endocarditis).

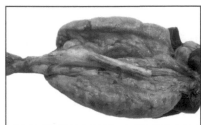

Fig. 1.208 Examine the tracheobronchial lymph nodes (PCV2-SD, porcine reproductive and respiratory syndrome).

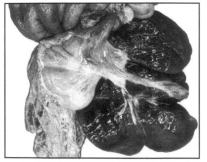

Fig. 1.209 Return to the abdominal viscera. Examine the gallbladder.

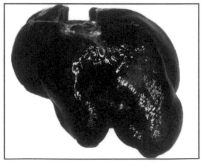

Fig. 1.210 Examine the liver (white spot, Aujeszky's disease).

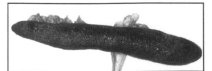

Fig. 1.211 Examine the greater omentum and examine the spleen (Aujeszky's disease).

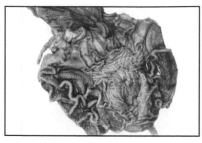

Fig. 1.212 Remove the stomach mid duodenum. Open the greater curvature (gastric ulceration).

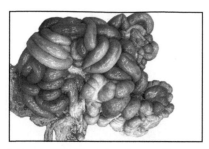

Fig. 1.213 Examine the small intestines with multiple incisions; examine lymph nodes (salmonellosis).

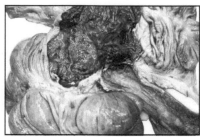

Fig. 1.214 Examine the distal ileum, caecum and colon (ileitis, swine dysentery, colitis).

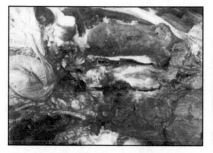

Fig. 1.215 Return to the carcase. Split the pelvis to allow removal of the urogenital tract and remaining rectum.

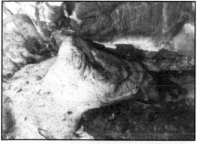

Fig. 1.216 Remove the urogenital tract from the caudal end to the bladder. Dissect from the kidneys to the bladder to retain the ureter intact.

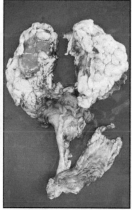

Fig. 1.217 Lay out the urogenital tract on a separate surface.

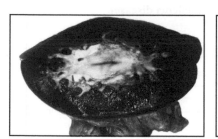

Fig. 1.218 Examine the kidneys, opening the pelvis from the lateral edge.

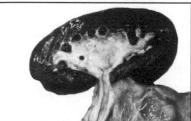

Fig. 1.219 Open the kidney to examine the pelvis and ureter (pyelonephritis).

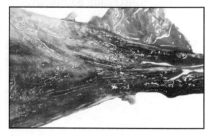

Fig. 1.220 Open and examine the bladder from the ventral surface taking care not to cut into the ureterovesical junction (cystitis).

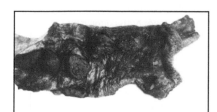

Fig. 1.221 Remove and examine the rectum (rectal stricture).

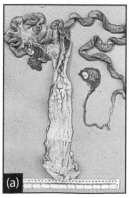

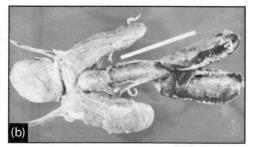

Fig. 1.222 Examine the genital tract noting reproductive status. Female reproductive tract (a), male reproductive tract (b); (brucellosis).

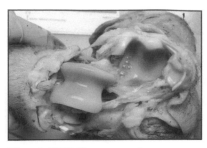

Fig. 1.223 Return to the carcase. Open and examine the elbow and carpus joints of both front legs. Open the stifle and hock joints of both hind legs (arthritis).

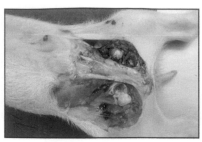

Fig. 1.224 Examine lymph nodes and incise superficial inguinal lymph nodes (PCV2-SD).

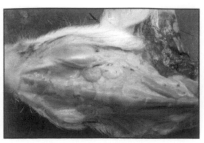

Fig. 1.225 Mandibular and parotid lymph node (tuberculosis). Note the large submandibular salivary gland.

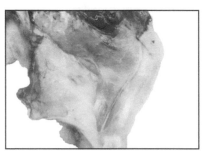

Fig. 1.226 Examine popliteal lymph node and any other lymph nodes demonstrating pathology.

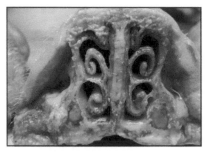

Fig. 1.227 Section the snout at the level of the lateral commissure of the mouth (atrophic rhinitis).

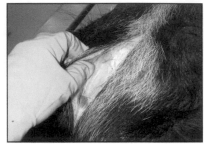

Fig. 1.228 Incise the skin over the forehead and look for oedema (oedema disease).

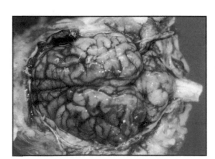

Fig. 1.229 Section or remove the skull and examine the cranial cavity.

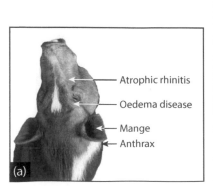

Atrophic rhinitis
Oedema disease
Mange
Anthrax

(a)

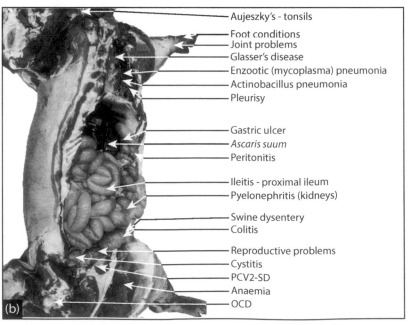

Aujeszky's - tonsils
Foot conditions
Joint problems
Glasser's disease
Enzootic (mycoplasma) pneumonia
Actinobacillus pneumonia
Pleurisy

Gastric ulcer
Ascaris suum
Peritonitis

Ileitis - proximal ileum
Pyelonephritis (kidneys)

Swine dysentery
Colitis

Reproductive problems
Cystitis
PCV2-SD
Anaemia
OCD

(b)

Fig. 1.230 (a, b) Summary of the post-mortem examination indicating the major locations where specific lesions indicative of the presence of a disease/pathogen may be particularly noted.

The post-mortem examination findings should be reviewed and any samples taken properly marked. There should be a systematic approach to describing your pathological findings. A morphological diagnosis includes the following: severity, time, distribution, anatomical site and lesion (for example, severe acute multifocal renal infarcts).

The following images (**Figures 1.231–1.283**) illustrate what might be seen when undertaking a post-mortem examination. (See Clinical Quiz 1.2 on page 52.)

Severity

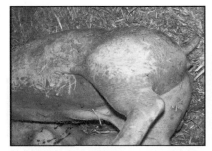

Fig. 1.231 Peracute.

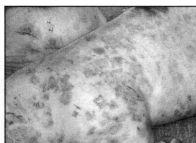

Fig. 1.232 Acute.

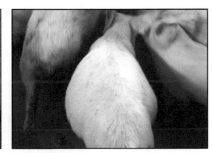

Fig. 1.233 Chronic.

Distribution

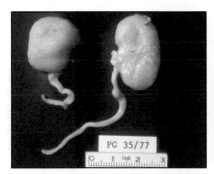

Fig. 1.234 Bilateral.

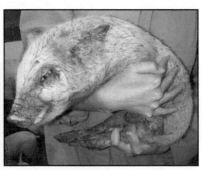

Fig. 1.235 Diffuse.

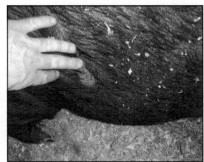

Fig. 1.236 Focal.

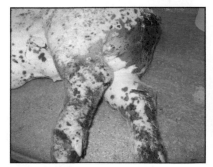

Fig. 1.237 Multifocal.

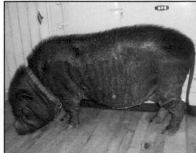

Fig. 1.238 Patchy.

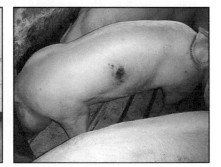

Fig. 1.239 Unilateral.

Colour

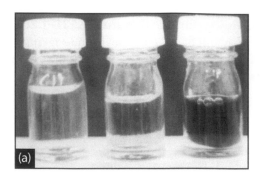

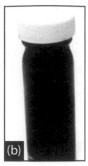

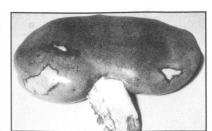Fig. 1.240 (a, b) Variety of urine colours.

Shape

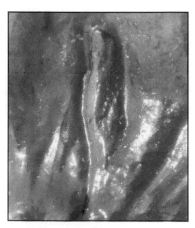

Fig. 1.241 Botryoid – shaped like grapes.

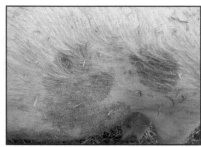

Fig. 1.242 Circular.

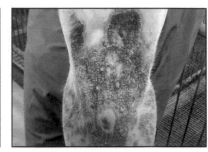

Fig. 1.243 Irregular.

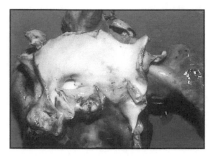

Fig. 1.244 Oblong.

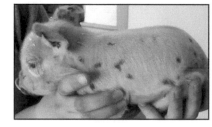

Fig. 1.245 Ovoid.

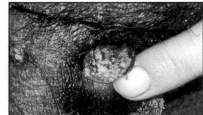

Fig. 1.246 Polypoid.

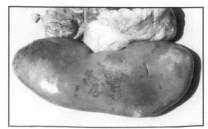

Fig. 1.247 Reniform – shaped like a kidney.

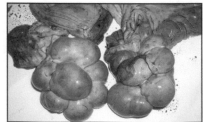

Fig. 1.248 Spheroid.

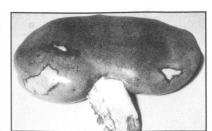Fig. 1.249 Wedge shaped.

Surface changes

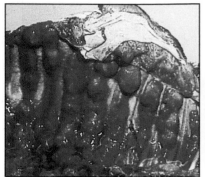

Fig. 1.250 Bulging.

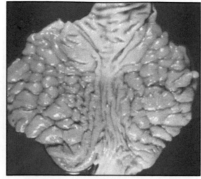

Fig. 1.251 Cobblestoned.

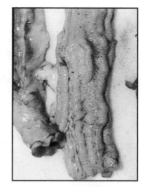

Fig. 1.252 Corrugated.

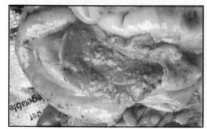

Fig. 1.253 Crusted.

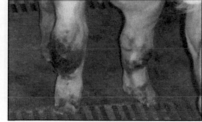

Fig. 1.254 Erosion.

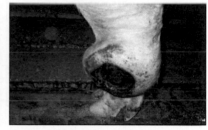

Fig. 1.255 Granular.

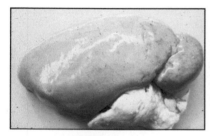

Fig. 1.256 Pitted.

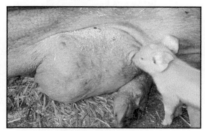

Fig. 1.257 Rough.

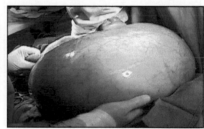

Fig. 1.258 Smooth.

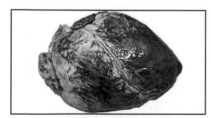

Fig. 1.259 Striated.

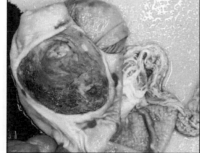

Fig. 1.260 Ulcerated.

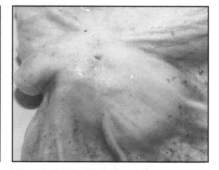

Fig. 1.261 Umbilicated.

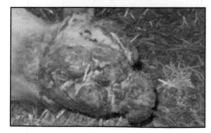

Fig. 1.262 Verrucous.

Margins of the lesion

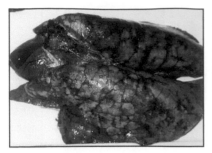

Fig. 1.263 Indistinct.

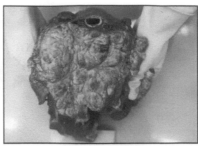

Fig. 1.264 Infiltrative.

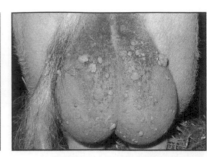

Fig. 1.265 Papillary.

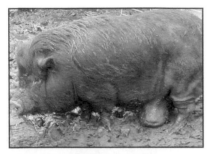

Fig. 1.266 Pedunculated.

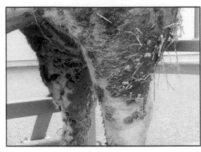

Fig. 1.267 Serpinginous – wavy.

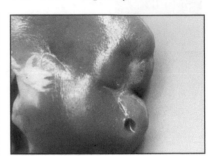

Fig. 1.268 Serrated.

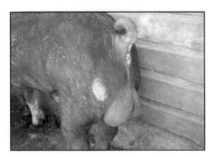

Fig. 1.269 Sessile – broad-based attachment.

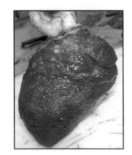

Fig. 1.270 Villous – finger like.

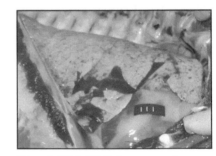

Fig. 1.271 Well demarcated.

Consistency

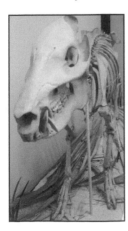

Fig. 1.272 Hard (e.g. bone).

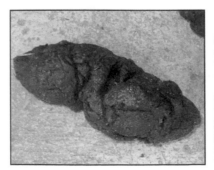

Fig. 1.273 Firm.

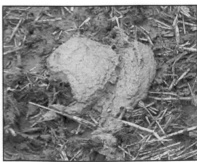

Fig. 1.274 Soft.

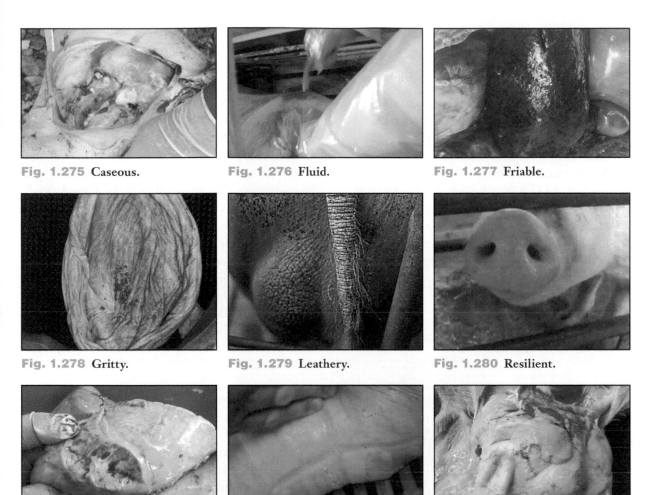

Fig. 1.275 Caseous.

Fig. 1.276 Fluid.

Fig. 1.277 Friable.

Fig. 1.278 Gritty.

Fig. 1.279 Leathery.

Fig. 1.280 Resilient.

Fig. 1.281 Rubbery.

Fig. 1.282 Spongy.

Fig. 1.283 Viscous.

SAMPLE COLLECTION AND SUBMISSION

Ideally, animals selected for laboratory analysis should be free from antimicrobial therapy and in an early or acute disease stage. Selected tissues should be collected as aseptically as possible. In addition, a meaningful history of the disease outbreak and a tentative diagnosis, based on clinical evaluation, should be included. Laboratory test results are directly affected by the selection, preparation, handling and shipment of selected specimens.

Identify tissue and samples
- Building or site.
- Animal identification number.
- Fluids, exudate/aspirates, tracheal washes, urine.

Preparation and collection of samples
Tissues – fresh

Collect approximately 6 to 12 cm² samples aseptically and place each into a plastic bag (e.g. Whirl-Pak® bags). Sample visible lesions with adjacent normal tissue. Double bag in Whirl-Pak bags. Do not mix tissues in one single bag. Transport with cold packs.

Eighteen to 24 cm of intestine should be carefully removed from the mesentery and tied to prevent leakage of intestinal contents. Collect sections of small and large intestine. The selected, clearly identified samples are double bagged and sealed in Whirl-Pak bags to prevent spillage. The samples should be refrigerated and cooled thoroughly prior to shipping.

Swabs

- **Aerobic culture**. Commercial swabs with Stuart or Amies transport medium are recommended to prevent desiccation.
- **Anaerobic culture**. Note that exposure to air for 20 minutes may destroy the sample. Transport in anaerobic transport medium (e.g. Clare Blair tubes).
- **Virus culture**. Collect blood in citrate tubes because EDTA may be detrimental to viral isolation. Dacron swabs are preferable over standard cotton swabs, which may contain bleach that can reduce the viability of the viruses. The swabs must be prevented from drying out.

Histopathology

Preparation of tissue for fixation: Multiple sites or types of lesions should be taken. The sections should be only 2 cm thick. The small size of the tissue results in rapid and complete penetration of the fixative. Present normal looking tissue with the pathological specimen (**Figure 1.284**).

Selected tissues should be cut with a scalpel since the squeezing action of scissors crushes and tears tissue. The tissue should be rinsed briefly with 0.85% NaCl to remove adherent blood since it will retard fixation. Autolysis or freezing will make samples unsuitable for proper evaluation. Place tissues in double Whirl-Paks. Identify bags if multiple animals are submitted. Do not use narrow mouth bottles to submit fixed tissue. **Note:** All hollow organs (intestine or uterus) should be gently flushed with 10% formalin without disturbing the mucosal lining before placing them in formalin.

Volume of fixative: The selected tissues should be fixed in 10% neutral buffered formalin (**Figure 1.285**). Use 10 times the volume of the tissues being fixed.

For tissue that floats in formalin, penetration is assisted by placing a small piece of card over the tissue (**Figure 1.285c**).

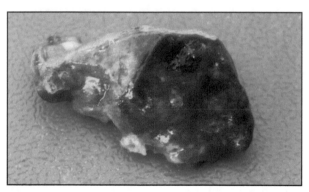

Fig. 1.284 The sample itself. Normal lung left portion with pathological area on the right.

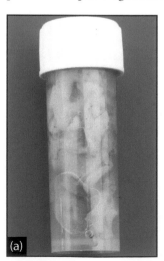 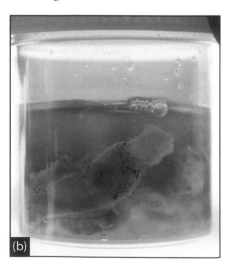 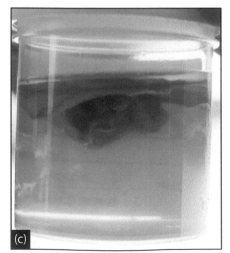

Fig. 1.285 How much fixative? (a) Wrong bottle for tissue. (b) Insufficient formalin. (c) Correct formalin to tissue ratio.

Collection of samples: Ideally, collect samples from all abnormalities recognised and from the draining lymph node. In addition, collect from the following organs: lung, heart, liver, spleen, kidney, small intestine, large intestine, tonsils and two lymph nodes (**Figure 1.286**).

In pigs less than 30 kg, a piece of brain and meninges can be helpful in reaching a definitive diagnosis.

Blood samples

- **Blood smear**. Prepare the blood smear on the slide at the farm. Allow to air dry and stain back at the laboratory.
- **Unclotted blood sample**. Collect in EDTA, heparin or citrate tubes. Pig blood clots relatively quickly so gently mix immediately after collection.
- **Clotted blood samples**. Serum is needed for biochemistry or measuring antibody titres

When sending paired sera, identify the acute samples from the convalescent samples on the tube and on the request form.

Packing specimens

To avoid leaking in transit, double bag the samples; Whirl-Pak bags work well for this purpose. Wrap sample bags and 2–4 ice packs in absorbent paper (e.g. newspaper) to absorb any fluid in the event of leakage. Place the package into a styrofoam container. Completed submission forms should be inserted into the envelope on the inside cover of the cardboard box.

Mailing

Samples should be submitted by the fastest means possible to avoid deterioration of specimens (**Figure 1.287**). Next day or overnight delivery is preferred over others. Discuss with the mailing system selected for any specific requirements. Ideally, take the samples to the diagnostic laboratory personally or by courier. Try to avoid Friday or Holiday samples. Ensure that all samples are adequately identified and that a suitable history is provided.

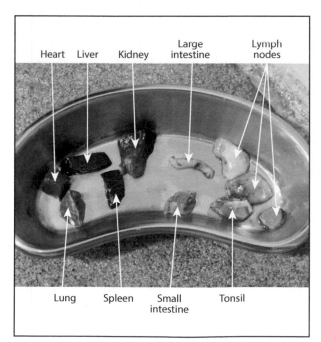

Fig. 1.286 **Which samples to take.**

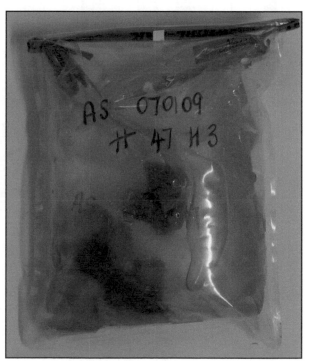

Fig. 1.287 **Posting the sample.**

SUMMARY OF THE DISEASES OF PIGS

Recognition of disorders by age: | Rare | Possible | Common |

CONDITION	2	4	6	8	10	12	14	16	18	20	22	24	26	GILT	SOW	BOAR
Abrasions	Common	Common	Possible	Possible	Possible	Possible	Possible	Possible	Possible	Possible	Possible	Possible	Possible	Possible	Possible	Common
Abscesses	Common	Common	Common	Common	Common	Common	Common	Common	Common	Common	Common	Common	Common	Common	Common	Common
Actinobacillus suis infection	Common															
Ascariasis	Possible	Possible	Possible	Possible	Possible	Possible	Possible	Possible	Possible	Possible	Possible	Possible	Possible	Possible	Possible	
Atrophic rhinitis: sneezing		Common	Common	Common												
Atrophic rhinitis: twisted					Possible	Common	Common	Common	Common	Common	Common	Common	Common	Common	Common	
Aujeszky's disease (pseudorabies)		Common	Common	Common	Common	Common	Common	Possible	Possible							
Bacterial arthritis	Common	Common	Possible	Possible	Possible	Possible	Common	Possible	Possible	Possible	Possible	Possible	Possible	Possible	Common	
Borrelia granuloma							Possible	Possible	Possible	Possible	Possible	Possible	Possible		Common	
Bursitis							Common	Common	Common	Common	Common	Common	Common	Common		
Carpal abrasion	Common	Common	Common													
Clostridium difficile infection	Common	Possible														
Clostridium perfringens infection	Common	Possible														
Coccidiosis	Common	Common														
Colitis			Possible	Possible	Common	Common	Common	Common	Possible	Possible	Possible					
Congenital tremor																
Cystitis														Possible	Common	
Dermatosis vegetans	Common	Common	Common													
Escherichia coli infection	Common	Possible	Possible	Possible												
Epiphysiolysis														Common	Common	
Epitheliogenesis imperfecta	Common	Common	Possible	Possible												
Erysipelas: arthritis				Possible	Possible	Common	Common	Common	Common	Common	Common	Common	Common	Common	Common	Common
Erysipelas: skin			Possible	Possible	Possible	Possible	Common	Common	Common	Common	Common	Common	Common	Common	Common	Common
Facial necrosis	Common															
Flaky skin															Common	Common
Foot and mouth disease	Common	Common	Common	Common	Common	Common	Common	Common	Common	Common	Common	Common	Common	Common	Common	Common
Gastric ulceration			Common	Common	Common	Common	Common	Common	Common	Common	Common	Common	Common	Common	Common	Possible

CONDITION	AGE IN WEEKS													ADULTS		
	2	4	6	8	10	12	14	16	18	20	22	24	26	GILT	SOW	BOAR
Glässer's disease		░	▓	░	░									░		
Greasy pig disease		░	▓	▓	░											
Haemorrhagic bowel				░	░	▓	▓	▓	▓	░				▓		▓
Hernia	▓			▓	▓	▓	▓	▓	▓	▓	▓	▓	▓	▓	▓	
Ileitis				░	░	▓	▓	▓	▓	▓	▓	▓	▓	▓		
Insect bites		░	░	░	░	░	░	░	░	░	░	░	░	░	░	
Joint ill	▓	▓														
Leptospirosis													░	▓	▓	
Meningitis	░	░	░	░	░	▓	▓	▓	▓	▓				░		
Mulberry heart			░		░											
Mycoplasma hyosynoviae infection				░	▓	▓	▓	▓	▓	▓						
Mycoplasma hyopneumoniae infection						▓	▓	▓	░	░						
Mycoplasma suis infection	░	░	░	░	░	▓	▓	▓	░					▓	▓	
Overgrown feet														▓	▓	▓
Parakeratosis						░	░	░			░					
Parvovirus														░		
Pasteurellosis			░	░	░	░	▓	▓	▓	▓						
Pityriasis rosea				░	░	░	░									
Porcine dermatitis and nephropathy syndrome					░	▓	▓	▓	░							
Porcine circovirus type 2-systemic disease					░	▓	▓	▓				░				
Porcine epidemic diarrhoea	░				░	▓	▓	▓	░	░	░	░	░	▓	░	▓
Porcine pleuropneumonia					▓	▓	▓	▓	░	▓	▓	▓	▓	▓		▓
Porcine reproductive and respiratory syndrome				░	░	▓	▓	▓	▓	▓	▓	▓	▓	▓	░	▓
Prolapsed rectum															▓	
Pulmonary bordetellosis			▓	░											░	
Pyelonephritis															▓	
Ringworm						░	░	░								▓
Rotavirus	▓															
Salmonellosis				░		▓	▓	▓	▓	▓	▓	░		░	░	▓
Sarcoptic mange				░										▓	▓	▓

| | AGE IN WEEKS | | | | | | | | | | | | | ADULTS | | |
CONDITION	2	4	6	8	10	12	14	16	18	20	22	24	26	GILT	SOW	BOAR
Shoulder sores																
Spirochaetal colitis																
Splayleg																
Streptococcal arthritis																
Sunburn																
Swine dysentery																
Swine fever (African and classical)																
Swine influenza																
Swine pox																
Tail biting – vices																
Transmissible gastroenteritis																
Thrombocytopaenia																
Trauma																
Trichuriasis																

Clinical signs as an indication of common disease problems on a pig farm. This list is not all inclusive; it is only intended to give the clinician a starting point

Abortions	Aujeszky's disease/pseudorabies Leptospirosis PRRS Swine fever		Diarrhoea – yellow	Coccidiosis *Escherichia coli* Salmonella
Abscess	*Actinobacillus pleuropneumoniae* serotype 3 Streptococcal infection *Trueperella pyogenes*		Diarrhoea – red blood	Clostridia enteritis Swine dysentery
			Diarrhoea – black	Ileitis - PIA Ulcer
Anaemia	Gastric ulceration Ileitis Iron deficiency *Mycoplasma suis* Swine dysentery		Diarrhoea – clear	Porcine epidemic diarrhoea Rotavirus TGE
			Diarrhoea – grey	Colitis *Escherichia coli* Ileitis
Breathing; heave line evident	Enzootic (mycoplasma) pneumonia Glässer's disease *Pasteurella/Streptococcus* pneumonia PCV2-SD PRDC *Salmonella*		Discharge – nasal	*Actinobacillus pleuropneumoniae* – blood Progressive atrophic rhinitis - blood Swine influenza
			Discharge – anal	See causes of diarrhoea
			Discharge – aural	Mange
Deep breathing	Lice – through anaemia *Pasteurella/Streptococcus* pneumonia Porcine pleuropneumonia Salmonella Swine fever Swine influenza		Discharge – mouth	*Actinobacillus pleuropneumoniae* – blood Foot and mouth disease
			Discharge – ocular	Oedema disease Progressive atrophic rhinitis Swine influenza
Breaths/ minute – increased	Heat stress PCV2-SD Porcine pleuropneumonia		Discharge – vulva	Brucellosis Cystitis 14–21-day post-service vulval discharge *Leptospira bratislava*
Bush foot	Bush foot		Granuloma	Granuloma
Coughing	*Actinobacillus suis* Aujeszky's disease/pseudorabies Enzootic (mycoplasma) pneumonia Gastric ulcer Porcine pleuropneumonia Porcine respiratory coronavirus PRDC Swine influenza		Greasy skin	Greasy pig disease
			Haematoma	Aural haematoma
			Lame high up	Glässer's disease *Mycoplasma* arthritis
			Lame low down	Erysipelas Foot and mouth disease Glässer's disease Lame sows
Deviation of nose	Acquired deviation Progressive atrophic rhinitis		Limb misshapen	Conformation
Diarrhoea	Clostridia Coccidiosis Colitis Dysentery *Escherichia coli* Ileitis - PIA Porcine epidemic diarrhoea Rotavirus Salmonella TGE		Loose faeces	Colitis Ileitis - PIA *Salmonella*
			Lymph nodes swollen	Lymphosarcoma PCV2-SD PRRS

(*Continued*)

(*Continued*)

Mastitis	*Actinobacillus suis* Coliforms *Streptococcus* species
Meningitis	Glässer's disease Streptococcal meningitis
Mucoid diarrhoea	Colitis Dysentery Ileitis- PIA
Mummified fetuses	Parvovirus PRRS PCV2-SD
Neurological problems	Aujeszky's disease/pseudorabies Congenital tremor Middle ear disease Stroke
Noise (vocal) change	Oedema disease Streptococcal meningitis
Oedema swellings	Oedema disease Glässer's disease
Orchitis	Brucellosis Japanese encephalitis virus
Paraplegia	Femoral epiphysiolysis Sow paraplegia Sow spinal abscess Splayleg
Parasites seen	*Ascaris suum* Lice
Pig conjugating	Salt poisoning - water deficiency
Pleurisy	*Actinobacillus suis* *Haemophilus parasuis* *Mycoplasma hyorhinis* Porcine pleuropneumonia *Streptococcus* *Trueperella pyogenes* (injury related) Origin – vice and foot injuries
Refusal of feed	Almost all conditions
Scratching	Allergy Lice Mange
Skin bluing	Septicaemia
Skin colour change (pallor)	Gastric ulcer Ileitis Leptospirosis
Skin erosions	Leg injuries
Skin necrosis	Glässer's disease Streptococci

Skin patchy lesions	Erysipelas PDNS Pityriasis rosea Ringworm Swine fever
Skin scaly	Essential oil deficient Lice Mange Zinc deficiency
Sneezing	*Pasteurella* Progressive atrophic rhinitis Swine influenza
Stillborn	Parvovirus PRRS
Sudden death	Aujeszky's disease/pseudorabies Clostridial enteritis Dysentery Erysipelas Glässer's disease Mulberry heart *Pasteurella/ Streptococcus* pneumonia Porcine pleuropneumonia Swine fever
Swollen abdomen	Glässer's disease Rectal stricture *Salmonella* Twist
Swollen joints	Erysipelas Glässer's disease *Mycoplasma* arthritis Streptococcal infections
Tumor	Tumours
Urine – blood	Pyelonephritis
Urine – smokey	Cystitis
Vesicles and blisters	Foot and mouth disease Seneca valley virus Swine vesicular disease
Vomiting	Hepatitis E virus Gastric ulcer *Salmonella* TGE
Vulva – necrotic	Mycotoxins
Vulva – swollen	Mycotoxins

PRDC, porcine respiratory disease complex; PCV2-SD, porcine circovirus type 2-systemic disease; TGE, transmissible gastroenteritis; PIA, porcine intestinal adenopathy; PRRS, porcine reproductive and respiratory syndrome.

(Continued)

Diseases by pathogen

PATHOGENIC AGENT	CLINICAL SIGNS	GROSS PATHOLOGY	MORBIDITY	MORTALITY	DIAGNOSIS	CONTROL
Adenovirus	Slight cough	Interstitial pneumonia			CFT; virus isolation	None
Actinobaculum suis	Urination of small volumes more frequently; dog squatting; vulvar discharges; lower fertility	Poor body condition; inflammation of the urinary tract	Variable – suggested to be 10–20%	Variable	Culture; histology	Broad-spectrum antibiotics; urine acidification through the water
Actinobacillus pleuropneumoniae	Acute death with epistaxis	Necrotic pneumonia; lung consolidation	Variable	Variable; can be >50% during initial stages	Gross	Individual and group therapy; elimination; vaccination
African swine fever virus	Incubation 2–6 days; pyrexia; dyspnoea; conjunctivitis; cyanosis; vomiting; diarrhoea	Septicaemia; petechiation; gastritis; enteritis; bronchopneumonia	Up to 100%	80–100% or mild	Clinical picture; gross lesions; histology; immuno-fluorescence	Eradication
Ascaris suum	None to active pneumonia 3–7 days after pigs are exposed when co-infection with influenza or *Mycoplasma*	Liver; severe eosinophil migration; lung interstitial pneumonia, bronchiolitis and oedema; white spots on liver	Variable	Minimal unless occurs with influenza or *M. hyopneumoniae*	Gross findings of milk spots; histology; faecal floats	Anthelminthic administered with appropriate timing
Aujeszky's disease virus (pseudorabies virus)	Incubation 5–7 days. Sows: abortions, stillborns, mummies. Weaners: neurological symptoms, diarrhoea, vomiting. Newborn: neurological symptoms, diarrhoea, vomiting	Rhinitis; pneumonia; lung consolidation; necrotic tonsillitis; liver necrosis	Suckling pigs high; variable in weaners and sows	Up to 100% under 3 weeks old	Clinical picture; histology; PCR; FA; IHC	Slaughter; eradication; vaccination; biosecurity
Blue eye disease (paramyxovirus)	Corneal opacity; nervous signs; fever; ataxia; reproductive losses with increased stillborns, mummification	Corneal opacity	Variable	High in those with clinical signs	Gross signs; PCR; histology; ELISA	No specific treatment; herd closure; cleaning/disinfection
Bordetella bronchiseptica	Active cough and persistent sneeze	Lobar pneumonia	High	Low	Culture; ELISA	Antibiotics and vaccination

(Continued)

PATHOGENIC AGENT	CLINICAL SIGNS	GROSS PATHOLOGY	MORBIDITY	MORTALITY	DIAGNOSIS	CONTROL
Brachyspira hyodysenteriae	Blood and/or mucus in faeces, often with straining	Lesions limited to the large intestine; oedema; congestion within the mucosa; patchy inflammation; continued flecks of fresh blood followed by fibrin in the necrotic debris	High	Variable	Identification of spiral-shaped organisms by dark field or crystal violet stains; culture with haemolysis control	Antibiotics
Classical swine fever virus (hog cholera)	Systemic lymph bleeding; button-like intestinal ulcers; spleen necrosis; multiple haemorrhages in the kidney; elevated body temperature (41–42°C); severe yellow/grey diarrhoea; reddening discoloration of the skin; anorexia; reproductive losses due to abortion, mummification	Recumbent pigs	High		Clinical picture; histology; PCR; ELISA antibodies	Eradication and vaccination
Clostridium perfringens	Diarrhoea in piglets 2–7 days of age	Yellow to pasty stools in one or more pigs within the litter	10–100% mortality	Variable, can be low or extremely high	Gram stain; toxin identification	Intensive sanitation; treat preventably with oral penicillin, bacitracin
Coccidiosis *Cystoisospora suis*	Occurs primarily in piglets between 7 and 15 days of age	Yellow to grey pasty diarrhoea; potbellied, long haired	Variable	Variable	Faecal or intestinal scrapings identifying the merozoites	Intensive sanitation; toltrazuril
Coliform mastitis	Agalactia or low milk output; elevated temperature	Inflammation of the mammary glands with increased oedema and firmness	Low	Low unless *Klebsiella* or toxigenic strains of *E. coli* present	Gross signs; culture	Intensive sanitation; high sow nutrition; antibiotics based on sensitivity; therapeutic anti-inflammatory support
Escherichia coli	Yellow, watery faeces	Fluid-filled jejunum	Affected litters high	Affected litters high	pH >8; culture; histology; toxin identification	Intensive hygiene; pre-farrowing vaccination against the strains present

(Continued)

PATHOGENIC AGENT	CLINICAL SIGNS	GROSS PATHOLOGY	MORBIDITY	MORTALITY	DIAGNOSIS	CONTROL
Foot and mouth disease virus and other vesicular disorders – Seneca valley virus	Vesicles or blisters at the hoof, mouth, lips, nose; elevated temperature	Vesicles or blisters	High	High	PCR; IHC	Eradication; vaccination against specific identified serotypes
Inclusion body rhinitis (Cytomegalovirus)	None; sneezing post weaning	Rhinitis	100%	None	Histology	None
Haemophilus parasuis	Dead pigs, lameness	Long haired; pneumonia; joint swellings, particularly of the hock and elbow	Variable	Variable	Culture; PCR	Individual antibiotic treatment; group treatment
Lawsonia intracellularis	Brown to black or red diarrhoea	Inflammation and thickening of the ileum	Variable	Variable	Clinical picture; gross changes; PCR; IHC	Sanitation or hygiene; vaccination; antibiotics
Leptospira spp.	Fever; jaundice; abortions; necrosis of skin and mucous membranes	Necrosis of skin; abortions	Variable	Variable	PCR, FA, histology	Tetracycline antibiotics; vaccination
Menangle virus	Fetal death leading to mummified fetuses, stillborns, and reduction in farrowing rates		Low	Low	PCR	None available
Mycoplasma hyopneumoniae	Chronic, non-productive cough	Lobar pneumonia in the dependant lobes	High	Low except when introduced into a naïve herd	Gross; histology; PCR; IHC	Antibiotics; vaccination, elimination
Mycoplasma hyorhinis	Sudden death; elevated temperature; respiratory distress	Extensive pleuritis	High	Variable	Extensive pleuritis; PCR; culture	Antibiotics
Mycoplasma hyosynoviae	Lame pigs; hind legs	Synovitis	Moderate	Low	Serology, PCR	Tiamulin
Nipah virus	Often asymptomatic; acute febrile; respiratory signs; muscle tremors	Incoordination; recumbency	Variable	Variable	PCR	None advised
Parvovirus	Infertility; increased mummification and stillborn rate	Varying lengths of mummified fetuses	Variable	Often high for 3–6 weeks in gilt litters	FA; PCR	Planned exposure; vaccination

(Continued)

PATHOGENIC AGENT	CLINICAL SIGNS	GROSS PATHOLOGY	MORBIDITY	MORTALITY	DIAGNOSIS	CONTROL
Pasteurella multocida	Wet cough; pneumonia	Lobar pneumonia	Variable	Variable	Culture	Control; vaccination; antibiotics to which it is susceptible
Porcine adenovirus	Diarrhoea	Epidemics of diarrhoea primarily in 7–28-day-old pigs	Naïve herds high	Naïve herds high	PCR; FA	Natural planned exposure
Porcine circovirus type 2	Stillborns; weak pigs; infertility	Multisystemic syndrome	In unvaccinated pigs quite high	10–20% in unvaccinated pigs	PCR; IHC	Vaccination; hygiene
Porcine delta coronavirus	Diarrhoea and vomiting	Watery, yellow diarrhoea; shortening or absence of the villi	Affected litters 100%	Affected litters 10–100%	PCR; histology, IHC	Intensive hygiene; natural planned exposure pre-farrowing or whole herd
Porcine epidemic diarrhoea	Diarrhoea and vomiting	Fluid-filled small intestine; absence of villi	90+%	90+% naïve herds	PCR	Natural planned exposure; vaccination
Porcine reproductive and respiratory syndrome virus	Incubation couple of days; respiratory distress; unthrifty pigs; increased secondary disease; naïve herd; reproductive losses; early farrowings	Interstitial pneumonia	100%	Low on its own, high when complicated	Clinical signs; serology (not detected for 3 weeks post infection); histology; PCR (DNA)	None; good nursing; secondary protection with antibiotics; elimination; good gilt introduction; biosecurity; management
Porcine respiratory coronavirus	None; dyspnoea	None	100%	None	Histology; serology	None
Rotavirus	Diarrhoea and vomiting depending on the type	Watery, yellow diarrhoea. Shortening or absence of the villi	Affected litters 100%	Affected litters 10–100%	FA; histology; pH <8	Intensive hygiene; natural planned exposure pre-farrowing or whole herd
Sarcoptes scabiei var *suis*	Extreme pruritus or itching	Thickened skin/inflamed skin, particularly in the soft areas above the udder; inguinal flank	High	Low	Acaricides	Herd elimination
Selenium toxicosis		None	Variable	Variable	Chemistry or histology	Remove the excessive selenium

(Continued)

PATHOGENIC AGENT	CLINICAL SIGNS	GROSS PATHOLOGY	MORBIDITY	MORTALITY	DIAGNOSIS	CONTROL
Staphylococcus hyicus	Generalised epidermitis	Dark, greasy appearance, generally around the face but can be generalised		Generally low mortality; high only if litters infected during the suckling phase are clinical during the suckling phase	Culture of *S. hyicus*	Clip needle teeth; treat with broad-spectrum antibiotics to which it is sensitive; spray pigs with broad-spectrum animal-safe disinfectant; intensive hygiene
Streptococcus suis	Pneumonia. CNS with paddling and incumbency	Lobar pneumonia. Oedema of the eyelids. Oedema of the brain	Low	Low	Culture	Individual animal therapy; vaccination
Swine influenza (influenza A virus)	Incubation hours to 4 days; anorexia; pyrexia; cough; prostration; dyspnoea; rapid spread; reproduction problems	Pneumonia; lung consolidation; enlarged mediastinal lymph nodes	High	Low	Clinical picture; virus isolation; histology; serology	None; good nursing; secondary protection with antibiotics; good gilt introduction; vaccination
Teschovirus	Polioencephalomyelitis; reproductive losses; pneumonia	Paralysis	Variable	Variable	Clinical signs; virus isolation from the CNS; PCR	None; natural planned exposure
Togaviruses	Newborn piglets: depression, tremors and diarrhoea	Diarrhoea; tremors; arthritis	Variable	Variable	FA	Minimise mosquito exposure
Torque teno virus	None		Variable	Variable	PCR	Natural planned exposure
Transmissible gastroenteritis virus	Vomiting and diarrhoea	Diarrhoea; fluid-filled small and large intestine; villus atrophy	100% naïve herds	90–100% naïve herds	PCR; FA; histology	Natural planned exposure; hygiene; vaccination
Tuberculosis (*Mycobacterium* sp.)	None to enlarged lymph nodes	Enlarged cervical and thoracic lymph nodes	Variable	Low	PCR; culture; acid-fast stain	Remove the contaminated source, which is generally associated with bird faecal contamination

CFT, complement fixation test; PCR, polymerase chain reaction; FA, fluorescent antibody (test); ELISA, enzyme-linked immunosorbent assay; IHC, immunohistochemistry; CNS, central nervous system.

CLINICAL QUIZ

1.1 Look at the clinical signs shown in **Figures 1.21–1.105**. Can you identify what condition or conditions, where applicable, are illustrated.

1.2 **Figures 1.231–1.283** illustrate what might be seen when undertaking a post-mortem examination. Can you identify the different conditions that may be associated with these findings?

The answers to these questions can be found on pages 471 and 472.

CHAPTER 2

REPRODUCTIVE DISORDERS

SIGNIFICANT ANATOMY OF THE REPRODUCTIVE TRACT

Before being able to understand reproductive abnormalities, it is first necessary to recognise what is normal. Integral to the recognition of a normal presentation is an understanding of the underpinning anatomy and physiology.

Boar

The reproductive anatomy of boars includes the testes and the epididymides, with each testis being inverted so that the tail of the epididymis is dorsal. The vas deferens connects the epididymis with the urethra. At the vas deferens/urethral junction and beyond are the accessory sex glands: the prostate, seminal vesicles, and bulbourethral gland (**Figure 2.1**). These accessory sex glands produce fluid, fructose, and gel, respectively.

The boar's prepuce has a bilobed diverticulum that can retain urine and preputial secretions. Emptying this diverticulum reveals a foul smelling fluid. This fluid is of significance as if it enters semen during collection,

it will kill or at least reduce the viability of the collected semen. It also will contaminate mid-stream urine, making a clean urine sample difficult to obtain.

Female – gilt and sow

The reproductive anatomy of the gilt/sow includes the ovaries, the oviducts which connect to the uterine horns at the uterotubal junction (UTJ), the uterine horns, the cervix, the vagina/vestibule and the vulva (**Figures 2.2, 2.3**).

The appearance of a normal porcine ovary will vary according to physiological status. Prepubertally, surface follicles remain no larger than 1–2 mm. As gilts enter their prepubertal follicular phase, these surface follicles grow under the influence of the gonadotropins, follicle-stimulating hormone (FSH) and luteinising hormone (LH), to the 4 mm stage. From the 4 mm stage to ovulation at 8–10 mm, follicle growth becomes progressively more LH dependent. Following ovulation, the follicles transition from red corpora haemorrhagica to pink corpora lutea, their size being related to follicle diameter at ovulation (**Figure 2.4**) but average 10 mm in size.

Fig. 2.1
The normal mature boar reproductive tract. The prostate is below the vesicular glands.

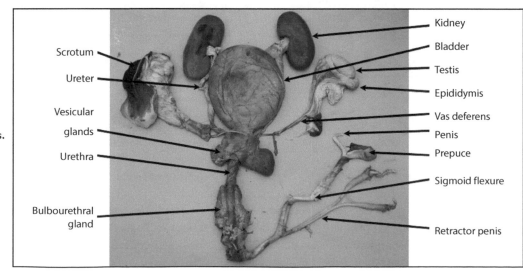

Scrotum
Ureter
Vesicular glands
Urethra
Bulbourethral gland

Kidney
Bladder
Testis
Epididymis
Vas deferens
Penis
Prepuce
Sigmoid flexure
Retractor penis

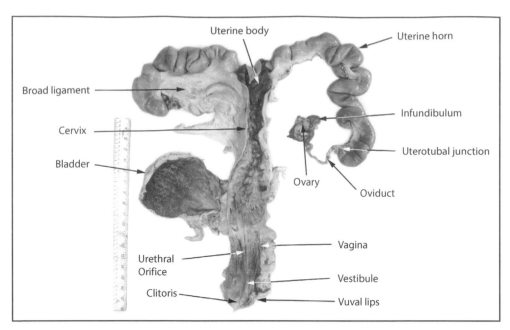

Fig. 2.2 The normal non-pregnant female reproductive tract.

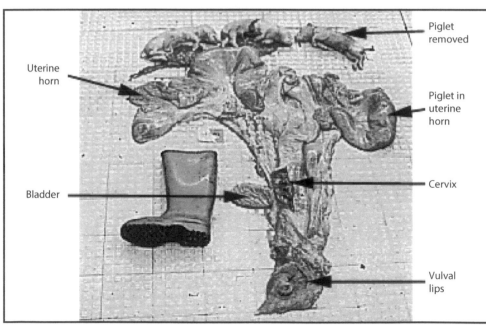

Fig. 2.3 The normal gravid (pregnant) reproductive tract.

OESTROUS CYCLE AND PREGNANCY IN THE PIG

Oestrous cycle ▶ VIDEOS 1 and 7

An understanding of the oestrous cycle is essential before reproductive interventions are considered.

The 21-day (18–24) porcine oestrous cycle is composed of an approximately 15-day luteal phase, a 4-day follicular phase and a 2-day oestrous period.

Ovulation occurs approximately 70% of the way through the oestrous period. After ovulation, the remains of the ovarian follicles are luteinised to become the progesterone secreting corpora lutea (hence 'luteal' phase).

During the luteal phase, corpora lutea production of progesterone limits the secretion of LH and FSH and thus restricts follicular development to the medium follicle stage and prevents the onset of oestrus.

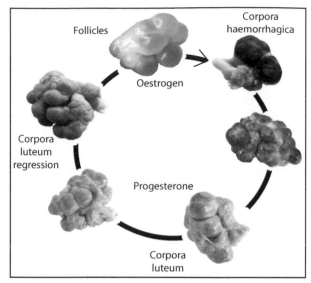

Fig. 2.4 **The changes in the ovary at different reproductive phases.**

At about 12–14 days of the luteal phase in the non-pregnant female, uterine (endometrial) production of prostaglandin F2 alpha ($PGF_{2\alpha}$) causes regression of corpora lutea and so terminates progesterone production. This allows resumption of appropriate secretory patterns of the pituitary gonadotropins, particularly LH, which stimulates ovarian follicular development to be completed (the follicular phase).

In weaned sows, the 4–5 day wean-to-service interval (WSI) (wean-to-estrus interval [WEI] in the USA) is equivalent to the follicular phase. Renewed follicular development produces oestrogen, ultimately resulting in behavioural oestrus. Approximately coincident with the onset of oestrus, there is an oestrogen-induced surge release of LH, which causes a cascade of events within the follicle including a switch from oestrogen to progesterone production and culminating with a new ovulation approximately 40 hours after the start of the LH surge.

Cycles continue unless interrupted by culling or pregnancy.

Signs of oestrus ▷ VIDEOS 1 and 7
Pro-oestrus
- In gilts, the vulva swells, but this is not consistent in the sow.
- The vulva becomes congested or red.
- The udder develops in gilts.
- The female becomes nervous and easily disturbed and climbs up gates and walls.

- She is ridden by other sows, but does not stand.
- Vaginal walls become reddened (congested).
- Clitoris becomes more prominent.
- Vaginal fluids thicken, produce strands between fingers.

Oestrus
- The vulval reddening starts to subside.
- There is a slight mucus vulval discharge.
- The female starts to mount other sows, and if mounted starts to stand.
- Emits a characteristic high-pitched grunt.
- She actively seeks boars.
- Has a decreased appetite.
- Stands to back pressure, particularly in the presence of a boar.
- In a Large White, pricks her ears.
- Stands with tail upright and flicking up and down.
- Rub marks.
- Has a clean vulva in outdoor units (post service).
- Rubs and is attracted to stockpersons.
- Has glazed eyes.
- Allows coitus.
- During oestrus the sow will stand for 10–15 minutes and will be refractory for 45 minutes before standing again.

Conception
Achieving successful pregnancy in pigs is dependent on appropriate breeding management and, conversely, depressed reproductive performance may be traced to poor breeding management.

Globally, most commercial sows are bred by artificial insemination (AI), the basic principles of which are simple; place enough viable spermatozoa in the right place at the right time, and keep it clean. Using current insemination technology, 2 to 3 × 10^9 spermatozoa in 70 mL semen diluent are deposited in the cervix. This large number is needed to compensate for sperm loss due to back-flow of semen, as well as entrapment and death of spermatozoa in the cervix and uterus. It also provides some compensation for less than optimal timing of insemination.

It is not the number of spermatozoa deposited into the cervix or uterus that ultimately controls fertility, it is the number of spermatozoa that enter the oviduct that is important. The proportion of inseminated spermatozoa that actually get to the oviduct is variable, but will be <2% of the spermatozoa deposited in the cervix.

Fresh spermatozoa are not capacitated and so are capable of attaching to the epithelium in the first 2 cm of the oviduct and enter an arrested state. However, capacitated spermatozoa are unable to attach to an ova. Capacitated spermatozoa, on the other hand, cannot attach to the oviduct epithelial cells and so fail to produce an effective spermatozoa reservoir but are able to attach to the ova. The local microenvironment in the spermatozoa reservoir is low in bicarbonate, which inhibits capacitation, and these spermatozoa constitute the spermatozoa reservoir potentially available to fertilise ova.

Capacitation status is particularly important in the fertility of frozen-thawed spermatozoa because, once thawed, 60% of the spermatozoa will have undergone a capacitation-like reaction and so result in a much smaller spermatozoa reservoir. Therefore, to improve fertility to insemination with thawed semen, spermatozoa deposition must be much closer to the time of ovulation (i.e. 4–6 hours).

The effective fertile life of non-frozen spermatozoa in the reservoir is about 24 hours. In order to reach the oviduct, the spermatozoa must traverse about 1 metre of uterus and get through the UTJ and enter the oviduct. Spermatozoa transport in the uterine horn is facilitated by uterine contractions. Most oestrous sows will have some spontaneous uterine contractility, which is improved by boar stimuli. If uterine contractions are reduced (e.g. if a boar is not present), spermatozoa transport may be poor, the spermatozoa reservoir reduced and thus fertility lowered. Uterine contractility cannot be monitored on-farm so ensuring good spermatozoa transport involves implementing techniques known to enhance uterine contractility. The key to good uterine contractility is stimulation of the sow during and after cervical insemination. Aim for 5 minutes of boar contact after insemination. If the boar has to be moved, have a second boar come behind him to continue the stimulation. If a breeding belt or other similar accessory is employed, do not remove it for about 5 minutes. This makes the whole breeding experience around 10–15 minutes, which mimics the normal breeding behaviour. Remember, once the semen dose has been taken up by the sow, a lot of the spermatozoa are in the body of the uterus and still need to be transported towards the oviducts.

It is known that as the site of spermatozoa deposition gets deeper into the female reproductive tract (deep uterine insemination), fewer spermatozoa per insemination dose are required to maintain fertility. Insemination catheters allowing for transcervical semen deposition into the uterine body are commercially available and allow for spermatozoa numbers to be reduced to 1×10^9 per AI dose. This technique is still dependent on reaching an adequate spermatozoa reservoir at the UTJ.

Signals arriving near the time of ovulation cause the release of spermatozoa from their arrested state in the spermatozoa reservoir and allow them to redistribute along the oviduct towards the site of fertilisation (isthmus-ampulla junction). Once spermatozoa leave the reservoir, the higher environmental bicarbonate triggers a calcium influx and initiates capacitation which, on average, takes about 6 hours to complete. The number of functional spermatozoa available for fertilisation (which will impact sow fertility) will be dependent on the number originally entering the spermatozoa reservoir (which is influenced by spermatozoa transport) and the interval between spermatozoa entry to the reservoir and their redistribution at the time of ovulation (which is influenced by timing of insemination relative to ovulation).

Sow fertility following AI (i.e. fertilisation rate, farrowing rate, litter size) is affected by the time of insemination relative to ovulation. If insemination occurs at or soon after the time of ovulation, by the time capacitation has occurred the eggs may be too old; their fertility decreases by about 6 hours after ovulation. Depending on how old the eggs are, the result could be an effective failure of fertilisation or, if fertilisation does occur, it may result in increased embryo mortality and smaller subsequent litters. Late inseminations are also associated with an increased risk of urogenital disease and reduced sow performance because of the low oestrogen at this time. Oestrogen positively affects uterine immunocompetence by increasing blood flow through the reproductive tract (hence the swelling and reddening of the female vulva), bringing more leucocytes and facilitating leucocyte entry to the uterine lumen if needed. Late oestrus/metoestrus is a time of reduced uterine immunocompetence, which can negatively affect uterine (and hence conceptus) health if females are inseminated at this time.

A component of the uterine immune response is an inflammation designed to eliminate the excess spermatozoa. This will commence within 2 hours of insemination and a second insemination performed less than 6 hours after the first will result in spermatozoa deposition into a hostile environment, the net effect of which will be a reduced fertility. This is not a problem with natural breeding as the seminal plasma has an anti-inflammatory effect.

If inseminated too far in advance of ovulation, too many spermatozoa die before ovulation occurs, the net effect being the same as inseminating too few spermatozoa to begin with, which results in increased regular returns and smaller litter sizes.

To maximise fertility, deposition of fresh-extended spermatozoa into the sow should occur during the 24 hours before ovulation. Assuming good quality semen within 4 days post collection, inseminations need only be performed once 24 hours after the first insemination.

An alternative is to ensure insemination occurs 6–12 hours before ovulation as fertility would be maintained even when fewer viable spermatozoa are available, but this would require hormonal control (e.g. exogenous gonadotropin-releasing hormone [GnRH] treatment). The administration of GnRH 80–96 hours post weaning results in the ability to do single fixed-time insemination on the entire weaning sow batch.

The time from detection of oestrus to ovulation is variable. It is accepted that sows having a short WSI (e.g. 3–5 days) will tend to exhibit a longer duration of oestrus and, conversely, sows having a long WSI (e.g. >5 days) will tend to have a shorter duration of oestrus. Ovulation usually occurs at about 70% through oestrus, independent of the duration of the oestrous period. The effect of this is that sows having a short WSI will tend to be late ovulators while sows having a long WSI will tend to be early ovulators. Parity 1 (P1) sows will normally have a WSI 1 day longer than multiparous sows.

In commercial practice, it has been observed that the fertility of sows inseminated following a WSI of 6 or more days is less than for sows inseminated following shorter WSIs. As many as 5% of lactation sows may have an oestrus while in lactation. This can complicate the WSI as the lactation oestrus may be missed and the normal cycle seen 18–24 days later – around 16 days post weaning for example. Lactation oestrus is particularly a problem in sows suckling litters of less than eight piglets. If breeding records indicate a high incidence of 16–20 days WSI, sows may require oestrus suppression during late lactation.

Pregnancy

Following fertilisation in the oviducts, the conceptus/developing embryos continue their journey, arriving in the uterus on day 2–3. The developing embryos migrate freely throughout both uterine horns during days 3–14. The blastocyst hatches from the zona pellucida about day 7.

On about day 10–11 the developing embryos produce oestrogen; this is the first signal for maternal recognition of pregnancy (MRP) and initiates luteal support by redirecting the luteolytic $PGF_{2\alpha}$ from the uterine vein to the uterine lumen.

Between days 11 and 16, the embryonic placental tissue elongates to 1 metre. Placentation occurs between day 17 and about day 24. During the period of placentation, the embryos produce more oestrogen, which constitutes the second signal of MRP. It is generally believed that a minimum of two embryos per uterine horn are needed to ensure an adequate signal is produced.

Impact of the maternal recognition of pregnancy signals

If the sow does not receive the first signal (due to fertilisation failure or loss of the litter prior to day 11), she will exhibit a regular return to oestrus (18–24 days); this is considered a failure of conception.

If she receives the first but not the second signal, she will exhibit an irregular return to oestrus (25–38 days); this is considered a failure of pregnancy as it results from an initial luteotrophic signal (hence, pregnancy) but a failure of ongoing support (hence pregnancy failure).

If the sow loses her litter after receiving both signals, she may become pseudopregnant with oestrus occurring around day 63 post mating (**Figure 2.5**).

Until about day 14 the corpora lutea are considered autonomous and are very resistant to the luteolytic effects of $PGF_{2\alpha}$. However, beyond 14 days the corpora lutea require endocrine support, particularly LH, and are also more sensitive to the luteolytic effects of $PGF_{2\alpha}$.

Organogenesis is complete by 24 days. Skeletal mineralisation commences by 35 days; skeletal

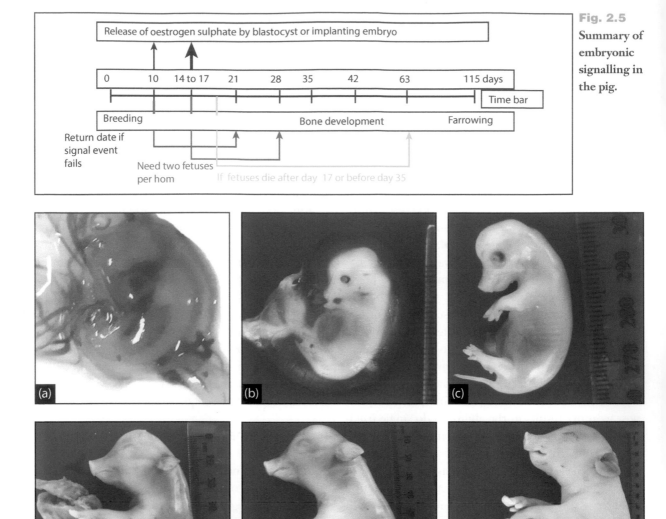

Fig. 2.5
Summary of
embryonic
signalling in
the pig.

Fig. 2.6 Changes in the physical appearance of the fetus with age. (a) 20 days; (b) 25 days; (c) 35 days; (d) 45 days; (e) 60 days; (f) 90 days.

absence from fluid accumulations in ultrasound scans of 'pregnant' sows is indicative of pseudopregnancy. The developing fetuses become immunocompetent at day 70 of gestation. Changes in the physical appearance of the fetus are shown in **Figure 2.6**.

Growth of the piglet is reasonably predictable and this allows the estimation of fetal age using mummified or aborted fetuses, which can be very useful in reproductive disease diagnoses (*Table 2.1*). An easy calculation of fetal age can be obtained using the formula below (**Figure 2.7**):

$$(\text{crown–rump length [mm]})/3 + 21 = \text{age of fetus in days}$$

Table 2.1 **Estimating the age of a fetus through crown–rump measurement.**	
CROWN–RUMP (mm)	**DAYS OF PREGNANCY**
20	30
50	40
88	50
130	60
167	70
200	80
232	90
264	100
200	110

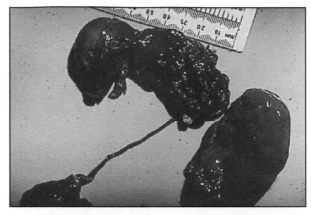

Fig. 2.7 Measuring a mummified piglet to determine its age at death. Crown–rump = 80 mm, therefore age is approximately 48 days.

Pregnancy diagnosis

Pregnancy diagnosis in the commercial pig farm should be completed over four distinct phases:

- 1–110 days post mating. The sow should be exposed once a day to a boar to assist the stockperson to see any signs of oestrus and thus non-pregnancy.
- 18–48 days post mating. The lack of the behavioural signs of oestrus when the 'pregnant' sow is in the presence of a mature male boar. This will detect regular and irregular returns.
- Around 28 days. Real-time ultrasonography (**Figures 2.8–2.13**) is highly effective (95%) at determining the state of pregnancy. Any questionable sow can be rechecked at 35 days.
- At 8 weeks of pregnancy. The sow's abdomen will become visibly pregnant and this should be used as the final 'pregnancy check' (**Figures 2.14, 2.15**).

Fig. 2.8 Interpretation of ultrasound. Not pregnant.

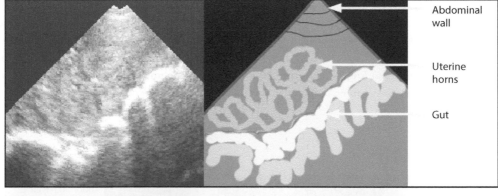

Fig. 2.9 Interpretation of ultrasound: 17 days pregnancy – difficult to see the uterine vesicles.

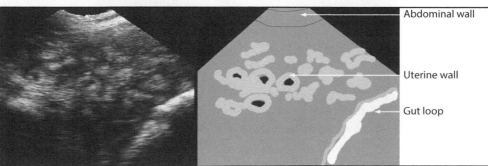

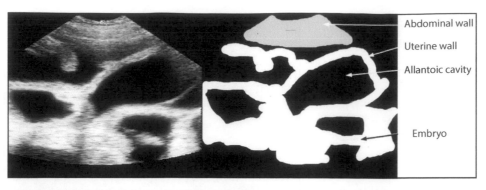

Fig. 2.10
Interpretation of ultrasound: 28 days pregnancy – vesicles easy to see, but note the embryo.

Abdominal wall
Uterine wall
Allantoic cavity
Embryo

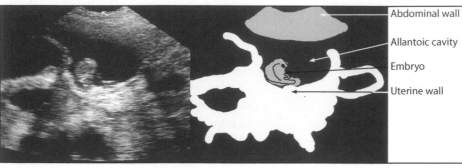

Fig. 2.11
Interpretation of ultrasound: 35 days pregnancy – note the uterine vesicles are easy to see with prominent embryo.

Abdominal wall
Allantoic cavity
Embryo
Uterine wall

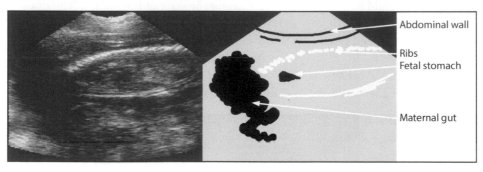

Fig. 2.12
Interpretation of ultrasound: 80+ days pregnancy. Bone in the fetus becomes more obvious, but the fetus can be difficult to see against the general mother background. Note

Abdominal wall
Ribs
Fetal stomach
Maternal gut

that maternal gut can look like uterine vesicle but there is no distinct edge. It can become difficult to see the fetus against the maternal abdomen as the allantoic fluid reduces in prominence.

Complications
See **Figures 2.13–2.15**.

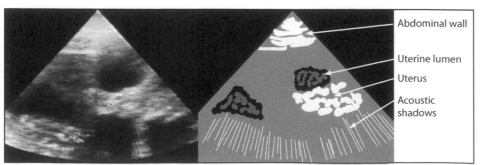

Fig. 2.13 Interpretation of ultrasound pseudopregnancy around 35 days. Note that while there appear to be black holes, there are no embryos. Sometimes the uterine lumen may be filled with 'grains'.

Abdominal wall
Uterine lumen
Uterus
Acoustic shadows

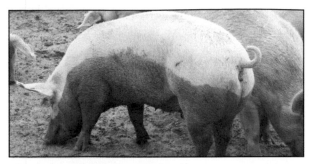

Fig. 2.14 Non-pregnant gilt.

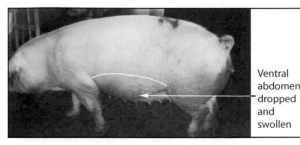

Ventral abdomen dropped and swollen

Fig. 2.15 Pregnant shape. Note the dropped ventral abdomen (white line) at about 8 weeks of gestation.

Gestation length

Gestation length varies from 112–120 days. It is calculated from the first mating. However, gestation commences on the day of fertilisation, therefore gestation length should be calculated from the last mating, which will be closer to the time of ovulation and subsequent fertilisation. Functional corpora lutea are required for maintenance of pregnancy and luteolysis at any time during gestation (after day 12) will terminate the pregnancy. Gestation lengths less than 112 days are classified as abortions.

HORMONAL CONTROL OF REPRODUCTION

Control of oestrus and ovulation

If because of a seasonal effect boar exposure of gilts is not effective for stimulating puberty onset, or if an induced gilt oestrus is required to fill a gap in the breeding target, exogenous gonadotropins can be administered. Common preparations include 1,000 IU equine chorionic gonadotropin (eCG) or the combination of 400 IU eCG and 200 IU human chorionic gonadotropin (hCG). These products are labelled for the induction of fertile oestrus in prepubertal gilts. However, when eCG/hCG combinations are administered to prepubertal gilts, up to 30% do not exhibit behavioural oestrus and about 30% of those that do exhibit behavioural oestrus may fail to cycle regularly. Although breeding at a subsequent natural oestrus will improve fertility, the poor predictability of cycling beyond the induced oestrus means that gilts should be bred at the induced oestrus. However, if historical data for a particular farm indicates that >90% of gilts show regular cyclicity following gonadotropin injection, then breeding should be delayed until the next natural

oestrus. If puberty appears delayed and the response to gonadotropin treatment is poor, it is likely that the gilts are cycling but their first (and possibly second) oestrus was missed; cyclic gilts will not exhibit oestrus in response to gonadotropin treatment.

Prolonged WSIs (>5 days) are associated with reduced sow performance and increased likelihood of early culling. A delayed oestrus is more likely in primiparous sows, especially as a component of seasonal infertility. A primary driver of prolonged WSI is inadequate lactation nutrient intake. Primiparous sows have a lower appetite than older sows and will thus also have a disproportional reproductive response to environmental factors that reduce sow appetite.

Boar exposure of weaned sows is likely not necessary until day 4 after weaning. However, where records analysis indicates a problem of prolonged WSIs, an appropriate initial response is more strategic boar exposure (e.g. exposure during cooler times of the day, starting the day after weaning). If this is not sufficient, exogenous hormonal stimulation of oestrus may be needed (i.e. eCG/hCG). Several studies have shown that gonadotropin treatment results in a shorter and more synchronous onset of the post-weaning oestrus. A more cost-effective use of gonadotropins would be to inject only problem sows, with treatment limited to sows anoestrus on day 7 after weaning. The response obtained will depend on the accuracy of non-oestrus detection in weaned sows because if a sow is cycling (but her oestrus was missed), she will not respond to hormone treatment.

Oestrus suppression/synchronisation

If gilts are known to be cyclic, the options for oestrus control are limited to the feeding of the progestogen altrenogest. Unlike cattle, a single injection of $PGF_{2\alpha}$ will not induce luteolysis before day 12 of the pig oestrous cycle so is of little value in oestrus synchronisation programmes.

Altrenogest is orally active and mimics the biological activity of progesterone by suppressing endogenous gonadotropin secretion, which limits ovarian follicle growth to medium follicle size. In gilts, altrenogest does not prevent normal luteolysis but will continue to suppress final follicular growth and oestrogen production after luteolysis because of its negative feedback on LH release, and so blocks oestrus onset. Ideally, gilts should be individually fed so that they consume at least 15 mg/day (but we suggest 20 mg/day); underdosing altrenogest (<13 mg/day) is associated with cystic follicles. However, oestrus suppression is needed only from the time of luteolysis, so if cycle dates are known, altrenogest feeding can be minimised by only providing it from day 13 of the oestrous cycle until 5 days before gilts are scheduled to be bred. Expect 90–95% of gilts to achieve oestrus on days 4–8 after last feeding.

Altrenogest can be also used to enhance the fertility of primiparous sows after weaning by providing a longer period for metabolic recovery from lactation. This results in a longer but predictable WSI and a likely increased subsequent litter size. The first altrenogest feeding must be on the day of weaning (or before) and most sows (>85%) will likely be in oestrus 5–7 days after the last feeding. With older parities of some genotypes, if records indicate a likelihood of lactation oestrus or very short WSI, altrenogest feeding can be initiated during late lactation.

Another use of altrenogest is the blocking of oestrus in zero-weaned sows or sows experiencing very short lactations, and it may be necessary if a sow herd experiences coronavirus enteric disease (transmissible gastroenteritis or porcine epidemic diarrhoea). Zero-weaned or very short lactation sows are likely to experience significant fertility problems, which may include cystic ovarian follicles and very poor farrowing rates and litter sizes. To increase the time for uterine recovery after gestation a period of oestrus suppression is indicated. This can be achieved with the feeding of altrenogest but, similar to breeding in late oestrus/metoestrus, the circulating progesterone (or progestogen such as altrenogest) compromises uterine immunocompetence. So, while potentially effective, if any residual uterine contamination exists, the feeding of altrenogest during the periparturient period may facilitate uterine disease, indicated by abnormal vulval discharge. As with any abnormal vulval discharge, these sows should be culled.

Controlling time of ovulation – single fixed-time insemination

The development of fixed-time insemination of gilts and sows allows for fewer timing mistakes and a reduction in labour requirements for oestrus detection and inseminations. Both eCG and eCG/hCG combinations are effective for induction of oestrus and the duration of this induced oestrus is longer, making it more amenable to controlling the time of ovulation. Ovulation will occur in 85–90% of sows about 42 hours after injection of hCG and at about 38 hours after GnRH or LH. If ovulation is predicted to occur >40 hours after detection of oestrus, as is likely with short WSI or gonadotropin-induced oestrus, treatment with hCG or GnRH will induce a predictable time of ovulation and if time of ovulation is known, timing of insemination is simple. This in turn allows for single fixed-time inseminations.

An alternative strategy, assuming a high proportion of spontaneous oestrus by day 4 after weaning, is to administer hCG or GnRH at about 80 hours after weaning and breed oestrous sows 24–36 hours after injection.

Number of inseminations required

Most farms will adopt a two insemination programme am/am at 24 hour intervals for sows in oestrus. There are no improvements in farrowing rates or litter size with more inseminations. With weaned sows, single insemination to sows in oestrus post day 5 also demonstrates no loss of farrowing rate or litter size.

FARROWING – PARTURITION

Control of farrowing ⏵ VIDEO 2

Farrowing induction can be employed to simplify piglet colostrum management and cross-fostering management. Once litters start suckling the antibody content of colostrum as well as the piglet's ability to absorb antibodies drops precipitously; anticipate a 40% drop in both variables by 6 hours after farrowing. Therefore, donor and recipient sows should have farrowed no more than 2 hours apart. Further, piglets should remain on their sow for at least 12 hours to allow transfer of immunoglobulins and immune cells;

piglets absorb antibodies from any sow but immune cells only from their own sow.

The administration of $PGF_{2\alpha}$ or its analogues has long been known to be effective for the induction of farrowing in sows. However, a large range in the interval between treatment and parturition can still be expected. Experience has shown that only 50–60% of induced sows are likely to farrow during the following working day and so be candidates for farrowing supervision. If sows receive $PGF_{2\alpha}$ but are not supervised during farrowing, then the cost of the $PGF_{2\alpha}$ is borne by those sows that are supervised, effectively increasing the cost of treatment per sow. The dose, and hence cost, of farrowing induction can be reduced by 50% if injected into the vulva, at the vulva–cutaneous border. If this route of injection is chosen, use a 12.7 mm 20 gauge needle, or smaller.

A further refinement for improving predictability of farrowing is a double injection of $PGF_{2\alpha}$ ('split dose'). With this technique, an injection of $PGF_{2\alpha}$ is given in the morning and then a second $PGF_{2\alpha}$ injection is given about 6 hours later. This results in a higher proportion of sows farrowing the next day during working hours, which facilitates farrowing supervision. Split-dose injection does not affect earlier farrowing sows but promotes farrowing of sows likely to have a longer treatment-to-farrowing interval. The second $PGF_{2\alpha}$ dose increases the likelihood of inducing terminal luteolysis with an initial fall in circulating progesterone concentrations, but then luteal recovery occurs with renewed production of progesterone and pregnancy maintenance.

Other treatments used in attempts to improve the predictability of parturition following $PGF_{2\alpha}$ injection include oxytocin, which has been associated with an increased myometrial contraction frequency, intensity and duration. The injection of 10 IU oxytocin approximately 20–24 hours after the injection of $PGF_{2\alpha}$ causes a more rapid and synchronous onset of parturition but it also often causes an interrupted farrowing (i.e. one piglet may be delivered rapidly but then farrowing stops, possibly for an hour or more, necessitating manual assistance). This may be due to pain associated with forced delivery through an incompletely dilated cervix causing a release of adrenalin that binds to uterine adrenergic receptors and stops contractions. Stillborns associated with oxytocin treatment tend to occur among the first born pigs of the litter rather than the norm, where stillborns occur in the last few pigs of the litter. The reason for this is that oxytocin causes stronger and more prolonged uterine contractions, which traumatise the umbilical cords causing fetal anoxia, as evidenced by more piglets being born with meconium staining. Also, stronger, longer lasting uterine contractions reduce uterine blood flow with associated fetal bradycardia and acidosis. Therefore, oxytocin should not be used at farrowing except therapeutically in cases of individual slow farrowing sows. If a sow has not delivered a piglet in more than 30 minutes, consideration should be given to oxytocin injection (2.5–5 IU intravulva). Similarly, if the farrowing is quite prolonged, especially with older sows if records indicate greater stillborn rates, then consider oxytocin use after the 6th or 7th pig has been born.

Midwifery in the farrowing area

Piglets may present in a variety of positions at the point of farrowing. Most of the time the piglet will still be born without assistance, but the following may help a stockperson understand what their fingers are telling them when manual assistance is deemed necessary.

Protocol for assisting farrowing

A sow or gilt that presents with a farrowing problem should already be in the farrowing area. If standing, encourage the female to lie down by rubbing her udder line. It is very dangerous to attempt to farrow a sow while standing, especially if there is a rear bar on the farrowing place.

Wash your hands carefully (**Figure 2.16**). Ensure your fingernails are short. Dry your hands. Place an arm length glove over each hand. It is sometimes best to try and learn to be able to use either

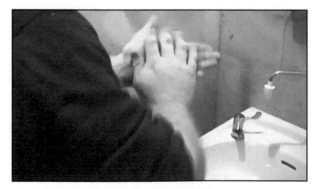

Fig. 2.16 **Wash your hands carefully.**

hand to assist farrowing. Ensure you apply plenty of lubricant to your hand and arm (**Figure 2.17**). Place extra lubricant onto the palm of your hand. Bring your fingers together and carefully enter the vulval lips and start exploring the vulva and vagina.

It should not be necessary to break sweat when farrowing a sow. Consider patience and use of oxytocin. Do not overreach into the sow to retrieve every piglet you can feel; give nature a chance (**Figures 2.18, 2.19**).

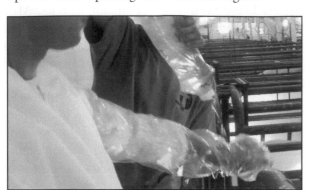

Fig. 2.17 Wear gloves and apply plenty of lubricant.

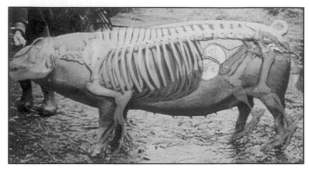

Fig. 2.18 General relevant anatomy of the sow at farrowing.

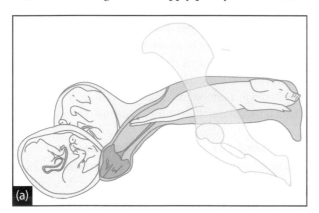

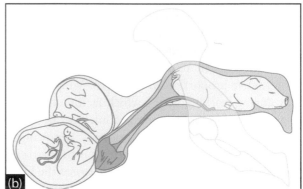

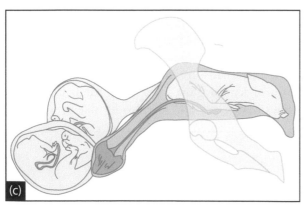

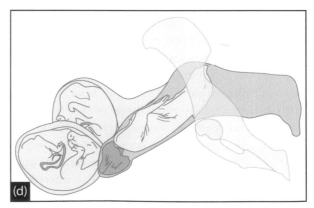

Fig. 2.19 Various fetal positions at farrowing and their necessary correction to facilitate delivery. (a) Normal (ideal) presentation. If piglet slightly oversized, place rope on both front feet and assist farrowing. (b) Front legs back – retrieve front legs, pull forward and remove piglet. (c) Forward but front feet back, possibly hind feet forward. Push piglet back into pelvis and pull front feet forward. Place head rope onto head and rope onto front feet and remove piglet. If still difficult, may be necessary to push hind feet backwards before pulling on piglet. (d) Piglet upside down. It may be possible to pull the front feet forward and by applying head rope and rope of feet, pull the piglet out. If still difficult, it may be necessary to rotate the piglet. *(Continued)*

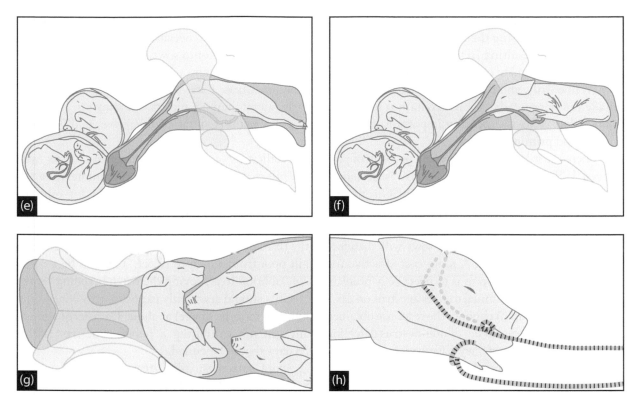

Fig. 2.19 (Continued) Various fetal positions at farrowing and their necessary correction to facilitate delivery. (e) Backwards with back feet backwards. Place rope around back feet of piglet and remove piglet. If removing piglet is difficult, check shoulder position; may be necessary to manipulate front legs into forward position. (f) Breech. Use fingers to hook onto rear hock and manipulate leg backwards until foot visible. Repeat with other leg. Apply ropes to the feet and remove piglet. (g) Most difficult position. Push piglet back into uterine body and bring head forward. Place head rope onto piglet. Retrieve legs and place rope on legs and remove piglets. Often other pigs will rapidly follow; several may be stillborn. (h) Placement of head rope. The rope goes behind both ears and is looped into the mouth. It is then tightened against the mouth. Thus with gentle traction, varying between legs and head, the piglet can be eased through the pelvis.

STIMULATING POST-WEANING OESTRUS

Prolonged WSIs (i.e. >5 days) are associated with reduced sow performance and increased likelihood of early culling (**Figure 2.20**). Indeed, infertility is more likely in sows returning to oestrus between days 6 and 12 after weaning.

A delayed oestrus is more likely in primiparous sows, especially as a component of seasonal infertility. A primary driver of prolonged WSIs is inadequate lactation nutrient intake. Primiparous sows have a lower appetite than older sows, and will thus also have a disproportional reproductive response to environmental factors that reduce sow appetite.

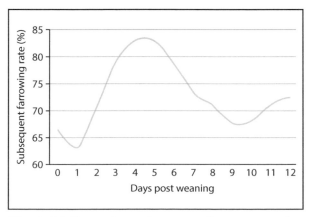

Fig. 2.20 Future farrowing rate and wean-to-service interval.

In particular, an inadequate lysine intake results in young sows mobilising their lean tissue to obtain the needed lysine, resulting in post-weaning infertility. A reasonable estimate of sow requirements is 60 g of total lysine daily, and to facilitate an adequate lysine intake the lactation diet should contain at least 1.1% total lysine. This is especially important in hyper-prolific and primiparous sows.

Where records analysis indicates a problem of prolonged WSIs, an appropriate response is hormonal stimulation of oestrus using an eCG/hCG combination. Treatment results in a shorter and more synchronous onset of the post-weaning oestrus and the oestrus duration will be longer; sows will therefore tend to be late ovulators. A more cost-effective use of exogenous gonadotropins is to inject only problem sows, with treatment limited to sows anestrus on day 7 after weaning. In all likelihood, the response obtained will depend on the accuracy of non-oestrus detection in weaned sows since if they have had a missed oestrus, they will not respond to hormone treatment.

SELECTION OF FUTURE BREEDING STOCK

Gilt selection must emphasise body conformation, particularly their legs/feet and the mammary chain. However, a key component of successful pig farming is maximising the productivity of sows through the first and second parities, as these two parities predict performance for the rest of the sow's life. A herd objective is to have 60% of sows in parities 3 to 6. Suggested benchmarks are shown in *Table 2.2*.

The numbers weaned may have little to do with the numbers born because of cross-fostering the additional piglets onto sows, especially parity 1 (P1). The farm should aim to have one piglet weaned per functional teat. Each batch farrowing place should wean more than 12 piglets and aim for 100 kg of weaners per batch farrowing place at 27 days of lactation.

Facilitating a productive longevity starts with the gilt rearing and selection programme. The target oestrus and breeding age/weight for gilts are minimum of second oestrus at about 220 days of age (190–240 days) and 130 kg live weight. Waiting for the third oestrus allows for the farm to have a bigger gilt pool from which to select. This can be a major contribution to achieving the batch breeding target.

Gilts should start daily exposure to a boar (minimum 10 months of age) at about 175 days of age and any gilt not exhibiting a pubertal oestrus within 28 days should be culled.

Avoid extremes; gilts greater than 130 kg live weight at less than 175 days of age are likely to be culled early for feet/leg problems, while gilts less than 130 kg live weight at more than 240 days of age will be too small to survive normal herd management.

A target backfat depth at farrowing of 18 mm at the P2 position (65 mm off midline at last rib) may be achieved by modifying gestation feeding; there is little evidence that high-plane feeding of parity 1 sows or sows during pregnancy is a problem unless such feeding makes them fat.

During lactation, sows require 26 g total dietary lysine/kg litter average daily gain (i.e. about 60 g/day). Lysine deficiency results in sow lean tissue mobilisation and reduced post-weaning fertility. Therefore, dietary lysine for primiparous sows should be a minimum of 1.1%.

Parity 1 lactation lengths should not be less than 18 days and these young sows should nurse at least 12 piglets. Mammary glands that work during the first lactation produce more milk in subsequent lactations. If nurse sows are required to extend the suckling period of low weight-for-age piglets, choose primiparous sows (this does not include obviously diseased fall-back pigs). For example: in a 4-week lactation system, wean litters of primiparous sows at 4 weeks of age and then replace them with 1- or

Table 2.2 **Suggested benchmarks of sow productivity with increasing parity.**				
	1ST PARITY	**2ND PARITY**	**3–6 PARITIES**	**7+ PARITIES**
Total born	12.5	13.8	15	14.5
Born alive	11.8	12.8	14.2	12.8
Stillborn	0.5	0.7	0.7	1.5
Mummified	0.2	0.2	0.1	0.2
Weaned	12+	12+	12+	12+
Farrowing rate %	80	85	87	82
Parity distribution %	20	18	60	2

2-week-old vigorous but light weight pigs and allow them to lactate for a further 2 weeks. The piglets will be weaned at 3–4 weeks of age but the primiparous sows will have lactated for 6 weeks. Expect these sows to deliver 1.5 extra pigs in their second litters. These nurse sows need to be housed outside of the batch farrowing system.

SEMEN ANALYSIS

Semen can be examined microscopically to determine spermatozoa concentration and to assess motility and morphology as measures of semen quality (**Figures 2.21–2.29**). The use of a vital stain such as nigrosine/eosin will aid these assessments.

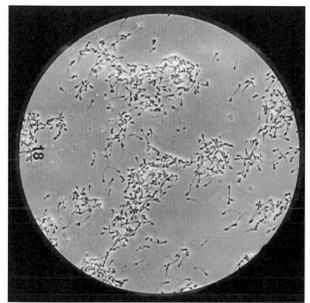

Fig. 2.21 Semen down the microscope. The spermatozoa should be seen to be active with forward motion. In very good samples wave motion is seen.

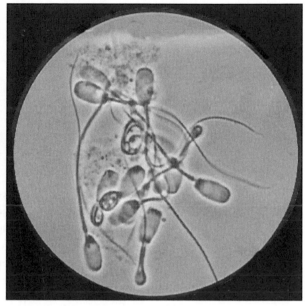

Fig. 2.22 Clumping of semen. In contaminated samples clumping of spermatozoa can be seen. This may also occur with chilling.

Fig. 2.23 Normal seminal appearance. The normal sperm with a tail central to the head. The tail is straight without any kinks. The head is smooth and even.

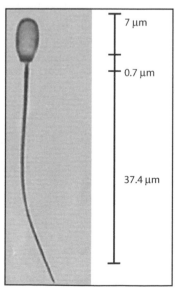

7 µm

0.7 µm

37.4 µm

Figs 2.24, 2.25 Seminal proximal (2.24) and distal (2.25) cytoplasmic droplets. These may have little significant impact on fertility and are more common in immature sperm. The droplet comes from the acrosome/ head cover, which uncovers at ejaculation and then runs down the tail.

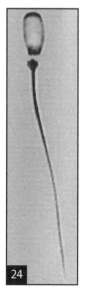

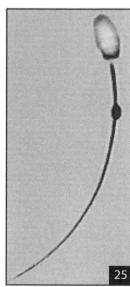

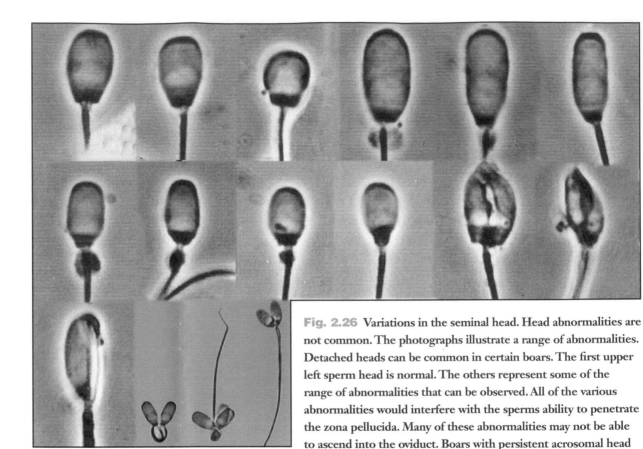

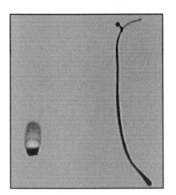

Fig. 2.26 Variations in the seminal head. Head abnormalities are not common. The photographs illustrate a range of abnormalities. Detached heads can be common in certain boars. The first upper left sperm head is normal. The others represent some of the range of abnormalities that can be observed. All of the various abnormalities would interfere with the sperms ability to penetrate the zona pellucida. Many of these abnormalities may not be able to ascend into the oviduct. Boars with persistent acrosomal head defects over 5% should be culled.

Semen with a motility of less than 50% and with abnormalities greater than 30% should be rejected. However, before a boar is rejected review the semen on multiple days. In addition, note that none of the visual assessments (aside from aspermia or death of the sperm) have any correlation with reproductive performance.

Fig. 2.27 Detached head appearance.

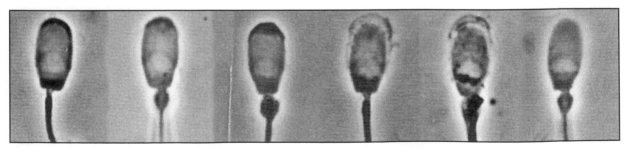

Fig. 2.28 Variations in seminal cytoplasmic droplets. The left hand sperm head is normal. The others represent some of the range of abnormalities that can be observed. The impact of the presence of droplets on fertility is debatable, as many of the droplets (without head defects) are part of the normal maturation process of sperm post ejaculation.

Fig. 2.29 **Variations in the seminal tail. Some of the variety of tail defects that can be visualised are illustrated. Deformities of the tail interfere with the sperm's ability to swim in the oviduct and through the zona pellucida.**

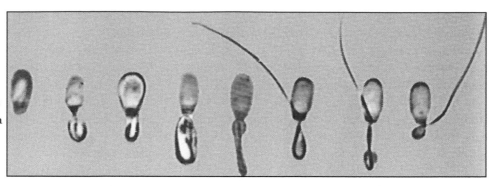

REPRODUCTIVE DISORDERS

Abortions

There are a range of causes of abortion in the pig, the majority being non-infectious and the aetiology of about 90% not definitively diagnosed (**Figure 2.30**). It is not unusual for 1.5% of all services to fail-to-farrow due to abortion. Abortion associated with luteolysis can occur at any time of pregnancy (after day 12) but the loss of embryos around day 20 without the loss of the corpus lutea will not result in abortion; the sow will enter a period of pseudopregnancy and recycle after day 63 post mating.

Non-infectious abortion

Environmental/seasonal effects: About 70% of all abortions fall into this category. In the wild, sows

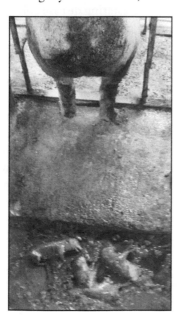

Fig. 2.30 **Aborted litter associated with African swine fever.**

would normally farrow in the spring and, therefore, some residual seasonality can be expected with a tendency for pregnancies to be lost in the summer and autumn. Many factors are believed to be involved in the summer infertility/autumn abortion, including photoperiod, heat stress, variable daily temperatures and temperature-linked reductions in appetite. In outdoor farms, white pigs are particularly prone to sunburn in the summer, which is likely to cause an abortion due to heat stress and pain. To minimise the potential for abortion, provide outdoor sows with wallows to allow them to cool themselves and also apply mud as a sunscreen.

Inadequate nutrient intake during lactation requires the sow to mobilise too much of her body reserves, particularly lean tissue, to support milk production. Following weaning and breeding, pregnancy maintenance can be impacted by the interaction of poor body condition (due to low lactation nutrient intake) and various environmental effects. The incidence of autumn abortion may be higher on farms with sows in lower body condition and provision of supplemental heat to gestating sows may reduce the incidence of abortion. Autumn is associated with warm days but potentially very cold nights. If supplemental heat or extra feed energy is not supplied, then sows have to divert feed energy from production to heat generation and they can become catabolic. If already in poor body condition, this extra stress on the less robust corpora lutea may trigger luteolysis and abortion. When investigating autumn abortion pay particular attention to the thermal environment. Confined sows on concrete cannot huddle for warmth. Hang a maximum–minimum thermometer and determine whether the area is wet or if there are broken windows resulting in draughts. Investigate if other aspects of ventilation are causing disruption in air flow patterns resulting in draughts. With sows housed in groups, those lower in the hierarchy may suffer restricted access to the feeder in addition to the stress of bullying, potentially resulting in pregnancy loss. (See Chapter 10 and review thermal control.)

Non-environmental effects: Vaccinations can also result in abortions; their function is to induce an immune-mediated inflammatory reaction, which may cause pyrexia and sufficient $PGF_{2\alpha}$ production to trigger an abortion.

Although difficult to prove, mycotoxins have long been suspected as being responsible for abortions. In particular, zearalenone is a phytoestrogen and can mimic maternal recognition signals, resulting in embryo losses and pseudopregnancy. It is possible that zearalenone reduces LH, which would adversely affect luteal function. Never feed mouldy feed to animals. Mouldy straw can also play a significant role in the causes of abortion. Ensure good feeder hygiene at all times. Manage feed bins so they are thoroughly cleaned 2–3 times a year. Add mycotoxin absorbent/deactivation agents to the feed of adults and developing gilts.

Infectious abortion

There are a range of infectious causes of abortion. Refer to the section dealing with these specific diseases for more detailed information. Disease agents can cause abortion through one of two major routes:

1 Indirectly via luteolysis, likely through a high temperature releasing endogenous prostaglandins. Pathogens include swine influenza virus, African swine fever virus and *Erysipelothrix rhusiopathiae*.
2 Directly via disease of the reproductive system resulting in fetal death and/or placentitis. Pathogens include ADV (pseudorabies), CSF virus (CSFV), porcine reproductive and respiratory syndrome virus (PRRSV), PCV2, *Leptospira* spp. and *Brucella* spp.

Investigation into an abortion and sample submission

- Optimal specimens: chilled, not frozen.
- Two or three intact fetuses and placentas; include the freshest fetus.
- If there are mummifed fetuses, submit three mummies –small and largest.
- Submit 5 mL of sow serum.
- Placenta fresh.
- Do bacterial culture on the lung, stomach contents, liver and placenta.
- Fluorescent antibody tests on lungs for parvovirus and PCV2 and tissue homogenate for *Leptospira* spp.

Aujeszky's disease (pseudorabies)
Definition/aetiology
Suid herpesvirus 1 is the cause of Aujeszky's disease (AD) or pseudorabies (PR). The virus is an enveloped DNA herpesvirus. This infectious agent displays a wide host range, infecting almost all mammals (except higher primates). Aujeszky's disease virus (ADV) does not affect man. Pigs are considered the natural host; the other potential hosts usually are dead-end hosts. Dogs present with rabid signs, hence the name pseudorabies. Cattle and sheep and, rarely, horses present with a mad itch. In cats, rats and mice the effects of ADV are rapidly fatal and this may be a useful indicator for the presence of the disease.

Although field isolates may differ in virulence, AD is a devastating disease able to cause a myriad of clinical signs at all ages, including reproductive, neurological and respiratory outcomes. Genetic resistance to AD has been described but the mechanisms are unknown. There are very efficient vaccines (manufactured with deleted genes) able to provide immunological responses that can be differentiated from those elicited by the natural infection. This characteristic of the gene deleted vaccines has allowed for the eradication of AD in many parts of the world.

Transmission occurs within a herd by nose to nose contact and through mating, both natural and AI. Transplacental infection can occur. The virus, typical of a herpesvirus, is latent in the pig. However, outside the pig the virus can survive short periods in the air, up to 7 hours with the relative humidity higher than 55%. The virus is rapidly inactivated when exposed to drying. Between farms, infection of wild animals also help to spread the disease. The pathogen can spread up to 2 km by air under the correct conditions. Transmission can occur between trucks during transport, therefore tailgating of trucks should be avoided. Also, parking next to other pig trucks at service stations is to be avoided. The incubation period of the disease is 2–4 days.

Clinical presentation

Infection of swine with ADV at early ages (suckling and nursery pigs) may cause high fever, anorexia, depression, dyspnoea, hypersalivation, vomiting, incoordination, paddling and death (**Figure 2.31**). At these ages, the dominating clinical picture is of neurological origin accompanied with very high mortality rates (**Figures 2.32, 2.33**); the older the pig, the less the incidence of central nervous clinical signs.

In growers and finishers, the usual dominating clinical outcome is respiratory, with tachypnoea, sneezing and coughing, but concurrent respiratory tract infections are very common and death is the result of severe bacterial pneumonia. In recovered cases, the animals show rough hair and growth retardation.

In breeding stock clinical signs depend on their physiological and reproductive status. Clinical signs may include fever, dyspnoea, irregular return-to-oestrus (due to embryonic death and embryo resorption), abortions (**Figure 2.34**), stillborns and fetal mummification.

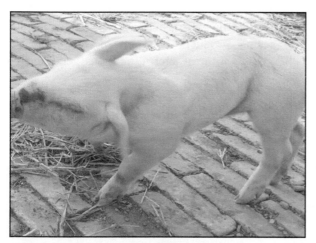

Fig. 2.31 Piglet showing clinical signs of incoordination due to Aujeszky's disease, displaying lateralisation of the head and body.

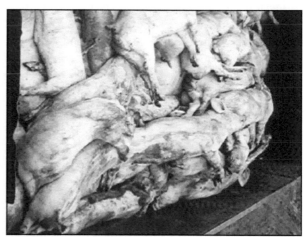

Fig. 2.32 High mortality in growing pigs with Aujeszky's disease.

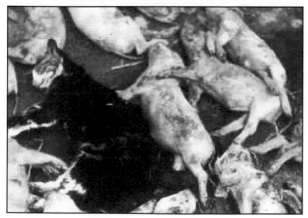

Fig. 2.33 Farm cats rapidly die in cases of Aujeszky's disease.

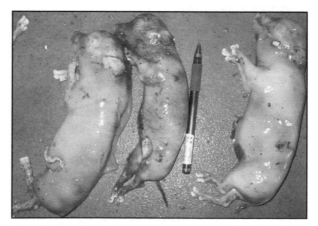

Fig. 2.34 Abortion in pregnant sows with Aujeszky's disease.

Differential diagnosis

Differential diagnosis of AD is wide, since it can cause a variety of clinical signs. However, the presence of neurological signs in suckling pigs associated with reproductive problems in sows is highly compatible with AD. When the dominant clinical signs are neurological, Teschen-Talfan disease (teschovirus infection), Japanese B encephalitis, haemagglutinating encephalomyelitis, porcine encephalomyocarditis, classical swine fever (CSF), blue eye disease (in Mexico), streptococcal meningitis, oedema disease, hypoglycaemia and arsenical and mercurial poisoning should be ruled out. Reproductive disease also has a wide differential diagnoses list, including CSF, teschovirus infections, encephalomyocarditis virus, Japanese B encephalitis virus, porcine circovirus type 2 (PCV2), porcine cytomegalovirus and leptospirosis. The respiratory side is more complicated to differentiate from other diseases since these signs are usually a consequence of concurrent diseases and not just ADV infection. In all cases, final diagnosis must be established by laboratory confirmation.

Diagnosis

Besides compatible clinical signs, diagnosis of ADV infection is established by detection of the virus in different tissues of the pig. Postmortem studies are unlikely to be suggestive since most cases display no gross lesions. Multifocal necrosis, with 1–2 mm. small foci, may be seen in very young animals (**Figures 2.35, 2.36**).

Microscopically, multifocal systemic necrosis can be seen in multiple organs, sometimes with intranuclear and intracytoplasmic inclusion bodies. Moreover, the most typical lesion in neurologically affected pigs is non-suppurative meningoencephalitis, sometimes with multiple necrotic foci of the brain. Aborting sows may also display histopathological findings of endometritis, vaginitis and placentitis; occasionally, multiple necrotic foci can also be seen in parenchymatous organs of the fetus. In these areas with necrosis and brain inflammation, there is plenty of virus, which is easily detectable by means of immunohistochemistry or in situ hybridization techniques. Alternatively, the virus can be detected by polymerase chain reaction (PCR) from different tissues. The most important tissues to test are brain, tonsils and lungs, and placenta and fetuses in cases of reproductive failure. Detection of antibodies (usually by enzyme-linked immunosorbent assay [ELISA] tests) is very important, especially to differentiate antibodies elicited by the vaccine (results should be positive against gB protein and negative against gE protein) and those generated by natural infection (seropositivity against both proteins).

Management

Current ways of preventing ADV infection are based on the use of vaccine viruses that are gene deleted. Natural or artificial deletion of protein gE provided live viruses with replicative capacity but with a high degree of attenuation. Therefore, they were included in vaccine products and proved very efficient. The combination of such efficacious gene deleted

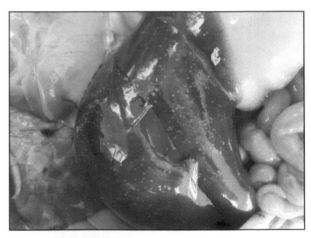

Fig. 2.35 Multifocal necrotic foci in a liver of a piglet affected by Aujeszky's disease.

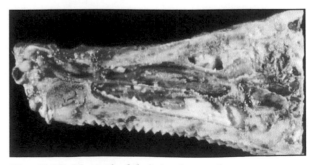

Fig. 2.36 Necrotic debris in the nasal passageways and tonsils.

vaccines, together with the differential ELISA tests to detect both gE and gB proteins, facilitated the eradication of ADV from most parts of the world in a practical and feasible manner.

Control: To maintain a naïve herd status requires good biosecurity and the purchase of breeding stock only from ADV-free herds.

Eradication: Vaccination and elimination of animals positive to the field virus leads to ADV-free farms and areas. Depopulation followed by 30-day no pigs is recommended.

Brucellosis
Definition/aetiology
Brucellosis is an infection characterised by impaired reproduction. Infections occurring near breeding can result in total embryo loss and irregular returns to oestrus (25–35 days after breeding) while exposure during late gestation can result in abortion, stillborns or weak liveborn pigs.

Infection with *Brucella suis* biotypes 1 and 3 results in the organism colonising various sites including regional lymph nodes with subsequent continuous or intermittent bacteraemia. The bacteria then colonise and persist in various organs including placentas, mammary glands, testes and boar accessory glands.

Clinical presentation
If evident, clinical signs can include sows maybe aborting, become infertile and or having a severe metritis. Boars may exhibit orchitis (**Figures 2.37, 2.38**) and infertility. Piglets and weaners may present with lameness and posterior paralysis.

Differential diagnosis
Although various diseases can result in small litters with increased mummies or stillborn piglets, the most likely differentials include leptospirosis (regular and irregular returns, with possible vulval discharge, late-term abortions, mummies, stillborns, and weak piglets) and brucellosis (if pigs have access to feral/wild pigs).

Diagnosis
A diagnosis of brucellosis is based on clinical evidence and serological testing.

Management
If only a few sows are infected, a test and slaughter programme can be attempted, although this often fails. Therefore, in the event that brucellosis enters a herd, the most appropriate and safe procedure is a total depopulation with rigorous cleaning and allowing facilities to remain empty for 2–3 months before restocking.

Congenital abnormalities
Congenital abnormalities occur in the pig and they can appear to be alarming (*Table 2.3*). Organogenesis is complete by 24 days of gestation and this can be used to provide a timing for the occurrence of the abnormality. More abnormalities are seen in late winter, probably associated with the feeding of mycotoxins in the new harvest of the previous autumn.

Some of the conditions listed in *Table 2.3* are illustrated in **Figures 2.39–2.54**.

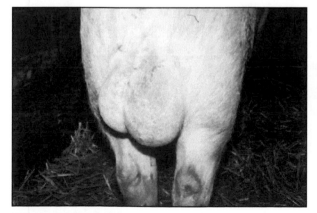

Fig. 2.37 Boar with *Brucella* orchitis of the right testis.

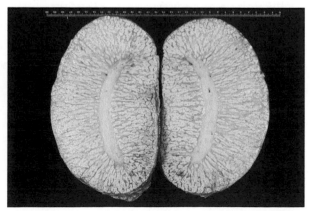

Fig. 2.38 Cross section of a testis with *Brucella* orchitis.

Table 2.3 **Congenital abnormalities that can occur in pigs.**

CONDITION	LEVEL*	POSSIBLE CAUSE	COMMENTS
Arthrogryposis	0.2	Hereditary	Euthanase piglets
Atresia ani	0.4	Hereditary	Low heritability Environmental influences
Bent legs		Unknown	Possibly exposure mid-pregnancy to toxic agents
		Hereditary	Auto recessive gene
		Poisons	Hemlock Black cherry
		Vitamin A	Excess dietary levels or by injection
Cleft palate	0.2	Hereditary	Destroy piglets
Congenital tremor		Classical swine fever virus	Type AI
		Congenital tremor virus (atypical porcine pestivirus)	Type AII
		Sex linked in male Landrace	Type AIII
		Recessive gene in the Saddleback	Type AIV
		Trichlorfon poisoning	Type AV
		Aujeszky's disease virus	Demonstration of virus
		Organophosphorus poisoning	Overdosing
Dwarfism		Hereditary	Rare
Epitheliogenesis imperfecta		Hereditary	Destroy if large
Hermaphrodite		Hereditary	Low levels
Inguinal hernia	1.5	Hereditary	Method unknown Environmental influences
Inverted teats	20	Hereditary	Ensure good teat selection in boars and gilts
Kinky tail	1.5	Hereditary	Common
Lymphosarcoma		Hereditary	Seen in young adults
Malignant hypothermia		Hereditary	Associated with lean genes
Meningocoele		Hereditary	Low incidence
Naval bleeding		Unknown	Associated with shavings
Pietrain creeper syndrome		Hereditary	Uncommon
Pityriasis rosea	1	Hereditary (Landrace)	Common – resolves without treatment
Porcine stress syndrome		Hereditary	DNA test and eliminate
Thrombocytopenic purpura	1	Antibody–antigen reaction	Uncommon
Splay leg	1.8	Hereditary	Common in the Landrace
		Fusarium toxin	Mouldy feeds
		Environmental	Slippery floors, chilling of piglets
Umbilical hernia	1.5	Hereditary	Environmental influences Navel tearing

* Refers to occurrence in a population.

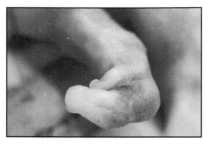

Fig. 2.39 Arthrogryposis. A soft tissue defect causing contraction of joints.

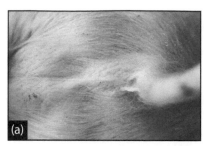
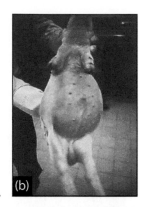

Fig. 2.40 Atresia ani. (a) The anus is missing. (b) The blockage results in abnormal swelling. Females can survive by creating a cloaca. Males die.

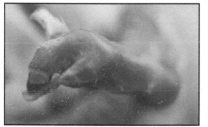

Fig. 2.41 Bent legs. The abnormality occurs in the bone skeleton, causing deformation of the leg.

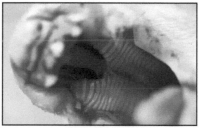

Fig. 2.42 Cleft palate. A range of conditions with defects of both the hard and soft palate. The piglets cannot drink properly and die.

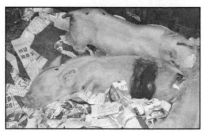

Fig. 2.43 Epitheliogenesis imperfecta. A full-thickness defect of the skin present at birth. Some cases are able to survive to finish with scarring.

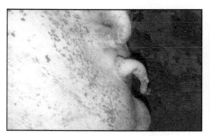

Fig. 2.44 Hermaphrodite. The pig has both male and female reproductive organs; a range of abnormalities, classically enlarged clitoris. VIDEO 8

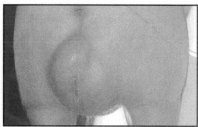

Fig. 2.45 Inguinal hernia. Failure of the inguinal ring and presence of intestinal contents in the inguinal region. Need to be careful at castration.

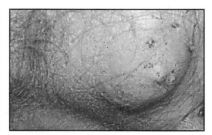

Fig. 2.46 Inverted teats. The teat can be manipulated out of the mammary gland but will invert again; piglets cannot suckle.

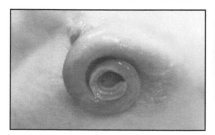

Fig. 2.47 Kinky tail.

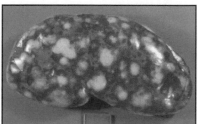

Fig. 2.48 Lymphosarcoma. Picture shows lymphosarcoma in a kidney. Generally seen in young adults to 16 months.

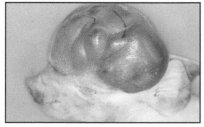

Fig. 2.49 Meningocoele. Defect of the cranium resulting in a prolapse of the meninges under the skin; generally fatal.

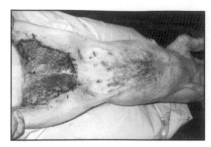

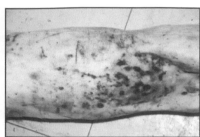

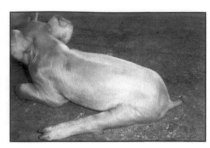

Fig. 2.50 Pityriasis rosea. Skin disorder seen in pigs weighing 30–60 kg. While quite dramatic, the pig is not sick and spontaneously recovers.

Fig. 2.51 Thrombocytopenia purpura. Autoimmune condition. The colostral antibodies attack the piglet, resulting in generalised haemorrhage.

Fig. 2.52 Splay leg. Defect of the development of the lumbar muscles. Management can assist these pigs. Improve floor footing.

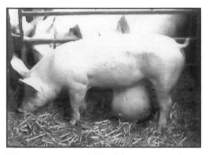

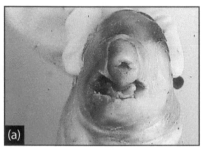

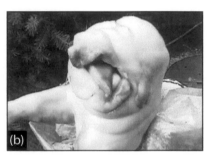

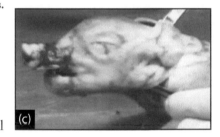

Fig. 2.53 Umbilical hernia. Defect of the body wall in the umbilical region. If larger than 30 cm circumference, destroy the pig.

Fig. 2.54 Three facial abnormalities. (a) Underdeveloped upper and lower jaw and proboscis-like nose; (b) underdeveloped upper and lower jaw; microtia and micropthalmia; (c) inferior brachygnathia.

A range of other abnormalities, including inversion of abdominal contents and specific organ defects, are all recognised but the genetic or specific cause has not been determined (**Figures 2.55–2.63**).

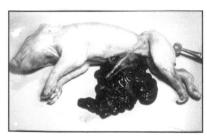

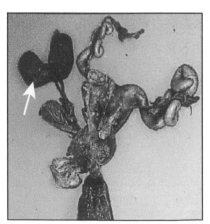

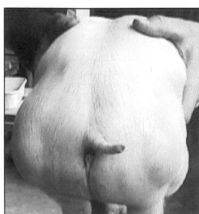

Fig. 2.55 General multiple abnormalities: ompahalocele, hind leg defects, spinal dysraphrism and kinky tail.

Fig. 2.56 Defect of the kidneys – horseshoe kidneys (arrow).

Fig. 2.57 Muscle defect.

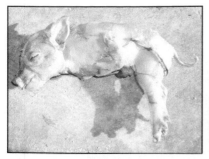

Fig. 2.58 Limb defects.

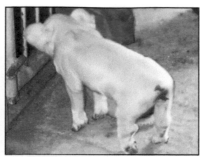

Fig. 2.59 Blocky legs.

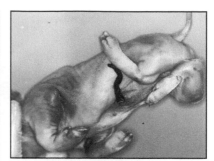

Fig. 2.60 Missing tibia.

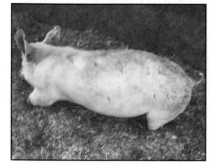

Fig. 2.61 Missing limbs.

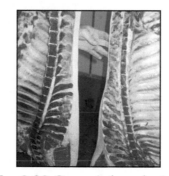

Fig. 2.62 Congenital porphyria on left; normal right.

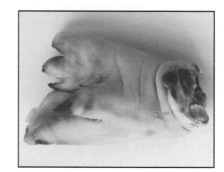

Fig. 2.63 Toe defects.

Leptospirosis

Definition/aetiology

Leptospirosis is caused by infection with one or more *Leptospira* serovars, which penetrate mucous membranes or skin lesions, circulate in the blood and settle in various sites, especially the kidneys, leading to shedding in the urine (**Figures 2.64, 2.65**). Also, more chronically, male and female reproductive tracts become colonised by leptospires (**Figures 2.66, 2.67**).

Reproductive disease can be caused by various *Leptospira* serovars but is most likely due to *L. interrogans* serovars *pomona* or *bratislava*. After localising in the uterus during the last half of gestation, developing fetuses are killed, although the mechanisms involved are not known.

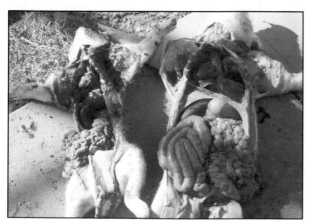

Fig. 2.64 Grower with *L. icterohaemorrhagica* with the characteristic jaundice (right).

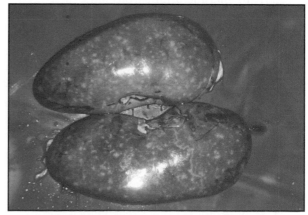

Fig. 2.65 *Leptospira pomona* associated with interstitial nephritis.

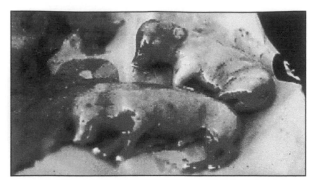

Fig. 2.66 Abortion in pigs associated with leptospirosis. The specific species was not determined.

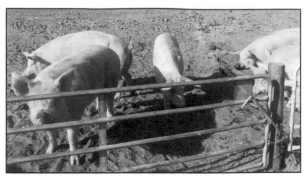

Fig. 2.67 Infertility and returns to oestrus may be associated with leptospirosis. These sows are 'talking' to the boar through the fence line.

Further, *L. bratislava* can localise in the oviduct and uterus in non-pregnant sows.

Clinical presentation

Reproductive signs associated with infection with *L. pomona* in particular, but also with *L. bratislava*, include late-term abortions. Infection with *L. bratislava* is also associated with premature litters, increases in stillborns and mummies, and a mixture of live poor pigs and dead piglets at birth. *In-utero* infected fetuses may survive to become infected piglets that grow to become adult carriers, which can perpetuate disease or transmit the disease if sold to other farms.

By colonising the reproductive tract of non-pregnant sows, *L. bratislava* infection also exhibits as early pregnancy loss, often associated with a copious vulval discharge. Repeat breeders are common, particularly in gilts and primiparous sows.

Differential diagnosis

The clinical signs of leptospirosis can be mistaken for other causes of infertility, so other infectious causes such as PRRS or 14–21 days endometritis/vulval discharge should be eliminated. The clinician also needs to eliminate non-infectious causes of infertility such as seasonal infertility or management failures, especially poor breeding management.

Diagnosis

Analyse the date of any abortions, repeats, stillborns, weak piglets and the age of occurrence in sows and gilts. It is more likely that reproductive signs will be seen in young sows (parity 1 or 2). Look for risk factors such as access to wildlife or untreated surface water.

Perform serology on suspicious animals and repeat 2–3 weeks later looking for rising antibody titres. In chronic disease, antibody titres are quite low and their significance is difficult to assess. Test aborted fetuses and the urine or kidneys and oviducts of slaughtered gilts.

Management

Control of leptospirosis will require that the pigs be confined. It is unlikely that all infected carriers can be eliminated, although vaccination using a bacterin containing the appropriate serovar in conjunction with antimicrobial treatment (e.g. tylosin phosphate or oxytetracycline hydrochloride) and a clean water supply will minimise the impact of disease. An excellent rodent control programme is also indicated as rodents will cycle disease on the farm.

Mycotoxicosis abortion and mummification

Mycotoxicosis is often blamed for mummification, abortion and reproductive problems on pig farms, but it can be very difficult to prove. When mycotoxins affect a pregnant sow it will generally be a point event, so all the affected fetuses will die at the same time and thus be the same size (**Figure 2.68**). This is different from viral agents where the fetuses die over time and are thus of different sizes.

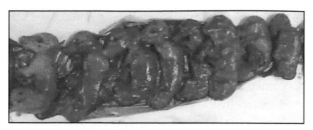

Fig. 2.68 A mummified event possibly associated with mycotoxicosis. Note the mummified fetuses are all approximately the same length and thus the same age.

Porcine circovirus 2

PCV2 infection can lead to various clinical outcomes, including reproductive failure. Fetal infection results in a non-suppurative myocarditis (**Figure 2.69**) with fetal death, mummification and abortions. When PCV2 is associated with reproductive disease it is referred to as PCV2-RD (see Chapter 8).

The clinical presentation of PCV2-RD infection will likely depend on when the female is infected, resulting in a stillborn, mummified, embryonic death and infertility (SMEDI) virus effect. The virus can replicate in hatched blastocysts and embryos at any stage of gestation. Infection occurring later will result in mummies with the virus moving from fetus to fetus and hence delivering mummies of various gestational ages. In one study, fetuses infected at 75 days were stillborn while those infected at 92 days were lesion free. At the herd level, there may be a sudden increase in regular and/or irregular returns to oestrus and, classically, an increase in the incidence of mummies, which will be of various gestational ages at the time of death. At the herd level, although not recorded, early infections will presumably present similar to parvovirus infection, with increased regular and irregular returns. Abortion may also occur if the fetal mortality is high enough.

Porcine parvovirus
(See also SMEDI agents)

Definition/aetiology

Porcine parvovirus (PPV) causes reproductive problems, most obviously an acutely increased number of mummies, particularly in non-vaccinated gilts and sows. Embryo or fetal death results from transplacental infection with parvovirus. The source of the virus is faeces and other body secretions from an infected animal contaminating the environment. Virus can also be introduced via fomites or rodents. The virus is very hardy and can survive for months in the environment.

Clinical presentation

The clinical presentation will depend on when the female is infected (**Figure 2.70**). Infection occurring between:

- the blastocyst hatching and 10 days will result in an increase in regular returns;
- 10 day embryos and implantation (17–20 days) will result in an increase in irregular returns;
- implantation to 35 days will result in an increase in pseudopregnancies;

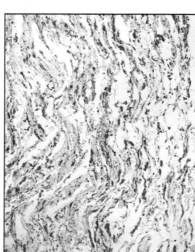

Fig. 2.69 Fetal myocarditis associated with PCV2-RD illustrated by immunohisto-chemistry.

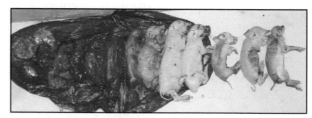

Fig. 2.70 Parvovirus infection in a parity 1 sow with nine various sized mummies, two stillborn and three neonatal deaths. There were four liveborn piglets, making a total of 18 born, which would have been a great litter for a parity 1 sow.

- from 35 to 70 days will result in mummification. The mummies will be of various gestational ages at the time of death;
- after 70 days, the fetus is capable of mounting an immune response, resulting in stillborns or live birth with poor or normal neonatal viability.

Abortion is not usually associated with parvovirus.

Differential diagnosis

Although various diseases can result in small litters with increased mummies or stillborn piglets, the most likely differentials include PCV2-RD (mimics PPV but more likely to involve abortion), leptospirosis (regular and irregular returns, with possible vulval discharge, late-term abortions, mummies, stillborns and weak piglets), teschoviruses (Enterovirus) and brucellosis (if pigs have access to feral/wild pigs).

Diagnosis

The clinical presentation of increased returns with birth of normal pigs and mummies of different gestational ages is very suggestive. Confirm by presence of viral antigen in mummies of less than 70 days gestational age. Serum antibody titres are of limited value since even if vaccinated, a field virus can still infect and replicate, causing high titres normally associated with disease but without clinical consequence.

Management

Vaccination of gilts is the control method of choice for parvovirus. Maternal antibodies can interfere with the immune response of gilts to vaccination and these antibodies may be present until 6 months of age. Therefore, incoming gilts need to be vaccinated after this age and at least 2 weeks prior to breeding. There is no requirement to vaccinate boars.

Feedback programmes will assist immunological stability of the herd.

Proplase of the reproductive tract
Clinical presentation

- **Vaginal prolapse** (**Figure 2.71**). Prolapse of the vagina is a common presentation in older fat sows around farrowing. The prolapse may be associated with large litters. The condition is difficult to predict on an individual sow basis, but the cause is associated with stretching and relaxation of the pelvic ligaments. Thus the condition is more common in larger litters, in sows housed on floors with excessive slope where the risk is increased, and if there is a high feed intake, especially with fermentable feed. These factors can lead to increasing abdominal pressure.
- **Uterine prolapse** (**Figure 2.72**). Uterine prolapse is a rare problem, which infrequently occurs after farrowing. The sow will present with the whole uterus prolapsed. The majority of sows will die of shock. It is possible to replace the uterus but the condition is generally fatal. Once the uterus is replaced, high concentrations of potassium in the compromised tissues may lead to heart failure in the sow. If the sow survives replacement or amputation, culling should occur.
- **Bladder prolapse** (**Figure 2.73**). Extremely rare, but dramatically presents during farrowing as a large sack visible at the vulval lips and interferes with the farrowing process. Emergency euthanasia and caesarean section should be performed to save the other piglets. It is occasionally possible to drain the bladder and replace it through the urethra. The sow normally dies.

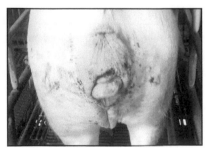

Fig. 2.71 Vaginal/cervical prolapse.

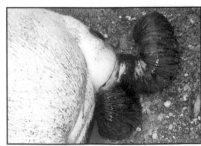

Fig. 2.72 Uterine prolapse.

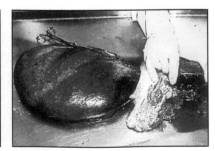

Fig. 2.73 Prolapse of the bladder at post-mortem examination.

Treatment of vaginal prolapse

Replace the prolapsed vagina and retain with a purse-string suture. Equipment required to replace a rectal or vaginal prolapse: large curved needle (5 cm) and scissors; suture tape or nylon suture material for growing pigs; warm water and antiseptic; obstetrical lubricant.

Method

- Clean the area around the prolapse and remove all faeces.
- Carefully return the prolapse into the vagina. This may take a little time. Be patient and push gently. With vaginal prolapses the wall can become very oedematous (jelly like) and it is easy to push your fingers through the outer wall. Do not worry if this happens once or twice.
- Infiltration with local anaesthesia around the anal or vaginal ring may be used.
- Covering the prolapse in sugar will help to reduce the oedema and the size of the prolapse.
- Once the prolapse has been returned, start stitching using a purse-string suture (**Figure 2.74**). The prolapse is likely to be pushed out again but do not worry, continue stitching, replacing the prolapse when it gets in the way.
- Start the purse-string suture under the tail and move round taking reasonable bites with the needle. It will take 6–8 in and out moves to go all the way round.

- At the end 'over sew' so the area to be tied will be strong.
- Push the prolapse back in again and hold it in.
- Pull the two ends of the suture closed. Place three fingers (depends on the size of the animal) into the vagina and pull the sutures tight around your fingers. There has to be sufficient room for the animal to urinate.
- Inject the animal with a suitable antibiotic (e.g. penicillin/streptomycin – note withdrawal times).
- Put some liquid paraffin (0.75 L per adult sow) into the mouth or feed to help soften the faeces, which reduces straining and the likelihood of a repeat prolapse.

'Riding' in the finishing herd

As the finishing pigs mature, they may become reproductively active (**Figure 2.75**). With entire males being present, this can lead to an explosion of fighting and aggression associated with the developing sexual drive. In the event of increased sexual activity, pigs may become traumatised and even killed. Food conversion and growth rates can be significantly affected. The boars may be more interested in fighting than eating. The trauma may lead to carcase damage and condemnation. In future breeding stock the penis can become damaged and permanently traumatised. Separation of males and females may assist some of this aggression, but groups of males will still fight among themselves. The use of chemical castration (GnRH agonist) may be considered as part of the control programme.

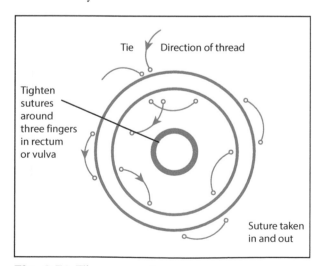

Fig. 2.74 The purse-string suture.

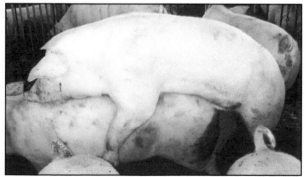

Fig. 2.75 Boars riding each other as they mature.

Stillborn, mummified, embryonic death and infertility agents

There are a number of agents, mainly viral, that can result in loss of a fetus. These are broadly termed SMEDI agents. The clinician needs to make an accurate diagnosis of the cause of the problem before recommending a suitable control programme.

Many agents only affect the neighbour piglet, others spread rapidly throughout the uterine environment (**Figure 2.76**, *Table 2.4*). This feature can be important in determining the aetiology of the problem. Often the problem cannot be accurately determined. Having an immunologically stable herd through feedback programmes is often the only way to remove the batch destabilising features of these SMEDI agents.

Stillborns and mummification

Definition/aetiology

Non-infectious causes of mummified and/or stillborn pigs include high environmental temperatures and carbon monoxide poisoning. Large litters may experience increased mummies due to uterine overcrowding. Prolonged deliveries are likely to increase stillborns as is the use of oxytocin to stimulate piglet delivery.

Infectious causes of mummies and stillborns include PPV, PCV2, leptospirosis and brucellosis. Other pathogens can also cause reproductive problems, including ADV (pseudorabies) and PRRSV, but these pathogens will be associated with other clinical signs and are dealt with elsewhere.

Diagnosis

It is important to differentiate between those piglets that are stillborn and those that died shortly after being born alive, and are thus pre-weaning mortality (**Figures 2.77, 2.78**).

Many piglets who die shortly after birth may be incorrectly assigned as stillborn (**Figures 2.79, 2.80**). Differential diagnosis can be achieved by looking at the slippers covering the feet, which are worn down within 15 minutes of life (**Figures 2.81, 2.82**). Look for the presence of a long umbilical cord and meconium (piglet faeces on skin) (**Figures 2.83–2.85**).

Management

Supervision: To reduce the number of stillborn piglets, observe the farrowing sow every 30 minutes. If no piglets are born it may be necessary to manually intervene to assist the sow. Medicines such as intravulval oxytocin injection (2.5–5 IU) can be given. There are factors that may allow the farm team to predict that an individual sow will have more stillborn pigs than normal. Monitor the following features:

- **Age of the sow**. Stillborns increase after parity 7.
- **Increase in litter size**. Stillborns increase after 12 total born.
- **Recognise the problem sow**. From the previous litter and age etc.

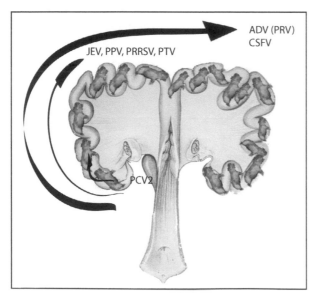

JEV, PPV, PRRSV, PTV

ADV (PRV)
CSFV

PCV2

Fig. 2.76 Potential spread *intra utero* of pathogens between fetuses within the uterus.

Table 2.4 **Spread of the SMEDI agents throughout the uterine environment.**

PATHOGEN	SPREAD TO NUMBER OF ADJACENT FETUSES
Porcine circovirus 2	Next fetus
Japanese encephalomyelitis virus	Next 2 to 5
Porcine parvovirus	
Porcine teschovirus	
Porcine reproductive and respiratory syndrome virus	
Aujeszky's disease virus (pseudorabies)	Can affect all embryos rapidly
Classical swine fever virus	

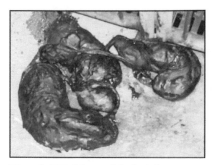

Fig. 2.77 Mummified piglets.

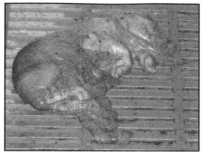

Fig. 2.78 Pre-partum stillborns can be easily recognised if partially autolysed, as shown. PRRSV is a major cause.

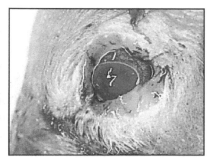

Fig. 2.79 Check the opacity of the cornea. Freshly dead (less than 24 hours), the cornea will still be clear.

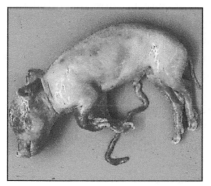

Fig. 2.80 A stillborn piglet will be wet with a long wet umbilical cord.

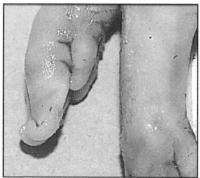

Fig. 2.81 Check the feet for 'slippers', which protect the uterus from the sharp piglet's nails.

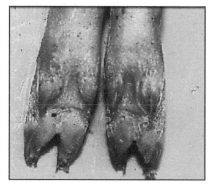

Fig. 2.82 A live piglet will rub off its slippers in about 15 minutes.

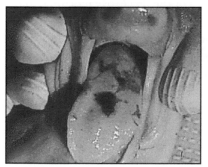

Fig. 2.83 Meconium will be present on the skin and in the mouth, trachea and stomach. The meconium is the faeces in the unborn piglet's large bowel, passed when they go anoxic.

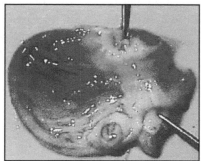

Fig. 2.84 The stomach will only contain fluid with some meconium; there will be no milk or colostrum.

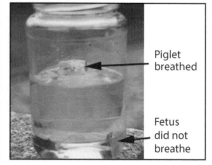

Piglet breathed

Fetus did not breathe

Fig. 2.85 A stillborn piglet's lung will sink in water, whereas if the piglet breathed, its lungs will float.

- **Slow farrowings**. Normal farrowing less than 5 hours. If longer, consider low iron or calcium blood levels (normal blood serum concentrations: iron >9 µmol/L; calcium >1.9 mmol/L).

- **Sow feeding/condition**. Overfat sows have longer farrowings. Lack of exercise results in longer farrowing times. High parasite levels or disease will increase farrowing times or result in poor uterine tone.

- **Nutrition/water**. Water flow rate needs to be greater than 2 L per minute. Increase fibre before farrowing. Both help to reduce constipation. Do not overfeed before farrowing as it can lead to oedema.
- **Farrowing place design**. Allow sufficient room for stockpersons to comfortably attend to the sow at farrowing time. Reduce stress and do not have sows cramped when lying down. No draughts, monitor door closure policy. Having lights dimmed and playing music will help to settle sows. Intermingle sows and gilts.
- **Temperature of farrowing house**. Keep below 22°C. Monitor placement of rear heat lamp to reduce stress on the farrowing sow.
- **Management of piglet tasks**. To reduce stress try not to teeth clip, tattoo etc. piglets within hearing of sows still farrowing.

Control of stillborn and mummified piglets: If the stillborn or mummified numbers are too high and the clinician believes that there may be a pathogen associated with the problem, consider control of parvovirus and PRRSV in particular. There are many other pathogens that may be associated with stillborn piglets (SMEDI viruses – porcine teschoviruses or PCV2, for example) and immune stabilisation of the herd's gilts using feedback materials is required in order to control these pathogens.

Seasonal infertility

The most common manifestations of seasonal infertility are reduced ovarian activity and a reduction in farrowing rates (**Figure 2.86**). Although reductions in litter size are occasionally observed, there is no correlation year on year with the seasons. The reduced ovarian activity is expressed as a delayed oestrus both in gilts (i.e. delayed puberty) and in sows after weaning (i.e. longer WSIs). The seasonal increase in the mean WSI is especially evident in primiparous sows.

Infertility is most likely the result of high ambient temperatures reducing lactation feed intakes. Under conditions of inadequate nutrient intake, hormonal consequences include reduced basal circulating LH concentrations in lactation, which limits follicular

recovery prior to weaning, and a smaller ovulatory LH surge at the post-weaning oestrus, which likely results in more stress-sensitive corpora lutea and an increased likelihood of pregnancy failure. The low feed allowance normally provided to gestating sows magnifies the adverse effects of poor lactation nutrient intake on basal LH concentrations and fertility, suggesting that early gestation feed allowances should be increased whenever low lactation feed intakes are encountered.

Interestingly, feed restriction to 60% of *ad libitum* caused a marked increase in circulating melatonin concentrations in pigs subjected to a long photoperiod (i.e. summer), but not in those subjected to a short photoperiod. This suggests a possible role for photoperiod in seasonality.

Seasonal increases in anoestrus and/or delayed oestrus should initially be addressed by:

- Increasing the number of animals bred at times of year when seasonal problems occur.
- Increasing lactation nutrient intakes. Things to consider include cooling the farrowing facility, increased feeding frequency, provision of cooled water, increased dietary lysine (minimum 1.1%).
- After weaning, employ daily boar exposure in the cooler times of the day (early morning) and, if all else fails,
- Injection of gonadotropins. However, be aware that such injections result in short WSIs and longer oestrous periods, which may require changes in breeding management.

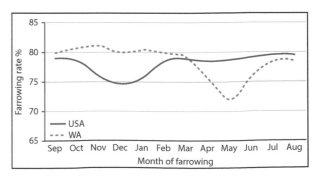

Fig. 2.86 The farrowing rate in the Northern Hemisphere (USA data) and Southern Hemisphere (WA – Western Australian data).

Seasonal effects on farrowing rate have been treated in several ways. One approach involves injection of GnRH or hCG at the onset of oestrus or 12 days after insemination. Injection at oestrus onset may improve the synchrony between sperm deposition and ovulation and/or improved quality of corpora lutea. The former effect would enhance fertilisation rates and the latter effect may enhance early luteal progesterone production. In reality, an effect on sow fertility would be evident only if either of the measures were limiting. Injection 12 days after insemination would provide additional luteal support by inducing follicle growth and secretion of oestrogen and increased uterine PGE_2, both of which are luteotropic in pigs.

Tumours of the reproductive tract of pigs

As pet pigs become older a range of tumours are being recognised affecting the reproductive tract and mammary glands. These should be approached with the normal clinical skills provided to any pet animal.

Ovarian carcinoma

Large, generally single, occasionally bilateral, ovarian tumours infrequently found at post-mortem examination (**Figure 2.87**).

Uterine leiomyoma VIDEO 9

Tumours of the older female reproductive tract are being increasingly reported, particularly associated with the broad ligament and uterus (**Figure 2.88**). This is in line with the increasing age of pet pigs.

Testicular tumours

Tumours of the testes may be seen and removed through castration (**Figure 2.89**).

Scrotal haemangioma

Scrotal haemangiomas are very common, with little or no significance to the boar's fertility (**Figure 2.90**).

Vulval discharge VIDEO 10

A discharge from the vulva may be classified as normal during the 3–4 days after farrowing (a serous blood tinged lochia) or within 7 days of breeding. A small volume of discharge associated with urination indicates a urinary tract infection. Small discharges may be seen on any day of gestation and may not indicate any significant pathology.

A copious purulent discharge, which may be malodorous, may originate from the vagina (vaginitis)

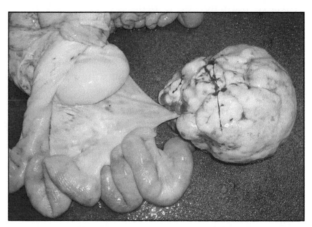
Fig. 2.87 Ovarian tumour.

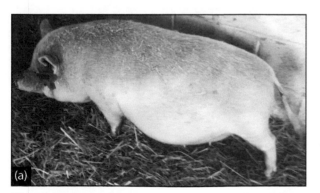

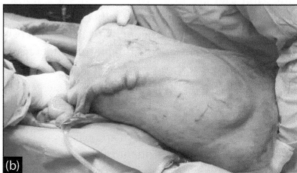

Fig. 2.88 Large leiomyoma pre-surgery (a) and the tumour exteriorised during surgery (b).

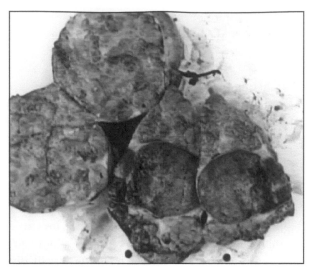

Fig. 2.89 Cut surface of a Sertoli cell tumour of the testis.

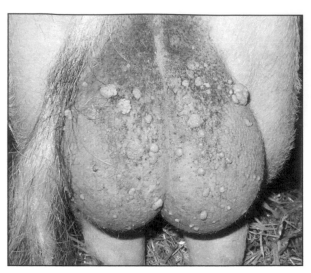

Fig. 2.90 Multiple scrotal haemangiomas in a working boar.

or uterus (endometritis). Vaginitis may be observed independent of the stage of the oestrous cycle and initially may not be a problem. However, if not resolved promptly, it may ascend and progress to endometritis. If the discharge occurs during pro-estrus or oestrus, it is more likely to be of uterine origin and becomes evident when the cervix opens in readiness for breeding.

If vulval discharge is observed in more than 2% of sows, it is a problem herd since if, say, 4% of sows are observed to have a discharge, it is highly likely that many more are discharging but simply are not observed. Vulval discharges or tacky vulval mucous membranes 14–21 days post breeding indicates endometritis (**Figure 2.91**), which is associated with a marked reduction in farrowing rates. Discharges involve an ascending urogenital infection and are more likely if sows are housed under poor hygiene and especially if immunocompromised, such as may occur with mycotoxicosis. However, although environmental considerations are very important, sow management may also need careful evaluation.

If discharges are evident associated with the post-weaning oestrus, successful conception is unlikely and a regular return to oestrus is highly likely. If a discharge is evident in the WSI, farrowing management needs to be critically evaluated.

In particular, some farrowing attendants have a tendency to manually intervene excessively and the interventions may not be hygienic. However, even if all care is taken to be hygienic when intervening during farrowing, a risk of uterine infection exists and the risk increases with the number of interventions. There is a need to educate the attendants and to develop a rational intervention standard operating procedure that will detail when intervention is warranted (i.e. evidence of dystocia) and post-farrowing treatments to minimise risks if intervention is needed (i.e. 10 IU

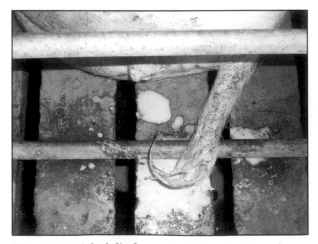

Fig. 2.91 Vulval discharge 14–21 days post service.

oxytocin at the end of farrowing with possibly a follow-up luteolytic dose of $PGF_{2\alpha}$ 24 hours later). Antibiotics are unlikely to be rewarding.

Vulval discharges may occur more frequently from 16 days after mating at a time when the sow or gilt is approaching a return to oestrus. Indeed, a discharge during this time usually is followed by a regular return to oestrus. However, in cases of endometritis, returns may also be irregular, abortion rates may increase and the number of failure-to-farrow sows may increase. Even if farrowing successfully, placental involvement may result in compromised piglets and increased neonatal mortality. The origin of these discharges may be a non-observed post-weaning discharge sow. However, it is more likely to involve a problem at breeding. Poorly timed inseminations can introduce contamination at a time of relatively poor uterine immune competence, and oestrus detection management and insemination techniques need critical evaluation. Natural breeding is more likely to induce a 14–21 day post-service vulval discharge.

Successful treatment of discharging sows is unlikely. If sow retention is a priority, then discharging sows should not be bred but be allowed to cycle normally. The immunogenic effect of oestrogen during the subsequent proestrus may permit a self-cure. If a sow does not exhibit a discharge at the next oestrus, breeding may be successful but be aware that performance will be that of a 'return' sow. Since not all discharging sows will be detected, it may be more appropriate to put in place a strict culling policy; any sow that exhibits a discharge and is not pregnant is culled as is any sow having two repeats – no exceptions.

Zearalenone mycotoxicosis ▶ VIDEO 11

Zearalenone is an oestrogenic mycotoxin that will result in disturbance of the reproductive pattern in females and demonstration of reproductive traits in young growing animals; for example, enlarged nipples and vulva. Zearalenone produces toxic signs at more than 1 ppm and ideally the feed should contain less than 0.3 ppm to minimise the risk of clinical signs. Zealalenone is produced in the field on damp/damaged corn.

Note: Oestrogen is produced naturally by the sow as part of the parturition process. This will result in the female piglets being born with enlarged vulvas and both male and female piglets having enlarged nipples (**Figures 2.92, 2.93**). These enlarged nipples can result in nipple necrosis (see **Figure 2.105**). This will resolve in 3–5 days.

Many mycotoxin events are controlled by the addition of clays and other absorbents to the feed. (For details on other mycotoxins see Chapter 8.)

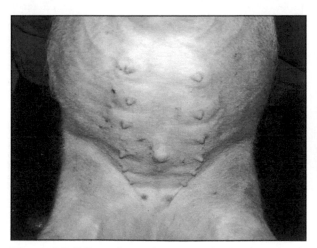

Fig. 2.92 Effect of zearalenone in the finishing herd. This pig has enlarged nipples.

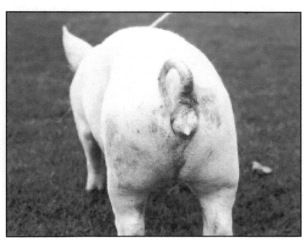

Fig. 2.93 Weaner gilt with an unusually enlarged vulva.

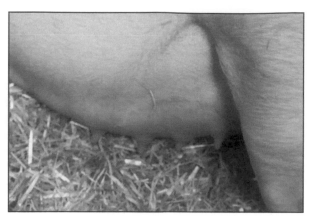

Fig. 2.94 Non-lactating mammary glands. A gilt should have a minimum of eight paired teats. The sow shown is 1 week pre-farrow. Note that the nipples are enlarged.

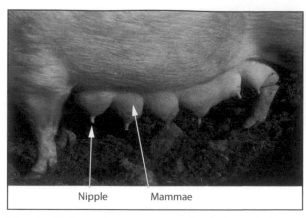

Fig. 2.95 Lactating mammary glands, lateral view. It is not unusual to have no functioning glands. It is essential for piglet survival that the mammary glands are full. Note the size of the nipples when selecting sows as a potential nurse animals.

MAMMARY GLAND HEALTH AND DISORDERS

Anatomy

The pig has many mammary glands running along her ventral surface. In commercial pigs it is advised to have a minimum of two rows of eight nipples resulting in 16 functioning mammary glands (**Figures 2.94, 2.95**).

The important feature of mammary anatomy is that each nipple will be supplied by two or even three separate functioning mammae (**Figures 2.96, 2.97**). Milk is stored in the mammae as there is no true teat cistern. Milk production is controlled by several hormones, including the interactions of prolactin (increased milk yield) and serotonin (feedback inhibitor of lactation); milk let-down is induced by oxytocin.

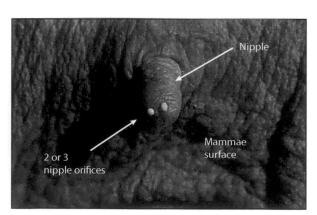

Fig. 2.96 Detail of the nipple and one mammae. Milk has been expressed to demonstrate the location of the teat openings.

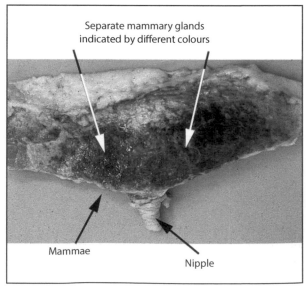

Fig. 2.97 Cross-section of the mammary gland, with ink injected post-mortem to delineate each of the two mammary glands supplying the common nipple. The anterior glands may have three mammary glands supplying the one common nipple.

Cyclic nursing and suckling ▶ VIDEO 2

It is important to understand and appreciate the normal nursing pattern of the sow and her piglets (*Table 2.5*). Suckling occurs approximately once every hour.

Ergot poisoning

Ergot (*Claviceps purpurea*) tends to occur on small grains (e.g. wheat [**Figure 2.98**]). Ergot poisoning results in a sow having an immature udder, resembling the udder about 5 days pre-farrowing, at the point of farrowing. This is because ergotamine interferes with prolactin production. Sows present with a flaccid udder and milk production is sparse and non-responsive to oxytocin. The piglets are starving as the sow cannot produce milk. If contaminated feed is fed to finishing pigs, circulation problems and end-arterial thrombi may occur, resulting in gangrene of the feet, tail and ears.

Mastitis – acute

Definition/aetiology

Acute mastitis is primarily associated with Enterobacteriaceae (e.g. *Klebsiella* spp. and *Escherichia coli*) but *Staphylococcus*, *Streptococcus* and *Clostridium* spp. may also be involved. Accurate diagnosis of the causal agent is complicated by the difficulty in obtaining a suitable sample to investigate, and each nipple is supplied by two or even three mammae and only one may be may be diseased.

Clinical signs

Mastitis may be concurrent with udder congestion and free flow of milk, which is an excellent bacterial growth medium. The sow is obviously ill and probably toxic; she may have discoloured ears. The udder is hard and reddened, particularly in the area infected (**Figures 2.99, 2.100**). She will be pyrexic

Table 2.5 **The normal nursing pattern.** ▶ VIDEO 2	
SOW	**PIGLETS**
Slow grunting	Assemble at udder
Increased grunt rate	Nosing and teat location
Rapid increase in grunt rate	Slow suckling
Milk flow (15 sec)	Rapid suckling
Grunting declines	Slow suckling or nosing
Sleep or change position	Fall sleep

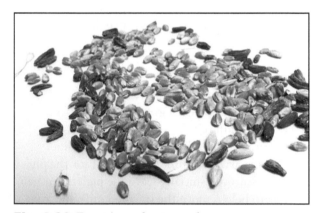

Fig. 2.98 Ergot in a wheat sample.

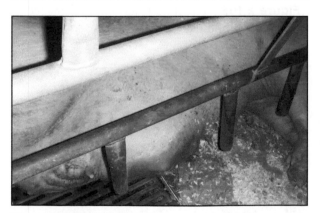

Fig. 2.99 Hard udder with an acute mastitis.

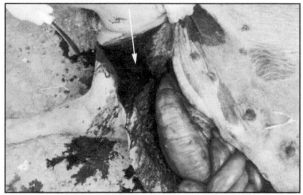

Fig. 2.100 Haemorrhagic mastitis in a dead sow associated with *Clostridium perfringens* mastitis (arrow).

with a rectal temperature of 40–42°C. Her piglets will be hungry and unsettled. The sow may be extremely depressed and if the milk is blood stained and the udder is cold, this may indicate a clostridial mastitis

Differential diagnosis

Swollen painful mammary glands may also occur in udder oedema. A condition called MMA (mastitis, metritis and agalactia) is commonly quoted. However, this condition/diagnosis should be avoided and the separate parts recognised and treated appropriately.

Diagnosis

Accurate diagnosis can be difficult. Clinical signs and especially the presence of hungry piglets are suggestive. Obtaining a milk sample from the affected mammae may be difficult as the adjacent mammae will supply milk to the teat. If the milk is blood stained, this may indicate a clostridial toxic mastitis. If the sow dies, diagnosis of the mastitis can be demonstrated post-mortem.

Management

- Inject the sow with 10 IU oxytocin.
- Inject antibiotic with gram-negative effect.
- Provide pain relief.
- Ensure excellent hygiene of the udder line.
- Provide artificial milk replacement for the piglets. However, initially leave the piglets on the sow to help remove the infected milk and give her a will to live.
- Provide the sow with excellent water supplies and consider providing some fresh food.

Control

- Review late gestation feed management. Reduce feed from day 110 of gestation and provide bran on day 115 to relieve constipation.
- Critically examine farrowing house hygiene practices, especially the water supply.
- Ensure adequate fly controls are in place.
- Cull infected sows if a herd problem exists.

Mastitis – chronic   ▶ VIDEO 12

Chronic mastitis is associated with a range of bacteria (*Staphylococcus* spp., *Streptococcus* spp., *Trueperella pyogenes* and *Actinobacillus suis*). The sow presents with large and often multiple lumps in the mammary gland (**Figure 2.101**). The swelling is classically first seen at the end of lactation or in the newly weaned sow. Sows will generally show no other clinical signs. In the next lactation the infected gland will be non-functional. Once observed there is no effective treatment. Review the number of remaining functional teats and programme the sow to enter the cull pool.

Teat disorders
Supernumerary teats

These can occur sporadically (**Figure 2.102**). They should be avoided in replacement breeding stock.

Teat damage

Teats can be damaged by piglet teeth. However, teeth clipping is not required to stop damage to the mammary glands. Ensuring the sow produces plenty of milk will reduce or eliminate the damage (**Figure 2.103**). The hind teats can be damaged by the hind legs and slats (**Figure 2.104**).

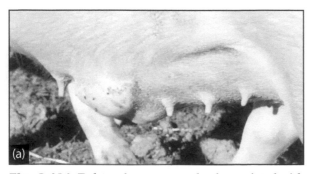
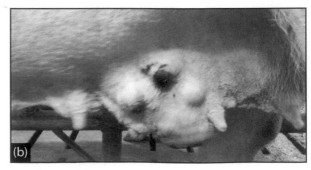

Fig. 2.101 Enlarged mammary gland associated with a chronic mastitis.

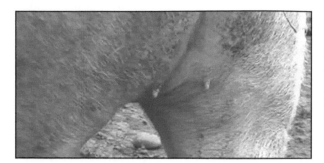

Fig. 2.102 Supernumerary teats.

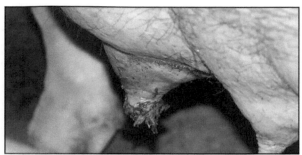

Fig. 2.103 Teat damage from piglets associated with inadequate milk supplies.

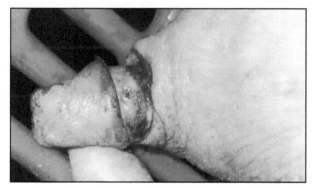

Fig. 2.104 Teat damage associated with overlong hind toes.

Teat necrosis

All new born piglets are born with swollen, naturally enlarged teats and vulvas associated with maternal oestrogen production during the later stages of pregnancy (**Figures 2.105, 2.106**). If the piglets rub their teats on rough flooring, teat necrosis occurs.

This damage can result in poor mammary development and is particularly significant in selection and productivity of future breeding stock, both male and female. The presence of zearalenone mycotoxicosis in future breeding stock can result in enlarged nipples in the growing area and subsequent nipple necrosis.

Udder oedema
Definition/aetiology

Udder oedema involves fluid accumulation in the mammary glands and may be evident in the dry/gestating sow up to 20 days prior to farrowing (95 days of gestation).

Clinical signs

There is a build up of fluids in the mammary gland with little or no milk let down (**Figure 2.107**). The sow shows some discomfort with the glands, which

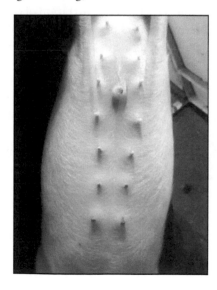

Fig. 2.105 Teat necrosis in a 10-day-old piglet.

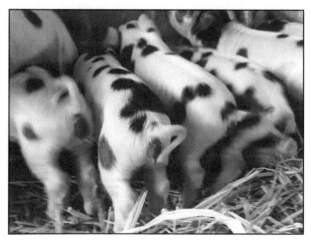

Fig. 2.106 Enlarged vulvas in a Gloucester Old Spot litter.

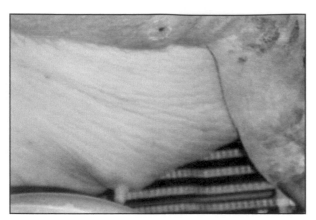

Fig. 2.107 Udder oedema with the lines of the floor imprinted on the udder.

may be large enough to interfere with locomotion. Piglets attempting to use the affected teats will not thrive and may require fostering. Palpation of the gland will reveal that when a thumb is pressed into the udder the depression will take a long time to disappear. The majority of udder oedema cases are associated with overweight sows that receive too high a feed intake while pregnant. This high feed intake then continues after day 110.

Management

Individual sow treatment: Treatment can be difficult and unresponsive. Attempt to get milk flow to occur by administering intramuscular oxytocin (5 IU every 4–6 hours). Pain relief for the full mammary glands may be required. Provide milk replacer for the piglets, who will struggle to feed. Be aware that the piglets may also have received too little colostrum. Replace the struggling litter with a litter of good piglets who will 'force' the milk to flow. Split suckling may also help.

If scant faeces are evident, the constipation may facilitate transfer of endotoxin into the circulation, which can result in hypogalactia. To help counter constipation, exercise sows in the immediate post-partum period to facilitate defecation. Orally administer 10 g of magnesium oxide to a normal sized sow.

Control on a herd basis: Review feeding practices in the later stages of pregnancy and condition score the sows. Ensure the water supplies are excellent (minimum 2 litres per minute). Avoid constipation by providing more fibre before farrowing.

REPRODUCTIVE SURGERY IN THE PIG

Introduction

Pet pigs have established themselves as a popular but unusual pet. They are generally more intelligent than a dog and relatively easy to train. Pigs kept in a caring home environment present with few behavioural problems. However, puberty and its subsequent reproductive requirements can present with unpleasant and potentially dangerous behavioural traits. Pigs come well-armed with four very sharp teeth in their mouths and a powerful neck and bite. Even pet varieties of pigs can weigh 100 kg and they may out run most humans when provoked. Micropigs are generally created by gross underfeeding of otherwise normal pigs.

Note: Any medicines described below are only suggestive and it is important to check the legal availability of any product. All pigs are considered food animals.

The surgical procedure
Pre-surgery
If the surgery is elective, it may be necessary to get a movement license before moving the pig to the surgery. The pig should be starved for 12 hours prior to surgery and water removed 6 hours before surgery. Pigs are very prone to gastric ulceration, which can start within 24 hours of not eating.

Premedication
Depending on the pig, premedication can start at home with the administration of acepromazine maleate oral tablets provided via a small apple or chocolate bar at a rate of 1–2 mg/kg. Alternatively, the pig can be premedicated with 0.1 mg/kg acepromazine maleate injection intramuscularly. Intramuscular injection of ketamine (20 mg/kg) and xyalzine (2 mg/kg) has proven to be extremely good at knocking the pig down.

Azaperone is a sedative used commercially in pigs. However, while it is good for calming sows at mixing and farrowing, it is unsuitable as a premedication as the pig will go into an excitable phase on handling, making intravenous injection difficult and possibly dangerous. With many sedatives, penile prolapse (paraphimosis) can occur and owners need to be warned that this can be permanent.

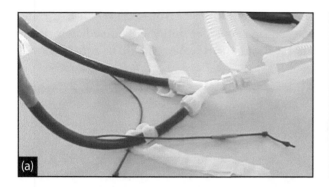

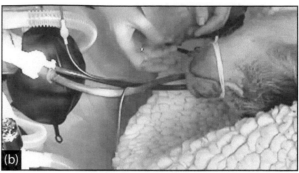

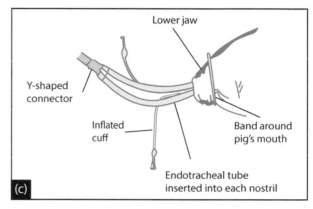

Fig. 2.108 (a–c) Intranasal intubation.

A convenient method of sedation is using an intramuscular injection of a Telazol® or Zoletil® (250 mg tiletamine plus 250 mg zolazapam)/xylazine-ketamine mixture ('TKX'). Reconstitute powdered Telazol® with 250 mg ketamine (2.5 mL) and 250 mg xylazine (2.5 mL) ('TKX'). Dose at 1 mL/25–35 kg.

Anaesthesia

Anaesthesia can be achieved using thiopental sodium intravenously (approximately 10 mg/kg to effect) via an ear vein. The pig should be restrained at all times. While the pig may squeal, the easiest and least stressful technique for both pig and operator is the snout restraint.

The sedated pig's ear veins are raised by applying pressure at the base of the ear. Using a surgical swab the ear veins are visualised. A needle (butterfly catheter) is inserted but drawback is not performed as the ear vein normally collapses. Injecting a very small amount of anaesthetic will indicate if the needle is properly placed. **Note:** A large amount of barbiturate injected into the perivascular tissues can lead to a degree of necrosis and potentially permanent damage to the ear.

Once the pig is anaesthetised, the anaesthesia is maintained using gaseous isoflurane on a circle. Intubation of the pig is quite complex as the larynx is anatomically difficult to visualise because of the large epiglotitis (see Chapter 3) and masking poses a risk of not achieving a good seal.

The technique of intranasal intubation can be utilised (**Figure 2.108**). A 90 kg pig will take a 9 mm endotracheal tube, while 60 and 30 kg pigs will take 7 mm and 5 mm endotracheal tubes, respectively. Once inserted

with a twisting action past the nares, the cuff can be inflated and the mouth closed with tape. The pig will then breathe normally through the nose. Anaesthesia can be easily maintained using this technique. The large epiglotitis closes off the oral cavity. This technique has allowed surgeries of over 4 hours without incident.

MALES

All non-breeding pet boars should be castrated. The male pet pig is generally fine until 2 years of age but after this he becomes 'male' and dominant and his tusks rapidly develop. Castration is the only answer. Chemical castration methods are available. The ideal time for castration is 5–7 days of age when the operation can be completed with minimal fuss. Pain management is required. Castration of the mature pig demands surgery and a general anaesthetic. Castration over the age of 3 weeks has to be carried out by a veterinary surgeon and under this age only an owner who has received training from a vet should castrate their piglets. Only a veterinary surgeon should castrate a piglet with a scrotal hernia.

Castration – piglet

Depending on the local legal issues, generally, no anesthesia is required if the piglet is castrated before 7 days of age (**Figures 2.109–2.114**). Once castrated the piglet should be returned immediately to his mother. Pain management should be provided.

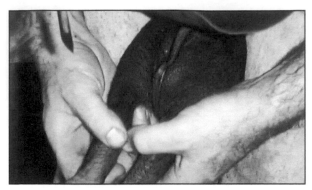

Fig. 2.109 Place the piglet between your legs with the chest held by the legs. The piglet will stop struggling quickly.

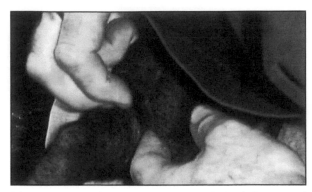

Fig. 2.110 Push the testicles up and check for scrotal hernias. Do not continue with open castration if a hernia is suspected.

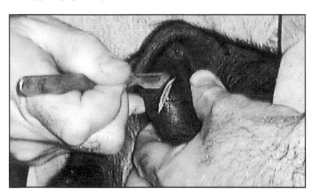

Fig. 2.111 With a surgical blade incise over the midline of the scrotum.

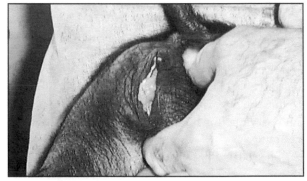

Fig. 2.112 The testes will prolapse through the cut.

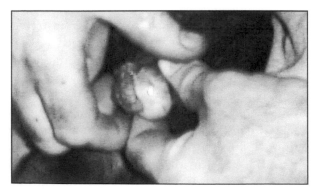

Fig. 2.113 Grasp the testis between finger and thumb. Push the testis out of the cut and remove it from the piglet with a pulling and twisting action.

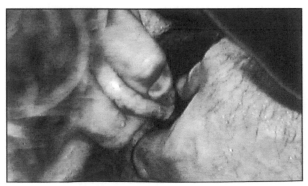

Fig. 2.114 Ensure no remnants of the vaginal tunic remain on the outside of the piglet. Remove the other testis and then return the piglet to his mother.

Castration – adult boar

The procedure for castrating adult boars is described in **Figures 2.115–2.120**.

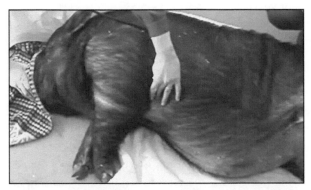

Fig. 2.115 Check the pig over as part of the normal anaesthesia requirements.

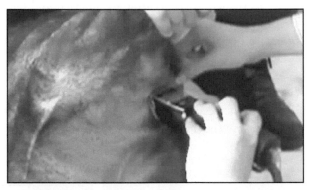

Fig. 2.116 Clip the area of the scrotum and inner groin.

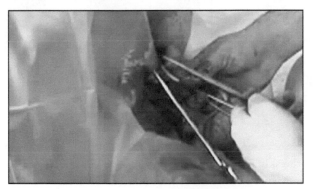

Fig. 2.117 Make an incision midline just in front of the scrotum. Push the top testis through the incision.

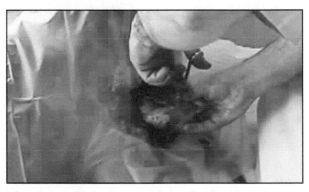

Fig. 2.118 Twist the testicle cord. Clamp and ligate the vaginal tunic. Pull to separate the tunic above the ligation. Push the other testis through the midline incision and remove.

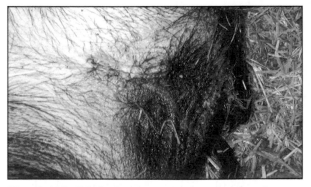

Fig. 2.119 Stitch the two vaginal tunics closed. Close the subcutaneous tissues and finally the skin.

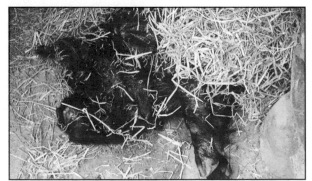

Fig. 2.120 Allow recovery from the anaesthesia. Provide pain management as appropriate.

Chemical castration – male and female

An anti-GnRH vaccine may be administered to entire males and female pigs. As the technique is to vaccinate the pig against its own GnRH, two or three injections at 2–4 week intervals will be required. The vaccine will wear off after about a year and subsequent yearly vaccination is advised. This can be very useful to reduce riding behaviour in entire boars in the finishing herd and as an alternative to surgical ovariohysterectomy in the female pet pig.

Scrotal hernia repair

Repair of a scrotal hernia is described in **Figures 1.121–2.126**. Anaesthetise the pig using a suitable method (e.g. general anaesthesia).

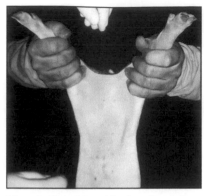

Fig. 2.121 Identify the pig with the scrotal hernia. A separate operator is required to hold the pig.

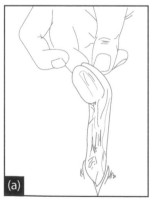

Fig. 2.122 Push the scrotal hernia up into the groin.

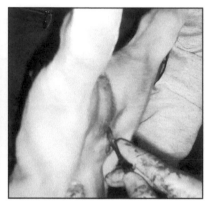

Fig. 2.123 Incise the skin over the hernia. Do not puncture the vaginal tunic – closed castration.

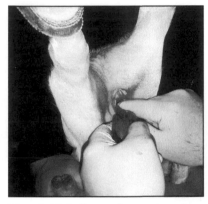

Fig. 2.124 Grasp the testis and free it by blunt dissection.

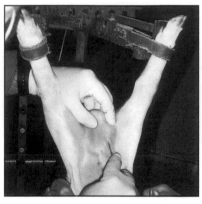
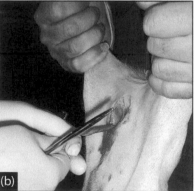

(a)   (b)

Fig. 2.125 (a, b) Twist the testis and vaginal tunic, pushing any intestinal contents back into the abdomen.

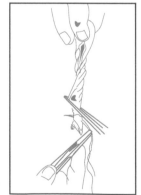

Fig. 2.126 Tie off the base of the twist using 0 Vicryl®, placing a stay stitch into the base of the twisted vaginal tunic. It may be possible to knot the twisted vaginal tunic. Do not use an electrical tie, which will be found at slaughter.

Cut the cord above the Vicryl® stitch or vaginal tunic knot. Place a mattress stitch into the skin to close the wound. Allow the piglet weaner to recover in a warm box. Provide pain management as appropriate.

Epididectomy – adult pig

It is possible to carry out a similar procedure on piglets up to 7 days of age without anaesthetic but with pain management (**Figures 2.127–2.135**). This would be a partial castration. Ideally, carry out the procedure on day 3 of age.

Assuming that the epididectomy is successful, castrate the pig on the other side. Allow the pig to recover from the anaesthetic. Provide pain management as appropriate. Check the absence of semen before using the boar on a sow.

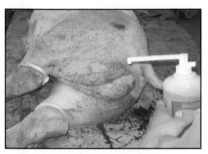

Fig. 2.127 Place the pig in left lateral recumbency. Clean and prepare the scrotal area.

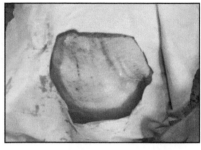

Fig. 2.128 Drape over the two testes.

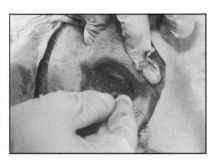

Fig. 2.129 Incise over the right (upper) top of the testis (i.e. over the tail of the epididymis).

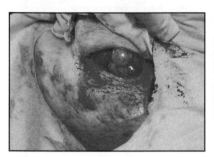

Fig. 2.130 The tail of the epididymis will be visible through the incision.

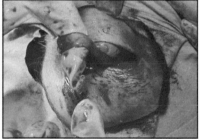

Fig. 2.131 By blunt dissection pull the tail of the epididymis and push your fingers through the mesentery between the testis and epididymis.

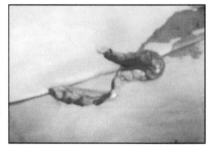

Fig. 2.132 Pull the epididymis free from the testis by breaking down the testicular ligament and pull on the epididymis until the vaginal tunic breaks.

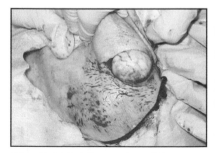

Fig. 2.133 The testis will be seen exposed.

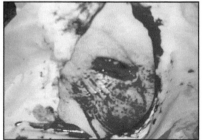

Fig. 2.134 Close the wound, the vaginal tunic, the subcutaneous tissue and the scrotal skin.

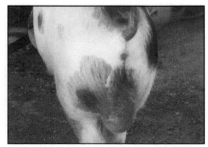

Fig. 2.135 Post recovery. Note the monorchid testis. The other testis was removed.

Ventral vasectomy – adult pig

The procedure is described in **Figures 2.136–2.144**.

Allow the pig to recover from the anaesthesia. Provide pain management as appropriate.

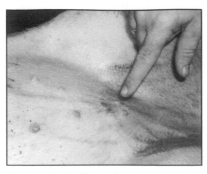

Fig. 2.136 Place the pig on its back and prepare the area between the groin.

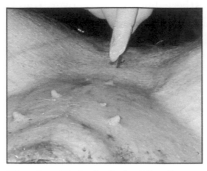

Fig. 2.137 A single incision is made midline or two incisions in the groin groove. Note the large blood vessels in the groin.

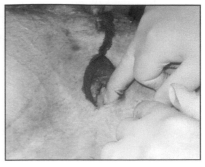

Fig. 2.138 Cut down through the skin and muscle layers. The vaginal tunic will be felt under the finger as a mobile tube.

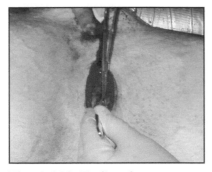

Fig. 2.139 Finding the vas deferens can be assisted by the assistant pushing up on the testis.

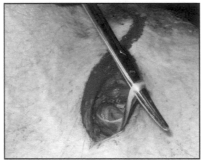

Fig. 2.140 Carefully cut through the vaginal tunic. The vas deferens will be seen as a white tube. Release the vas deferens by pushing an artery forceps through the interstitial tissues. Pulling on the released vas deferens will pull on the testis.

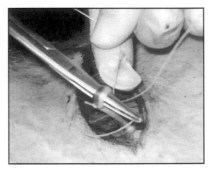

Fig. 2.141 Once you are sure the vas deferens is released, place sutures and ligate the vas deferens at the proximal end. Use 0 Vicryl®. Nylon may be found at slaughter and should be avoided.

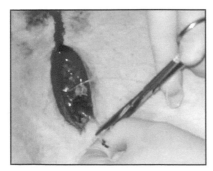

Fig. 2.142 Repeat the ligature at the distal end of the vas deferens – about 9 cm further down the vas deferens.

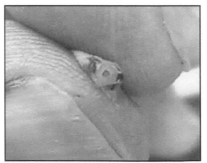

Fig. 2.143 The vas deferens can be confirmed by rolling the removed duct and seeing the central hole, as shown. Place the removed vas into 10% formaldehyde.

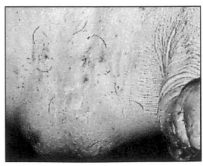

Fig. 2.144 Repeat the procedure on the opposite side. Close the incision: the vaginal tunic, muscle, submucosal layers and skin layers.

FEMALES

Introduction

The sow/gilt can present with a variety of behavioural 'problems' that we associate with her reproductive cycles. The sow cycles every 21 days (18–24) and the signs of oestrus can be quite bizarre. Off feed, slight temperature, vulval discharge, rubbing, searching, mounting of objects, including children, and a change in aggression level and loss of house training are all seen regularly. These problems can be readily resolved through spaying (ovariohysterectomy) of the sow/gilt.

Ovariohysterectomy

The procedure is described in **Figures 2.145–2.153**.

Provide pain management as appropriate. Examine the pig 2 weeks post operation and examine the scar.

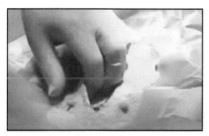

Fig. 2.145 Place the pig in dorsal recumbency. Make a midline incision through the skin and subcutaneous tissues. The linea alba will become visible. Incise through the linea alba just caudal to the umbilicus. The incision should be about 6 cm long.

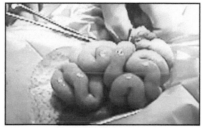

Fig. 2.146 The uterus is normally very easy to find. Retract the horn. Follow the uterine horn forward to the ovary. Identify the ovary. Ligate the ovarian artery and incise.

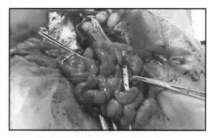

Fig. 2.147 Ligate and incise through the broad ligament vessels. These can be very large. The uterine body will need to be ligated in sections.

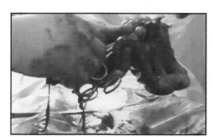

Fig. 2.148 Cut through the body of the uterine horn.

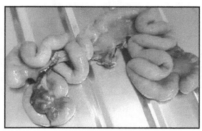

Fig. 2.149 The uterus and ovaries are removed.

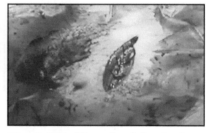

Fig. 2.150 Close the abdominal incision. Suture the linea alba with Vicryl® or PDS® III. The muscles and subcutaneous layers are closed with catgut, Vicryl®, PDS® or Dexon™.

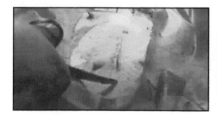

Fig. 2.151 Close the skin incision. (Subcutaneous closure with absorbable suture so that there are no sutures to remove later.)

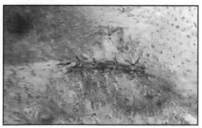

Fig. 2.152 The skin incision after subcutaneous sutures.

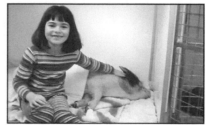

Fig. 2.153 Postoperative care to ensure comfortable recovery.

Caesarean section

The procedure is described in **Figures 2.154–2.166**.

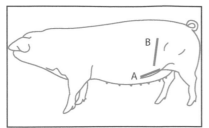

Fig. 2.154 Drawing showing two positions for the incision to gain access to the abdomen. In commercial breeds (Landrace or Large White) position A is preferred. The incision is made some 12 cm above the teat line (one hands width). This access is used to minimise the amount of subcutaneous fat. In addition, the three abdominal muscle layers have merged into one layer. During the subsequent suckling the wound is away from the piglets.

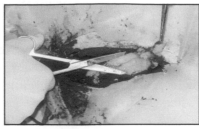

Fig. 2.155 Incise through the skin and muscle layer to the peritoneum. Penetrate the peritoneal layer with a scalpel blade and then, using scissors, extend the incision.

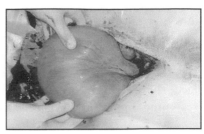

Fig. 2.156 The uterus is normally very obvious within the abdomen. Remove part of a uterine horn with a piglet inside.

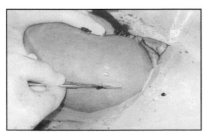

Fig. 2.157 Incise the uterus over the back of the piglet. Take care not to incise into the piglet.

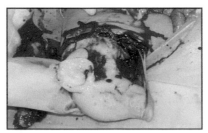

Fig. 2.158 Remove the piglet and pass to an assistant to encourage respiration. Clear the airways and if necessary use a respiratory stimulant.

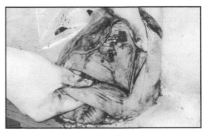

Fig. 2.159 Hold the edges of the incised uterus.

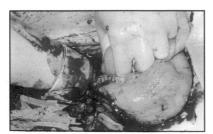

Fig. 2.160 Remove adjacent piglets, higher and lower from the incision. Do not attempt to remove all the piglets through the one hole. Three piglets per uterine incision are adequate. Repeat over another piglet.

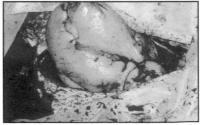

Fig. 2.161 Close the uterine incision using an inverted Lembert stitch and absorbable suture such as PDS® II or catgut.

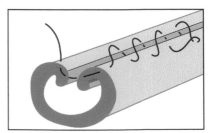

Fig. 2.162 An inverted Lembert stitch.

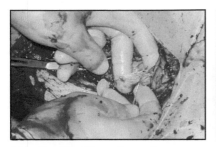

Fig. 2.163 Close the peritoneum cavity with Vicryl® or PDS® II.

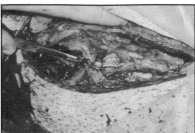

Fig. 2.164 Close the muscle layer as one layer. Close the subcutaneous layer.

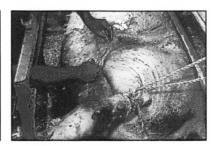

Fig. 2.165 Close the skin with Vicryl® using a subcutaneous pattern.

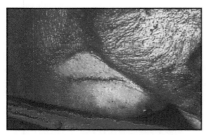

Fig. 2.166 The healing skin incision 2 days post caesarean.

Provide pain management as appropriate. Do not allow the piglets to suckle until the sow has reasonably recovered. Provide the piglets with warmth and syringe feed them with a small amount of warm water. Do not provide any milk products as this may interfere with colostrum antibody gut transfer, which decreases rapidly after 6 hours of first milk access. Providing the piglets with colostrum from another sow may be useful.

CLINICAL QUIZ

2.1 In the middle of oestrus how long does a sow stand for mating?

A 3 days	C 6 hours	E 15 minutes
B 1 day	D 1 hour	F 1 minute

2.2 In the middle of oestrus, after being in standing heat, how long will it take for an average sow to respond to a boar by standing again?

A Immediately	C 25 minutes	E 1 hours
B 10 minutes	D 45 minutes	F 1 day

2.3 Some reproductive viruses are classified as SMEDI viruses. What is the meaning of this acronym? Give two examples of porcine viruses that may create these clinical signs.

2.4 Which mycotoxin is a phytoestrogen?

The answers to these questions can be found on page 472.

CHAPTER 3

RESPIRATORY DISORDERS

INTRODUCTION

Disorders and diseases affecting the respiratory system are some of the most frequent problems in pig production worldwide. Their prevalence is higher when pigs are raised in closed environments with high stocking densities since such scenarios facilitate transmission of airborne pathogens within and between herds. Respiratory disorders can usually be observed as herd outbreaks with variable morbidity and mortality rates. They range from mild clinical signs with a reduced feed intake to severe respiratory and/or systemic diseases with a high mortality rate. Economic losses result from increased mortality, decreased weight gain, increased condemnation at slaughter and increased cost for treatments and vaccinations, as well as increased labour costs.

The majority of pig upper and lower respiratory disorders are caused by infectious agents (alone or in combination) but environmental factors and management practices, together with the immune status of the pig, play a significant predisposing role. The negative impact of some infectious agents (mainly viruses) and environmental factors on the mucociliary barrier of the airways and the phagocytic capacity of alveolar macrophages facilitate the invasion of the respiratory tract by other microorganisms. Importantly, this microbial invasion may take the form of subclinical colonisation, local respiratory disorder or widespread systemic disease. Although still poorly investigated in pigs, it is very likely that the respiratory microbiome (totality of microorganisms and their collective genetic material present in the respiratory tract) plays a key role in modulation of the immune system as well as clinical expression of disease – this is referred to a metagenomics.

Primary infectious agents may cause disease and lesions alone, but several pathogens are frequently involved in a respiratory disease outcome. Moreover, usually it is not feasible to distinguish clinically, or by gross pathology, the different infectious agents involved in a given problem, which has led to the use of the term porcine respiratory disease complex (PRDC) or enzootic (mycoplasma) pneumonia (EP). PRDC refers to a clinical respiratory disease of multifactorial origin in grow/finish pigs. In consequence, PRDC represents a clinical diagnosis that does not preclude a particular infectious agent being involved in the disorder. Agents most commonly involved in PRDC are *Mycoplasma hyopneumoniae*, porcine reproductive and respiratory syndrome virus (PRRSV), swine influenza virus (SIV) and porcine circovirus type 2 (PCV2). These pathogens may further predispose to concomitant bacterial pneumonia or even to systemic bacterial infections. The main infectious and non-infectious causes of respiratory disorders in pigs are listed in *Table 3.1*. On the other hand, EP is the result of *M. hyopneumoniae* infection, together with other respiratory bacteria.

Note that systemic pathogens not primarily targeting the respiratory tract may also cause respiratory clinical signs, such as Aujeszky's disease virus (pseudorabies virus) (see Chapter 2), the swine fever viruses – classical and African (see Chapter 9), Nipah virus (see Chapter 8), *Salmonella enterica* serotype *choleraesuis* (see Chapter 4), *Erysipelothrix rhusiopathiae* (see Chapter 9), *Mycoplasma suis*, as well as various

Table 3.1 Most frequent infectious and non-infectious causes of respiratory disorders in pigs and associated clinical signs.

AGENT (DISEASE)	CLINICAL SIGNS
Actinobacillus pleuropneumoniae	Productive cough, dyspnoea, fever, variable mortality rate, bloody nasal discharge, growth retardation
Actinobacillus suis	Sudden death, dyspnoea, cutaneous signs
Ammonia and dust	Sneezing, coughing and growth retardation
Ascaris suum	Dyspnoea (associated with larva migrans), coughing
Bordetella bronchiseptica (non-progressive atrophic rhinitis)	Deviation of snout, sneezing, nasal and ocular discharge
Chlamydia spp.	Conjunctivitis, dyspnoea, fever; most often subclinical
Haemophilus parasuis, Streptococcus suis, Mycoplasma hyorhinitis, Actinobacillus suis	Polyserositis, dyspnoea, growth retardation, mortality
Metastrongylus spp.	Coughing
Mycoplasma hyopneumoniae (enzootic [mycoplasma] pneumonia)	Non-productive cough, reduced feed intake, growth retardation
Pasteurella multocida (pneumonic pasteurellosis)	Productive cough, fever
Porcine circovirus type 2 (PCV2-SD)	Hacking cough, dyspnoea, growth retardation, subcutaneous lymphadenopathy
Porcine cytomegalovirus (inclusion body rhinitis)	Subclinical or mild rhinitis in baby pigs, ubiquitous, sneezing
Porcine reproductive and respiratory syndrome virus (PRRS)	Hacking cough, dyspnoea, growth retardation, subcutaneous lymphadenopathy
Porcine respiratory coronavirus	Subclinical, ubiquitous
Swine influenza virus (swine influenza)	Non-productive cough, fever; often subclinical
Toxigenic *Pasteurella multocida* (progressive atrophic rhinitis)	Deviation of snout, reduced growth, sneezing, nasal and ocular discharge, bloody nasal discharge.
Water shortage	Coughing and growth retardation

Table 3.2 Herd factors with significant influence on the outcome of respiratory disorders.

GENERIC FACTORS	SPECIFIC FACTORS THAT MAY FACILITATE RESPIRATORY DISORDERS
Production system	High stocking density Variable stocking density Continuous flow Introduction of pigs from different sources or from herds with low sanitary status
Housing	Poor insulation and/or ventilation Open partitions between pens Large rooms Slatted floors
Nutrition	Insufficient energy intake Insufficient amounts of macro- and micronutrients in feed
Management	Poor monitoring of disease signs Incorrect vaccination plans and other preventive measures Poor caretaking of diseased pigs Poor hygiene Poor biosecurity Excess of cross-fostering Poor water availability Poor cleaning Lack of all-in/all-out (AIAO)

toxins (e.g. organophosphates, carbon monoxide, carbamate) and mechanical problems such as gastric ulceration (see Chapter 4). The mechanisms involved in causing respiratory problems are very diverse and depend on the aetiology, but usually include replication in endothelial or epithelial cells throughout the body, generation of anaemia, alteration of the blood oxygen partial pressure, cardiac insufficiency, neuromuscular disorders and central neurological conditions affecting the respiratory centre of the brainstem.

Herd factors significantly influence the outcome of respiratory disease. Therefore, when evaluating respiratory problems, it is essential to consider the issues noted in *Table 3.2*.

GENERAL CLINICAL SIGNS OF RESPIRATORY DISORDERS

Clinical signs (*Table 3.3*, see p. 110) may include sneezing, nasal and ocular discharge, productive or non-productive coughing, tachypnoea (rapid breathing)

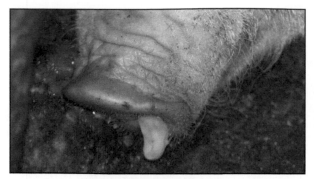

Fig. 3.1 Nasal discharge.

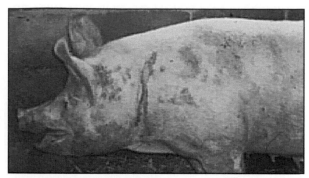

Fig. 3.2 Coughing. The injection was given too far caudally. ▶ VIDEO 13

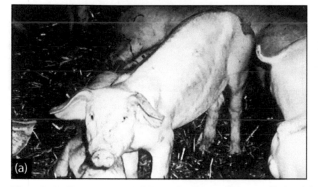

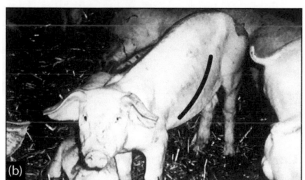

Fig. 3.3 Dyspnoea. (a) Note the heave line outlining the diaphragm. (b) Heave line illustrated.

and dyspnoea (laboured breathing) (**Figures 3.1–3.3**). Fever, anorexia, cyanosis and sudden death may occur in cases of severe disease. Some infectious agents may cause subclinical and/or mild disease, eventually associated with growth retardation and increase in feed conversion efficiency. Conversely, other pathogens may lead to severe respiratory signs (with dyspnoea and/or tachypnoea) but also to a systemic disease with a variety of signs that are not restricted to the respiratory system.

Eventually, some infectious agents or their combination with other pathogens or non-infectious risk factors may lead to the death of the animal. The aetiological clarification of respiratory disease episodes requires proper clinical and epidemiological investigations as well as a pathological examination (necropsy). In some more demanding cases, laboratory investigations will be very useful.

When dealing with PRDC, laboratory investigations will be necessary due to its multi-aetiological and multifactorial nature. It should also be remembered that the majority of pigs do not display clinical signs associated with infection with these 'pathogenic' agents.

GENERAL DIAGNOSIS OF RESPIRATORY TRACT DISORDERS

A holistic diagnostic approach must be practiced, including proper historical, clinical and epidemiological assessments at the herd level and pathological examination of affected pigs. To enable a good pathological examination, a good knowledge of the normal clinical anatomy of the pig is crucial since the accurate identification and location of lesions may suggest more than one disease/ condition. It is important to assess the respiratory tract with the cardiovascular system, which circulates the oxygen and removes the carbon dioxide. Issues with the cardiovascular system or with the lungs results in pressure issues and cardiovascular failure. The two systems should be considered in partnership with each other.

CLINICAL ANATOMY OF THE RESPIRATORY TRACT AND THE CARDIOVASCULAR SYSTEM

Nose

See **Figures 3.4, 3.5**.

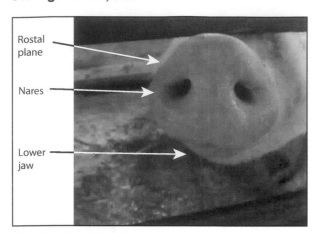

Rostal plane

Nares

Lower jaw

Fig. 3.4 Detail of the nose.

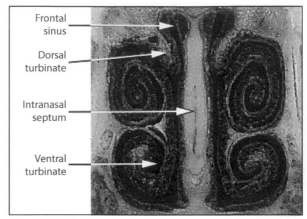

Frontal sinus

Dorsal turbinate

Intranasal septum

Ventral turbinate

Fig. 3.5 Cross-section of the nose at the level of the premolars.

Larynx, trachea and bronchial system

See **Figures 3.6–3.8**.

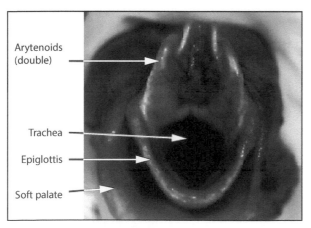

Arytenoids (double)

Trachea

Epiglottis

Soft palate

Fig. 3.6 Entrance to the larynx.

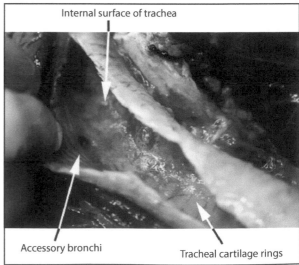

Internal surface of trachea

Accessory bronchi

Tracheal cartilage rings

Fig. 3.7 The accessory bronchus on the right-hand side.

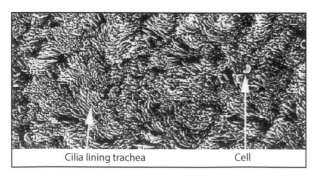

Cilia lining trachea   Cell

Fig. 3.8 The mucociliary escalator scanning electron microscope view.

Lungs

It is important to note that the right lung comprises four lobes (apical, cardiac, diaphragmatic and intermediate lobes), the right apical lobe being mainly ventilated by an accessory bronchus (**Figures 3.9, 3.10**). This anatomic organisation facilitates the usual finding of bacterial pneumonia in the right lung apical lobe.

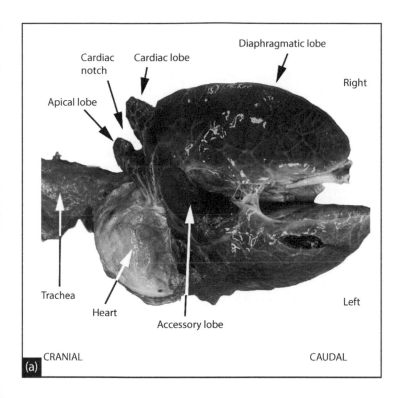

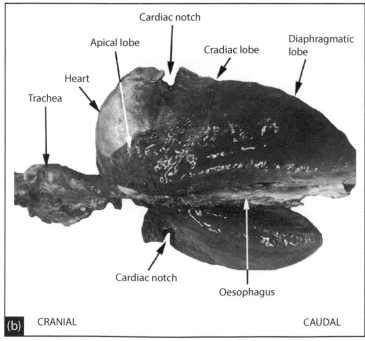

Fig. 3.9 Lungs. (a) **Dorsal view.** (b) **Ventral view.** *(Continued)*

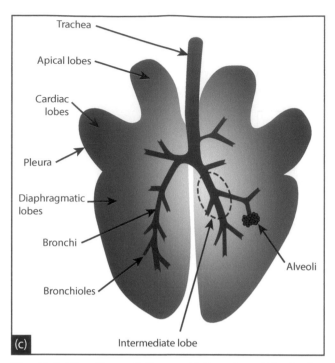

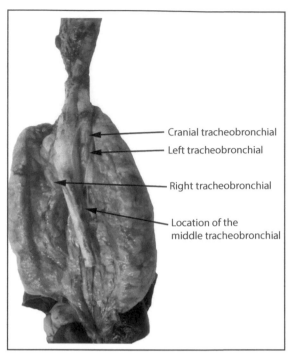

Fig. 3.9 (Continued) Lungs. (c) Drawing of the basic pig lung – useful to indicate the location of pathology.

Fig. 3.10 The bronchial lymph nodes. (See also Chapter 8.)

Cardiovascular system
See **Figures 3.11–3.13**.

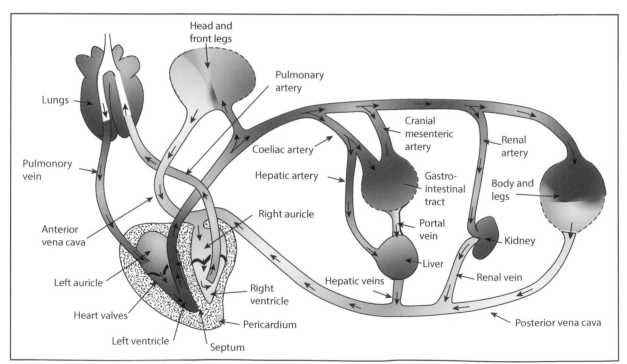

Fig. 3.11 Overview of the cardiovascular system. Red, oxygen-rich blood; blue, carbon dioxide-rich blood.

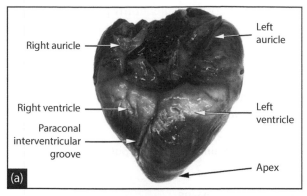

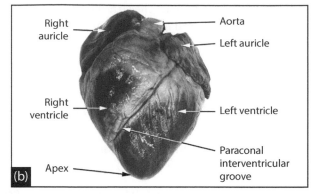

Fig. 3.12 (a) Parietal surface of the heart, dorsal view. (b) Parietal surface of the heart, ventral view.

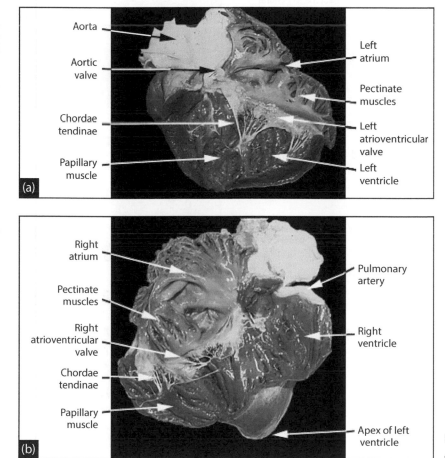

Fig. 3.13 (a) Heart opened, left side. (b) Heart opened, right side.

GROSS PATHOLOGY OF THE RESPIRATORY SYSTEM

Upper respiratory lesions can be mainly found in the nasal cavity and larynx. Most of these lesions are of an inflammatory nature (rhinitis and laryngitis), but other possibilities can be found such as atrophy of nasal turbinates and haemorrhages in the nasal cavity and larynx.

Atrophy of nasal turbinates should be studied by examining a transverse cut of the snout performed between the first and second upper premolars (the cut is at the level of the labial commissure). Also, the conjunctiva may be affected in some infections, with lesions of an inflammatory nature (conjunctivitis).

Inflammation of the trachea (tracheitis) and bronchi (bronchitis) as well as haemorrhages are unusual in pigs.

Most lesions of the lower respiratory tract grossly affect the lung tissues themselves. It should be remembered that there are only a limited number of changes that are possible in any organ and gross pathology assessment only provides a description of lesions, not a diagnosis of the presence of a pathogen.

A description of the different pneumonic types and pleuritis found in pigs can be found in *Table 3.3*. The normal pneumonic patterns within a lung are illustrated in **Figure 3.20**.

Table 3.3 **Description of the different pneumonia types and pleuritis found in pigs and potential generic or specific causes.**

PATHOLOGY	GROSS APPEARANCE	CAUSES	IMAGE
Catarrhal-purulent or suppurative bronchopneumonia	Part of or the whole cranial and middle lobes are bilaterally consolidated*. Pleural surface not affected. Typical image of enzootic {mycoplasma) pneumonia (**Figure 3.14**)	Bacteria in general	Fig. 3.14
Fibrino-haemorrhagic-necrotising pleuropneumonia	Fibrinous exudation on the pleura. Lung can be consolidated due to inflammation and/or necrosis. Haemorrhagic appearance of the necrotic area (**Figure 3.15**)	Very virulent bacteria (APP, *A. suis*, some strains of *P. multocida*)	Fig. 3.15
Interstitial pneumonia	Lack of lung collapse and with a rubbery consistency. Multifocal to diffuse tan-mottling. Potential interstitial oedema (**Figure 3.16**)	Viruses, *Salmonella enterica* serotype *choleraesuis*	Fig. 3.16
Bronchointerstitial pneumonia	Pulmonary cranioventral consolidation but with a multifocal distribution in apical and middle lobes and, to a lesser extent, in diaphragmatic lobes (**Figure 3.17**)	SIV, *M. hyopneumoniae*	Fig. 3.17

(Continued)

PATHOLOGY	GROSS APPEARANCE	CAUSES	IMAGE
Embolic pneumonia	Abscesses or necrotic lesions randomly distributed throughout the lung parenchyma (**Figure 3.18**)	Opportunistic systemic bacteria disseminated haematogenously	Fig. 3.18
Pleuritis	Fibrinous exudation on the pleura without affecting the lung parenchyma (**Figure 3.19**)	APP, *H. parasuis*, *Streptococcus suis*, *M. hyorhinis*, *Escherichia coli*	Fig. 3.19

Table 3.3 *(Continued)* **Description of the different pneumonia types and pleuritis found in pigs and potential generic or specific causes.**

* Cranial part of diaphragmatic lobes may also be affected.

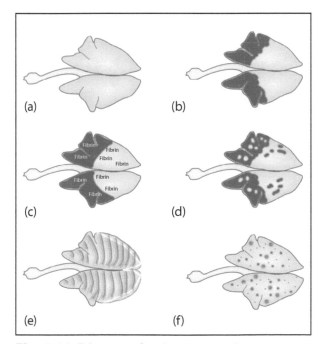

Fig. 3.20 Diagrams showing pneumonic patterns within a lung. **(a)** Normal lung. **(b)** Suppurative bronchopneumonia. **(c)** Fibrino-necrotising pleuropneumonia. **(d)** Bronchointerstitial pneumonia. **(e)** Interstitial pneumonia. **(f)** Embolic pneumonia.

LABORATORY INVESTIGATION OF RESPIRATORY DISORDERS

Assessment of the specific cause of a respiratory disease outbreak may require the aid of laboratory analyses. The main objective is to confirm or rule out the potential involvement of infectious agents or toxins with the respiratory disorder.

Several laboratory techniques are available:

- Determine the presence of particular lesions (histopathology).
- Pathogens in lesions (immunohistochemistry [IHC], immunofluorescence, in situ hybridisation [ISH].
- Isolation of an infectious agent (bacteriology or virus isolation).
- Antimicrobial susceptibility of a bacterial agent (antibiogram).
- Genome of the pathogen (polymerase chain reaction [PCR], reverse transcription [RT]-PCR, including real-time PCR methods).
- Antibodies against an infectious agent (mostly by enzyme-linked immunosorbent assay [ELISA] tests).

Table 3.4 **Sample types to be selected depending on the laboratory technique.**

LABORATORY TECHNIQUE	SAMPLE TYPE	PURPOSE
Histopathology	Lung pieces from damaged and non-damaged areas; skip tips of the lobes; fixation in formalin	Detection of microscopic lesions; usually very orientative on the nature of the lesion
IHC/ISH	Same as for histopathology	Detection of a pathogen in the site of the lesion; detects antigen (IHC) or genome (ISH) of a pathogen
Bacteriology/virology	Nasal, laryngeal, tracheal and bronchial swabs, oral fluids via rope; lungs (complete lung is preferred); refrigeration*	Isolation of bacteria or viruses; can be done for monitoring purposes
Antibiogram	Same as for bacteriology	Antimicrobial susceptibility of isolated bacteria
PCR/RT-PCR	Swabs from involved parts of the respiratory tract, oral fluids; lung pieces; serum**; can be refrigerated or frozen	Detection of pathogen genome; can be done for monitoring purposes
Antibody detection (ELISA)	Serum and oral fluids	Detection of antibodies against a pathogen; usually done for monitoring purposes

* Frozen samples are not a problem for virological tests.
** For those systemic pathogens causing respiratory disorders.

Into such a wide laboratory analysis scenario, the clinician must contribute to the reliability of the techniques by selecting appropriate samples and guaranteeing prompt delivery to the laboratory (*Table 3.4*).

BACTERIOLOGY OF THE MAJOR BACTERIA ISOLATED FROM THE RESPIRATORY TRACT

Actinobacillus suis
See **Figures 3.21–3.24**.

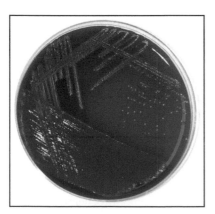

Fig. 3.21 Blood agar – wide zone of β haemolysis.

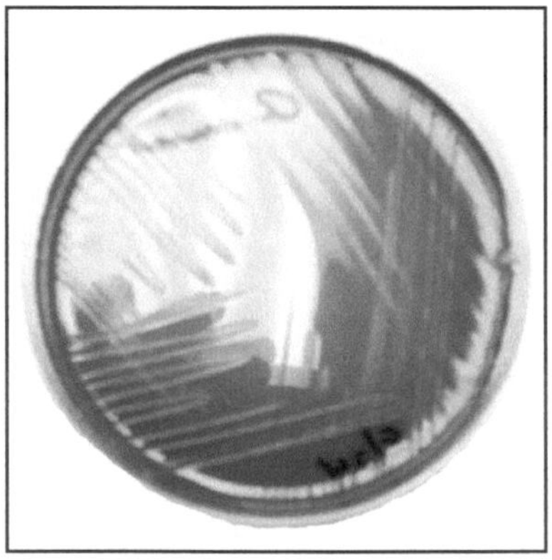

Fig. 3.22 MacConkey's – no growth. Sometimes very small.

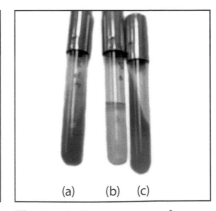

(a)   (b)   (c)

Fig. 3.23 Tests – no growth on MacConkey's, an important differential from *E. coli*. (a) Kligler's: lactose +ve, dextrose +ve red; (b) Simm's: difficult, little reaction; (c) Urease +ve, red.

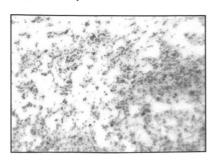

Fig. 3.24 Gram-negative rod.

Actinobacillus pleuropneumoniae

See **Figures 3.25, 3.26**.

Organism generally requires nicotinamide adenine dinucleotide (NAD) to grow. This is also called V factor and is supplied by the staphylococcus streak.

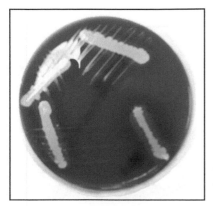

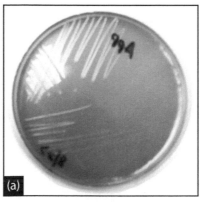

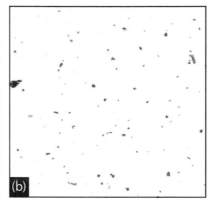

Fig. 3.25 Blood agar. Requires *Staphylococcus* streak. Haemolytic – satellitism.

Fig. 3.26 (a) MacConkey's. No growth. (b) Gram-negative rods and coccobacillary forms.

Bordetella bronchiseptica

See **Figures 3.27–3.30**.

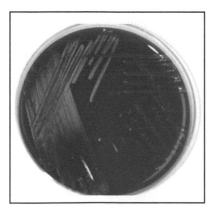

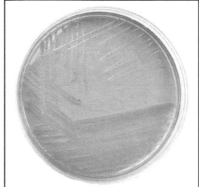

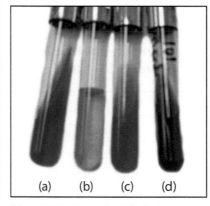

Fig. 3.27 Blood agar. Incubate for at least 48 hours.

Fig. 3.28 MacConkey's – non-lactose fermenter.

Fig. 3.29 Tests. (a) Kligler's: –ve red; (b) Simm's: poor reaction little growth; (c) Urease: strong positive – pink slant; (d) Simmon's citrate agar; positive – blue colour.

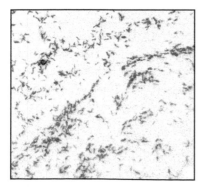

Fig. 3.30 Small gram-negative coccobacilli.

Haemophilus parasuis

See **Figures 3.31–3.34**.

Reputedly grows best under CO_2 on chocolate agar. It is urease negative – yellow; useful to distinguish from *Actinobacillus pleuropneumoniae*, which is urease positive – blue.

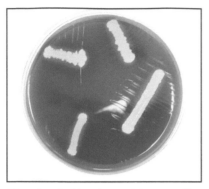

Fig. 3.31 Blood agar. Very small colonies around the *Staphylococcus* streak.

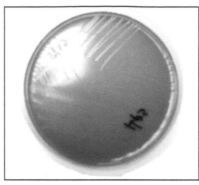

Fig. 3.32 MacConkey's. No growth.

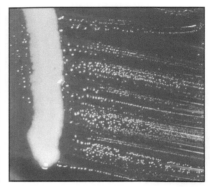

Fig. 3.33 Can be difficult to grow – requires NAD. (See also Fig. 6.14.)

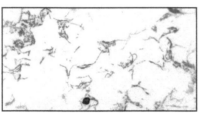

Fig. 3.34 Gram-negative coccobacillus.

Mycoplasma hyopneumoniae

Mycoplasmas require special media. *M. hyopneumoniae* requires a long incubation period and a specialised laboratory to grow the organism, which even then is frequently overgrown with other *Mycoplasma* spp. Its isolation is not performed for routine diagnostic purposes, and it is substituted by techniques detecting its DNA.

Pasteurella multocida

See **Figures 3.35–3.38**.

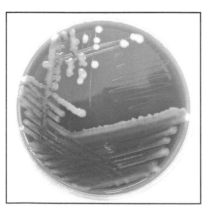

Fig. 3.35 A mucoid colony - may run together.

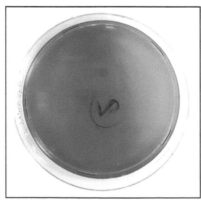

Fig. 3.36 MacConkey's. No growth.

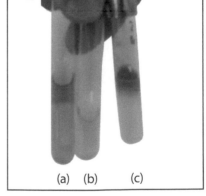

Fig. 3.37 Tests: note distinctive odour – musky. **(a)** Dextrose broth: +ve – red, no gas; **(b)** Lactose: –ve – yellow; **(c)** Indole: positive – red. In addition, urease negative.

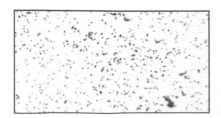

Fig. 3.38 Small gram-negative rod or coccobacillus.

Streptococcus suis

See **Figures 3.39–3.41**.

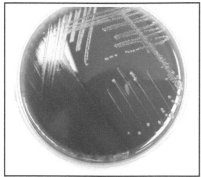

Fig. 3.39 Blood agar.

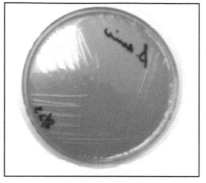

Fig. 3.40 MacConkey's. No growth.

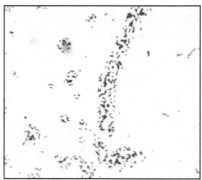

Fig. 3.41 Colony.

Trueperella pyogenes

See **Figures 3.42–3.44**.

The basic bacteriology of respiratory diseases of pigs is shown in *Table 3.5*.

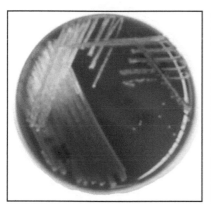

Fig. 3.42 Blood agar. Catalase −ve.

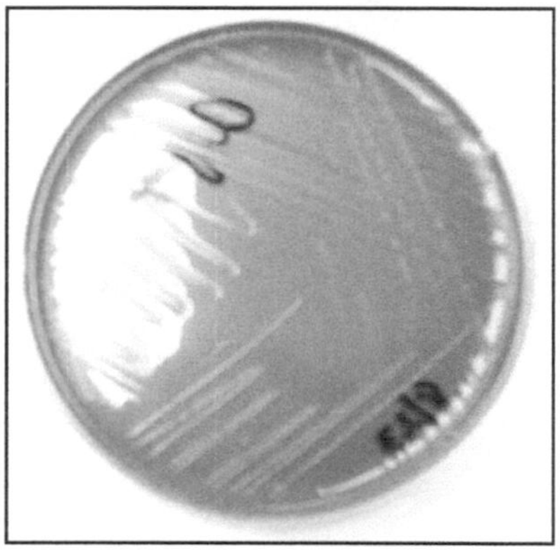

Fig. 3.43 MacConkey's. No growth.

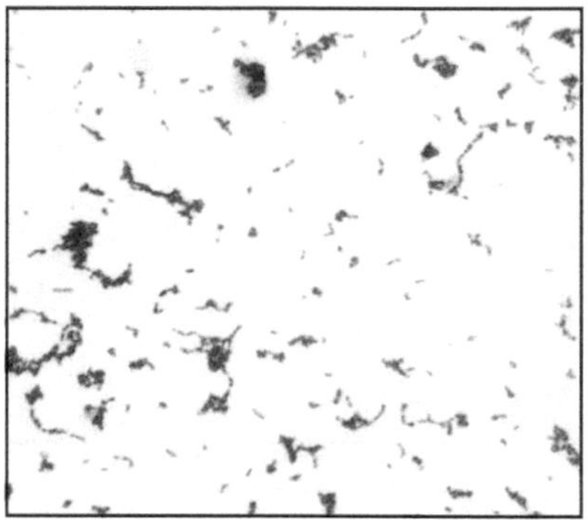

Fig. 3.44 Gram-positive pleomorphic rods – 'Chinese letters'.

Table 3.5 **Basic bacteriology of respiratory diseases.**

ORGANISM	GRAM STAIN	GROWTH				SUGARS AND REACTIONS									
		ANAEROBE ONLY	HAEMOLYTIC BLOOD AGAR	MACCONKEY	TERGITOL	CATALASE	OXIDASE	DEXTROSE BROTH	KLIGLERS	KLIGLER'S IRON	LACTOSE	LYSINE	SIMMS	SIMMS CITRATE	UREASE
Actinobacillus pleuropneumoniae	−CB		Y	−	−	V	V								+
Actinobacillus suis	−B		β	−	−	+	V	+			+			P	+
Bordetella bronchiseptica	−CB		N	+NL	+NL	+	+		−				P		+
Haemophilus parasuis	−CB		N	−	−	+	−								−
Pasteurella multocida	−CB		N	−	−	+	+	+			−			+	−
Streptococci	+C		α/β	−	−	−	−								
Trueperella pyogenes	+B		N	−	−	−	−								

Code: + and green = positive; − and red = negative.
Gram stain: B = bacillus/coccobacillus; C = coccoid; CB = coccobacillus.
Sugars and reactions: V= variable; P = poor.
Haemolytic: Y = yes and type α or β; N= no.

INVESTIGATION INTO RESPIRATORY DISORDERS

Sample submission

Two or more euthanased pigs with early clinical signs should be submitted plus a freshly dead pig, if available.

Individual animal investigation

With regard to pet pig management, further investigation into respiratory disorders may be required.

Radiography of the pig chest
See **Figure 3.45**.

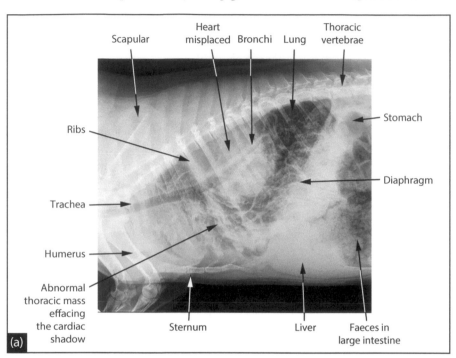

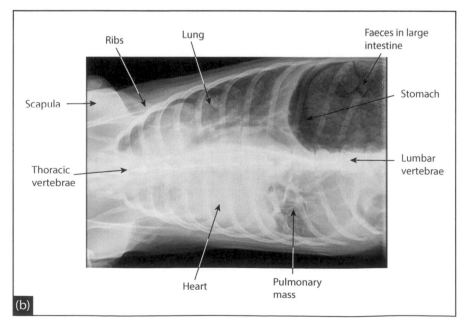

Fig. 3.45 Lateral (a) and ventrodorsal (b) radiographs of the chest. In this case the heart is displaced away from the diaphragm by a thoracic mass.

Computed tomography of the pig chest
See **Figure 3.46**.

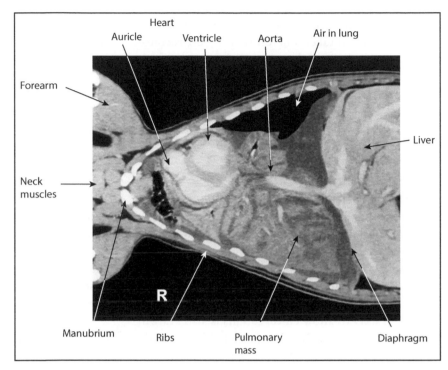

Fig. 3.46 CT scan of a 1-year-old pig with a very large chronic pulmonary mass, possibly a resolving abscess. The pig was in extreme respiratory distress.

GENERAL MANAGEMENT OF DISORDERS OF THE RESPIRATORY TRACT

The management of a respiratory disease outbreak depends on the specific cause or causes that initiated it. Therefore, therapeutics of respiratory disorders must focus first on diagnosis. Once this is achieved (clinical, pathological etc.), the nature of the intervention measure will adjust to the following actions:

- **Immediate actions:**
  - Antibiotic treatment in case of bacterial respiratory infections; use of anti-inflammatory drugs.
  - Urgent vaccination in case of certain viral infections (e.g. Aujeszky's disease [pseudorabies]).
  - Removal of feed or water in case of toxicity.
  - Report to the appropriate government department for reportable pathogens (e.g. African swine fever).

- **Short-term actions:**
  - Change from immediate actions based on laboratory results.
  - Revision of the vaccine planning and strategic medications.
  - Improve the most significant herd factors influencing the particular respiratory disorder affecting the farm (those not depending on structural or building issues).
  - Review and improve the pig's environment.
- **Mid-/long-term actions:**
  - Impose a batching programme and achieve all-in/all-out (AIAO) pig flow.
  - Improve herd factors depending on structural or building issues.
  - Partial or total depopulation.

The most frequently implemented actions against overt respiratory disease outbreaks include the use of antibiotics and non-steroidal anti-inflammatory drugs (NSAIDs). NSAIDs also have antipyretic and analgesic activity.

The general practice is provision of antibiotics in the feed or water, but this metaphylactic approach might not be adequate since the most clinically affected animals usually have reduced feed and water intake. Therefore, the best recommendation is to include parenteral antimicrobial medication of sick animals and the ones in direct contact with them.

DISORDERS OF THE RESPIRATORY TRACT

Actinobacillus (porcine) pleuropneumonia VIDEO 14
Definition/aetiology

Actinobacillus pleuropneumoniae is the aetiological agent of actinobacillus (porcine) pleuropneumonia (APP), a severe contagious respiratory disease distributed worldwide. *Actinobacillus pleuropneumoniae* is a gram-negative coccobacillus that generally requires NAD to allow culture. This is also known as the V factor. The NAD is provided by a streak of *Staphylococcus* on the blood agar plate. There are a total of 15 serotypes currently recognised. They present with very variable virulence patterns; some of them are considered non-virulent (causing subclinical infections) while others are able to cause death of pigs in less than 24 hours. Interestingly, the same serotype may exhibit different virulence in different parts of the world. North America considers serotypes 1 and 5 most severe, whereas Europeans consider serotypes 2, 9 and 11 as most significant.

There are three significant toxins:

- Toxin I is cytotoxic and haemolytic.
- Toxin II is mildly cytotoxic and weakly haemolytic.
- Toxin III is cytotoxic.

Although *A. pleuropneumoniae* is considered a primary pathogen able to cause disease by itself, concurrent infections may promote disease severity linked to its infection.

The economic importance of this disease relies on mortality, loss of overall performance and medical (antimicrobial and vaccine) costs. Moreover, *A. pleuropneumoniae* is another significant pathogen able to participate in PRDC.

Airborne spread is possible but only over very short distances. *A. pleuropneumoniae* is classically a nose-to-nose spread infection. Survival in the environment, unless the bacteria is protected by mucus, is very short.

Clinical presentation

The disease can take any of four major clinical forms (subclinical, peracute, acute or chronic) even within the same batch of animals in a major outbreak (**Figures 3.47–3.51**).

- **Subclinical**. (Normal, no clinical signs). *A. pleuropneumoniae* is a normal inhabitant of the nasopharynx in pigs, mainly in the tonsils. The organism occurs on most farms and in about 25% of the pigs on the farm at any one time. The clinical signs of this 'infection'

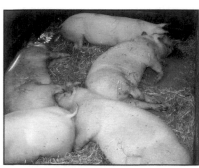

Fig. 3.47 This pen of pigs with porcine pleuropneumonia dyspnoea are quiet and have difficulty moving.

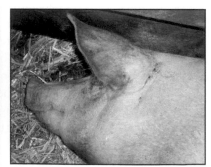

Fig. 3.48 Cyanosis of the ears in a peracute porcine pleuropneumonia case.

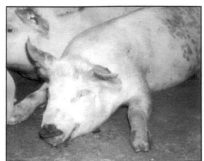

Fig. 3.49 Epistaxis and blood from the mouth are typical of porcine pleuropneumonia outbreaks.

Fig. 3.50
Many dead finishing pigs are typical of an acute porcine pleuropneumonia outbreak.

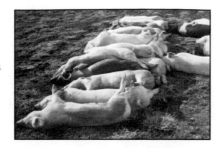

Fig. 3.51
Ventral cyanosis is typical of death associated with porcine pleuropneumonia.

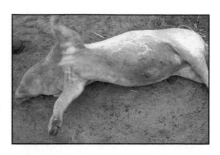

is nothing or subclinical. These subclinically infected animals are considered carriers of the infection and the major source of potential introduction of *A. pleuropneumoniae* serotypes into recipient farms, which may be negative (rare) or have a different spectrum of serotypes.

- **Percacute**: Pigs with the peracute presentation may present as dead pigs with other pigs presenting with an acute phase, even for a very short period of time, often overlooked under farm conditions (and perceived as sudden death), together with a foamy bloody nasal or oral discharge just before death. With the peracute form, the clinician needs to become concerned if when entering the building the pigs are non-vocal and reluctant to move. Morbidity of the batch of pigs may be over 80%.

- **Acute**: In an acute outbreak, the main clinical signs of APP are observed in late nursery pigs and/or in grow/finish animals. They consist of fever (41.5°C), vomiting, anorexia, tachypnoea, dyspnoea and some coughing/sneezing.

- **Chronic**: Animals that survive the acute phase of the disease may become chronically affected, showing little or no fever, mild coughing, inappetence and perhaps a reluctance to move.

The severity of the clinical signs may vary depending on the age of the animals, the infecting *A. pleuropneumoniae* serovar and specific bacterial strain, environmental conditions, genetic line susceptibility, pig immune status and magnitude of the exposure to the bacterium. Farms with clinical APP and ongoing respiratory problems (PRDC) tend to display a worse clinical outcome.

Differential diagnosis

For sudden death in grow/finish pigs, differential diagnoses would include African swine fever,

classical swine fever, erysipelas, salmonellosis, streptococcal septicaemia, acute Glässer's disease and a toxin release from the slurry pit (H_2S).

In cases of severe fibrino-necrotising pleuropneumonia, *A. suis* and pleuritic strains of *P. multocida* are differentials.

In chronic situations, multiple bacterial pulmonary infections can mimic the clinical signs. In most of the cases, gross pathology (necropsy or slaughter check) allows a strong suspicion of APP due to the presence of pleuropneumonic lesions at different levels of evolution. When only pleuritis is seen without damage of lung parenchyma, infection with this bacterium is unlikely and other systemic bacterial pathogens should be considered (*H. parasuis*, *S. suis* and/or *M. hyorhinis*).

Diagnosis

At necropsy, dead pigs show haemorrhagic necrotising pneumonia and fibrinous pleuritis, usually in a dorsocaudal distribution (rarely in cranioventral locations) (**Figures 3.52–3.55**).

The presence of animals with different disease presentations within a batch makes diagnosing APP challenging. In acute or peracute stages, presence of APP compatible clinical signs and/or lesions (haemorrhagic necrotising pneumonia and fibrinous pleuritis) is usually sufficient to establish the diagnosis. Isolation of the bacterium in these lung lesions is confirmatory.

Antibody detection by ELISA tests (serum or saliva) and PCR or bacterial isolation (lung, tonsils or nasal/tonsillar swabs) are needed for the detection of chronically or subclinically infected animals. Isolation of *A. pleuropneumoniae* is interesting since it allows its serotyping and, eventually, the possibility of preparing autogenous vaccines (*Table 3.6*).

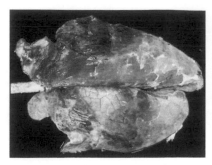

Fig. 3.52 Fibrino-haemorrhagic-necrotising pleuropneumonia associated with an experimental infection with *A. pleuropneumoniae*. Note the marked interstitial oedema close to necrotic areas.

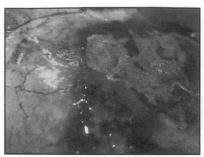

Fig. 3.53 The interface between the porcine pleuropneumonia lesion and normal lung. Note the haemorrahgic zone and small forward haemorrhages with the necrotic area behind the haemorrhagic lesion.

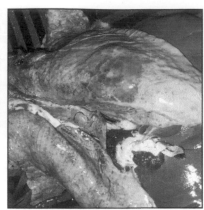

Fig. 3.54 Discrete porcine pleuropneumonia lesion in the diaphragmatic lobe.

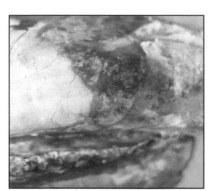

Fig. 3.55 Porcine pleuropneumonia lesion with overlying pleuritic lesion.

Table 3.6 ***Actinobacillus pleuropneumoniae* typing by toxin analysis.**

SEROTYPE	APX 1	APX II	APX III	APX IV
1	■	■		■
2		■	■	■
3		▨	■	■
4		■	■	■
5	■	■		■
6		■	■	■
7		■		■
8		■	■	■
9	■	■	■	■
10	■			■
11	■	■	■	■
12		■		■
13		■		■
14	■			■
15		■	■	■
A. porcintonsillarum				
A. suis	■	■	■	

Red, toxin present; orange, toxin variably present.

Management

Treatment in an outbreak: During pleuropneumonia outbreaks the priority is to stop mortality by treating affected pigs with antimicrobials. Most antibiotics are active against *A. pleuropneumoniae*, although resistance against beta-lactams and tetracyclines is common. Tulathromycin, florfenicol and amoxycillin are good first-choice antibiotics. Antibiotic therapy is effective in acutely affected pigs and reduction of mortality is the most immediate observable effect. In fact, the success rate of the treatment influences the immune response of pigs, since the higher the efficacy the lower the antibody response, and the more likely the possibility of reinfection. Therapeutic success also depends on the earlier detection of clinical signs and intervention. Parenteral is the preferred route for antibiotic administration since in the acute phase of the disease pigs are anorexic and significantly decrease their water intake.

Pleuropneumonia is extremely painful and suitable pain relief is an essential part of the treatment programme.

Control: Good environmental management (e.g. temperature, ventilation, stocking density, excellent water supplies) is crucial to minimising the impact of outbreaks.

Vaccination allows prevention of porcine pleuropneumonia, with the existence of bacterins that are serotype-specific (there are some cross-reacting serotypes) and subunit vaccines (which include the three major exotoxins, ApxI, ApxII and ApxIII). However, vaccination response can be disappointing

and appropriate timing of the vaccination programme (two doses 3–4 weeks apart, the first one at
around 5–6 weeks of age) programme is essential.

Elimination: Eradication of the infection at herd
level based on age segregation and medication is possible, although the most effective method is depopula-
tion/repopulation (see Chapter 11).

However, elimination is not easy. Colonisation
of tonsillar crypts by the bacterium makes it
very difficult to eliminate by means of antibiotic
treatment.

Summary

A check list to help deal with an outbreak of porcine
pleuropneumonia is shown in *Table 3.7*.

Table 3.7 **A check list that may be helpful in understanding an outbreak of *A. pleuropneumoniae*.**

FARM: DATE:		CHECK
Undisturbed group of pigs	Examine and record lying pattern of undisturbed pigs – photo/video	
	Behaviour of pigs around the water supply – photo/video	
	Behaviour of pigs around the feeders – photo/video	
Stock	Clinical pigs respond to tulathromycin, ceftiofur, penicillin	
	Is tilmicosin used in-feed or water medication	
	Record post-weaning antibiotic use	
	Any porcine pleuropneumonia vaccine used?	
Check for PRRSV	Blood results – note 21 days antibody delay	
PCV2-SD	Were pigs vaccinated at weaning against PCV2	
	Check vaccine purchases correspond to weaning numbers	
	Check medicine storage is 2–8°C	
Post-mortem	Ensure diagnosis correct – photo/video	
	A. pleuropneumoniae actually isolated – which type is isolated	
	Slaughterhouse reports	
Sick pigs	Treatment of sick pigs	
	Movement of recovered pigs	
	Collect true mortality and morbidity figures	
Check weaning age and weight	Age at weaning	
	Weight at weaning	
Immunology	Vaccine programme	
Pig flow	Collect true weaning/farrowing/breeding and gilt numbers by batch	
AIAO	AIAO by pigs, water, feed, floor, air and medicine	
Medicines	Ensure needles and syringes not used between different batches	
Water	Flow – 700 mL/min minimum	
	Height suitable for the pigs	
	Number of drinkers	
	Cleaning programme between batches	
Floor	Stocking density	
	Cleaning programme between batches	

(Continued)

Table 3.7 *(Continued)* **A check list that may be helpful in understanding an outbreak of *A. pleuropneumoniae*.**

		CHECK
Air	Temperature variation	
	Relative humidity (50–75%)	
	High dust and endotoxin issues	
	Note level of slurry under slats – air flow from underneath slats?	
	Draughts in the 'proposed sleeping area'	
	Examine defecation pattern of pigs	
	Smoke buildings and record air movement patterns – photo/video	
	Cleaning programme between batches	
Feed	Feed space and feeder management	
	Problem coincides with a change in diet/feed type and feed size	
	Cleaning programme between batches	
Other problems	PRRSV, PCV2-RD and mange are classic examples of problems	
	Eliminate any additional stressors – weighing, tagging, bleeding	

Actinobacillus suis

Definition/aetiology

Actinobacillus suis is a ubiquitous opportunistic pathogen usually found colonising the upper respiratory tract of pigs. Under specific but not well-defined circumstances, it can cause septicaemic disease, usually in piglets but also in older pigs. Most disease cases are described in high health farms. Globally, it is considered that *A. suis* causes sporadic disease. It may be isolated from cases of polyserositis. *A. suis* is a gram-negative rod bacteria.

Clinical presentation

This bacterium has been associated with a variety of clinical signs including sudden death, dyspnoea, coughing, lameness, fever, wasting, abscesses (**Figures 3.56, 3.57**), neurological signs and abortions.

Three major clinical pictures are defined. The first is sudden death due to septicaemia in young piglets (<5 weeks of age) with multiple haemorrhages in the body and serofibrinous exudate in body cavities. Histologically, bacterial thromboemboli are found.

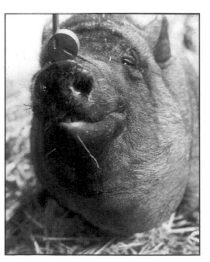

Fig. 3.56 Abscess in a pet pig associated with *Actinobacillus suis*.

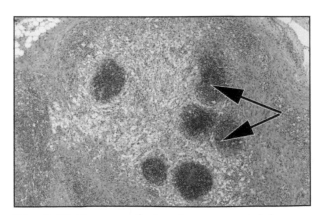

Fig. 3.57 Presence of microabscesses containing thromboemboli of *Actinobacillus suis* colonies (arrows) in its centre in a lymph node. H&E.

The second clinical form consists of severe respiratory signs (cough, fever, dyspnoea) with fibrino-haemorrhagic-necrotising pleuropneumonia. This may be associated with a polyserositis (Glässer's disease).

The third clinical form is an acute septicaemia in adult pigs, showing erysipelas-like lesions on the skin; abortions may occur.

Differential diagnosis

Different diseases can be clinically confused with *A. suis* infection, depending on the dominant clinical picture. On the respiratory side, the most important diseases to rule out are porcine pleuropneumonia and pleuritis/pneumonia associated with *P. multocida*. If only pleuritis and/or other serositis are seen, without damage to lung parenchyma, systemic bacterial pathogens should be considered (*H. parasuis*, *S. suis*, *M. hyorhinis*).

Diagnosis

Diagnosis is based on clinical signs and culture and identification of *A. suis*. The most appropriate samples will depend on the clinical presentation, but lung tissue is recommended as well as other parenchymatous organs (spleen, liver, lymph nodes) due to the septicaemia caused by the bacterium.

Management

Antibiotic treatment is recommended at the onset of clinical signs. Pain relief is an essential part of the treatment programme. Autogenous vaccines have been used sporadically with variable results.

Anaemia

Anaemia may be recognised in a pale looking pig. The vulva is a good place to look for anaemic pallor (see Chapter 9). Blood sample examination will confirm the presence of anaemia (see Chapter 7). Other skin colour changes can be exhibited (e.g. cyanosis), especially after exercise. The pig may cough with severe anaemia – a cardiac cough. Pulmonary oedema may be seen at post-mortem. Anaemia can be associated with iron deficiency in weaner pigs, *Mycoplasma suis* in weaned pigs (see Chapter 9) or chronic gastric ulceration (see Chapter 4).

Ascaridiosis (see also Chapter 4) ▶ VIDEO 13

The roundworm *Ascaris suum* is the most common nematode infecting pigs and it causes mainly hepatic lesions due to larvae migration. However, in heavy infestations, and because of migration through the lungs (**Figure 3.58**), respiratory clinical signs may develop. Adult worms are found in the small intestine. Dead adult worms may be seen in the faeces.

Atrophic rhinitis ▶ VIDEO 15

Atrophy of the nasal turbinates can be caused by a number of conditions. There are two forms: progressive atrophic rhinitis (PAR) and non-progressive atrophic rhinitis (AR).

Progressive atrophic rhinitis
Definition/aetiology

PAR is a severe and irreversible form of turbinate atrophy associated with toxigenic strains of *Pasteurella multocida*, either alone or in combination with *Bordetella bronchiseptica*. The most frequent capsular subtype of *P. multocida* causing PAR is type D.

Although PAR is fairly well controlled by means of vaccination, when the condition is new or is out of control on a farm, its negative impact on growth and feed efficiency represents a devastating disease.

P. multocida is passed from the sow to her offspring within the first week of life. If the pig is affected after 9 weeks of age, no clinical signs are exhibited as the nose has already developed.

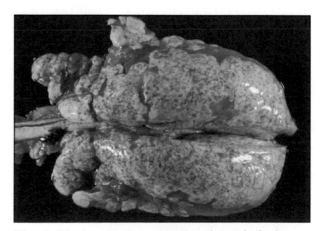

Fig. 3.58 *Ascaris suum* **migration through the lung indicated by the haemorrhages.**

Clinical presentation

Sneezing in baby pigs or epistaxis is often the first clinical sign that the farm is starting an outbreak of PAR (**Figures 3.59, 3.60**).

At a population level, the animals may continue sneezing, snuffling and snorting at almost any age, sometimes with a mucopurulent nasal and ocular discharge. Often, there is a bloody nasal discharge in the early stages of the condition.

The most characteristic finding is deformation of the snout (superior brachygnathia), with lateral

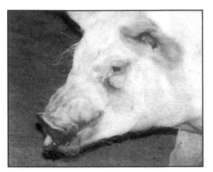

Fig. 3.59

Epistaxis in a weaned pig.

deviation if nasal septum deviation also occurs (**Figures 3.61–3.63**). The prevalence of this deformity varies among herds, as does the degree of growth retardation and reduction of feed efficiency.

Tear staining caused by the occlusion of the nasolacrimal duct occurs almost always. However, this is not pathognonomic as pigs will have excessive lacrimation under other stressful conditions (**Figure 3.64**). Tear staining may be used as an indicator of stress in pigs.

Reoccurrence, failure of vaccination or even severe clinical signs in previously normal herds may occur when the unit is severely stressed by viruses such as PRRSV, PCV2 or SIV.

Differential diagnosis

Sneezing in pigs can be also caused by porcine cytomegalovirus (inclusion body rhinitis) and *B. bronchiseptica* infections. Superior brachygnathia is typical of certain pig breeds and should not be confused with PAR. Environmental contaminants such as ammonia, dust, pollen and irritants should be ruled out. Physical

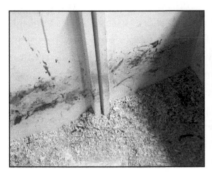

Fig. 3.60 Blood on the walls should alert the farm team to the possibility of a breakdown in health associated with PAR.

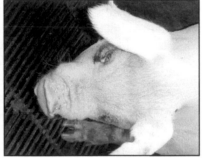

Fig. 3.61 Deformation of the snout with lateral deviation in a pig severely affected by PAR. Tear staining at the medial canthus of the eye is noted.

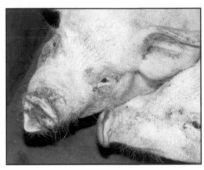

Fig. 3.62 Shortening of the upper jaw (superior brachygnathia) is common.

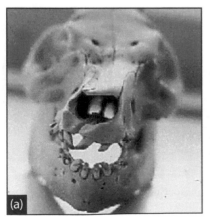

(a)

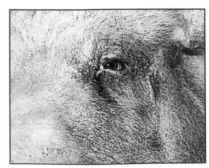

Fig. 3.63 (a, b) Deformation of the snout is part of a whole skull deformation.

(b)

Fig. 3.64 Lacrimal staining is not always associated with PAR.

changes may occur because of genetics or environmental challenges such a feeder or drinker design.

Lacrimal staining/conjunctivitis may be seen in a number of condition including PRRS. There may be congenital deformities of the face resulting in poor lacrimal duct placement.

Diagnosis

A definitive diagnosis depends on clinical and pathological findings as well as demonstration of toxigenic *P. multocida* in the nasal cavity (nasal swabs). The pathological lesions can be scored from zero to 5 with or without nasal septum deviation.

A snout scoring scheme where there is progressive reduction of the nasal turbinates is shown (**Figure 3.65**).

A herd's status can be determined by detection of the toxigenic *P. multocida* in nasal and/or throat swabs;

test pigs at 4, 8 and 12 weeks of age. ELISA tests to detect antibodies against the dermonecrotoxin in serum (if not vaccinated), and isolation of the bacterium from nasal swabs and performance of a subsequent PCR to detect the toxin gene, are the most commonly used diagnostic laboratory techniques.

Management

Treatment of individuals:

* Reduce the prevalence and load of *P. multocida* in young pigs by means of sow vaccination or in-feed medication (tetracycline or florfenicol), and antimicrobial treatment of piglets (tulathromycin).
* Treat growing pigs showing clinical signs symptomatically. Note that the lesions will not 'heal' but the impact of the secondary infections can be reduced.

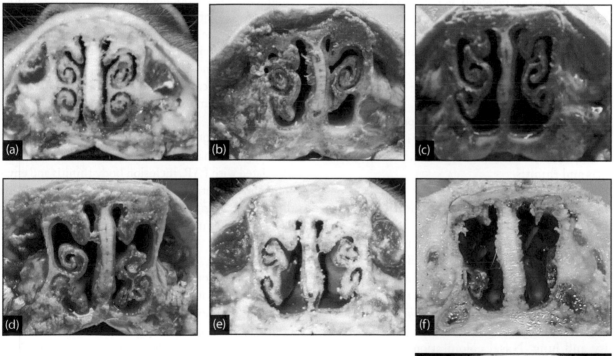

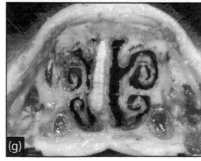

Fig. 3.65 Gross pathology of a cross-section of the nasal passages at the level of premolar 1. (a) Score 0; (b) score 1; (c) score 2; (d) score 3; (e) score 4; (f) score 5; (g) atrophy of nasal turbinates (score 1) and deviation of the nasal septum in a pig affected by PAR.

- Modify housing, ventilation and management to improve the environment. Putting the pigs onto liquid feeding will mitigate almost all the clinical effects of PAR.

Control:
- Vaccination of the sow, especially the pregnant parity 1 (P1) sow, will provide colostrum protection to the piglets.
- Ensure that colostrum intake is maximised. Develop a formal pig flow model to achieve AIAO.

Elimination:
- Depopulation and restocking from a herd known to be free of PAR is the only possible option. Clean, disinfect and fumigate all buildings and leave for 8 weeks. Eliminate mice and rats.
- The pathogens may rarely be transmissible over 1,000 metres, probably due to fomite transfer.
- It is possible to save genetic material by a segregated early weaning programme to set up a new unit followed by depopulation and restocking of the old unit.

Zoonotic implications

It is possible that humans may become infected with toxigenic *P. multocida* and this may result in a variety of upper respiratory tract diseases, including tonsillitis and rhinitis.

Non-progressive atrophic rhinitis
Definition/aetiology

Bordetella bronchiseptica is the primary aetiological agent of non-progressive AR (mild and reversible atrophy of nasal turbinates) and suppurative bronchopneumonia. One of its toxins, the dermonecrotoxin (different from that of *P. multocida*), plays a key role in inducing lesions in both the nasal cavity and lung. Nasal colonisation by *B. bronchiseptica* also promotes colonisation of toxigenic strains of *P. multocida*, leading to PAR. Non-progressive AR is not considered a significant economic problem. There may also be genetic and physical reasons for non-progressive AR. Modification of the shape of the head and nose may also occur because of difficulties with the drinker or feeder (**Figure 3.66**).

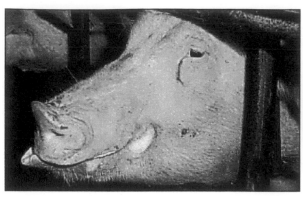

Fig. 3.66 Acquired AR and deviation of the snout associated with a misplacement of a nipple drinker.

Clinical presentation

Sneezing, nasal and ocular discharges and a non-productive cough with dyspnoea are the major clinical signs linked to non-progressive AR and suppurative bronchopneumonia, respectively. More severe forms of *B. bronchiseptica*-associated pneumonia occur in suckling piglets. Pneumonia can also occur secondarily to respiratory/systemic viral infections. In most of these cases, pigs are infected subclinically. Tear staining caused by the occlusion of the nasolacrimal duct also occurs frequently.

Differential diagnosis

Sneezing and nasal and ocular discharges are also associated with PAR, inclusion body rhinitis and environmental pollution. Suppurative bronchopneumonia differential diagnoses can be established with many bacteria, including *P. multocida*, *H. parasuis* and *S. suis*.

Diagnosis

Clinical conditions linked to *B. bronchiseptica* infection are diagnosed with a combination of clinical data and isolation/detection of the bacterium from the nasal cavity (nasal swabs) or lung (tissue or bronchial swab). However, detection of the pathogen in the nasal cavity might not be diagnostic in a number of cases due to its ubiquitous nature colonising the turbinates.

Management

Bordetella bronchiseptica is usually susceptible to tetracyclines and enrofloxacin, but resistant to ceftiofur. Antibiotics can ameliorate the pneumonic severity, but total clearance of the bacterium from the nasal cavity is almost impossible. Therefore, the major objective is to control disease when present but not to avoid colonisation. *B. bronchiseptica* is a ubiquitous organism and present on all pig farms.

Zoonotic implications
B. bronchiseptica is also a human pathogen.

Barbiturate overdose
It may be necessary to euthanase a pig with barbiturate via an intracardiac injection.. The heart muscle may demonstrate crystals associated with the extra-vascular barbiturate (**Figure 3.67**). These will be dissolved in the preparation of histological sections.

Cardiac failure
The clinician is often faced with the problem of a dead pig with no obvious gross pathology. The time from death to post-mortem examination may be too long or it may not be economically feasible to carry out histological examination to assist the clinician make a diagnosis. If there is no gross pathology evident, this needs to be reported. However, if the heart is empty of blood, it may be that cardiac failure occurred (**Figure 3.68**). This is often associated with bullying and excessive stress on the pig. Puberty is a major stress time in many animal's lives and pigs are no different.

Chlamydiosis
Several *Chlamydia* spp. can affect pigs, namely *Chlamydophila abortus*, *C. pecorum*, *C. psittaci* and *Chlamydia suis*. The first three infect multiple species while the pig is the natural host for the latter. The most important *Chlamydia* species causing respiratory problems in swine are *C. psittaci* and *C. suis*. However, the organisms are ubiquitous, complicating a possible role of *Chlamydia* in any clinical problem.

Chlamydial respiratory disease in pigs includes conjunctivitis and dyspnoea. Since it causes a systemic infection, fever and inappetence are usual; diarrhea and neurological clinical signs are sporadically observed. At necropsy, lesions compatible with bronchointerstitial pneumonia are seen. Pleuritis has been described from clinical cases.

Several antimicrobials are active against chlamydial organisms, but the most used ones are tetracyclines.

Conjunctivitis
Definition/aetiology
Conjunctivitis of grow/finish pigs can be very common on farms. There is no specific infectious agent. A combination of *B. bronchiseptica* and *C. psittaci* and an interaction with environmental factors such as high ammonia concentrations (>15 ppm).

Clinical signs
The pigs present with sneezing and runny eyes in late lactation and in the nursery. This progresses to a moderate to severe conjunctivitis, which may interfere with vision. The conjunctiva of both eyes become injected and inflamed (**Figures 3.69, 3.70**). In severe cases the

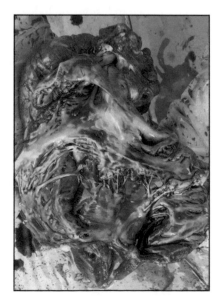

Fig. 3.68 All the chambers of the heart are empty of blood, which may be associated with cardiac failure.

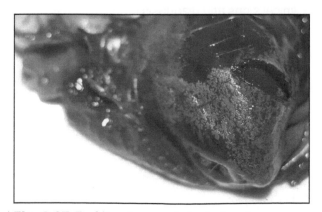

Fig. 3.67 Barbiturate crystals in the heart.

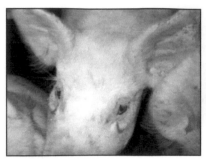

Fig. 3.69 Growing pigs with conjunctivitis.

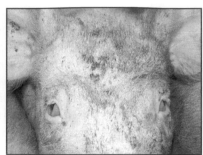

Fig. 3.70 Both eyes are equally affected with conjunctivitis.

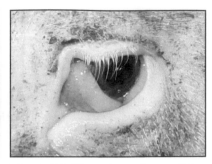

Fig. 3.71 Note the prolapse of the third eyelid.

third eyelid prolapses (**Figure 3.71**). Once prolapsed, the condition seems to become established and may be difficult to resolve. The problem may persist into adult life.

When walking the pens the clinician may see individuals affected; the pigs otherwise do not seem affected by the condition, but on some farms all pigs in the pen are affected.

Differential diagnosis

The major differential diagnoses are AR and swine influenza (SI). Conjunctivitis may be commonly seen in nursery cases of PRRS.

Diagnosis

Clinical signs are very characteristic. *Chlamydia* may be suspected as a secondary invader of a swollen exposed conjunctiva.

Post-mortem lesions include severe conjunctivitis with prolapse of the third eyelid, but the sclera and cornea are unaffected. As the condition progresses there may be tear staining on the face. Young pigs may present with a moderate to severe purulent/fibronecrotic rhinitis.

Management

Treatment: On farms with PAR, review the vaccine programme. On negative farms, test and eliminate toxigenic *P. multocida* as a problem. Minimise the clinical effects of PRRSV, but note the condition occurs on PRRSV-negative units.

Antimicrobial treatment appears to have little effect; indeed, an overuse of antimicrobials may be part of the problem by encouraging *Chlamydia*. Provide pain management.

Control: Review environmental management of the farm buildings. For example:

- Avoid chilling and draughts.
- Reduce ammonia concentrations in the air.
- Reduce dust levels in the grow/finish house – cover feeders, consider wet feeding.

Endocarditis
Definition/aetiology

Vegetative valvular endocarditis lesions develop on the endocardial valves, in particular the mitral valve. These lesions result in impaired cardiac function and can act as a nidus for further bacterial seeding from these damaged valves. Many organisms can be associated with endocarditis. The most common are *S. suis*, *Erysipelothrix rhusiopathiae* and *Staphylococcus* spp. The problem is seen in the late nursery to finishing pig and is often an end stage of nursery respiratory and polyserositis issues.

Clinical signs and diagnosis

The pig presents in distress with dyspnoea and its ears and tail are often cyanotic (**Figure 3.72**). The feet may be cold from the poor blood circulation. At post-mortem examination there will be signs of heart failure with possible ascites, pericarditis and pulmonary oedema. Examination of the heart reveals the endocardial lesions (**Figures 3.73–3.75**).

Management

There are few treatment options available. Euthanasia should be considered.

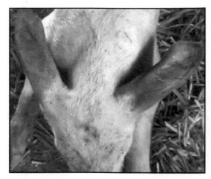

Fig. 3.72 Cyanotic ears of a pig with endocarditis.

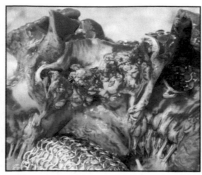

Fig. 3.73 Vegetative valvular endocarditis.

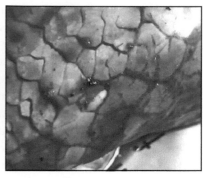

Fig. 3.74 Pulmonary oedema in a pig with endocarditis.

Fig. 3.75 Infarct in the epicardium from an endocarditis lesion.

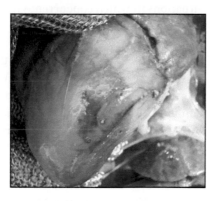

Control:

- Practice clean piglet processing protocols.
- The control of nursery respiratory and polyserositis issues need to be addressed.
- Avoid damaged floors, which can injure feet and allow the introduction of bacteria via the damaged coronary band.
- Ensure erysipelas vaccination is current for adults.

Enzootic (mycoplasma) pneumonia ▶ VIDEO 13 ▶ AUDIO 10

Definition/aetiology

The uncomplicated infection with *Mycoplasma hyopneumoniae* is known as mycoplasmosis and is characterised by development of a bronchointerstitial pneumonia. However, under field conditions, concurrent bacterial infections occur leading to a final result of suppurative bronchopneumonia, referred to as enzootic pneumonia (EP) in Europe and as mycoplasma pneumonia in North America. Moreover, this bacterium is considered to be one of the key pathogens in the context of another clinical syndrome, PRDC. Many of these different definitions of pneumonic conditions in finishing pigs around 16–24 weeks of age are merely semantics.

M. hyopneumoniae is widespread globally and considered a major source of economic losses due to respiratory disease and poor growth. The bacteria can spread over medium distances and a farm needs to be at least 3 km from a positive pig enterprise to remain negative in the long term. Pathogen aerosol spread can be affected by numerous other features: population size, wind direction and general weather conditions. Note that most pathogens are not spread by aerosol. There is no transmission of *M. hyopneumoniae* via semen.

Mycoplasma bacteria do not have a cell wall. They are very small and the lack of a cell wall renders all mycoplasmas resistant to the beta-lactam antimicrobials.

M. hyopneumoniae is a fastidious microorganism and may be difficult to grow in culture. Culture of *M. hyopneumoniae* is complicated by the natural presence of other mycoplasma organisms in the nasopharynx and mucociliary escalator. These would include *M. hyorhinis*, *M. flocculare*, *M. hyopharyngis* and a number of other mycoplasmas including many that are yet to be identified.

Pathogenesis of enzootic pneumonia

M. hyopneumoniae is spread by nose-to-nose transmission and the infection is generally spread from the sow to her offspring at around 14 days of age. The infected piglets then slowly infect a larger number of pigs in the nursery. The number of piglets infected at weaning is a good indication of a future problem in the finishing herd. Note that the piglets will not present with clinical or gross pathological signs.

M. hyopneumoniae bacteria then bind and colonise the cilia of the epithelial cells of the nose, trachea, bronchi and bronchioles. The adherence to and colonisation of the cilia reduces the efficiency of clearance offered by the mucociliary escalator. As a result of this, a descending infection can occur from 'pathogens' in the nasopharynx microflora. The pattern of pathology of the lung is then determined by the descending infection. The anatomy of the porcine lung and the right apical bronchi is therefore important. The right apical lobe is closest to the nasopharynx and it is generally the first lobe to demonstrate gross pathological changes of atelectasis. The actions of *M. hyopneumoniae* also reduce the effectiveness of macrophages recruited to help control the infection.

Clinical presentation

Enzootic (mycoplasma) pneumonia is clinically characterised by a high morbidity and low mortality. Pigs of all ages are susceptible to *M. hyopneumoniae* infection, but EP is usually not observed in animals younger than 6 weeks of age (25 kg liveweight) due to protection by maternally derived immunity. The major prevalence of EP occurs from mid-finishing to market weight with the classic 18-week wall (60–80 kg liveweight), and major clinical signs become evident in this period.

The severity of clinical signs depends on the presence of secondary infections (bacterial, viral and parasitic), infection pressure, environmental conditions and possibly the strain involved in the outbreak (**Figures 3.76, 3.77**). When *M. hyopneumoniae*

infection is not complicated with concurrent pathogens (mycoplasmosis scenario) the disease follows a subclinical course with mild clinical signs consisting of chronic, non-productive cough and reduced average daily weight gain (ADG) and feed efficiency. These lesions are associated with hyperplasia of peribronchiolar lymphoid tissue and are most often seen in outdoor herds.

When concurrent infection with other bacterial pathogens occurs, clinical signs such as a productive cough, laboured breathing, fever and even death may be seen. These clinical signs can become worse in situations in which concurrent viral infections occur together with *M. hyopneumoniae*.

The pattern of mortality in EP-positive and EP-negative herds is shown in **Figures 3.78, 3.79**.

If a naïve herd breaks with *M. hyopneumoniae*, clinical signs will be seen in all age groups including adults. In adults, pregnant sows may abort and even die while boars may become transiently (6 weeks) infertile following the pyrexia.

Differential diagnosis

Enzoonotic (mycoplasma) pneumonia can be clinically confused with swine influenza (SI). Importantly, dyspnoea due to pulmonary cranioventral consolidation can be caused by a number of bacteria (*B. bronchiseptica*, *P. multocida*, *H. parasuis*, *A. suis* and *S. suis*). These are particularly important in the nursery, where EP is uncommon. Finishing pneumonic scenarios (PRDC) can also occur without the presence of *M. hyopneumoniae*, but it is important to rule out its presence.

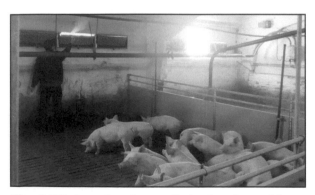

Fig. 3.76 **Assessing the ventilation in a farm with active EP.**

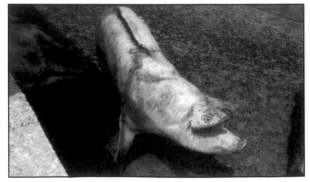

Fig. 3.77 **Introduced gilt recently infected by** *M. hyopneumoniae*. **The pig was coughing.**

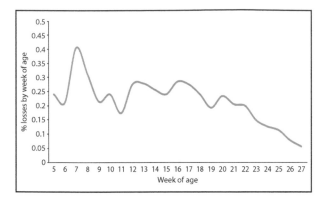

Fig. 3.78 Finishing mortality in a *M. hyopneumoniae*-negative herd.

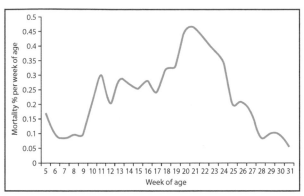

Fig. 3.79 Finishing mortality in a vaccinated *M. hyopneumoniae*-positive herd. Note the '18-week wall'.

Environmental factors such as poor water availability and high ammonia concentrations (>15 ppm) may mimic the actions of *M. hyopneumoniae*.

Inhalation pneumonia will look like EP at gross pathology and can lead to a misdiagnosis even in the farrowing house.

Individual pigs can cough for a wide variety of reasons (e.g. dusty feed).

Diagnosis

Strong suspicion of *M. hyopneumoniae* infection is justified when a persistent non-productive cough in the grow/finish area is evident. The final diagnosis is established by means of detection of *M. hyopneumoniae* (usually by ELISA and confirmed by PCR). Confirmation by culture is difficult since it is a fastidious microorganism to grow.

In EP-negative farms, the infection should be monitored through ELISA tests, measuring serum antibodies against *M. hyopneumoniae* in the finishing pig.

Post-mortem examination reveals the characteristic cranioventral lung consolidation. The severity of lung lesions at slaughter has been linked with the prevalence of *M. hyopneumoniae* colonisation at weaning. The consolidation of the lungs reduces their capacity and can be demonstrated to the farm health team by the fact that affected lung tissue does not float in water (**Figures 3.80–3.84**).

Pulmonary screening at the abattoir is a useful diagnostic aid that allows correlating the existence of cough at the herd level with the percentage and extent of cranioventral lung consolidation (**Figure 3.85**). However, acute cases may present with very severe consolidation. The lesions in the slaughterhouse are

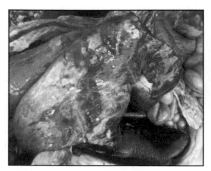

Fig. 3.80 Pulmonary cranioventral consolidation affecting multifocally the apical and middle lobes in a case of EP. Note the concurrent pleuritis.

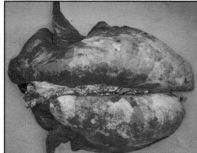

Fig. 3.81 EP of the cranioventral portion of a finishing pig lung.

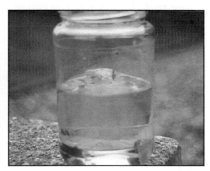

Fig. 3.82 Inflated lung floats on water whereas consolidated lung (hepatinisation) sinks.

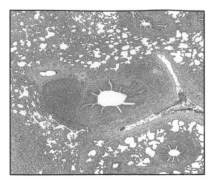

Fig. 3.83 Histological examination of the lung indicates a cuffing bronchopneumonia.

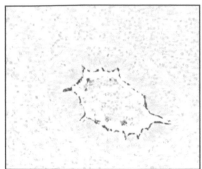

Fig. 3.84 Immunohistochemistry revealing the presence of *M. hyopneumoniae* (brown positive stain) on the surface of the bronchi.

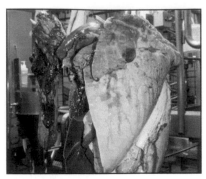

Fig. 3.85 Slaughterhouse examination revealing the degree of enzootic pneumonia in a herd.

only indicative of the stage of the infection at the point of death and may have only been present for a very short period of time. Ensure that the lungs examined belong to your client's pigs.

Lung scoring systems

A variety of scoring systems can be used.

A simple recording system that can easily be used in the slaughterhouse is based on a visual scoring system recording the amount of consolidation out of a maximum score of 55. To score, estimate the percentage of the area affected by consolidation and assign a score. Therefore, if 50% of the right apical lobe is consolidated, this scores 5. The apical and cardiac lobe degree of compromise areas score up to 10, the top of the diaphragmatic lobe scores up to 5 and the intermediate lobe scores up to 5 (**Figure 3.86**). Note that there are many different scoring systems all with a similar preconception.

The approximate relationship between lung damage/scoring system at slaughter at 100 kg and daily liveweight gain and food conversion ratio (FCR) is shown in *Table 3.8*.

Treatment

Strategic medication with antimicrobials active against *M. hyopneumoniae* and other concurrent bacteria may be useful during periods when the pigs are at risk for overt respiratory disease. Note that any bacteriology carried out with a subsequent antibiogram is going to examine the secondary infections (e.g. *P. multocida* or *S. suis*) not the primary cause. Pain relief is an essential part of the treatment programme.

Control

Vaccination: The main effects of vaccination include reduced clinical signs, lung lesions and medication use, as well as improved performance including ADG and FCR. However, bacterins provide only partial protection and do not prevent colonisation by the organism. The efficiency of the *M. hyopneumoniae* vaccines in controlling EP is high (**Figures 3.87, 3.88**). Using the above vaccination system reduces the score from 25 to 5.

Vaccination schedules (timing of vaccination, vaccination of sows, vaccination combined with antimicrobial medication) depend on the type of herd, the

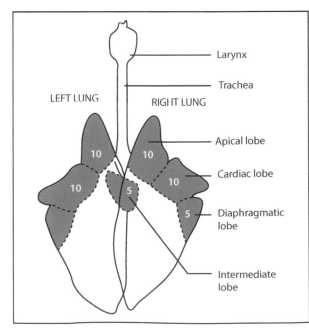

Fig. 3.86 A post-mortem lung scoring system to compare EP severity between pigs.

Table 3.8 **Approximate relationship between lung damage/scoring system at slaughter at 100 kg and daily liveweight gain and food conversion ratio.**

LUNG LESION	DLW REDUCTION		FCR INCREASE	
	%	G/DAY (APPROX)	%	VALUE
0/55 Negative	0	0	0	0
2/55 Mild	4	25	0	0
10/55 Mild	7	50	5	0.15
15/55 Moderate	11	75	8	0.25
20/55 Moderate	15	100	11	0.35
30/55 Severe	20	125	14	0.40
55/55 Severe	22	550	17	0.50

DLW, daily liveweight gain; FCR, food conversion ratio.

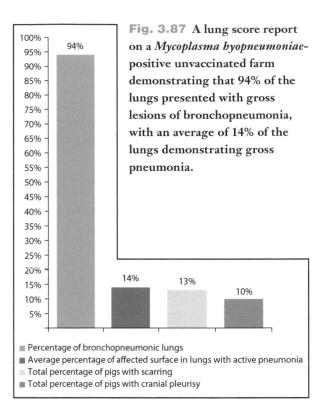

Fig. 3.87 A lung score report on a *Mycoplasma hyopneumoniae*-positive unvaccinated farm demonstrating that 94% of the lungs presented with gross lesions of bronchopneumonia, with an average of 14% of the lungs demonstrating gross pneumonia.

■ Percentage of bronchopneumonic lungs
■ Average percentage of affected surface in lungs with active pneumonia
■ Total percentage of pigs with scarring
■ Total percentage of pigs with cranial pleurisy

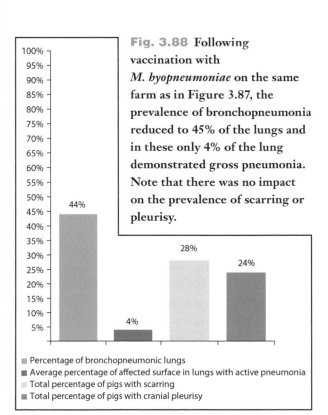

Fig. 3.88 Following vaccination with *M. hyopneumoniae* on the same farm as in Figure 3.87, the prevalence of bronchopneumonia reduced to 45% of the lungs and in these only 4% of the lung demonstrated gross pneumonia. Note that there was no impact on the prevalence of scarring or pleurisy.

■ Percentage of bronchopneumonic lungs
■ Average percentage of affected surface in lungs with active pneumonia
■ Total percentage of pigs with scarring
■ Total percentage of pigs with cranial pleurisy

production system and management practices, the infection pattern and the preferences of the pig producer. In general, piglets should be vaccinated at or around weaning.

It is advisable to vaccinate gilts during their introduction programme, especially if the gilts come from *M. hyopneumoniae*-negative multiplication farms.

Management

Management practices and housing conditions in the herd should be optimised, including batching and AIAO production:

- Avoid destabilising herd immunity by sudden changes in parity structure (the introduction of a large number of gilts for example).
- Provide pigs with the appropriate stocking densities – avoid overstocking.
- Prevent other respiratory diseases.
- Provide optimal housing and climatic conditions.

Eradication

Eradication of *M. hyopneumoniae* can be achieve through a variety of methods, based on vaccination of the adults, age segregation and medication, but the risk of reinfection is relatively high, so biosecurity measures must be in place. Depopulation and repopulation with negative gilts is the popular method of elimination.

The farm must be at least 3 km from potential sources to have a reasonable chance of staying negative for 18 months or more.

Glasser's disease (polyserositis in general) ▶ VIDEOS 16–18 and 36
Definition/aetiology

Fibrinous polyserositis of pigs is a condition that normally occurs in nursery pigs but can affect any age group. When polyserositis is observed, this lesion evokes a suspicion of Glässer's disease in the first instance, but not exclusively. If laboratory analysis is carried out and *Haemophilus parasuis* isolated, the veterinary surgeon will have confirmation of Glässer's disease. If, however, another pathogen is isolated, then a diagnosis of polyserositis caused by *S. suis*, *M. hyorhinis* or other agents is reached.

There are at least 15 serotypes of *H. parasuis*; many are non-virulent and the serotypes have little immunological similarity. However, one common virulence factor that may be recognised is virulence-associated trimeric autotransporter.

The clinical entity is influenced by the concurrent presence of other pathogens, notably PRRSV, PCV2 and SIV in the grow/finish herd. Mismanagement of the environment of the pig also increases the prevalence of the clinical signs in a group of pigs.

Clinical presentation

Nearly all herds are positive to some of the strains of *H. parasuis*.

Naïve herds - peracute: It is extremely rare to find a naïve herd. However, a herd or group of pigs (often newly introduced gilts or boars) may have different strains of *H. parasuis* and be naïve to the native strains.

Within 48 hours, the adults demonstrate severe pneumonia, depression, anorexia and pyrexia of 42°C. Terminally, the animal demonstrates incoordination, prostration and meningitis and dies. Death can occur very quickly after arrival without any preceding clinical signs.

Normal herds:
Subclinical: Most pigs present with no clinical signs of infection with the causal agents.

Peracute: Quite often the animal presents only as a sudden death. Eventually, petechial haemorrhages in the kidney may be seen.

Acute: The pig may, however, display depression, anorexia and with the rectal temperature rising to 40.5°C. The clinical signs are complex and determined by which serosal membrane is affected. The animal may appear as if walking is painful. If pericarditis becomes prominent, cyanosis may appear on the extremities and the pig is ear bitten. Terminally, meningitis may be evident.

Chronic: If the pig survives, it will waste and become hairy (**Figures 3.89, 3.90**). Loss of part of the ear associated with failure of the circulation supply to the ears (**Figure 3.91**).

In the grower pig herd, otherwise normal pigs may present with sudden death. At post-mortem

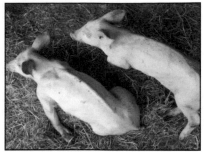

Fig. 3.89 Wasting in nursery pigs.

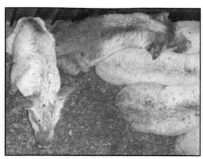

Fig. 3.90 Hairy poor weaners.

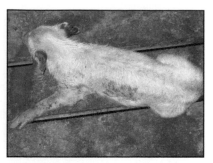

Fig. 3.91 Glässer's disease with septic pericarditis resulting in gangrene of the ear tips.

examination the pig presents with a well-organised polyserositis. This is most common when the farm is also affected by another condition, such as SI. The SI relevance is then missed or undervalued as the clinical examination is focused on the more dramatic pathology of the polyserositis.

Differential diagnosis

Actinobacillus pleuropneumoniae results in pleuritis, sometimes with a concurrent pericarditis, and this can resemble Glässer's disease, but the age group affected is normally older; moreover, this bacterium causes severe pleuropneumonia, which is not a feature of Glässer's disease. Vitamin E deficiency (mulberry heart disease) can also create a similar clinical picture in sudden death pigs. Other causes of polyserositis - *S. suis* and *M. hyorhinitis*.

Diagnosis

In peracute cases there may be no gross pathology, but on histological examination an acute meningitis is seen. If the pig has survived for a couple of days

at least, there will be a severe fibrinous pleuritis. In clinically sick pigs on a normal farm, diagnosis can be made from clinical and post-mortem signs.

Culture of *H. parasuis* is difficult compared with other organisms; in particular, *S. suis* may outgrow *H. parasuis*. Its isolation requires special media. The presence of antibiotics in the pig makes isolation of *H. parasuis* additionally difficult. *Mycoplasma hyorhinis* culture should be encouraged.

PCR for *H. parasuis* is available but may not differentiate pathogenic strains and as almost all pigs are positive anyway, a positive result may not be informative.

Post-mortem lesions: The organism may infect all serosal membranes and produces a polyserositis. The clinical signs are dependent on which serosal membrane is affected; for example: (**Figures 3.92–3.101**):

* **Heart.** The disease causes pericarditis with both tags and fluid around the heart (**Figures 3.92, 3.93**).

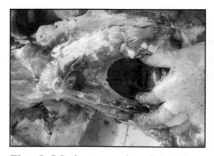

Fig. 3.92 Acute pericarditis. Note the pericardial fluid revealed on opening the chest.

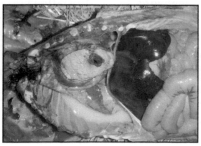

Fig. 3.93 Chronic pericarditis.

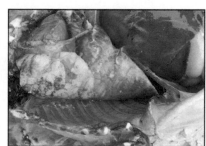

Fig. 3.94 Pneumonia and pleuritis.

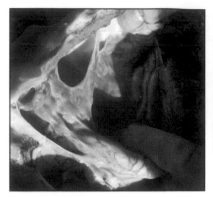

Fig. 3.95 Pleuritis.

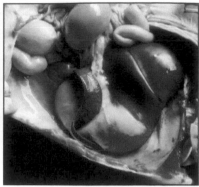

Fig. 3.96 Ascites.

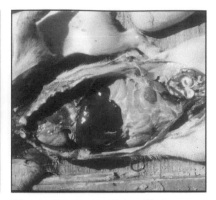

Fig. 3.97 Peritonitis – fibrinous.

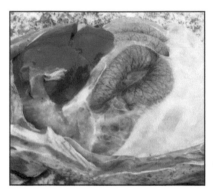

Fig. 3.98 Polyserositis – peritonitis.

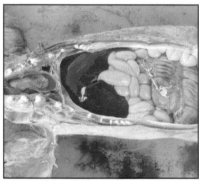

Fig. 3.99 Polyserositis in a growing pig with swine influenza.

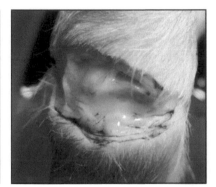

Fig. 3.100 Polyserositis – synovitis.

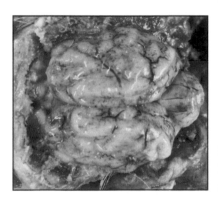

Fig. 3.101 Polyserositis – meningitis.

- **Joints.** When the joints become infected, synovitis and arthritis with swollen joints are seen (**Figure 3.100**).
- **Brain.** The meninges may become infected, resulting in meningitis (**Figure 3.101**).

Management

Treatment of individuals: Antimicrobial agents, in particular penicillin or amoxycillin, delivered initially via the water supply. However, death can be very rapid and occur before treatment can be initiated. Provide pain management in individual cases. Note that in cases of polyserositis associated with *M. hyorhinis*, fluorfenicol and tulathromycin may be useful in mixed infections.

Control: Since the introduction of PRRSV, Glässer's disease has become more common and the clinical signs are severe. Vitamin E deficiency is often associated with expression of clinical signs. Environmental stress can play a role, characterised by

- **Lungs.** The disease creates extensive pleuritis. As pleuritis can take 6 months or more to resolve, at slaughter pleuritis tags can still be present (**Figures 3.94, 3.95**).
- **Intestines.** The bacterium infects the abdominal cavity, resulting in peritonitis. Chronic peritonitis results in adhesions between intestinal loops and peritoneum (**Figures 3.96, 3.97, 3.98, 3.99**).

draughts, chilling and a damp environment. In particular, if the nursery environment is inadequate at entry, this places great stress on the newly weaned piglet as will variation in diurnal temperatures or poor adherence to cooling curves. It is essential that all rooms are suitable for the animals before arrival. This is an important area that the veterinary surgeon can audit. Monitor the number of gilts in a breeding batch and ideally keep to below 20% of the batch. Ensure that farm immunity is stable with good gilt introduction routines. Control can be difficult, but the clinician must recognise all of these factors:

- Ensure PRRSV is controlled.
- Ensure PCV2 is controlled.
- Vitamin E concentrations are recommended to be 125–200 ppm in nursery feed.
- Ensure that the farm is practicing batching and AIAO with the room cleaned, dried and well maintained between batches.
- Good gilt introduction routines to reduce PRRS and SI flare ups

Vaccination: Vaccination is possible. Currently, autogenous vaccines are often more effective owing to the large number of serotypes and little heterologous protection between the different serotypes. Note that a farm can be infected with multiple serotypes. If the problems start early in the nursery, vaccination of the sows pre-farrowing to boost piglet colostral protection may be beneficial. Vaccination of the weaned pig may help in cases later in the nursery or growing herd.

Inclusion body rhinitis

Porcine cytomegalovirus (PCMV) is a herpesvirus affecting swine that causes mostly subclinical infections. It is a DNA enveloped virus. However, in a proportion of cases this virus can cause reproductive problems (infertility and embryonic, fetal and neonatal mortality) as well as respiratory disease. The clinical respiratory form of PCMV infection is known as inclusion body rhinitis. The name comes from the characteristic histological lesions in different tissues, but mainly the nasal cavity. The virus is considered of ubiquitous distribution all over the world.

PCMV is a systemic infecting virus and, therefore, can be found in different tissues. However, because of its tropism for epithelial cells, the recommended post-mortem samples for histopathological analysis are nasal turbinates (**Figure 3.102**), lungs and kidneys. The typical microscopic observation of basophilic intranuclear inclusion bodies, cytomegaly and karyomegaly allows a definitive diagnosis of PCMV infection.

Lung worms
Definition/aetiology

Several species of *Metastrongylus* spp. can infect the pig. *M. apri* is the most common, but *M. pudendotectus* and *M. salmi* can also be found with some frequency. It is common in outdoor pigs and wild boar but infestation in intensively reared pigs is rare.

Clinical presentation

In most cases, the infestation is subclinical and only in heavy infestations are there clinical signs such as dyspnoea and a cough.

Fig. 3.102 Submucosal gland of a nasal turbinate of a pig with inclusion body rhinitis. The left gland shows bigger cells (cytomegaly) and nuclei (karyomegaly), as well as basophilic intranuclear inclusion bodies (arrows) caused by PCMV infection. HE stain.

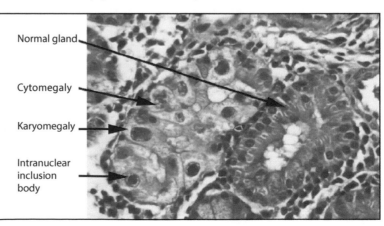

Normal gland

Cytomegaly

Karyomegaly

Intranuclear inclusion body

Differential diagnosis

Clinical signs are rather non-specific, therefore a large number of possibilities should be considered. From a lesion point of view, *Metastrongylus* spp. cause a bronchointerstitial pneumonia but its distribution tends to be dorsocaudal in the lungs, which is different from other causes of this pneumonia type in pigs.

Diagnosis

Detection of adult worms of 3–5 cm in length in the lumen of bronchi located mainly in the diaphragmatic lobes constitutes a definitive diagnosis. Microscopically, there is hypertrophy of bronchial muscle and epithelial hyperplasia as well as nodular lymphoid hyperplasia. Surrounding alveoli display granulomatous inflammation due to the presence of worm eggs (**Figure 3.103**). Although not very sensitive, egg flotation techniques of faecal material can be used to establish the diagnosis.

Management

Numerous commercial dewormers based on benzimidazoles, levamisole and lactones are very effective against adult parasites. Lactones are also effective against migrating larvae. There are no vaccines against *Metastrongylus* spp.

Mulberry heart disease
Definition/aetiology

Sudden death in the nursery, often of the biggest pig in the group. The problem is associated with vitamin E/selenium deficiency resulting in heart failure. The problem can be more common in start-up units where the pigs are growing very fast.

Clinical presentation

There are no or few clinical signs prior to death; the best pig in the group is found suddenly dead. The problem occurs in pigs about 15–30 kg bodyweight.

Differential diagnosis

Review other causes of sudden death in nursery pigs such as porcine pleuropneumonia, oedema disease and streptococcal septicaemia.

Diagnosis

Diagnosis can be difficult and is based on the clinical signs.

Post-mortem examination reveals large amounts of fluid around the heart and lung and fluid in the abdomen with filaments of fibrin. Examination of the epicardium reveals haemorrhage and pale areas in the heart muscle. The liver may be enlarged and mottled with areas of haemorrhage and possible rupture (**Figure 3.104**), called hepatosis dietetica. With rupture of the liver, there will be blood in the abdominal cavity. There may be pale muscle areas in the leg and back muscles.

Histological examination of the liver, heart or damaged muscle may be highly suggestive. With a vitamin E deficiency it is possible piglets will die from an oxidative crisis following the iron injection on day 4.

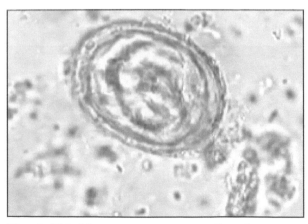

Fig. 3.103 *Metastrongylus* spp. egg. Note the embryonic larvae.

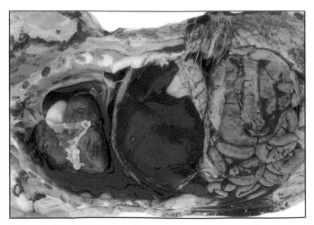

Fig. 3.104 Mulberry heart with a ruptured liver. The abdomen was full of blood.

Management

Treatment of affected group: Injection of 70 IU vitamin E. While vitamin E is a fat soluble vitamin, water soluble preparations are available. It may also need supplemental selenium, but note that selenium can be very toxic.

Control: Review vitamin E concentrations in the feed and increase to 250 g/tonne (ppm) if low. Check the nursery environment and address stress factors. Examine for Glässer's disease. Review feed storage as vitamin E is destroyed by high moisture and mycotoxins and this can result in a temporary acute shortage of vitamin E.

Review the genetics of the breeding stock source. Some lines of pigs have a greater demand for vitamin E, especially fast growing pigs. Note that start-up units can have a particularly high demand as the pigs are generally very healthy and the unit is clean and well prepared for the pigs, so growth rates can be spectacular.

Pasteurellosis ▶ VIDEO 18 ▶ AUDIO 10
Definition/aetiology

Pasteurella multocida is mainly considered a secondary pathogen, usually found in enzootic (mycoplasma) pneumonia as a concurrent infection. *P. multocida* is a gram-negative coccobacillus.

The most frequent capsular subtype of *P. multocida* causing pneumonia and/or pleuritis is subtype A. Very sporadically it has been linked with outbreaks of fatal and acute septicaemia. Toxigenic subtype D *P. multocida* is associated with PAR.

Clinical presentation

Clinical signs depend on the pathogens involved in the polymicrobial process where *P. multocida* is found. Coughing, intermittent fever, anorexia and thumping respiration are the most common signs associated with suppurative bronchopneumonia (**Figure 3.105**). In severe scenarios, cyanosis can be seen. These latter cases have been associated with strains able to produce abscesses and pleuritis.

Differential diagnosis

Pasteurellosis is usually involved in EP as a secondary agent and therefore other pathogens that are involved in EP should be included in the differential diagnosis (*B. bronchiseptica, H. parasuis, S. suis*).

In cases of pleuritic pasteurellosis, the major pathogen to rule out is *A. pleuropneumoniae*; however, with infections with *P. multocida* it is rare to have sudden death and the distribution of lesions is mainly cranioventral. Infection by *Trueperella pyogenes* can also cause lesions similar to those of pleuritic pasteurellosis.

Diagnosis

Since lung lesions caused by *P. multocida* are not specific to this bacterium, diagnosis must be established by clinical signs, presence of a suppurative bronchopneumonia and the corresponding bacterial isolation (lung tissue) (**Figures 3.106, 3.107**).

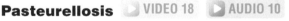

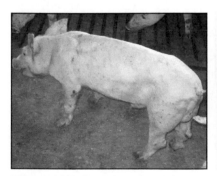

Fig. 3.105 Growing pig with pasteurellosis. Note the wide base stance of the front legs.

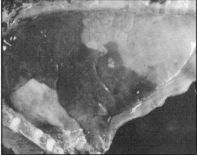

Fig. 3.106 Extensive pulmonary cranioventral consolidation (suppurative bronchopneumonia) due to a *P. multocida* infection. This pig was suffering from enzootic (mycoplasma) pneumonia.

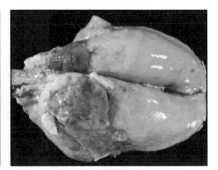

Fig. 3.107 Pulmonary cranioventral consolidation (suppurative bronchopneumonia) together with fibrinous pleuritis due to a *P. multocida* infection in a young pig.

Nasal swabs allow detection of *P. multocida* but, being a commensal infectious agent, its diagnostic significance is minimal.

Management

Treatment against *P. multocida* in well-established pneumonic lesions is difficult because of the difficulty ensuring proper antibiotic penetration in consolidated lung tissue. An antibiogram may be needed in some cases. Pain relief is an essential part of the treatment programme.

Control of primary pathogens within the EP complexes is the most effective measure to counteract the effects of *P. multocida*. No vaccination is carried out against this pathogen.

Pleuritis/pleurisy

Pleuritis is a common result of pathogens/foreign material gaining access to the pleural serosa. Organisms are moved to the pleural cavity as part of the respiratory systems defence mechanisms.

It is not possible to differentiate the cause of the pleuritis by gross examination of the carcase as the lesion is a healing scar tissue and generally sterile. Pleuritis can be present for several months before resolution, therefore pleuritis seen at the slaughterhouse may have occurred at any time in the previous 6 months (i.e. the entire life of the pig).

Slaughterhouse examination
See **Figures 3.108, 3.109**.

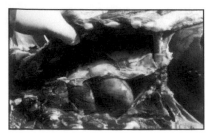
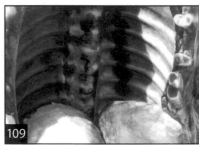

Figs. 3.108, 3.109 Pleuritis on the surface of the lung (3.108) or attached to the carcase rib cage (3.109).

Post-mortem findings associated with a variety of pleuritis causing pathogens
See **Figures 3.110–3.117**.

Pleuritis can also be associated with other pathogens (e.g. *Escherichia coli*) potentially introduced as a result of vices.

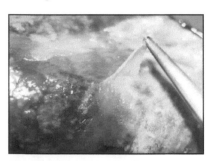

Fig. 3.110 *Actinobacillus pleuropneumoniae.*

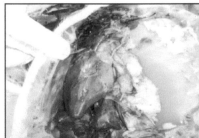

Fig. 3.111 *Streptococcus* spp.

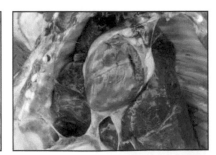

Fig. 3.112 *Haemophilus parasuis* – Glässer's disease.

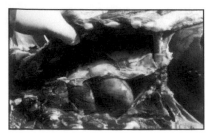

Fig. 3.113 *Mycoplasma hyorhinis.*

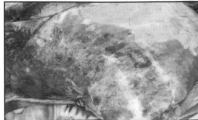

Fig. 3.114 *Actinobacillus suis.*

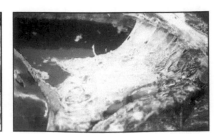

Fig. 3.115 *Trueperella pyogenes.*

Fig. 3.116
Septic pleuritis
(*Pseudomonas*)
from a puncture
wound.

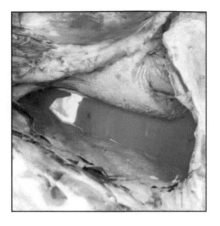

Fig. 3.117
Complicated
enzootic
pneumonia –
*Pasteurella
multocida.*

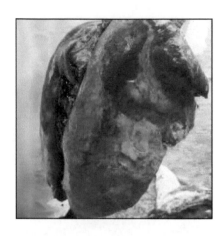

Causes
See **Figures 3.118–3.122**.

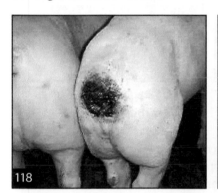

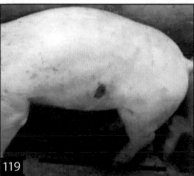

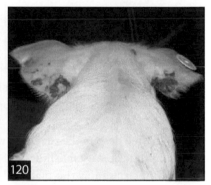

Figs. 3.118–3.120 Vices: (3.118) tail biting; (3.119) flank biting; (3.120) ear sucking.

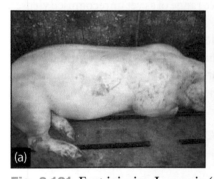

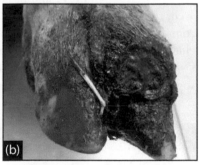

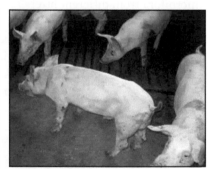

Fig. 3.121 Foot injuries. Lame pig (a), which on examination revealed severe ulceration of the foot (b).

Fig. 3.122 Respiratory infections.

Treatment and control
Review causes of vice and examine the flooring. Review post-weaning housing and stress factors, especially air quality and water supplies (**Figures 3.123–3.128**). Control Glässer's disease. Control clinical porcine pleuropneumonia – majority of farms are positive to at least one serotype of *A. pleuropneumoniae* but do not have any significant pleuritis issue. Pain relief is an essential part of the treatment programme.

Post-weaning sneezing AUDIO 9
Definition/aetiology
It is not unusual for pigs to start sneezing in the nursery within 10 days of weaning. The pigs are generally

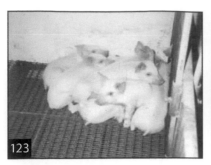

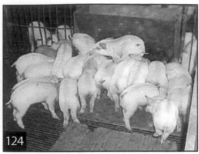

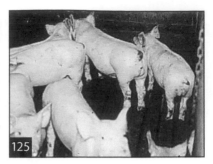

Figs. 3.123–3.125 To reduce the incidence of pleurisy, avoid: (3.123) draughts; (3.124) fighting over feed; (3.125) fighting over water.

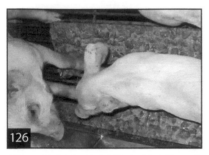

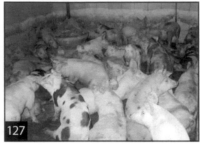

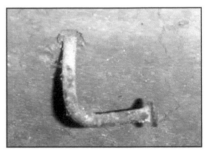

Figs. 3.126, 3.127 (3.126) Rough floors – note new floors can be particularly problematic; (3.127) poor pig flow.

Fig. 3.128 Remove any sharp objects within pig height.

clinically well despite the sneezing, with no fever. The sneezing indicates establishment of normal nasopharyngeal microflora as the maternal immunity of the individual pigs wane and the mixing of the different microflora from different litters.

Because different mothers are involved, the microflora isolated from different pigs can be complex. Typical isolates include a range of bacteria including *P. multocida*, *B. bronchiseptica*, *H. parasuis*, *A. pleuropneumoniae*, *A. suis*, *Streptococcus* spp., *Pseudomonas* spp., *Proteus* and other environmentally originating bacteria. A variety of *Mycoplasma* spp. can be isolated. *Chlamydia* spp. may be involved in any associated conjunctivitis. Viruses include PCMV (inclusion body rhinitis), PRRSV, PCV2 and a whole range of as yet unrecognised viruses.

Clinical presentation

A group of weaned pigs presents with mild to severe sneezing (**Figures 3.129, 3.130**). Conjunctivitis may be seen in several pigs. The symptoms will

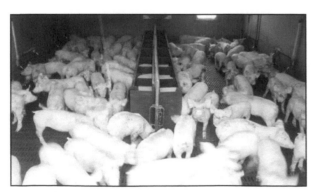

Fig. 3.129 Nursery pigs that have post-weaning sneezing.

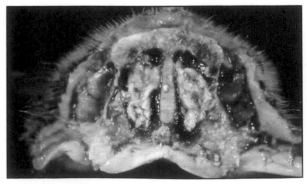

Fig. 3.130 Massive presence of a fibrinopurulent exudate within the nasal cavity (fibrinopurulent rhinitis).

progressively reduce within 2–3 weeks. The sneezing may progress to middle ear disease in a few individuals (head tilt). Morbidity is high but mortality low.

Differential diagnosis

If sneezing occurs in the farrowing house, review AR controls. SI is unusual in pigs younger than 6 weeks of age in established herds because of maternal immunity transfer via colostrum. However, a SIV serotype can be an acute problem when newly introduced into a herd.

Diagnosis

A non-progressive rhinitis with conjunctivitis. The nasal cavity may be filled with purulent material and this can on occasions be very severe.

Management

As this is a mixed infection, treatment is supportive and generally unrewarding, but clients can be very concerned. Post-weaning sneezing may be considered almost 'normal' on most farms, but it will still be necessary to critically review the management of the farm buildings, in particular to avoiding chilling and draughts.

If the farm is PPRSV positive, review the PRRSV stablisation programme.

The problem can be reduced by combining litters in late lactation so the piglet microflora becomes established pre-weaning.

Porcine reproductive and respiratory syndrome ▶ VIDEO 19

Definition/aetiology

PRRS is considered to be the most economically significant infectious pig disease worldwide. It is caused by a porcine arterivirus, which is further subclassified into two genotypes: European (type 1 also known as Lelystad) and American (type 2).

PRRSV is an enveloped RNA virus and is very susceptible to change and mutation. The immunity between strains may be poor and current vaccines may not provide protection against all strains on the farm. There may be multiple strains on the same farm complicating control.

Once infected, the pig enters a transient carrier state and is able to excrete the virus in body secretions. This excretion phase normally only last 35 days, but in some cases it can last 200 days, which again greatly complicates elimination and control programmes.

The two major clinical scenarios linked to PRRSV infection are reproductive failure in adults and respiratory disease scenarios in pigs of all ages. The greatest impact in post-weaning pigs is not just due to the direct effects of the viral infection; the immunomodulating effects of the virus facilitates the contribution of other pathogens to cause concomitant respiratory or systemic disease problems.

PRRSV detail

Understanding the detail of a virus can be very important in biosecurity design, tracking its epidemiology and understanding vaccine selection (**Figures 3.131, 3.132**).

There are seven regions of the positive sense RNA genome of PRRSV (*Table 3.9*). The GP$_5$ protein is the most variable structural protein, with only 51–55%

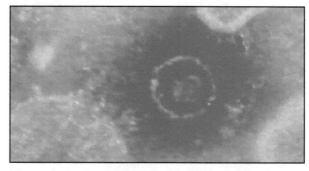

Fig. 3.131 The appearance of the virus down the electron microscope.

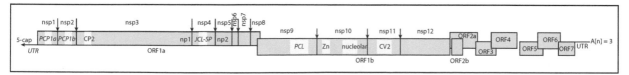

Fig. 3.132 The general layout of the 15 kb PRRSV genome, illustrating the two long open reading frames (ORF1 and ORF2) and the smaller other frames. Note that there is some overlapping between the ORFs.

Table 3.9 **The open reading frame (ORF) regions of PRRSV.**

ORF 1	RNA replicase ORF1a and ORF1b	No structural proteins
ORF 2	Minor membrane glycoprotein GP_{2a} GP_{2b}	Structural proteins
ORF 2–7	Nucleocapsid protein N, nucleolar localisation	
ORF 3	Membrane glycoprotein GP_3	
ORF 4	Membrane glycoprotein GP_4	
ORF 5	Major membrane glycoprotein GP_5	
ORF 6	Membrane associated protein - M	
ORF 7	Nucleocapsid protein - N	

amino acid homology between North American and European isolates, whereas the M protein is the most conserved protein with 78–80% amino acid homology.

Clinical presentation

Clinical presentation of the reproductive form of PRRS is characterised by a sow becoming off feed, pyrexic (40°C), return-to-oestrus, abortions, premature farrowing and, rarely, mortality of the sow (with concurrent infections) (**Figures 3.133–3.137**).

Note that the abortions tend to occur after day 60 of gestation.

Clinical presentation of the respiratory form of PRRS is highly variable, depending on the herd, ranging from subclinical infection to devastating disease. Such variability is influenced by the virus isolate, host immune status, host susceptibility, concurrent infections, environment and management.

Within an epidemic outbreak, all stages of production may be affected by respiratory disease. Often, the production stage that is under most stress is the most affected (e.g. an overstocked nursery).

In suckling pigs, besides increased pre-weaning mortality, evidence of emaciation, splay legged posture, tachypnoea and thumping respiration are observed. Other common clinical signs such as neurological disorders and diarrhoea (often associated with *Escherichia coli*) are mainly due to concurrent infections. The piglets may become infected from milk, which can carry the virus particles. Such a clinical picture in the farrowing area can last for 1–4 months, depending on the farm.

Nursery and grow/finish pigs mainly suffer from anorexia, dyspnoea without coughing, reduction of ADG and increased mortality due mainly to concomitant infections (**Figures 3.138–3.140**).

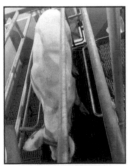

Fig. 3.133 Sow off colour.

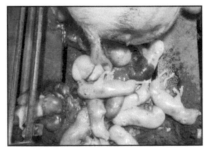

Fig. 3.134 Aborted sow.

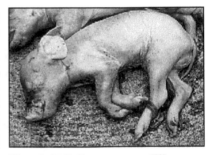

Fig. 3.135 Prepartum stillborn piglet.

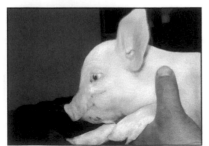

Fig. 3.136 Premature piglet with a dome head.

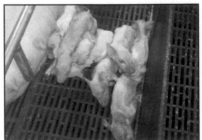

Fig. 3.137 Piglets with PRRSV infection piling in the farrowing house.

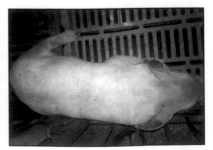

Fig. 3.138 Nursery pig with blue ears.

Fig. 3.139
Conjunctivitis in a nursery pig.

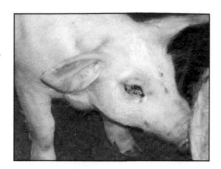

Fig. 3.140
Blue ears in a sow.

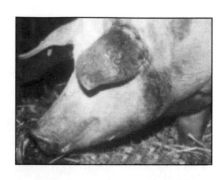

Endemic disease scenarios may replicate a PRRS outbreak at a lower intensity, mainly due to the introduction of susceptible gilts into the farm not appropriately or effectively acclimatised. This endemic situation mainly expresses as lower ADG and increased mortality in nursery to finishing pigs, generally due to concurrent bacterial/viral infections.

Highly pathogenic PRRSV (with two deletions in the ORF5 NPS2 region of the virus) has been associated with severe clinical signs and high mortality sporadically in North America and Europe. In Asia 'high path' PRRSV can be particularly problematic, although the diagnosis is also complicated by concurrent serious infections with uncontrolled PCV2-SD, classical swine fever and Aujeszky's disease.

Classification of a herd's status with regard to PRRSV

It is helpful to have a classification for a herd for each of the various pathogens in order to provide clarity to the veterinarian and farm team. As an example, for PRRSV the designation in *Table 3.10* can be used. Similar systems can be used to designate your other client's farms and their pathogens.

Table 3.10	**Farm PRRSV status classification scheme.**
1	Positive unstable
2fv	Positive stable. Ongoing field virus exposure (fv)
2vx	Positive stable. Live virus vaccinated (vx)
2	Positive stable
3	Provisionally negative
4	ELISA negative

Differential diagnosis

PRRS can be associated with most conditions able to cause respiratory distress (see *Table 3.1*), meaning a wide number of possible isolation opportunities. This is complicated by the fact that PRRSV infection can take place together with other respiratory pathogens and the clinical picture rarely allows confirming or ruling out PRRS. However, a broad differential diagnosis should include PCV2-SD, SI and EP.

Diagnosis

Observation of interstitial pneumonia at necropsy is suggestive of involvement of a viral infection in the respiratory clinical process (**Figures 3.141, 3.142**). Since this lesion is not unique to PRRS, laboratory confirmation is needed. This is achieved by a number of possibilities, including histopathological assessment (together with IHC, or in situ hybridisation to detect the virus) and viral detection in tissues or sera of pigs (usually by RT-PCR).

However, the usual diagnostic approach implies population monitoring, and this can be achieved by antibody detection by ELISA (evidence of seroconversion) or detection of the virus in samples of live pigs, such as serum or oral fluids. Note that it can take 2–3 weeks for the antibody level to rise sufficiently to create a positive test result. Also note that the antibodies may disappear 6 months after exposure, although this is not a problem in detection investigations.

In all cases, a global diagnostic approach, including PRRSV and other pathogens, is the best strategy to cope with a clinical picture, which is usually polymicrobial and multifactorial.

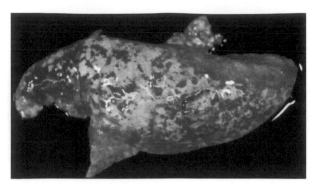

Fig. 3.141 Lung affected by a severe interstitial pneumonia, characterised by lack of pulmonary collapse, and darker areas in a lobular generalised pattern (coalescing in some areas) in a **PRRSV** infected pig.

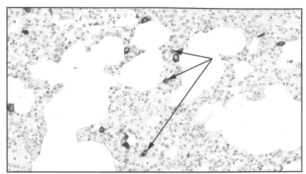

Fig. 3.142 Lung affected by a moderate interstitial pneumonia, characterized by thickening of alveolar walls. Moderate presence of macrophages containing PRRSV antigen (dark brown stained cells, arrows). Immunohistochemistry to detect **PRRSV**.

The epidemiology of an outbreak can be investigated using sequencing of the virus, which can then be compared between different sources. This may be beneficial in vaccine selection but is fraught with difficulties as vaccine sequence will generally not match the local virus strains.

Management

Treatment: PRRS is a viral infection and therefore there is normally no specific treatment possible with economic constraints. However, unusually, because PRRSV infects the macrophages, macrolides such a tiamulin fumate modify macrophage function and may interfere with PRRSV replication and infection of the alveolar macrophage. Thus, in an outbreak, tiamulin may provide a treatment option.

The outbreak results in pyrexia and this is largely the cause of the abortions. Therefore, control of the pyrexia through NSAIDs such as salicylic acid can ameliorate the clinical signs.

Control: There is no effective control programme currently available, therefore elimination and negative status is preferred. Prevention of PRRS is based on avoiding PRRSV entry. There are a number of issues to be considered; for a more detailed examination refer to Chapter 11.

Location: To have a reasonable chance of maintaining a PRRSV-negative status the farm must be more than 1 km from other pig enterprises or major roads.

Breeding stock: These measures usually include acclimatisation facilities and testing protocols for incoming negative breeding stock. This can be extremely difficult when considering artificial insemination since the virus can be introduced via semen. With regards to artificial insemination, gene transfer should occur through frozen semen where there is time to test the producing boars. Alternatively, the farm should practice on-farm artificial insemination collection.

Vehicle restrictions: Transportation vehicle sanitation, drying and movement control protocols are essential.

General biosecurity: Personnel entry protocols through removal of off-farm shoes before entry. General measures such as insect or bird entry control. Incoming air virus filtration systems have been designed, but they are difficult to maintain.

In seropositive farms: Pig management is considered key in order to ameliorate or prevent further disease outbreaks. Such management is devoted to reducing within-farm virus spread. The principle of control is to produce negative weaners from the farrowing area. This can only be achieved by having a stable adult herd. Gilt acclimatisation represents probably the most important factor. The greatest likelihood of introducing PRRSV into the breeding herd is through the introduced previously negative gilts becoming positive but still being carriers and excreting the virus when they enter the breeding pool. This may be prevented if negative gilts enter the farm around 60 kg liveweight and are then vaccinated and exposed to the farm's native virus. This allows at least 6 weeks for the gilt to stop excreting the virus before entering the breeding pool.

Management should include:

- Gilt acclimatisation programmes ensuring that the gilt enters the breeding herd positive to PRRSV but not excreting the virus.
- Biosecurity. This is still essential because the farm does not want to introduce a novel PRRSV, which may not be covered by the current immune status of the sows. In addition, the novel virus may recombine with the native farm virus strains, resulting in a new virus strain where protection is not immediately available.
- Batch farrowing and AIAO programmes.
- Restrict cross-fostering to the first 24 hours after birth.
- Control of concurrent diseases and early segregation/elimination of compromised and sick animals.

Vaccination: Vaccination is widely used, including vaccination of sow, piglet, or both. The most used products are modified live vaccines (MLVs). Killed vaccines in naïve animals do not provide any control but may be used post vaccination with a MLV to reduce the carrier and excretion phase.

Eradication: Eradication of PRRS can be achieved by means of total or partial depopulation, test and removal and herd closure. Regional eradication of PRRS from a wide geographical area or in a country (regional control) has been implemented with variable degrees of success. Farmer and veterinarian commitments are the cornerstones for regional/national disease control. Examples of possible eradication programmes are discussed further in Chapter 11.

Porcine circovirus type 2-systemic disease

PCV2 is considered a major factor in the development of many respiratory conditions of pigs (see Chapter 8 for more details).

Porcine respiratory coronavirus

Porcine respiratory coronavirus (PRCV) is a natural deletion mutant of transmissible gastroenteritis virus (TGEV), which infects the respiratory tract. Since PRCV infection is widely spread (ubiquitous in many areas of the world) and subclinical in nature, its more interesting effect relies on the cross-reactivity and cross-protection with TGEV. Globally, PRCV is nowadays considered a pathogen of very limited interest since it is believed that its clinical impact is minimal or negligible.

There are no special measures recommended to prevent or control PRCV infections. Moreover, persistence of this viral infection in the herd is considered positive since it cross-protects against TGEV infections, which can be extremely detrimental for pig production. There is no protection between PRCV and other coronaviruses of pigs such as porcine epidemic diarrhoea (see Chapter 4 for more details on TGEV).

Pulmonary miliary abscessation

Pigs are found at post-mortem examination with multiple abscesses throughout all the lung lobes (**Figure 3.143**). Abscesses that reach the pleural surface may rupture, leading to focal pleuritis. This is also referred to as embolic pneumonia.

Treatment involves identifying the nidus of the infection and resolving the cause. If the problem is associated with a vice (**Figure 3.144**), the causal stressors need to be resolved. If the nidus is the foot, management of the floor is essential.

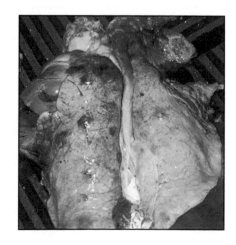

Fig. 3.143 **Miliary abscessation of the lung following a bacteraemia.**

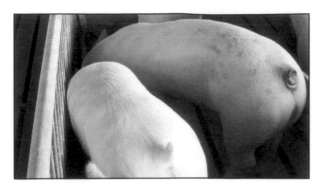

Fig. 3.144 Vice (in this case a tail bitten pig), the classic cause of miliary abscessation.

Swine influenza VIDEO 13

Definition/aetiology

Swine influenza viruses (SIVs) are some of the most important causes of acute respiratory disease outbreaks in pigs worldwide, but infections are mostly subclinical or in combination with other pathogens (causing subacute or chronic respiratory problems and EP). SIV is an orthoinfluenza type A virus (**Figure 3.145**). This is an enveloped RNA virus. It has eight segments to its genome and this allows for reassortment and recombination of the genome. The virus is defined by the H (haemagglutinin) and N (neuraminidase) antigens. There are 16 H and 9 N types known. All of the types exist in birds.

Three major subtypes of SIV have been described infecting swine based on their haemagglutinin and neuraminidase glycoproteins (H_1N_1, H_1N_2 and H_3N_2), each causing similar clinical signs and lesions. Importantly, pigs are also susceptible to the so-called pandemic H_1N_1 SIV strain that caused a human pandemic in 2009. This originated in man but spread to pigs and was given the nomenclature 'swine flu'. Note that there are seven different pig adapted influenza strains and more will appear.

SIVs have zoonotic potential and swine have traditionally been considered as a potential 'mixing vessel' (between human and avian species) host for genetic reassortment of the virus. In addition, most recent studies indicate that SIV epidemiology is much more complex than thought in the past, describing high frequencies of multiple strains/subtypes infecting the same batch of animals in some cases.

The virus multiplies in bronchial epithelium causing focal necrosis, bronchiolitis and atelectasis.

Clinical presentation

Subclinical infections are by far the most usual ones, but their impact has not been fully elucidated. SIV is also found frequently in pigs affected by EP, but it is difficult to reliably establish the specific contribution of the virus to the whole clinical picture.

Typical SIV infection is described as acute outbreaks characterised by sneezing and nasal discharges, a non-productive cough, tachypnoea, fever, anorexia and reluctance to move (**Figure 3.146**). The clinical signs spread around the farm rapidly and occur in multiple age groups. SIV infections can also cause reproductive disorders (abortions), mainly linked to the fever experienced by the sow, not by infection of the fetuses (**Figure 3.147**).

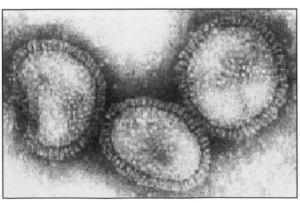

Fig. 3.145 Electron microscopy of swine influenza virus.

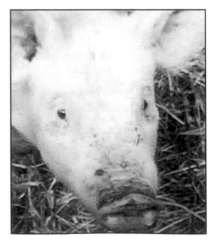

Fig. 3.146 Pig with a nasal discharge.

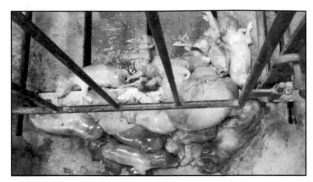

Fig. 3.147 **Abortion associated with SIV infection.**

Mortality is minimal if no concurrent infections are present. Recovery is quite fast, since the whole duration of the outbreak may vary between 5 and 10 days. Clinical signs are limited to susceptible, seronegative pigs.

As 90% of farms are *Mycoplasma hyopneumoniae* positive, SIV infection usually occurs in farms with concurrent infections and this complicates the outcome of the clinical signs. In these cases a significant spike in mortality can occur. When the dead pigs are necropsied it is not uncommon to find fibrinous polyserositis (Glässer's disease) as a common problem in the dead animals. These animals die because their heart is weakened. One feature of an infection is that when the clinician enters the barn the pigs are very quiet and reluctant to move. When the pigs get up, coughing and sneezing become apparent.

It is not possible to clinically distinguish between infection by one or other SIV subtypes. Following an outbreak of SI the finishing pigs become more susceptible to other concurrent pathogens, in particular APP.

Differential diagnosis

Swine influenza can easily be confused with EP, although it tends to display a more acute and rapidly spreading clinical picture. However, both pathogens cause a bronchointerstitial pneumonia as the basic lesion, with a typical cranioventral distribution. In SIV infection there is also a tendency for the diaphragmatic lung lobes to be affected multifocally. This may reflect the more extensive invasion of SIV into the lower airways.

Abortion can be associated with SI.

Diagnosis

Clinical diagnosis should be coupled with post-mortem findings and laboratory detection of SIV or antibodies against it. The lungs are affected by a bronchointerstitial pneumonia. The lesions are mainly distributed cranioventrally, in a multifocal (patchy) pattern, although the diaphragmatic lobes can also be affected (**Figures 3.148–3.150**).

SIV can be isolated from nasal and bronchial swabs and lung tissue in cell cultures or in embryonated fowl's eggs. However, routine practical detection of the virus is accomplished by RT-PCR

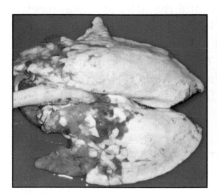

Fig. 3.148 **Lung affected by a bronchointerstitial pneumonia caused by SIV. The cardiac left lung lobe is completely consolidated, associated with a concomitant bacterial infection.**

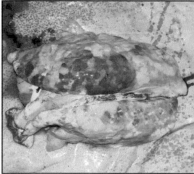

Fig. 3.149 **Note the checkboard pattern in this uncomplicated case of swine influenza.**

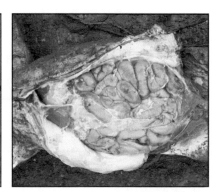

Fig. 3.150 **SIV can kill pigs that have an underlying condition – in this case polyserositis.**

from nasal swabs or oral fluids. In fact, SIV may be detected for a longer period in oral fluids than from nasal swabs.

The easiest and cheapest method to monitor infection dynamics, as well as to confirm subclinical infection, is through ELISA tests measuring serum antibodies against SIV. Seroconversion takes place quickly and evidence of it is found around 2 weeks after detection of clinical signs. It is important to remember that during the acute outbreak there will be no antibodies to SIV. After the outbreak, there may be antibodies but no virus particles.

Management

Treatment: There is no effective treatment for SI, although antimicrobials may be administered to control secondary concurrent infections from the descending nasopharyngeal microflora. Tetracycline is commonly used to provide control of these pathogens. However, while antimicrobials may provide no effective treatment, pain relief is an essential part of the management programme.

Even in outbreaks, it is important to review and resolve any environmental problems with water and ammonia, or overstocking, that are seen during the investigation.

Control: Since transmission of the virus is mainly by aerosols (aerogenic or from incoming subclinically infected pigs) and humans may act as vectors of transmission, virus entry into the farm is difficult to prevent. Natural infection provides lifelong immunity to the strain causing the infection.

Vaccination is considered the most effective way of preventing outbreaks of SI. Vaccines are traditionally based on inactivated H_1N_1, H_1N_2 and H_3N_2 viruses. Sows and/or pigs are usually administered two doses 2–3 weeks apart, although single administration products are available. Because protection through vaccination is for only 6 months the sows will need to be revaccinated each parity. Note that the virus may change and the vaccine will not cover new strains.

Zoonotic implications

Some influenza viruses can be transmitted between pigs and humans.

Swine influenza virus – a moving genetic target

SIV can change by two major methods:

1 Genetic drift. Here parts of the genetic code change with replication errors (**Figure 3.151**). This is typical of a RNA virus.
2 Genetic shift. Here recombination of different viruses occupying the same cell at the same time make a new type of virus (**Figure 3.152**).

Examples: In 2018 the SIVs of importance are H_1N_1, H_3N_2, H_1N_2 . There were seven different major types of SIV recognised. Note that there are differences between European and American strains; even with the same type of H or N they may originate from difference species (i.e. avian or mammal).

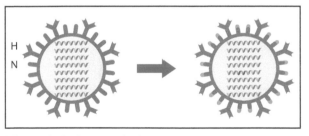

Fig. 3.151 Genetic drift.

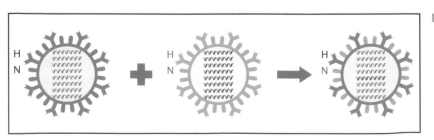

Fig. 3.152 Genetic shift.

CLINICAL QUIZ

3.1 Identify the other lesion/s in the lung in **Figure 3.58** (see p. 123) that are not associated with the *Ascaris* migration.

3.2 Why do ceftiofur, penicillin and amoxicillin have no effect on *Mycoplasma hyorhinis*?

3.3 The pig's anatomy affects the pathogenesis of enzootic (mycoplasma) pneumonia. Explain.

The answers to these questions can be found on page 473.

CLINICAL GROSS ANATOMY OF THE INTESTINAL TRACT

To understand any pathology it is vital to understand what is normal (**Figures 4.1–4.12**). The intestinal tract is defined here as being from the mouth to the anus and includes the contents of the abdomen. Post-mortem examination of pigs is discussed in Chapter 1.

Fig. 4.1 **General view of the head of the pig.**

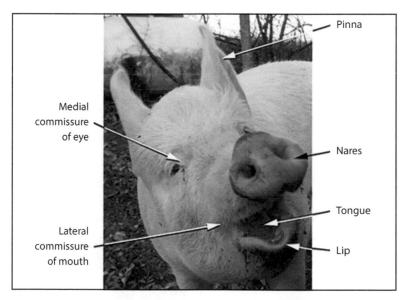

Pinna

Medial commissure of eye

Nares

Tongue

Lateral commissure of mouth

Lip

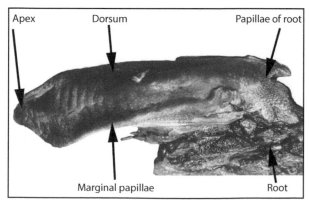

Apex   Dorsum   Papillae of root

Marginal papillae   Root

Fig. 4.2 **Dorsal view of the tongue.**

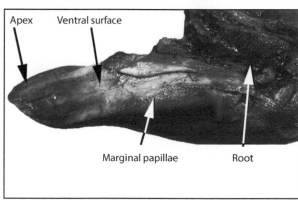

Apex   Ventral surface

Marginal papillae   Root

Fig. 4.3 **Ventral view of the tongue.**

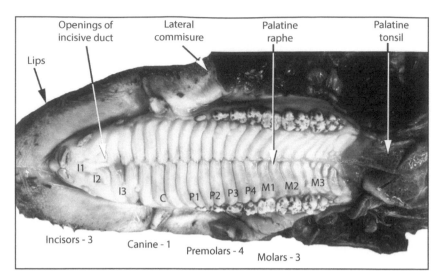

Fig. 4.4 Ventral view of the hard and soft palates.

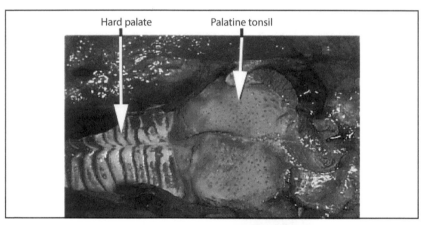

Fig. 4.5 Detail of the palatine tonsil.

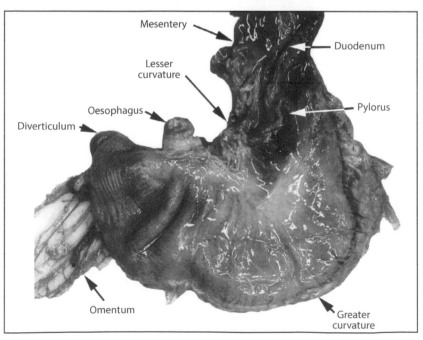

Fig. 4.6 The parietal surface of the stomach indicating major landmarks.

Fig. 4.7 The mucosal surface of the stomach opened along the greater curvature. The green colouration is associated with the reflux of bile post-mortem. Important features are the keratinised oesophageal entrance, the pouch-like diverticulum (which is more developed in other members of the Suidae family) and the pyloric torus, which protects the stomach from bile salts (in the pig, the bile duct entrance is very close to pyloric sphincter).

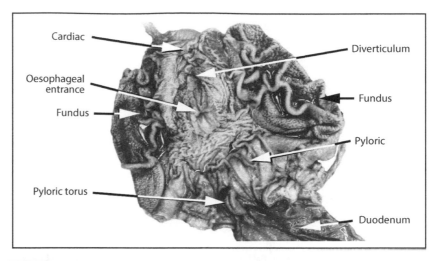

Fig. 4.8 Orientation of the small and large intestine can be assisted by recognising the ileocaecal ligament, which attaches the caecum (which is easy to recognise) with the distal ileum. It is important to examine the distal ileum at each post-mortem examination to check for ileitis. Photograph taken during surgery on a pet pig.

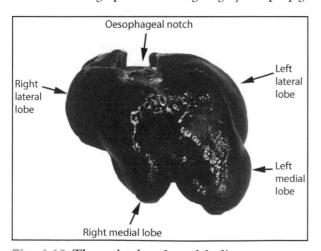

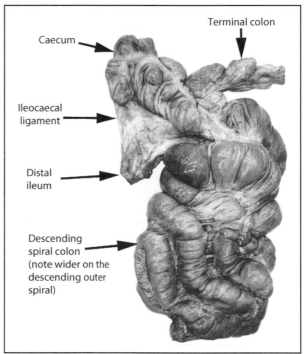

Fig. 4.9 The large bowel of the pig is a spiral with the wider descending colon on the outside and the narrower ascending colon on the inside of the spiral.

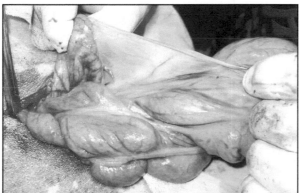

Fig. 4.10 The parietal surface of the liver.

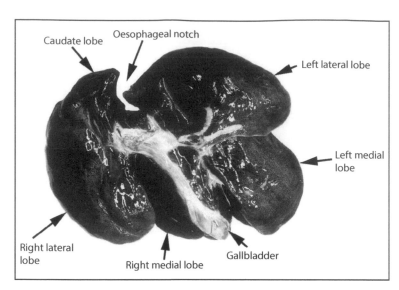

Fig. 4.11 The visceral surface of the liver.

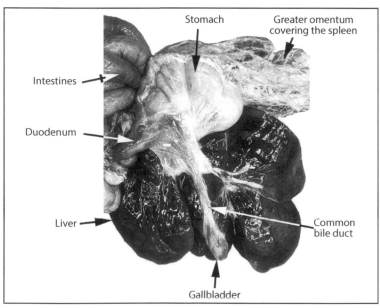

Fig. 4.12 The liver and stomach demonstrating the path of the common bile duct.

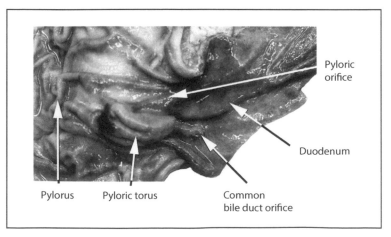

Fig. 4.13 The close proximity of the common bile duct orifice and the pyloric orifice in the stomach is shown.

INTESTINAL INVESTIGATION

Specimen collection

A pig with representative clinical signs should be euthanased, ideally within the acute phase of the condition. Collect one fresh dead pig if available.

Individual animal investigation

It may be necessary, mainly in pet pig medicine, to further investigate an abdominal problem using radiographs (**Figure 4.14**). Contrast studies with barium sulphate may be particularly rewarding when investigating constipation.

Observe and record the pig, especially defecation, if possible. Faecal changes might indicate disease.

Fig. 4.14 Lateral (a) and dorsoventral (b) radiographic views of the abdomen of a pig. This pig was constipated.

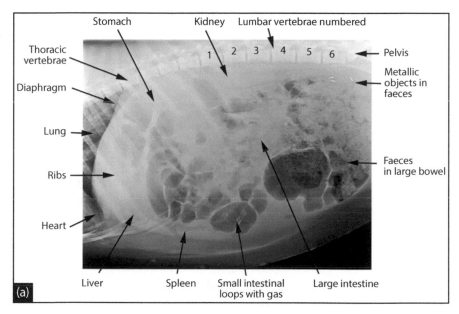

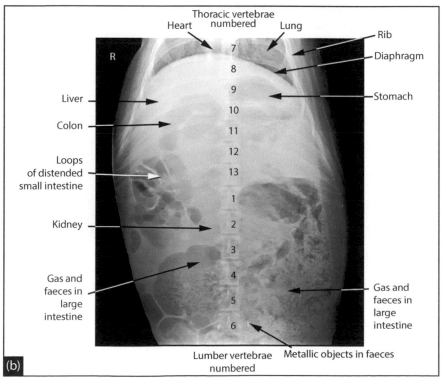

Faecal consistency

See **Figure 4.15**.

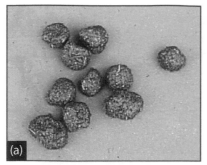

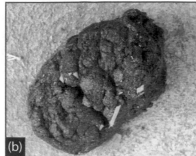

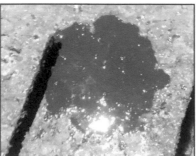

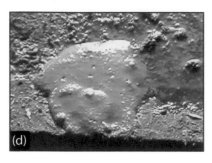

Fig. 4.15 The range of consistency of faeces: (a) constipated; (b) normal; (c) loose; (d) diarrhoea.

Faecal colour

The colour of faeces can be very varied and may occasionally be a clinical sign useful in making a diagnosis (**Figures 4.16a–4.16j**). (See Clinical Quiz 4.1 on page 206.)

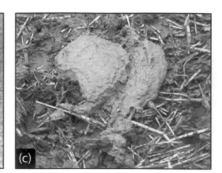

Fig. 4.16a Yellow.

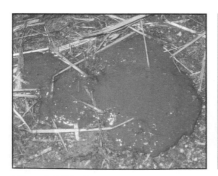

Fig. 4.16b Grey.

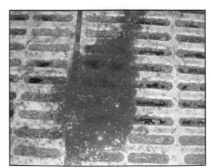

Fig. 4.16c Blood in faeces – dysentery.

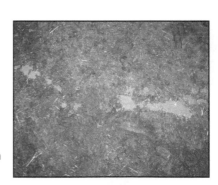

Fig. 4.16d Reddish with mucus.

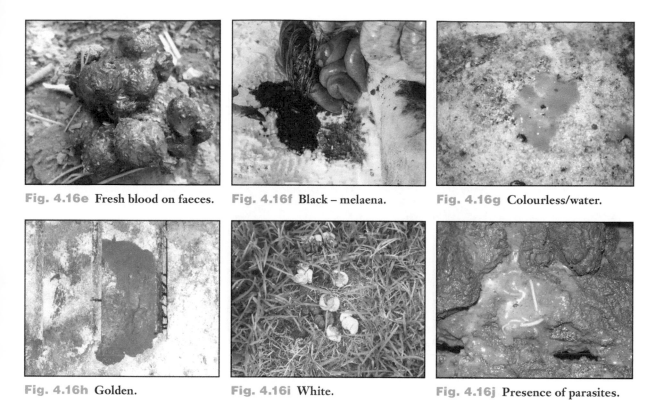

Fig. 4.16e Fresh blood on faeces.

Fig. 4.16f Black – melaena.

Fig. 4.16g Colourless/water.

Fig. 4.16h Golden.

Fig. 4.16i White.

Fig. 4.16j Presence of parasites.

Describing gross intestinal pathology

Some examples of gross intestinal pathology are shown in **Figures 4.17–4.26**. (See Clinical Quiz 4.2 on page 206.)

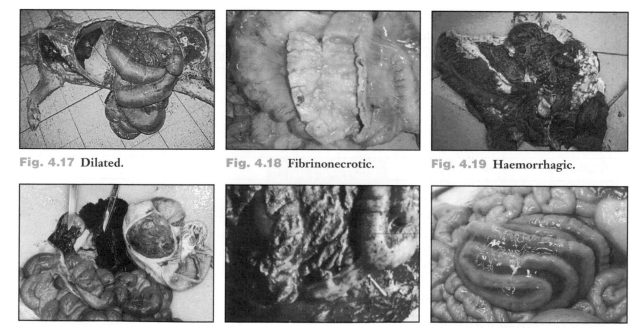

Fig. 4.17 Dilated.

Fig. 4.18 Fibrinonecrotic.

Fig. 4.19 Haemorrhagic.

Fig. 4.20 Ulcers.

Fig. 4.21 Mucoid.

Fig. 4.22 Oedema.

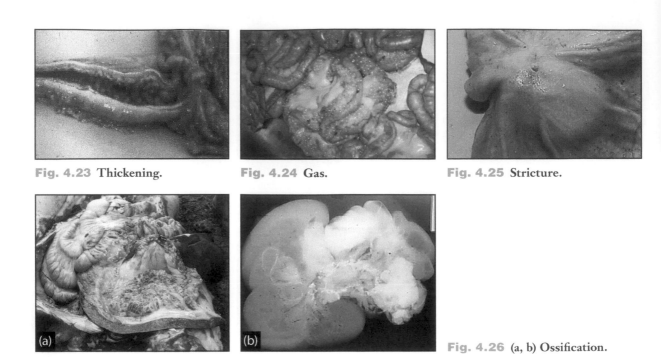

Fig. 4.23 Thickening.   **Fig. 4.24** Gas.   **Fig. 4.25** Stricture.

Fig. 4.26 (a, b) Ossification.

Basic intestinal bacteriology

Several intestinal conditions are associated with bacteria. A rectal or post-mortem swab can be taken and the species of bacteria grown and identified. This is combined with an antibiogram to assist treatment programmes. Many of these bacteria are also commensals or opportunistic pathogens of the intestines. The intestinal tract naturally should have a healthy microbiota, which acts as a major component of the defence mechanisms and assists digestion. *Table 4.1* describes the basic identification and characteristics of the major bacteria that may be isolated from intestinal disorders.

Table 4.1 **Basic intestinal disorder bacteriology: summary.**

ORGANISM	GRAM STAIN	GROWTH				SUGARS AND REACTIONS									
		ANAEROBE ONLY	HAEMOLYTIC BLOOD AGAR	MACCONKEY	TERGITOL	CATALASE	OXIDASE	DEXTROSE BROTH	KLIGLER'S	KLIGLER'S IRON	LACTOSE	LYSINE	SIMMS	SIMMS CITRATE	UREASE
Brachyspira spp.	+S	+	β	−	−	−	−								
Clostridium perfringens	+B	+	Y	−	−	−	−								
Escherichia coli	−B		N+β	+L	+L	+	−		+G		+		+		−
Salmonella spp.	−B		N	+NL	+NL	+	−			+	−	+			−
Streptococcus spp.	+C		α/β	−	−	−	−								
Trueperella pyogenes	+B		N	−	−	−	−								

+ and green = positive; − and red = negative.
Gram stain: B = bacillus/coccobacillus; C = coccoid; S = spirochaete.
Sugars and reactions: G = gas.
Haemolytic: Y = yes and type α or β; N = no.
L = lactose fermentation; NL = non-lactose fermentor.

Escherichia coli
See **Figures 4.27–4.30**.

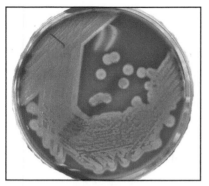

Fig. 4.27 Blood agar. Most pathogenic strains will show large colonies, which are β haemolytic, smooth and mucoid.

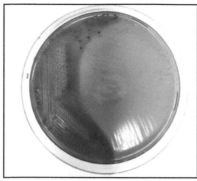

Fig. 4.28 MacConkey's. Pink colonies – lactose fermenter.

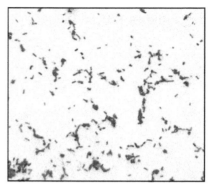

Fig. 4.29 Gram-negative rod.

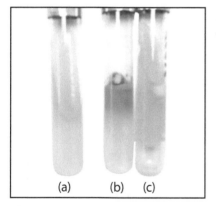

Fig. 4.30 Sugar tests to assist in confirming *E. coli*. (a) urease negative: yellow; (b) Simm's positive: red colour; (c) Kligler's positive: with gas.

Salmonella spp.
There are over 2,300 serotypes of *Salmonella*. See **Figures 4.31–4.34**.

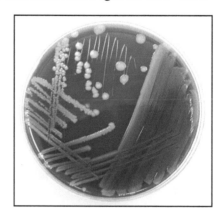

Fig. 4.31 Salmonella strains are large non-haemolytic smooth colonies on blood agar.

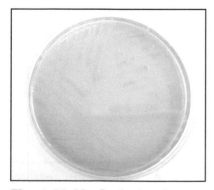

Fig. 4.32 MacConkey's pale colony – a non-lactose fermenter.

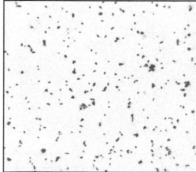

Fig. 4.33 Gram-negative rod.

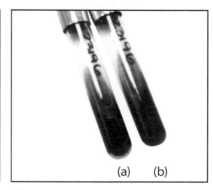

Fig. 4.34 Sugar tests to assist in the confirmation. (a) Kligler's iron agar; H₂S + lactose: blue colour; (b) Lysine iron agar positive: blue colour.

Brachyspira hyodysenteriae and
Brachyspira pilosicoli
See **Figures 4.35, 4.36**.

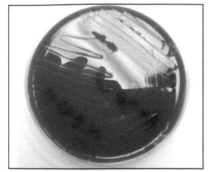

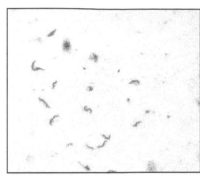

Fig. 4.35 *B. hyodysenteriae* culture on blood agar. Requires anaerobic culture and 42°C. A filmy surface growth is typical, rather than distinct individual surface colonies. β haemolytic bacteria lie under the surface.

Fig. 4.36 *B. hyodysenteriae.* Weakly gram-positive spirochaetes.

Clostridium difficile
See **Figures 4.37, 4.38**.

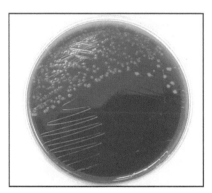

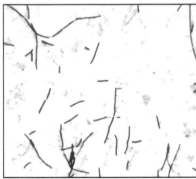

Fig. 4.37 *C. difficile* culture on blood agar. Requires anaerobic culture. Can be difficult to culture.

Fig. 4.38 Gram-positive rod.

Clostridium perfringens
See **Figures 4.39, 4.40**.

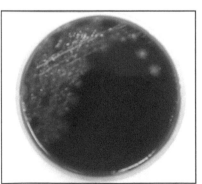

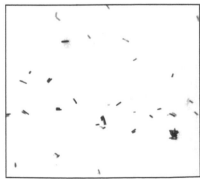

Fig. 4.39 *C. perfringens* on blood agar. Requires anaerobic culture. Note the flat spreading colony shape and double zone of haemolysis.

Fig. 4.40 Gram-positive rods with vegetative and solid rods; some spore formation.

Lawsonia intracellularis

L. intracellularis requires cell culture. It will not grow on agar media.

Worm egg count

Requirements

- McMaster slide – this provides a simple counting chamber.
- Make flotation solution:
  - Supersaturated sugar solution:
    - 200 mL water.
    - Heat to boiling.
    - Add sugar, until no more will dissolve.
    - Pour off the sugar solution into a glass container. This will keep.
  - Zinc sulphate solution: as above but with ZnSO$_4$
- 100 mL bottle with top and small glass beads to assist mixing.
- Fresh faeces.

The ZnSO$_4$ solution is used for *Ascaris suum* eggs, which do not float in saturated sugar solutions.

Examples of pig worm egg count results (not to scale): coccidia are small

See **Figures 4.41–4.45**.

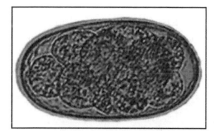

Fig. 4.41 Strongyle egg. Without further testing it is not possible to distinguish species down the microscope.

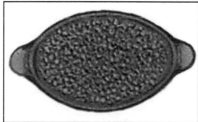

Fig. 4.42 *Trichuris suis* egg. Note the bipolar ends.

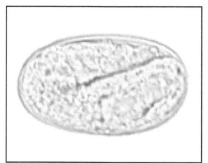

Fig. 4.43 *Strongyloides ransomi.* Has a larvae inside the egg.

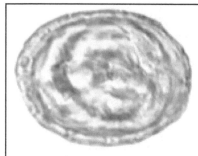

Fig. 4.44 *Metastrongylus* egg. Note the larva in the egg.

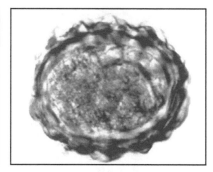

Fig. 4.45 *Ascaris suum* egg. Sticky and often covered in debris.

PRE-WEANING DIARRHOEA CONTROL MEASURES

Preparing the farrowing area

- Ensure there is efficient pig flow to achieve all-in/all-out (AIAO) at each phase.
- Move all the animals out of the farrowing area.
- Repair all broken equipment and facilities:
  - Water. Ensure all sows have adequate access to the water supply. A poorly placed drinker is shown (**Figure 4.46**). Disinfect water lines.
  - Air. Repair any broken vents. Ensure that the farrowing room ventilation system does not create chilling draughts (**Figure 4.47**).

- Check drip cooling system.
- Feed. Repair and replace any broken feeders. Check for sharp edges (**Figure 4.48**).
- Floor. Repair and replace any broken areas of the floor (**Figure 4.49**). A break in the floor can be both difficult to clean and very dangerous to the piglets and sow.
- Heated area. Ensure that the heated piglet creep area works properly. An infrared camera can be very useful (**Figure 4.50**).
- Review pressure washing protocols. Clean room thoroughly.
- Consider lime washing of farrowing places, especially the floor behind the sow. This not only assists the cleaning programme but helps to control splayleg. Lime washing is achieved by using one-third CaCO₃ mixed with two-thirds water by volume and painting onto the floor with a brush (**Figure 4.51**).
- Thoroughly clean all utensils and place in new disinfectant for at least 30 minutes. Each room should have its own utensils such as brush, scraper, etc. A poorly cleaned scraper in dirty disinfectant is shown (**Figure 4.52**) – this is a health risk to a clean farrowing room. In addition, the organic materials will deactivate the disinfectants quickly.
- Check the farrowing room is suitable for sows to enter; for example, water supplied at 2 litres a minute. Check piglet water supplies (**Figure 4.53**); air system – 18°C, no draughts. Check all heat mats

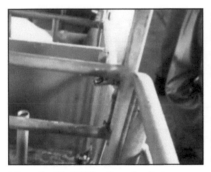

Fig. 4.46 Difficulty obtaining water.

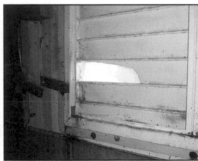

Fig. 4.47 Draught from a broken vent.

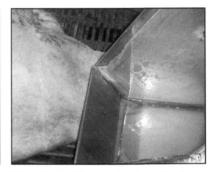

Fig. 4.48 Sharp edge in a feeder because the front of the feeder has eroded away.

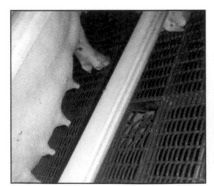

Fig. 4.49 Broken floor.

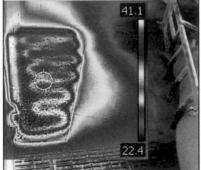

Fig. 4.50 Infrared image of the farrowing heat mat clearly indicating the edge of the heat mat and the working heated element within the mat.

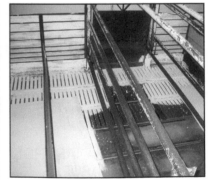

Fig. 4.51 Lime washed farrowing area.

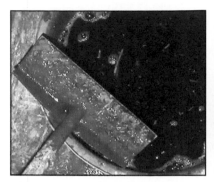

Fig. 4.52 Dirty scraper and disinfectant.

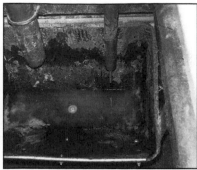

Fig. 4.53 Liquid feeding lactating sows.

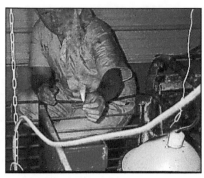

Fig. 4.54 Checking a farrowing area for draughts.

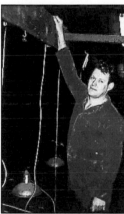

Fig. 4.55 Checking the farrowing area hygiene.

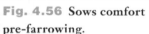

Fig. 4.56 Sows comfort pre-farrowing.

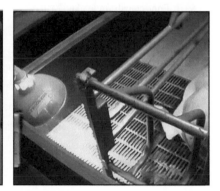

Fig. 4.57 Heat lamp pre-farrowing.

work as expected – 36+°C (**Figure 4.54**); floor hygiene – no evidence of faeces from the last group (**Figure 4.55**).

- Place sows into the farrowing room at 18°C.
- Day before farrowing. Turn creep light or heat mats on. Note the forward creep area (**Figure 4.56**). Night before farrowing. Place additional light behind sow. Raise room temperature to 20°C (**Figure 4.57**).

Colostrum

Pigs are born with a naïve immune system. A pig fetus starts to develop its immune system around day 70 of gestation. However, owing to the design of the placenta (epitheliochorial), prior to birth there is no passive transfer of antibodies. This fact dictates many of the production parameters required to raise pigs (**Figure 4.58**). A failure at this stage will significantly impact the performance of the pig for the rest of its life. For more information on colostrum see Chapter 8.

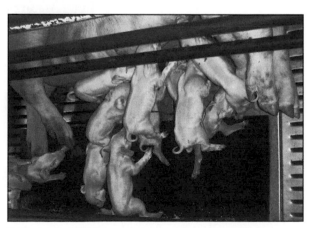

Fig. 4.58 Newborn piglets are immunodeficient.

Investigation protocol

Causes

Some possible causes of pre-weaning diarrhoea are listed in *Table 4.2*. This table can make a great evening training exercise for the farm health team.

Table 4.2 **Fourteen possible causes of pre-weaning diarrhoea in the pig.**

1	A range of pathogenic agents (e.g. *E. coli*, coronaviruses, *Coccidia* spp., *Clostridium* spp., rotavirus infection)
2	Almost any air movement is undesirable; >0.2 m/sec is a draught
3	Chilling of the piglets; check lying patterns and creep temperatures (ideally 36°C)
4	Variable temperatures in the creep
5	Damp floors, particularly in the creep area
6	Poor colostrum intake
7	No milk in the sows; check udder line; mycotoxins and management
8	Degree of cross-fostering
9	Piglet treatments are not clean enough; check cross-contamination between healthy and sick piglets
10	Infection transfer; is there a separate coloured and numbered brush and scraper for each room, foot baths, personal hygiene
11	Poor room cleaning between batches
12	Number of sows farrowing each batch, application of AIAO and pig flow
13	Presence of udder oedema
14	Vaccine storage protocols

Specific investigation

Examination of the pre-weaning room should be carried out (**Figure 4.59**) and pig-side diagnostic kits should be available (**Figure 4.60**).

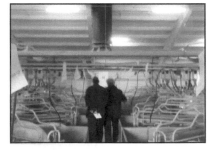

Fig. 4.59 **Environmental examination of the room.**

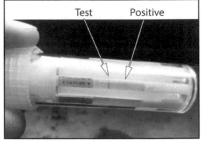

Fig. 4.60 **Pig-side diagnostic kits.**

Treatment protocols

Irrespective of the cause of the pre-weaning diarrhoea (**Figures 4.61, 4.62**), standard treatment protocols can be drawn up and implemented as a standard operating procedure (SOP) on the farm. An example is illustrated in *Table 4.3*.

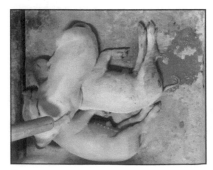

Fig. 4.61 **Watery diarrhea typical of rotavirus infection.**

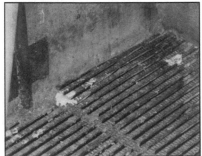

Fig. 4.62 **Yellow thicker diarrhoea typical of *E. coli* infection.**

Table 4.3 **Standard treatment protocols for pre-weaning diarrhoea.**

PIGLET TREATMENTS

1 Treat whole litter as soon as one piglet starts to show clinical signs

2 Place cube drinker (bucket with easy access for the piglets) filled with water, electrolytes (see *Table 4.4*) and glucose. This must be replaced at least four times daily. Keep clean

3 If creep feed is being provided, remove it

4 Ensure all piglets receive adequate colostrum within 6 hours of birth. Instigate a split suckling programme if necessary.

5 If the piglets are sick, administer antimicrobial measured doses once a day by mouth. Ensure you do not use this medication for healthy piglets

6 Inject with a suitable antimicrobial if the piglets are systemically sick. Pain medication may also be required

7 Clean up diarrhoea as soon as possible using paper. Use this material for immunological stimulation feedback to parity 1 sows 6 and 3 weeks pre-farrow and to gilts pre-breeding

8 All stockpersons must wash their hands after treating the piglets and dip their boots in disinfectant

9 Syringes or oral dosers must not be used on a sick piglet and then used on a healthy piglet

10 If diarrhoea occurs after day 10, consider coccidiosis and chilling draughts

CROSS-FOSTERING

Piglet movements must be carefully monitored. A lot of diarrhoea is associated with fostering. Review cross-fostering protocols

MOVEMENT OF UTENSILS AND PEOPLE FROM ONE ROOM TO THE NEXT

1 All rooms should have their own brush and shovel, which should be colour coded for the batch. Ensure that the rooms are thoroughly cleaned between batches. Consider lime-washing to enhance hygiene and disinfection

2 Each brush and shovel should be placed in disinfectant when not in use. Ensure disinfectant is still active

3 Piglet processing equipment must be thoroughly cleaned between rooms and batches

INVESTIGATION

Collect data on age of onset, parity, duration, morbidity and mortality. As soon as diarrhoea starts, submit rectal swabs or necropsy 1–3 acutely scouring piglets

LONG TERM

1 Pressure washing principles must be exemplary

2 Practice lime washing if possible

3 Practice AIAO pig flow

4 If diarrhoea is a persistent problem, have the environment examined in detail (i.e. for chilling draughts)

5 Ensure preventive protocols are adhered to (i.e. vaccination and immunological feed-back)

Table 4.4 **Home-made emergency electrolyte solution.**

Sugar (glucose)	8 teaspoons	40 g
Salt (NaCl)	1 teaspoon	5 g
Water	1 litre	

POST-WEANING DIARRHOEA
CONTROL MEASURES

Investigation protocol

A protocol for investigating post-weaning diarrhoea is outlined in *Table 4.5* (see also **Figure 4.63**).

Fig. 4.63
Home-made emergency electrolyte solution.

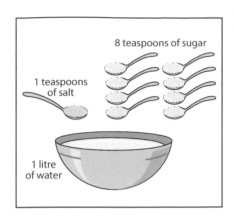

Table 4.5 **Investigation protocol for post-weaning diarrhoea.**

AREA OF CONCERN

1	Note the age of onset and day of onset of the diarrhoea post weaning. Many cases of diarrhoea actually start 5–7 days previously
2	Note the type of diarrhoea and appearance of the anal ring. Bloody, watery, yellow/pasty, mucoid. Alkaline faeces are generally *E. coli*. Acid faeces are generally viral aetiology
3	Carry out a post-mortem examination of a weaner. Euthanasia of acutely affected pigs and necropsy are generally more rewarding than chronically affected pigs with confusing secondary problems

ENVIRONMENTAL AND MANAGEMENT CHECKS ✓

1	Post-weaning feeding routines. Poor feed intake in the first week encourages gorging in the second week with protein overload of the gut and diarrhoea. Gruel feeding is essential, combined with little and often feeding routines
2	Hygiene of feeder, especially between batches. Is equipment colour coded?
3	Feeder space. Inadequate feeder space increases aggression. Note behaviour in first 3 days
4	Creep feeding and hygiene in the farrowing house
5	Mycotoxins in feed and feed storage. Mycotoxins damage vitamins such as vitamin E and can affect the palatability of the feed
6	Feed ingredients (e.g. presence of zinc oxide)
7	Is diarrhoea associated with a recent feed type change?
8	Water hygiene, especially between batches
9	Almost any air movement is undesirable; >0.2 m/sec is a chilling draught in the sleeping area
10	Chilling of the weaners; check lying patterns, sleeping area temperatures (initially, ideally >27°C) and defecation patterns
11	Variable temperatures and high humidity in the sleeping area
12	Damp floors/bedding, particularly in the sleeping area
13	Degree of cross-fostering pre-weaning
14	Number of sows farrowing each week disrupting AIAO and pig flow
15	Age of piglets at weaning and the variability in age and weight
16	Poor room cleaning between batches
17	Infection transfer. Is there a separate brush and scraper for each batch, foot baths, personnel hygiene
18	Review vermin and fly control
19	Weaner treatments have not been clean enough. Check cross-contamination between healthy and sick pigs
20	Type of iron injection utilised. Lack of sufficient iron may encourage more diarrhoea
21	Medication issues. Vaccine storage protocols
22	Review presence of other pathogens (e.g. PRRSV and PCV2)
23	Is a feed-back programme in place?
24	Check parity profile of the mother of weaners with diarrhoea

Treatment protocols

See *Table 4.6*.

Table 4.6 **Treatment protocols to control post-weaning diarrhoea.**

AIMS

Enhance pig's resistance to pathogens – or at least do nothing to reduce the pig's resistance

Reduce pathogen load

Note that most of the 'pathogenic' organisms are 'normal' in the environment

TREATMENT AND CONTROL PROTOCOLS

Reduce susceptible pigs

Remove bottom 10% (smalls) from the main group and house and manage differently

Review pig flow and ensure over- and understocking are not an issue

Review weaner age and weights

Review pre-weaning management to maximise health at weaning; review cross-fostering regimens in particular

Ensure adequate iron administration pre-weaning

Ensure all pigs are eating within 12 hours post weaning

Ensure adequate feed space available. Newly weaned pigs eat as a group. Restrict feeding even if feed is to be available *ad libitum*

Ensure a warm, draught-free sleeping area is available for all pigs

Provide warmer sleeping flooring – use of comfort boards etc

Enhance pig's resistance

Presence of zinc oxide for first 2 weeks post weaning. Concentration required depends on the amount of phytase. Note local legal constraints

Use acidifiers for the diet and water supplies

Use of probiotics – ensure milk and yogurt products are alive

Consider use of sterilised peat to act as an antitoxin/absorbent

Increase vitamin E concentration in feed to 250 ppm

Use suitable antimicrobial therapy

Ensure compliance with dose rate and treatment protocols. It may be necessary to treat whole groups of animals, including those not sick

Change genetics in cases of bowel oedema – *E. coli* F18

Consider vaccines for bowel oedema and *E. coli* F4

If vaccines are used, monitor and regulate storage requirements

Miscellaneous

If creep feeding is practiced pre-weaning, stop and review situation

Feed-back programmes using weaner faeces, including the diarrhoea, to gilts and sows 6 weeks pre-farrowing.

If gilt litter weaners are more prone, review management of gilt. Note particularly feed-back and immunity protocols

Review and possibly change creep/weaner feed type – meal, pellets, wet or dry size of pellets

---

(Continued)

Table 4.6 *(Continued)* **Treatment protocols to control post-weaning diarrhoea.**
Reduce pathogen load
Separate sick animals from main group as soon as possible – hospital area
Provide electrolytes in water supply to sick pigs
Do not move sick pigs back into previous week groups
Do not move recovered sick pigs back into main group until over 30 kg body weight
Practice rigid AIAO
Adequate hygiene between batches – use of lime washing
Ensure water lines are properly disinfected between batches
Ensure feeders are properly cleaned between batches
Ensure that there is no cross-contamination between batches through foot wear, brushes, scrapers or needles/syringes
Note hygiene of lying pads and comfort boards
Enhance vermin and fly controls
Monitor weaners rate and evenness of growth

DISORDERS OF THE INTESTINAL TRACT

Abdominal gastrointestinal misplacements

A common cause of sudden death in finishing pigs and adults is an abdominal catastrophe, characterised by a torsion/twist of the stomach or intestines (**Figures 4.64, 4.65**). The twist is commonly associated with the intestinal tract at the mesentery root or associated with a mesenteric tear (**Figure 4.66**). Occasionally, the spleen or a liver lobe can become associated with a twist (**Figures 4.67, 4.68**). Diagnosis is made at post-mortem. With scrotal hernias intestinal entrapment is common (**Figure 4.69**). With umbilical hernias intestinal entrapment is infrequent. Intussusception may occur in later weaners and young growers. Torsions may be associated with a change in feeding routines or feeding interruptions such as out of feed events. Therefore, variation in the time of feeding should be avoided, particularly over the weekend in the adult herd. Ensure feeder storage capacity is sufficient for overnight in case of feed delivery interruption.

Intestinal perforation is uncommon but can result in sudden death associated with release of abdominal contents into the peritoneum causing peritonitis (**Figure 4.70**). Hard plastic brush bristles have been found in a few cases. While rare, perforation of the stomach may occur associated with an overdose of NSAIDs.

Other possible causes of a gastrointestinal misplacement are illustrated in **Figures 4.71–4.74**.

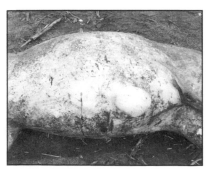

Fig. 4.64 General view of an abdominal twist. The abdomen may be more bloated.

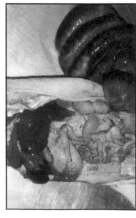

Fig. 4.65 Gross postmortem view of the pig in Figure 4.64 demonstrating the intestinal torsion.

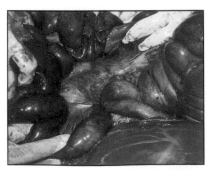

Fig. 4.66 A twist at the mesenteric root.

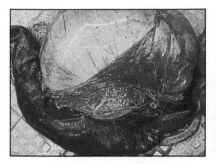

Fig. 4.67 Twist/torsion of the spleen at the greater omentum.

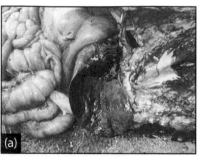

Fig. 4.68 Torsion of the liver lobe. (a) Appearance in the abdomen and (b) the liver laid out. Note the dark congested left lateral liver lobe.

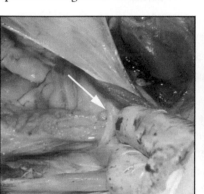

Fig. 4.69 Intestinal entrapment (white arrow) in a scrotal hernia.

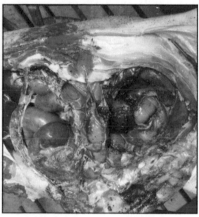

Fig. 4.70 Intestinal perforation.

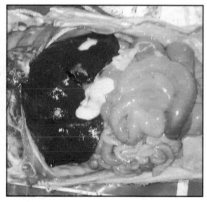

Fig. 4.71 Septic peritonitis. Acute peritonitis associated with abscessation in the peritoneal cavity.

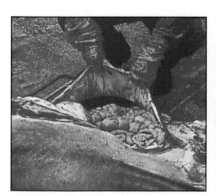

Fig. 4.72 Perforated gastric ulcer. Sudden death, which revealed a large perforating gastric ulcer releasing blood into the peritoneal cavity.

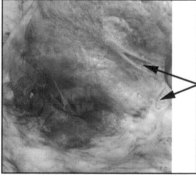

Fig. 4.73 Rupture of the ureterovesical junction. This may occur during mating; the boar enters the urethra rather than the anterior vagina. Tearing of the urethra and ureterovesical junction (arrows) occurs, with the sow dying due to haemorrhage and/or gangrene.

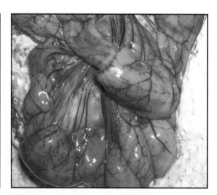

Fig. 4.74 Intussusception where one piece of intestine has invaginated (folded into) into another section of intestine.

Ascaris white spot liver ▶ VIDEO 13

Definition/aetiology

White spot liver is associated with the migratory phase of the large round worm *Ascaris suum*. The adult worm is large; the female is 20–40 cm long and the male slightly shorter at 15–20 cm with a curled tail. An adult female lives about 6 months. The adult female may lay 2 million eggs per day but egg production is extremely variable day on day. The eggs are very infective. The eggs are extremely sticky and will be easily transported onto the farm by pigs, insects, birds and equipment. Workers' boots are a significant means of spread of *A. suum* around the farm. They are extremely resistant and can survive for more than 7 years in the environment. Generally, disinfectants have little effect on the eggs. However, steam cleaning and direct sunlight will kill the eggs.

   A. suum has a typical roundworm life cycle (**Figure 4.75**, *Table 4.7*).

Clinical presentation

A. suum can affect any age of pig, although the adult worm is only seen in post-weaned pigs as it takes 15 days for the development of an adult.

   Ascaris larvae migrate through the lung but, usually, the pulmonary migration is without incident.

Table 4.7 **The life cycle of *Ascaris suum*.**

DAY	
Zero	Egg + L2 stage ingested and swallowed L3 hatch from egg in intestines
2–3	L3 penetrate intestinal wall and migrate to liver L3 develop in liver L3 migrate from liver to lung
3–7	L3 leave lung, coughed up and swallowed
8–10	L3 develop to L4 in intestines
10–15	Young adults develop
21–30	Eggs are passed
10	L1 develop in 10 days
13–18	L2 develop in 13–18 days
	Pre-patent period 40–52 days

This phase may result in an asthmatic cough and the pig may have problems breathing. Ascarids may exacerbate other pneumonic conditions, especially swine influenza. There are normally no clinical signs. In heavy or acute infestation there may be some reduction in growth rates due to competition between pig and worm for food. In severe cases this can be a 10% increase in food conversion ratio (FCR).

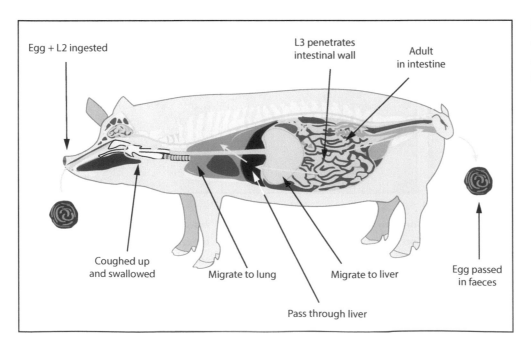

Fig. 4.75 The direct life cycle of *Ascaris suum* in the pig.

Egg + L2 ingested

L3 penetrates intestinal wall

Adult in intestine

Coughed up and swallowed

Migrate to lung

Migrate to liver

Egg passed in faeces

Pass through liver

In young weaned pigs there may be severe infestations associated with an acute massive infestation and this may result in intestinal blockage, rupture and death.

White spot (milk spot) liver

The normal economic concern of *A. suum* is the loss of liver in the slaughterhouse associated with the surface hepatic scarring associated with migration of the L3 larvae through the liver. These lesions are transient and the liver will completely heal within 25 days. The liver in a finishing pig is about 1.5% of the body weight.

Differential diagnosis

Stephanurus dentatus (kidney worm) in the early stages may result in a 'milk spot' liver. In later stages the liver damage is much more severe than *A. suum* involvement.

Diagnosis

Diagnosis of infestation with *A. suum* is made by the presence of the adult worm(s), which may be seen in the faeces or hanging from the anus, especially following worm treatment of the herd (**Figures 4.76, 4.77**). At post-mortem it may be possible to see adults in the intestinal lumen (**Figure 4.78**). It is very rare for a single resident worm to be seen. In weaners and young growing pigs, massive infestation of the intestinal lumen with adult worms may be rarely seen. The recent presence of the larval worm may be seen at post-mortem with characteristic lesions within the liver. Lesions of 'white spot' on the liver develop within days of infestation (**Figure 4.79**). However, they heal within 25 days. In the lung the recent presence of the L3 larvae may be indicated by small lesions, although these are easier to recognise as incidental findings on histology of the lung (**Figure 4.80**).

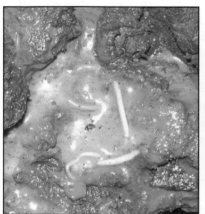

Fig. 4.76 Adult worms seen after worming the pig.

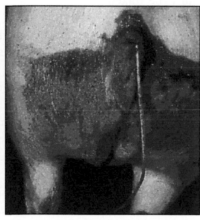

Fig. 4.77 *Ascaris suum* being passed from the anus.

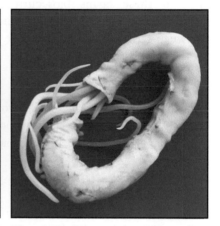

Fig. 4.78 Heavy worm infestation in the intestine – seen at slaughter in a 40 kg pig.

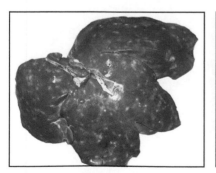

Fig. 4.79 'White spot' in the liver – severe case.

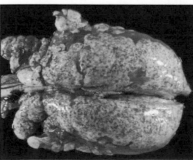

Fig. 4.80 Pig lung affected by *Ascaris suum* larvae migration. Lack of collapse typical of interstitial pneumonia (of granulomatous type in this case) and multiple haemorrhages due to larvae migration. Also, there is pulmonary cranioventral consolidation.

Laboratory diagnosis may be made during a worm egg count of the faeces or intestinal contents. Worm eggs are seen during faecal examination using the flotation technique. *Ascaris* eggs require ZnSO$_4$ flotation; normal sugar solution will not work. In addition, they may still be difficult to find as the production by the female is sporadic (see Worm egg count).

Management

Many anthelmintics work against *Ascaris* larvae and adults. The problem with treatment is the rapid reinfestation and the liver lesions heal within 25 days, with the result that medicine withdrawal times may preclude their use prior to slaughter. The adult worm in the gut also inhibits the development of future larval migration.

Specific *A. suum*-negative farms

In Australia some farms may be negative to *A. suum* and in these farms biosecurity must be taken extremely seriously; foot wear must not be moved between farms. Pathogen-negative farms elsewhere in the world are very unlikely.

Zoonotic implications

The human *Ascaris lumbricoides* worm is a separate species. There are no serious zoonotic implications. However, *A. suum* rarely may be found in children.

Clostridium difficile

Definition/aetiology

Clostridium difficile can be isolated from the intestines of scouring piglets that have often been pre-treated with antimicrobials.

Clinical presentation

In most pigs there are no clinical signs. If clinical signs are seen, they will become apparent in piglets before 21 days of age. The piglet presents with a yellow pasty diarrhoea that appears to be unresponsive to many antibiotics. Yellow pasty diarrhoea is extremely common in this age group (**Figure 4.81**). The piglets may present with a mild abdominal distension. In uncastrated males there might be scrotal oedema.

Differential diagnosis

Other causes of pre-weaning diarrhoea in piglets including *Escherichia coli*, transmissible gastroenteritis (TGE), rotavirus, porcine epidemic diarrhoea (PED) and *C. perfringens* A and C. Disease associated with *C. difficile* is often triggered by environment failings and therefore the ventilation system should be checked for chilling draughts. Review other causes of pre-weaning diarrhoea which have been discussed earlier in the chapter.

Diagnosis

At post-mortem, classic cases will present with mesocolonic oedema and fluid intestinal contents (**Figure 4.82**). Note the lack of other findings to help make the diagnosis. Microscopic examination demonstrates acute multifocal, diffuse erosive colitis with large gram-positive rods on the mucosa. It is important to detect the toxins to *C. difficile* before determining the relevance of an isolation.

Management

Treatment of individual litters: Supportive therapy. *C. difficile* is resistant to penicillin type antibiotics. Provide pain management as appropriate.

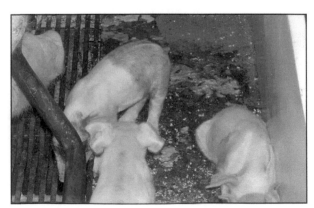

Fig. 4.81 Four-day-old piglets with a pasty diarrhoea associated with *C. difficile*.

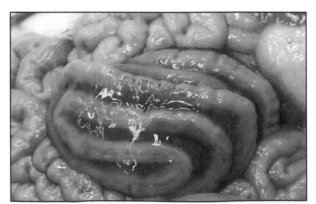

Fig. 4.82 Post-mortem findings of liquid intestinal contents and moderate oedema of the colonic loops.

Control on a herd basis: Review antimicrobial treatment programmes. In many cases note the previous possible overuse of antimicrobials. Initiate a feedback programme of piglet faeces and intestines of affected piglets to sows, especially parity 1, at 6 and 3 weeks pre-farrowing. If there is sufficient material, also introduce feedback materials to gilts in acclimatisation.

Zoonotic implications

C. difficile may cause serious problems in children and immunocompromised individuals.

Clostridial enteritis
Definition/aetiology
Clostridium perfringens is mainly type C and A, but occasionally other serotypes. While the problem is seen in all farming systems it is more often seen in outside/pasture farrowing accommodation, especially if the land has been used to farm sheep within the last couple of years, as the clostridial spores are very resistant. Clostridial organisms are very common in the environment.

Clinical presentation
With *C. perfringens* C, normal clinical presentations are acute (sudden death), subacute and chronic disease in piglets. Acute *C. perfringens* C is usually seen in piglets <3 days of age and the piglet's anus is often bright red. The intestines will be a fiery red with frank haemorrhage in the small intestine. Other piglets in the litter are very weak and pale. Subacute or chronic *C. perfingens* C presents with pasty diarrhoea lasting 2–4 days and the piglets often bloat before recovering. On necropsy, the intestine will be thickened and contain shreds of adherent material attached to it.

With *C. perfingens* A, the diarrhoea may be intermittent. Over time the piglets become emaciated but can remain active and alert. Eventually some piglets die.

Differential diagnosis
In the younger piglet with blood filled intestines, consider thrombocytopenia and other neonatal blood disorders. Trauma from the sow is common. In the older piglet/weaner with necrotic enteritis, consider coccidiosis and salmonellosis.

Diagnosis
Diagnosis is made on clinical signs and necropsy. At post-mortem, affected younger piglets present with their intestines full of blood (**Figure 4.83**) and gas bubbles may occur on the serosal surface; older piglets present with a chronic thickened enteritis (**Figure 4.84**). If the problem occurs post weaning, it can result in a thick diphtheritic membrane of chronic necrotic enteritis. Identification of clostridial organisms in the intestinal tract using a Gram stain is often possible.

Management
Treatment of affected piglets and littermates can be attempted by oral or injectable antibiotics that have

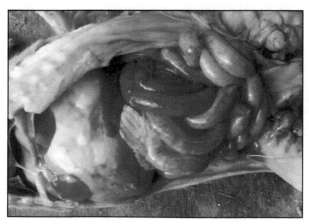

Fig. 4.83 Acute haemorrhagic enteritis in a 3-day-old piglet.

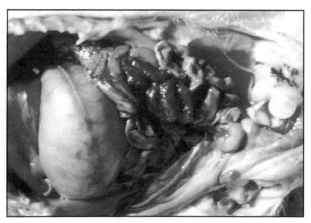

Fig. 4.84 Chronic enteritis with a thickened bowel. Note the intestines have gas bubbles visible on their surface.

demonstrated efficacy against clostridia. Provide pain management as appropriate.

Control of clinical signs in a herd involves practicing AIAO pig flow and effective farrowing house cleaning programmes. Vaccinate sows and gilts against clostridial organisms. Commercial vaccines do not contain *C. perfringens* A; however, autogenous vaccines can be made. Vaccines tend to be more effective against *C. perfringens* C and less effective against *C. perfringens* A. Inclusion of zinc bacitracin or virginiamycin in the diet 3 weeks pre-farrowing and in lactation is effective in reducing particularly *C. perfringens* C and to a lesser extent *C. perfringens* A shedding in the sow.

Coccidiosis (piglets)

Definition/aetiology

Coccidiosis is common in suckling piglets associated with infestation of the small intestine with the coccidial parasite *Cystoisospora suis* (**Figure 4.85**). Sows usually do not have *C. suis* but have other non-pathogenic coccidia (i.e. *Eimeria* spp.). It is possible to differentiate between these two different coccidial organisms microscopically as *Cystoisospora* oocysts contain two merozoites whereas *Eimeria* oocysts contain four (**Figure 4.86**). *Cystoisospora suis* is extremely common worldwide.

Oocysts are resistant to drying and most disinfectants and survive well in farrowing house environments. Infection from the sow plays only a small part in the pathogenesis. Most piglets are infected by oocysts carried over from previous litters. The oocyst infects young piglets by mouth with relatively heavy infestations needed to cause clinical disease.

Subclinical disease can be significant. After ingestion, the organisms move down to the small intestines where they invade the mucosa. In successive stages of a complex life cycle, they emerge from the wall at 5–9 days and again at 11–14 days after infection, and it is this emergence that causes diarrhoea (i.e. before the development of the oocyst) because of tissue damage.

The life cycle of coccidiosis in pigs is shown in **Figure 4.87**.

Clinical presentation

The incubation period is most commonly 3–5 days. The piglet may present with vomiting initially and then diarrhoea between 7 and 15 days of age. If the exposure dose is very high, the piglets can exhibit clinical signs within 48 hours. The diarrhoea ranges from white to pasty cream faeces through to a yellow watery scour. Over time, piglets with a significant infestation tend to be in poor condition, are hairy and grow more slowly than other piglets within the litter. Notably, a decline in weaning weights (0.5 kg at 28 days) is often the initial clinical sign.

In acute cases, mortality rates may reach 20%. Once the piglet starts with diarrhoea the intestinal wall is already damaged and treatment will not work effectively. In most cases, however, mortality is relatively low. Since *C. suis* is a protozoan, the diarrhoea is not responsive to antibiotic therapy.

Piglets that survive often become unthrifty finishers. A failure to recognise the disease leads to increased farrowing house mortality, poorer weaning weights and increased post-weaning problems.

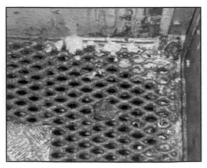

Fig. 4.85 Coccidial diarrhoea from piglets 14 days of age.

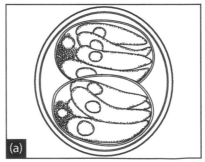
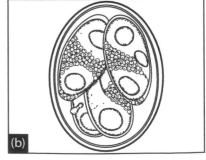

Fig. 4.86 Differentiation between (a) *Cystoisospora* (two merozoites within the oocyst) and (b) *Eimeria* (four merozoites within the oocyst).

Fig. 4.87
The life cycle of
Cystoisospora suis.

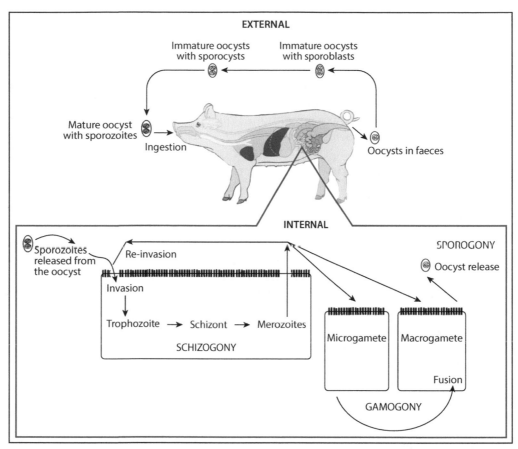

Differential diagnosis

Other causes of pre-weaning diarrohea, including *E. coli* and *C. perfringens*, and stress-induced diarrhoea, especially associated with draughts. In the post-weaning period, iron deficiency may exhibit similar signs.

Diagnosis

Diagnosis can be made through identification of the merozoite on intestinal scrapings or through faecal flotation. On necropsy, lesions vary from no gross lesions to a diphtheritic membrane in the jejunum or ileum. Steatorrhoea (increased fat in faeces) may be seen. Sometimes there is catarrhal enteritis. Identification of an inflamed section of the small intestine improves the success of diagnostic confirmation of merozoites. Coccidial oocysts are only excreted in the faeces long after the clinical disease has passed, so in the acute phase of the infestation faecal examination may be unrewarding.

Management

Treatment of affected litters: Treatment is supportive with electrolytes. Provide pain management as appropriate. Where possible, provide extra bedding, which might be shredded paper in controlled environments. This increases the heat to the piglets and reduces the effects of draughts. Stop creep feeding. Treat with an oral preparation of toltrazuril (or ponazuril) (7 mg/kg orally given at 4 days of age). This can make the pigs vomit. Sulpha-antibiotic medicines may also be used as treatment, although they are less effective than toltrazuril.

Control in a herd: Practice batch management and AIAO and ensure that the farrowing room pre-farrowing cleaning and preparation protocols are followed. Unless absolutely necessary, cease cross-fostering after 48 hours of age. Do not enter pens unless necessary. Prevent carryover of oocysts from previous litters by cleaning the farrowing house with an oocide disinfectant. Sows should be washed before entering the farrowing house. Enhance batch biosecurity by using separate coloured and numbered brushes, forks, shovels in each farrowing room/batch. Control flies as they may 'walk' the *Cystoisospora* between batches. Reduce draughts and other environmental stress factors. Oral administration of toltrazuril is highly effective as a prevention. Typically, piglets are dosed at or before 4 days of age.

Colonic spirochaetosis

Definition/aetiology

Colonic spirochaetosis (brachyspira colitis) is associated with a variety of species of *Brachyspira*, the most significant of which is *Brachyspira pilosicoli*. Pigs are infected by faecal–oral transmission. The organism causes intestinal mucosal damage and inflammation, resulting in enteritis/colitis reducing the surface area of the large intestine available, thus reducing the absorptive capacity of the intestine and the efficiency of feed utilisation. The large intestine is critical for absorption of fluids and nutrients and disruption will result in diarrhoea. Damage to the intestinal wall may also aid proliferation of other pathogens.

Clinical presentation

The organism is common/normal and generally results in no or few clinical signs. The condition classically affects 10–20-week-old grow/finish pigs (30–90 kg liveweight).

The clinical signs are more common 10–14 days after mixing and change of feed (i.e. to the grower diet or a pelleted diet). The incubation period is 6–14 days. In clinical cases a non-fatal wasting diarrhoea occurs in the growing pigs (**Figure 4.88**). In a group, about 50% of pigs may show transient to persistent watery to mucoid green to brownish diarrhoea without blood. The faeces resembles a cow pat. This will result in an increased days to finish and an increase in the FCR.

Brachyspira pilosicoli occurs in numerous other hosts such as dogs, mice, birds, guinea pigs, primates and probably also humans, although in man this might be a different type.

Differential diagnosis

Swine dysentery (*Brachyspira hyodysenteriae*), salmonellosis, TGE, PED, ileitis (porcine intestinal adenomatosis [PIA]), intestinal parasites (*Trichuris suis* or *C. suis*).

Diagnosis

Reviewing the health and feed usage records may be suggestive of a colitis problem. Focus the investigation on the time when the diet changes.

At post-mortem examination the colon and large intestine may demonstrate areas of liquid contents (catharral typhlo-colitis) (**Figure 4.89**). The spiral colon contains abundant watery green or yellow mucoid and frothy contents. Erosions in the colonic mucosa may be evident. Histological analysis by silver stains will reveal the *Brachyspria*.

Bacteriological culture will be needed for a positive diagnosis. Samples need to be transported in a media such as Amies transport media. Polymerase chain reaction (PCR) can identify the organism, but note that the organism is normal in most herds. Histopathology can confirm the tissue involvement.

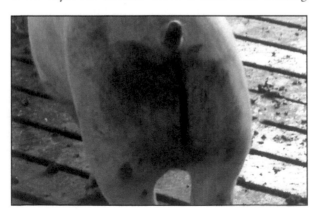

Fig. 4.88 Brachyspira colitis.

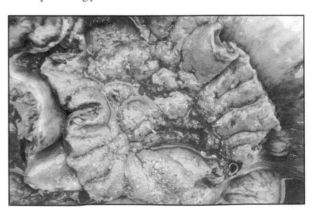

Fig. 4.89 Opened colon associated with colitis.

Management

Treatment of clinically affected groups: Reduce the number of subclinically infected carriers by treatment with antimicrobial therapy in both water and feed. Tiamulin fumerate is a useful antimicrobial. Provide pain management as appropriate. Reduce environmental contamination by improved sanitation.

Control at a farm level: Move towards an AIAO programme by batching. Reduce concurrent causes of enteritis/colitis. Eliminate all draughts and chilling. Reduce manure contamination of the pens. Enhance biosecurity by reducing access to wildlife, birds and rodents.

It is not practical to eliminate the organism, but it is essential to reduce the stressors to a level that the pigs will become non-clinical.

Zoonotic implications

It is possible that the disease may be similar to human colonic inflammation and may therefore have a human health significance.

Non-specific colitis

Definition/aetiology

By definition, non-specific colitis has no identifiable causal agent. The condition is more commonly seen in fast growing pigs on high density diets. Suspected causes are associated with the presence of trypsin inhibitors in peas, beans and soya. If there is an issue with fat quality, this may lead to diarrhoea. Where there is a fat quality issue there may also be a vitamin E shortage.

Clinical presentation

Diarrhoea can occur within hours of consuming a new batch of pelleted feed and it can dramatically cease within hours of the removal of the suspect feed. Nutrition, infectious agents and draughts are considered to be important factors. The problem classically will occur anytime in the nursery to finishing stage (20–110 kg) but most commonly in the early phase (25–30 kg).

In severe cases, the diarrhoea can have evidence of blood or mucus (**Figure 4.90**). There is a decrease in growth rates and increase in FCR. The problem may occur in pigs introduced to a new water supply with more than 1,500 ppm salt (NaCl). The problem normally last 3–5 days while the pigs acclimatise to the new water supply.

Differential diagnosis

Other causes of post-weaning diarrhoea.

Diagnosis

At post-mortem, the colon and small intestine may demonstrate areas of both acute and chronic inflammation (**Figure 4.91**). The spiral colon contains abundant watery green or yellow mucoid and frothy contents. In some cases there may be no gross lesions. The pig may present with raised rugae in the inside of the large bowel but few other lesions. Diagnosis can be based on the clinical signs and absence of other specific organisms.

Management

To treat and control an outbreak of colitis the farm health team needs to improve the environment.

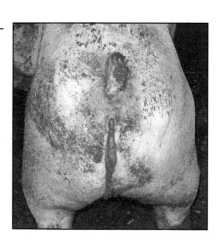
Fig. 4.90 Non-specific colitis.

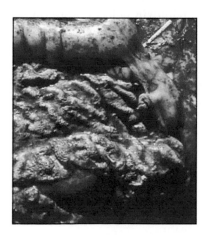
Fig. 4.91 Non-specific colitis findings at post-mortem.

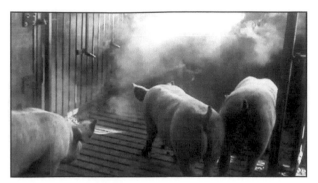

Fig. 4.92 **Checking for draughts using smoke.**

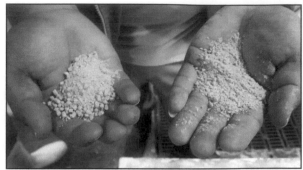

Fig. 4.93 **Poor quality pellet.**

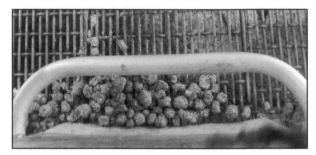

Fig. 4.94 **Constipation in the periparturient sow.**

Do not place pigs into buildings that are damp and cold. Check for and remove chilling draughts (**Figure 4.92**). Review the farm's batching programme to ensure that the stocking rate is correct and establish an AIAO programme. Check and clean the water supply. Ensure the correct pigs (i.e. weight and age) are placed in the building. If the feed is pelleted, change the feed to a meal (**Figure 4.93**). Some pellet quality can be very poor and the feed manufacturing programme may need to be reviewed.

Constipation

Constipation in sows is a particular problem in the periparturient phase, resulting in difficulties with parturition and subsequent milk production, especially of colostrum. The sow presents with small hard round pellets of faeces (**Figure 4.94**). These can become impacted in the rectum, reducing the available space in the pelvis and thus increasing the risk of stillborn piglets. The constipation reduces gut motility, which increases the absorption of endotoxin from gram-negative cell death. The absorbed endotoxin reduces prolactin production thus reducing milk output, which can appear as agalactia.

Check the water supply, reduce the periparturient feed intake and provide additional fibre (e.g. 0.5 kg bran in the diet), and exercise the sow. If a sow stops the farrowing process, consider allowing her to walk around; sometime defecation is required to clear the rectum of faeces.

In the pet pig, constipation can be extremely severe, resulting in impaction of the colon, which may be life-threatening. Medicate with enemas and oral laxatives such as mineral oil or magnesium oxide (5 g/100 kg) to soften the faeces.

If the pig is very dehydrated, several litres of fluid may be administer per-rectum.

Escherichia coli – overview
Introduction

Escherichia coli is an extremely important bacteria when considering the health of pigs. The majority of serotypes are beneficial and even vital for the normal function of the pig. However, a few strains are also associated with a variety of conditions from toxaemia in very young pigs, diarrhoea pre- and post-weaning and, in the adult sow, cystitis and mastitis.

How does an organism like *E. coli* cause disease?
Toxins: The bacteria can produce toxins that can modify its environment.

Exotoxins: Exotoxins are are produced by the live bacteria and are released into the environment. The exotoxins important in the pathogenesis of diarrhoea are:

• Heat-labile toxins (LT). There are two major types: LTI and LTII.
• Heat-stable toxins (ST). There are two major types: STa and STb.

- Enteroaggregative toxin (EAST1).
- Shiga-like toxin type II variant (SLT-IIe), also known as Stx2e or verotoxin oedema disease principle. These toxins act on the walls of the small arteries causing arteritis and resulting in oedema. The Stx2e toxin is a vasotoxin causing microangiopathy, leakage from the capillary vessels, which results in oedema due to the venous blood pressure increasing to 20 mmHg, resulting in oedema of the brain and neurological signs. This can create a toxic shock syndrome.
- Haemolysin toxins. Haemolysin toxins rupture erythrocytes and release iron, which the bacteria can use for reproduction. Many of the pathogenic *E. coli* are iron deficient and require an iron-rich environment. They therefore create a zone of β haemolysis on a blood agar plate (see basic intestinal bacteriology at the beginning of the chapter).

Endotoxins: The cell wall is referred to as O antigen. These endotoxins, which are made from the lipid polysaccharides of the cell wall, are released into the environment of the dying bacteria. In the gut, the toxins can be absorbed and result in a reduction in hormone production (e.g. prolactin in the periparturient sow). When in the air, dead bacteria and the resultant endotoxins are breathed in and the endotoxins can interfere with the action of the mucociliary escalator and affect bronchoconstriction, both reducing respiratory function.

Fimbriae: These are referred to as F antigens (previously K antigens) (**Figures 4.95, 4.96**): for example, F1, F4 (K88), F5(K99), F18 (F107), F6 (987P), F41 and FP. There are likely to be thousands of fimbriae types.

- F4 and F5 are important attachment fimbriae for enterotoxigenic *E. coli* (ETEC).
- F18 is the specific fimbriae found in *E. coli* associated with bowel oedema/oedema disease. There are pigs that are resistant to F4 because they have no attachment sites.
- F1 is a mannose sensitive attachment that is very common in *E. coli*, especially those involved in urinary tract conditions. Unfortunately, the immune system recognises β-mannans as potential pathogenic invaders and will divert food resources to mount an immune response. While this is useful to protect against bacteria such as *E. coli*, the body can also mount the same response towards plant food sources, especially soya containing high concentrations of β-mannans, and thus reduces their feeding value. Enzymes are available to digest these β-mannans into smaller sugars, which do not initiate an immune response.
- FP is present in some *E. coli* serotypes found in pyelonephritis cases in man and occasionally pigs.

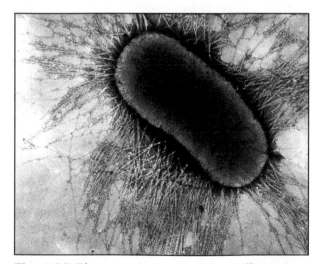

Fig. 4.95 Electron micrograph of *E. coli* illustrating the fimbriae.

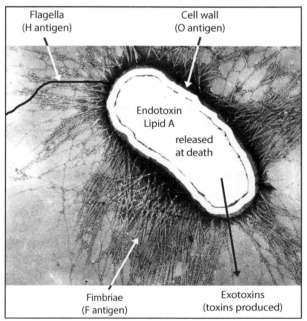

Fig. 4.96 Drawing of the major features of *E. coli*.

Flagellae: Some *E. coli* have the ability to create flagellae and if present, these are referred to as H antigens. The H antigens are not used to classify *E. coli*.

Capsule: Escherichia coli is surrounded by a capsule and this is referred to as the K antigen. Prior to the discovery of fimbriae this was a major classification distinction of *E. coli*. However, as fimbriae were discovered many of the 'K' antigens were reclassified as 'F'; for example, K88 became F4.

Thus the many thousands of different *E. coli* organisms can be classified; for example, *E. coli* O147, F4, F5. Its cell wall is classified as O147 and it has two significant fimbriae – F4 and F5. It may have many other fimbriae but they are not considered clinically significant.

Understanding this code is important in selection of the correct vaccine. However, there are still many strains of *E. coli* that will be isolated from the pig that cannot be typed by these methods.

How can *Escherichia coli* interact with the host cells

Various words are used to describe the pathogenic interactions of *E. coli* bacteria and the host:

- Enterotoxigenic *E. coli* (ETEC). This is a type of *E. coli* that produces enterotoxins. In order for the toxins to be effective the bacteria must attach to the surface of the enterocyte or the adjacent mucous layer. This attachment is made by the fimbriae.
- Enteropathogenic *E. coli* (EPEC). This is a type of *E. coli* that injects its toxins into the enterocyte. This involves a more intimate contact with the enterocyte. This is referred to as attaching and effacing lesion.
- Enteroinvasive *E. coli* (EIEC). This type penetrates through the enterocyte barrier, enters the blood stream and become systemic.
- Enteroadherent *E. coli* (EagEC). These bacteria adhere to the enterocyte.
- Enterohaemorrhagic *E. coli* (EHEC). These bacteria invade through the enterocyte barrier, resulting in haemorrhage.
- ExPEC – Extraintestinal pathogenic *E. coli*, for example with the P fimbriae affecting the urinary tract.

- STEC (or VTEC) – *Escherichia coli* which produce Shiga toxins. For example F18 bowel oedema *E. coli*.

Escherichia coli – pre- and post-weaning diarrhoea

Definition/aetiology

Diarrhoea in young pigs is often associated with *E. coli*. They are members of the family Enterobacteriaceae and are gram-negative rods/bacilli. *Escherichia coli* is a lactose fermenter and this allows easy differentiation from *Salmonella* spp., another significant cause of diarrhoea in young pigs. *Escherichia coli* are not significant pathogens in pigs older than 10 weeks of age. They are also a normal part of the microflora of the intestine. Many pathogenic *E. coli* are haemolytic and this can be used as part of the initial screening for the cause of the diarrhoea. Many *E. coli* organisms may even provide part of the microbiota protective screen for the pig.

Most *E. coli* problems are associated with management and environmental factors, in particular chilling draughts and sanitation. Examination of the environment is an essential component to any diagnosis. *Escherichia coli* diarrhoea is more prevalent in parity 1 litters.

Piglets with inadequate blood iron at weaning have an increased risk of post-weaning diarrhoea.

Clinical presentation

Escherichia coli can play a role in diarrhoea in the pig in three distinct phases.

0–3 days of age: Piglets present with watery yellow diarrhoea and often sudden death (**Figure 4.97**).

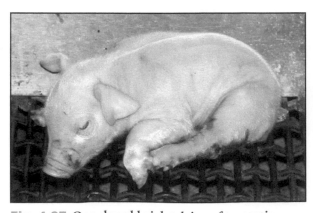

Fig. 4.97 **One-day-old piglet dying of toxaemia.**

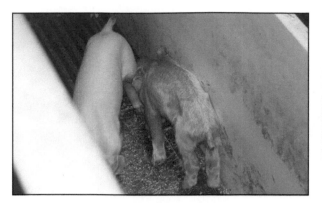

Fig. 4.98 Four-day-old piglet with diarrhoea.

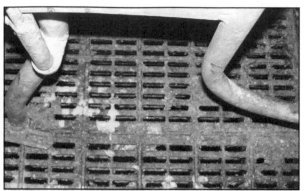

Fig. 4.99 Diarrhoea associated with *E. coli*.

4–10 days of age: Piglets present with a pasty yellow coloured faeces (**Figures 4.98, 4.99**). In the early stages of the clinical signs some vomiting may also be recognised. Piglets may be found dead, but most have clinical signs that lead to dehydration and ultimately death. If diarrhoea occurs after day 10 but before weaning, coccidiosis should be considered as part of the differential diagnosis.

Post weaning (normally starts 3–5 days post weaning): Pigs present with both acute and chronic diarrhoea (**Figures 4.100, 4.101**). The diarrhoea progressively leads to dehydration and death. Weaners may demonstrate ill thrift.

Differential diagnosis

Other causes of diarrhoea in piglets including *C. perfringens* A and rotavirus, PED, TGE and coccidiosis.

Diagnosis

There may be very few gross pathological findings. The small intestines, which are fluid filled, will be dilated and swollen. Sometimes congestion of the stomach or small intestines may be seen (**Figures 4.102, 4.103**). The intestinal contents will be alkaline while with viral diarrhoea the contents will be more acidic.

As soon as diarrhoea starts, submit rectal swabs and intestinal contents or tissues. If diarrhoea continues, submit live piglets before treatment (**Figure 4.104**).

Management

Treatment of individual litters and piglets: Treat the whole litter as soon as one piglet starts to show clinical signs. Place a trough drinker filled with water, electrolytes and glucose. In emergencies the use of cola drinks or lemonade may also be very beneficial. This must be replaced at least four times daily.

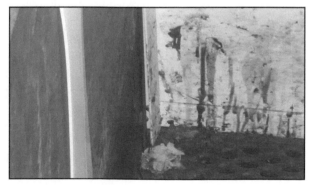

Fig. 4.100 Diarrhoea in post-weaned pigs. Note the faecal staining on the walls.

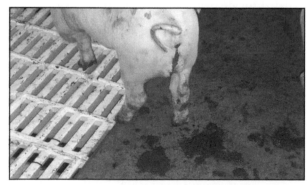

Fig. 4.101 The loose yellow/grey stools characteristic of diarrhoea associated with *E. coli* infection post weaning.

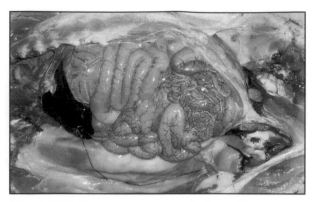

Fig. 4.102 Gross post-mortem findings. Congested small intestines and dilated large intestine full of fluid.

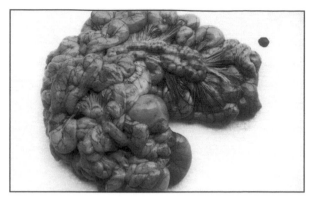

Fig. 4.103 Gross post-mortem findings. Congested and dilated small intestines.

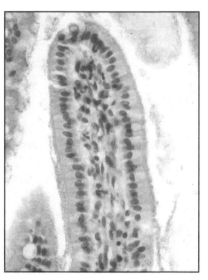

Fig. 4.104 Histological changes in an enterotoxigenic *E. coli* infection. Note the adherent bacteria.

Keep the bowl clean. Do not allow the bowl to become a toilet. If creep feed is being provided, remove the feed immediately.

Administer antimicrobial oral preparations once a day. Provide pain management as appropriate.

If the piglets have other clinical signs on top of the diarrhoea, in addition to oral treatment, inject with a suitable antimicrobial. Syringes or oral dosers must not be used on a sick piglet and then on a healthy piglet.

Clean up the diarrhoea as soon as possible with paper and use this material as part of the herd natural planned immunisation programme, especially for parity 1, at 6 and 3 weeks pre-farrowing. The use of medicated drying products pre-weaning directly onto the piglets can be beneficial. Take care not to get the drying agent into the piglet's eye. Potato starch can be very useful.

Stockpersons should wash their hands after treating the piglets and dip their boots in disinfectant. Ideally, wear gloves and have different boots for each affected room/batch. Each brush and shovel should be placed in disinfectant when not in use. Ensure disinfectant is still active.

Ensure that the rooms are thoroughly cleaned between batches. Consider lime washing ($CaCO_3$) to enhance hygiene and disinfection.

Control: Colostrum management is the key to management of *E. coli* diarrhoea. Review colostrum availability and adopt split suckling programmes with large litters.

Vaccines containing the common strains are highly effective in reducing *E. coli* pre-weaning diarrhoea. With parity 1 sows, primary and booster vaccinations will be required as an initial course. Normally, this is administered at 6 and 3 weeks pre-farrowing. Once these sows have been vaccinated, single booster vaccinations at 3 weeks pre-farrowing are all that is recommended.

Immune stabilisation (natural planned exposure/feedback) programmes are generally required to stabilise the farm's pre-weaning diarrhoea problems. This is administered to gilts at 6 and 3 weeks pre-farrowing using diarrhoea materials recovered from the farrowing house. However, once the farm becomes stable there is a shortage of material to use to achieve adequate immune stabilisation. Faecal material may be obtained post-weaning if the nursery is on the same farm.

Practice AIAO pig flow and review the batching programme. Ensure that the rooms are thoroughly clean before pigs enter the building. Pressure

Fig. 4.105
Colour code
each batch.

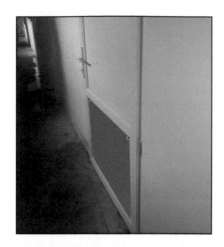

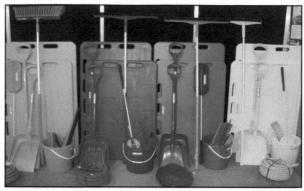

Fig. 4.106 **Different coloured equipment can be used for different batches/rooms of pigs.**

washing principles must be exemplary. Practice lime washing if possible.

Utensil movement and batch biosecurity protocols must be reviewed. All batches and rooms should have their own coloured and numbered brush and shovel (**Figures 4.105, 4.106**). With 3-week batches and 28-day weaning there will be two batches of lactating sows; with 1-week batch and 28-days weaning there will be five batches of lactating sows. Five-week batches utilise all the farm's farrowing places at one time (see Chapter 11).

All processing equipment (e.g. tattooing, notching and tail docking equipment) must be thoroughly cleaned between batches and rooms. Teeth clipping should cease.

Cross-fostering is a major cause of pre-weaning diarrhoea. Piglet movements must be carefully monitored. Review cross-fostering protocols and ideally stop cross-fostering after 1 day.

If diarrhoea is a persistent problem, have the environment examined in detail (e.g. for chilling draughts). Examine heat light/mat protocols and ensure that they are working within prescribed limits. Ensure preventive protocols are adhered to (i.e. vaccination and feed-back).

Genetic modification of the breeding stock may be considered; for example, F4 genetically resistant pigs are available but are not used commercially.

Zoonotic implications
E. coli has the potential to infect people.

Escherichia coli – bowel oedema/oedema disease
Definition/aetiology
E. coli with the Shiga toxin (STx2e) causes bowel or gut oedema (oedema disease). Normally, the bacteria has the F18 (rarely F4) fimbriae attachment. The *E. coli* is β haemolytic and is transmitted from pig to pig via the faecal–oral route. The Stx2e toxin is a vasotoxin causing microangiopathy resulting in leakage from the capillary vessels and so producing oedema. Venous pressure increases to 20 mmHg, resulting in oedema of the brain and neurological signs (see Chapter 5 for more details).

Gastric (stomach) ulceration
Definition/aetiology
Pigs with an ulceration of the *pars oesophageal* portion of their stomach. Stomach ulcers are very common and can occur in any age group. The condition can occur in 100% of groups of pigs with an incidence of 50% of sows and 60% of growers being common.

Stomach ulcers are often associated with feed interruption. Pigs that do not eat are very likely to develop stomach ulcers. Many stomach ulcers are perpetuated by (not caused by) stress/psychological effects, in particular transportation, crowding and mixing with unfamiliar pigs.

Once the ulcer is present, its healing can be complicated by the number of small particles in the feed below 500 μm (0.5 mm) acting as sandpaper on the ulcer. Pelleting or other feed related issues may also be associated with an increased incidence of stomach ulcers. An increase may be associated with the feeding of whey. Pigs fed with high concentrations of unsaturated fatty acids, especially if there is a vitamin E deficiency, are particularly prone to gastric ulceration. Mycotoxins may also play a role in gastric ulcers. Other factors that have been associated are a low protein diet, a high energy diet and diets containing more than 55% wheat. The wheat type may also have a role as high yielding wheat can have sharp spicules. Other associated conditions may be copper and zinc toxicity.

While bacteria and fungi are often found in association with ulcers, no specific infectious cause has been confirmed in pigs. In people, *Helicobacter pylori* is associated with duodenal ulcers.

Clinical presentation
Peracute: Death or collapse of apparently healthy animals (**Figures 4.107, 4.108**). The animal may be pale or, exceptionally, white.

Acute: Pigs present as weak, pale and wobbly on their legs. May be misdiagnosed as a neurological problem. The animals are anaemic with increased respiration and a cough, resulting in a diagnosis of respiratory disorders, which do not respond to antimicrobial therapy.

The pigs may grind their teeth and wag their tail in pain. Animals lie down and fidget while trying to find a comfortable position. The animal passes bloody tarry faeces (melaena). Vomiting may be noted. The pig is generally anorexic. Rectal temperature is normal; however, if subnormal it generally indicates a poor prognosis.

Chronic: Presents as an extended duration of acute clinical signs with weaker animals. This may be misdiagnosed as pneumonia in growers. In some chronic cases the oesophageal entrance becomes narrow and a stricture occurs. The pigs vomit/regurgitate shortly after feeding and lose weight rapidly.

Subclinical: No clinical signs and the lesion is an incidental finding at post-mortem. However, the chronic loss of blood will weaken the pig and increase the FCR.

Differential diagnosis
Swine dysentery, *Salmonella enterica* serotype *choleraesuis*, ileitis (PIA), torsion of the intestine, warfarin poisoning, copper poisoning and other causes of sudden death.

Diagnosis
A diagnosis can be reached based on clinical signs, which may include digested blood in faeces (melaena). This can be confirmed using a urine dipstick to detect blood. This supposition is then supported by post-mortem findings if the pig dies (**Figures 4.109–4.112**).

In peracute/acute cases the stomach may be filled with dark/black blood, sometimes with a large blood clot. In the more chronic cases there may be black streaks in the stomach contents. The large intestine is full of black tarry faeces. The ulcer varies from mild erosion to a large ulcer with a thickened scarred wall boundary. Chronic ulcers may bleed more than acute ulcers due to capillary blood vessels oozing blood over a long period of time. Acute death is associated with the ulcer invading an underlying large blood vessel.

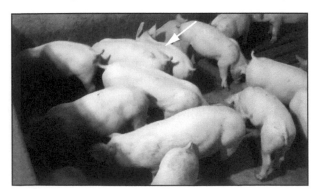

Fig. 4.107 Pale anaemic pig; one in particular is highlighted (arrow).

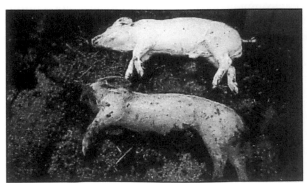

Fig. 4.108 Two dead pigs; the upper one is very white and is likely to have a gastric ulcer.

Fig. 4.109 The normal keratinised oesophageal opening in the pig.

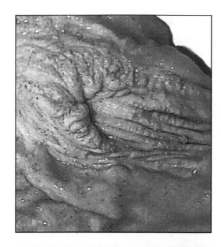

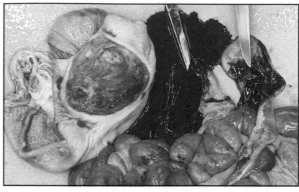

Fig. 4.110 A large chronic gastric ulcer with associated melaena in the large intestine.

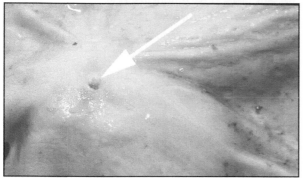

Fig. 4.111 In rare cases the gastric ulcer may heal inappropriately, resulting in a stricture (arrow) at the distal end of the oesophagus.

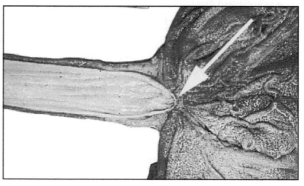

Fig. 4.112 The opened oesophagus and stomach illustrating the stricture.

Examine the feed, especially for particle size (**Figure 4.113**). If the particles are too small, encourage the farm to increase particle size. However, there is a conflict of interest. The farm health team would increase particle size as this may benefit gut health, whereas the farm production team would like to reduce the particle size to reduce FCR.

Management

Treatment of individuals: If individual pigs are recognised before death, get the pig to eat (e.g. use milk/rice/beer mix to encourage eating). Provide pain management as appropriate. Oral treatment with aluminum hydroxide or magnesium silicate can help to line the stomach and protect the ulcer from the stomach acids and thus healing can take place. Feeding straw/hay may help to increase the fibre content and may help to heal the ulcer. In pet pigs H_2 blockers or alternatives may be useful but are unrealistic in commercial situations.

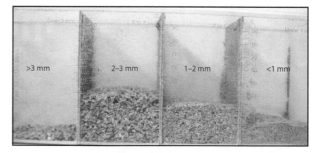

Fig. 4.113 Feed examination of particle size using a Byholm filter, which separates out the various particle sizes. Aim for few very small particles.

Control on a herd basis: Check feed sieve size is not less than 3.5 mm. Ensure that the feed mill is working properly; worn hammers and broken sieves can result in variable feed particle sizes. Increasing the feed particle size to a mean of 750 mm for 2 weeks may help the ulcer to heal. This may be useful to consider for new gilts as part of their introduction/

isolation protocol. Ensure feed is clean and stored appropriately. Reduce stress factors. Increase straw in diet. Vitamin E may be helpful at 100 g/tonne.

Ileitis VIDEOS 20, 21 and 46

Definition/aetiology

Ileitis (PIA, porcine enteropathies) is a thickening of the distal ileum associated with the organism *Lawsonia intracellularis*, an intracellular curved bacterium. The damage and thickening of the ileum results in a reduction of absorption of digesta, poor growth, poor body condition and an increase in FCR. *Lawsonia intracellularis* cannot be grown on normal blood agar.

The disease, even if subclinical, can affect 15–50% of the growing herd. The pigs are infected by oral contact with faeces from infected pigs. The incubation period is 13 days. The pathogen can be shed for at least 10 weeks and probably much longer. Nearly all farms have the organism present on the unit.

Clinically, the problem is recognised to be more severe in herds that are specific pathogen free, such as breeding nucleus and multiplication farms.

Clinical presentation

Normal: The affected pig has no clinical signs.

Peracute/acute

Regional ileitis: The young weaner or grower exhibits severe and rapid weight loss (**Figures 4.114, 4.115**). This may be misdiagnosed as PCV2-SD. Animals with regional ileitis may also present with a terminal peritonitis.

Haemorrhagic proliferative enterophathy: Young adults greater than 70 kg (may be seen in younger pigs). If the pig is peracute or acutely affected the pig may present dead. The hindquarters may be stained with bloody faeces (**Figures 4.116, 4.117**). If alive, it may be depressed, have a reduced appetite and be reluctant to move. There may be watery, grey, dark or bright red diarrhoea. Abortion may occur in recovering animals, often within 6 days of the onset of clinical signs.

Chronic – necrotic enteritis: Growing pigs with severe clinical signs and severe loss of condition and often persistent scour. Death is not uncommon. Major effect is increased FCR and thus feed costs.

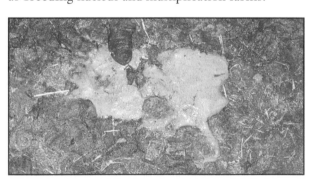

Fig. 4.114 Ileitis diarrhoea – 'cow pat'.

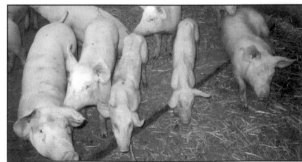

Fig. 4.115 Regional ileitis.

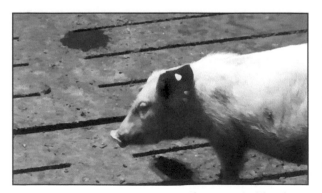

Fig. 4.116 The diarrhoea may also contain blood.

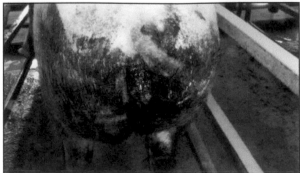

Fig. 4.117 Haemorrhagic proliferative enterophathy.

In chronically affected herds, days to slaughter may be extended by 14 to 30 days.

PIA clinical signs can be very slight with irregular periods of diarrhoea and anorexia. The reduced appetite may in more chronic cases present as retarded growth. The pigs may be very variable in weight (**Figure 4.118**). This may be found at post-mortem in finishing pigs in the slaughterhouse.

Differential diagnosis

Sudden death and haemorrhagic bowel in peracute and acute cases. An intestinal twist, haemorrhagic bowel syndrome (allergic), gastric ulceration, swine dysentery, salmonellosis, whipworms and the various coronavirus diarrhoeas of pigs post weaning may also be differentials.

The major differential of ileitis is swine dysentery. The important differential to remember is that *Brachyspira hyodysenteriae* is a strict anaerobe and therefore lives only in the large bowel. Lesions of swine dysentery are therefore not seen in the small intestine. *L. intracellularis* is microaerophilic and can exist in both the small intestine and the large bowel (caecum and colon) but primarily in the small intestine.

Diagnosis

The ileocaecal ligament is an important structure to identify in the diagnosis of ileitis as it allows the clinician to easily recognise the distal ileum and caecum (see **Figure 4.8**). Post-mortem examination allows the clinician to differentiate the four proliferative enterophathy syndromes.

Regional ileitis: The lower small intestine becomes thickened and ridged, often referred to as hose-pipe gut. Ulceration can be seen in the mucosa (**Figure 4.119**).

Haemorrhagic proliferative enterophathy: The small and large intestines are dilated and filled with a formed blood clot. The colon contains black tarry faeces. The intestinal contents are rarely liquid. The intestines bulge out of the abdomen once opened (**Figure 4.120**).

Necrotic enteritis: There is necrosis of the underlying PIA lesion resulting in a yellow/grey cheesy mass (diphtheritic membrane) that adheres tightly to the intestinal wall (**Figure 4.121**).

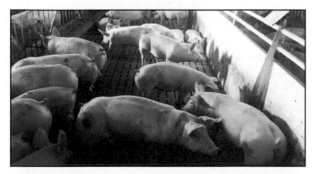

Fig. 4.118 Ileitis resulting in variability in finishing pigs.

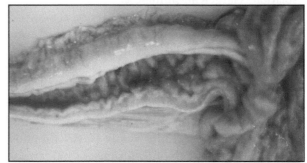

Fig. 4.119 Regional ileitis.

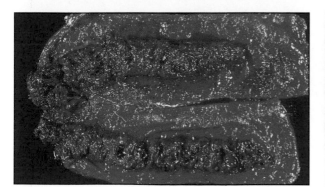

Fig. 4.120 Haemorrhagic proliferative enterophathy.

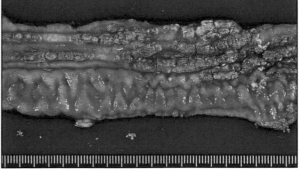

Fig. 4.121 Necrotic enteritis.

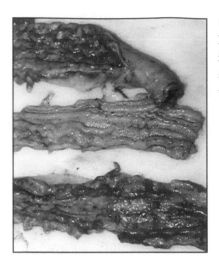

Fig. 4.122
Porcine
intestinal
adenomatosis in
the distal ileum.

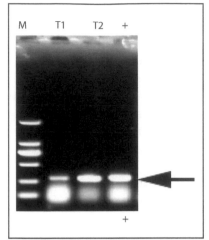

Fig. 4.123
PCR
examination for
the presence of
L. intracellularis.
Both test
samples are
positive.

Porcine intestinal adenomatosis: The intestinal wall thickens, often with oedema to varying degrees. The mucosa is thrown into folds and may result in sharply defined plaques or marked multiple polyp formation (**Figure 4.122**).

The bacterium does not grow in agar based media. Confirmation of the presence of *L. intracellularis* is by PCR analysis of faeces (**Figure 4.123**). However, the organism is normal on most farms and therefore its isolation is largely meaningless.

Histology of the intestine may be useful for a presumptive diagnosis, especially using immunohistochemistry (IHC) or silver staining (**Figure 4.124**).

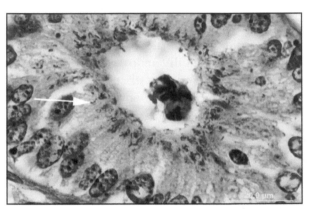

Fig. 4.124 *Lawsonia intracellularis* revealed by IHC. The numerous curved intracellular organisms stained (arrow) can be visualised in the apex of the enterocyte.

Management
Treatment of individual pigs and group: In affected pigs, antimicrobial therapy is very effective. Typical antimicrobials to consider would be tylosin phosphate, valnemulin, tiamulin, lincomycin and tetracyclines. Provide pain management as appropriate.

Control: Vaccines can be effective. Available vaccines are oral or injectable and can be administered to pigs in the farrowing house.

Use AIAO and batch management to reduce variation between batches. Batching helps to minimise mixing of pigs. Maintain appropriate pig density, water and feeder space, building temperature and ventilation. Wash and disinfect pens. Reduce scrape through passageways, which move faeces from one batch to the next. Match the health history of incoming pigs (gilts and boars) to those of the farm.

Zoonotic implications
L. intracellularis has been recognised in other mammals (horses and hares). There are concerns that this may be a pathogen in some chronic intestinal disorders of man.

Porcine epidemic diarrhoea VIDEO 22
Definition/aetiology
PED is caused by a specific enveloped RNA coronavirus. The virus particles are called 'corona' because of their appearance like a sun with the surrounding corona (**Figure 4.125**). The disease is reported in Asia, Europe and North and South America but not in Australia. Clinical signs can be seen in 12 hours or within 5 days of infection. The condition can occur at any time but is more severe in the winter/rainy season. Transmission is via the faecal–oral route.

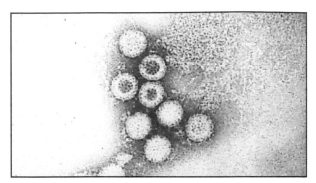

Fig. 4.125 Coronavirus in the electron microscope.

There are two forms of the disease:

- Type 1 affects all age groups including suckling piglets, but the effects are relatively mild and has a short impact on the farm.
- Type 2 affects all age groups with severe clinical signs, especially in piglets.

There are other related coronavirus pathogens such as porcine delta coronavirus. These are not specifically described as their clinical signs are similar but milder than PED. The other major coronavirus to note is TGE virus (TGEV), which is described later in the chapter.

PED is a notifiable condition in some European countries, including the UK, and also in Canada, USA and Australia and New Zealand.

The virus is present in massive numbers, especially in faecal material. The virus appears able to be transmitted up to 10 km airborne making biosecurity difficult as the infection wave moves through a district. However, when an area is threatened all efforts must be made by the whole district to control the spread and clean vehicles between the slaughter-house and finishing farms. Internal biosecurity is essential for eliminating the virus from the farm.

Clinical presentation

Acute: Explosive outbreak of diarrhoea in all age groups. Type 1 may take 10 days to move around the farm. In type 1, the mortality of piglets is between 20 and 80%.

Type 2 moves around the farm within hours. Mortality of piglets less than 10 days of age may be 100% (**Figure 4.126**). The clinical signs are acute vomiting followed by a watery diarrhoea. Piglets rapidly dehydrate and die within 4 days.

Type 1 problems persist for 4–6 weeks whereas type 2 may take 18 weeks to recover. Both types may become endemic on a farm, resulting in periodic clinical breaks, especially in offspring from parity 1 sows.

The finishing herd may lose 60 g/day growth rate and mortality increases by 1–2%. Sows at 25–30 days of pregnancy may abort in the initial outbreak (**Figure 4.127**).

The progression of PED on a farm's production is shown in **Figure 4.128**.

Endemic herd: The condition may create little or no problems and the virus progressively dies out. Unfortunately, the condition, especially type 2, may become a repetitive problem, especially in gilt litters, occurring every 3 months.

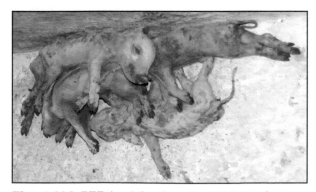

Fig. 4.126 PED in piglets less than 10 days of age. These piglets appeared healthy 2 days previously.

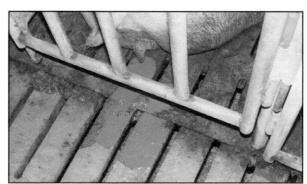

Fig. 4.127 PED in a adult sow.

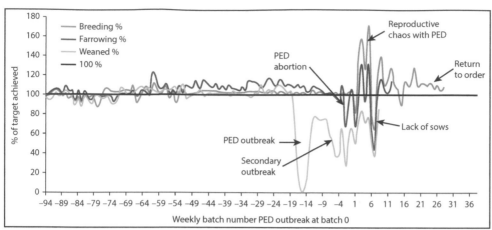

Fig. 4.128 The effects of PED on a farm's production. The infection occurred at batch 0 (a batch is defined as the time of the batch's breeding.) Therefore, the −16 and 17 batches are born and then die in the farrowing area. For more information on reading these graphs, see Chapter 11.

Differential diagnosis

Suckling pigs: TGE, rotavirus infection; growing pigs: salmonellosis, and ileitis in the grow/finish herd.

Diagnosis

Clinical signs and the speed of the infection spread around the farm is indicative of a viral diarrhoea.

At post-mortem, histological lesions are seen mainly in the jejunum and ileum (**Figures 4.129–4.131**). The duodenum is less affected. The lesions are villus atrophy. The pH of the intestine changes to acidic (c.f. *E. coli* infections where the pH becomes more alkaline).

The virus is distinct from TGEV and porcine respiratory circovirus (PRCV) (see Chapter 3). IHC of the infected intestines is very helpful. Antibody tests are useful, but virus and antibodies may be present without clinical signs. Pig-side lateral flow devices can be helpful in the diagnosis and determining the course of action to take (**Figure 4.132**).

PCR diagnosis from the faeces and then sequencing of the virus is definitive (**Figure 4.133**).

Management

Treatment of individuals or groups: There is no specific treatment available for affected pigs. Providing supportive electrolytes for affected piglets

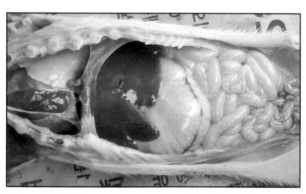

Fig. 4.129 Gross post-mortem view. Note the colourless small intestine.

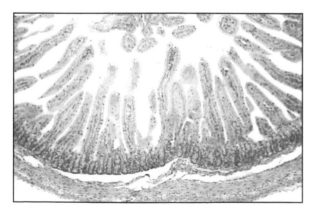

Fig. 4.130 Histology of the normal ileum. Note the lumen is almost full of the villi.

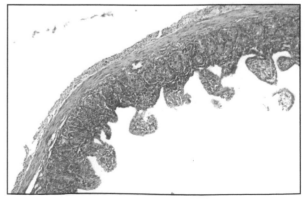

Fig. 4.131 Histology of an ileum affected with PED virus demonstrating severe villus atrophy.

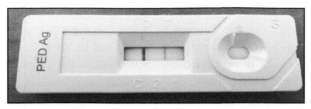

Fig. 4.132 PED lateral flow pig-side diagnostic kit. The brighter line (left) is the test and the other line (right) is a positive.

may be helpful. Charcoal may be useful as a binding agent in the gut. Older piglets and weaners may require continued supportive therapy for 2 weeks, until the intestinal tract heals. Live yogurt and probiotics may be useful to help restore gut function. Provide pain management as appropriate.

Control: Control of the condition requires colostrum management. Therefore, in the face of an outbreak on a naïve farm there is little the clinician can do for the first 3 weeks, until the sow's colostrum contains antibodies.

To ensure that all the sows produce adequate colostrum, an aggressive natural planned exposure programme is required. Feedback farrowing house diarrhoea and gut materials from infected piglets to sows from breeding to 3 weeks pre-farrowing. Ensure gilts in isolation receive this material as well. Immunity can be poor and may only last 12 weeks. Vaccination may help, but only boosts the natural immunity conferred from a field infection. Therefore, vaccination is only useful to control endemic conditions or during pathogen elimination.

Fig. 4.133 The genetic tree of PED viruses in 2015 (red square, China/USA varient; green square, Europe/China/old).

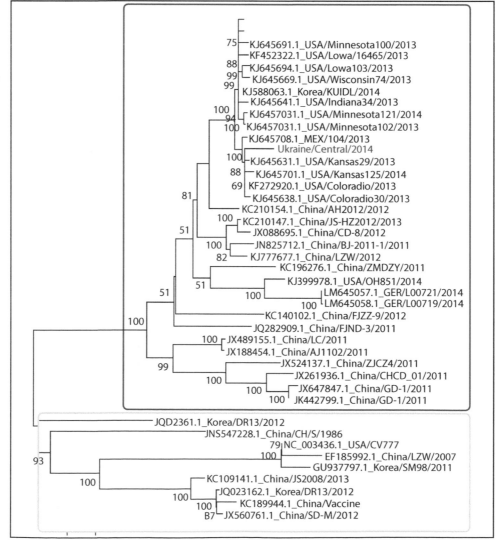

Ensure all piglets consume at least 200 mL colostrum (target is a minimum of 250 mL per pig).

Elimination: Elimination can be successful provided you have identified and mitigated the source of entry, have good biosecurity and practice AIAO. Although biosecurity may not stop the entrance of the pathogen, it is essential to reduce its movement around the farm.

Elimination should follow these four steps:

1. Stop introduction of new animals into the herd for 12 weeks to allow the virus to die out.
2. Ensure entire sow herd and on-site developing gilts receive natural planned exposure via feedback.
3. Remove 3 weeks of suckling pigs at or prior to birth by inducing abortions.
4. Thoroughly wash and disinfect all rooms and buildings.

After the condition has subsided, purchase gilts and boars from known negative herds. Collect colostrum from sows and provide to all piglets born from parity 1 sows.

Zoonotic implications
There are no zoonotic implications.

Periweaning failure-to-thrive syndrome/post-weaning ill-thrift syndrome
Definition/aetiology
Porcine failing to thrive syndrome is where pigs post weaning progressively fail and become thinner and will eventually die. This may appear as an outbreak and resemble pathogenic spread, but no pathogen has been identified. The piglets fail to learn to eat and drink post weaning. Starvation is the cause of the clinical signs.

Clinical presentation
The condition is seen within days of weaning and is exhibited by piglets who have not gained weight post weaning (**Figures 4.134, 4.135**). This is fundamentally different to PCV2-SD, where clinical signs are seen after the piglets have reached 10 kg body weight. The clinical signs are not dependent on weaning age but are more common when piglets are weaned before 17 days of age. The piglets present severely emaciated. Weaners progressively become gaunt, dehydrated and often uncoordinated and lethargic. Affected weaners often exhibit signs of vice including penile sucking and sham nursing.

Differential diagnosis
PCV2-SD, but here the clinical signs are seen in piglets that have usually been weaned for 3–4 weeks and would have a body weight greater than 10 kg.

Diagnosis
At post-mortem the stomach and small intestines may be empty of food (**Figure 4.136**). The stomach may be filled with fluid and possibly just straw (if housed on bedding). However, if the weaner has just figured out how to eat, there may be food in the stomach.

Absence of body fat and the superficial inguinal lymph nodes being more prominent can lead to a misdiagnosis of PCV2-SD.

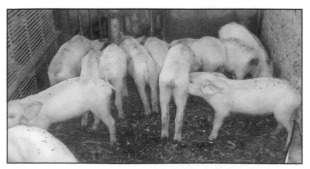

Fig. 4.134 Post-weaning piglets that are failing to thrive. Note the abnormal naval suckling of the weaners.

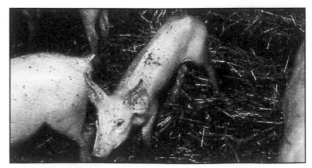

Fig. 4.135 A weaner that has failed to eat post weaning and is now dying.

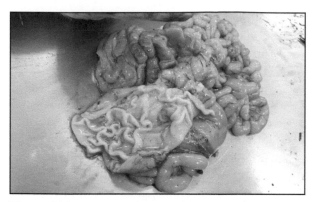

Fig. 4.136 Post-mortem examination of the intestine may reveal no food in the stomach or intestines.

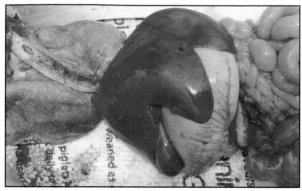

Fig. 4.137 The liver may be pale, with no other gross post-mortem findings.

The liver may be pale (**Figure 4.137**) and blood bilirubin concentrations are raised.

Histological changes in the small intestine include villus atrophy and fusion, which are indicative of starvation.

Always try and rule out other enteric and respiratory considerations. This is one condition where submitting a disciplined set of tissues is rewarding. Other tests that may be useful to consider include:

- Serum and whole non-clotted blood for haematology and biochemisty.
- Examine the pancreas when carrying out the post-mortem.

Management

Improve management during the post-weaning period, especially in the first 5 days. Practice manual gruel feeding 6 times a day. Ensure there is sufficient feeder space for each weaned pig and that gruel feeding does not continue beyond day 5 post weaning or a double weaning effect will occur. Examine pig flow, batching and weaning age. Increase weaning age if possible. Providing creep feed pre-weaning appears to have little impact on the progression of the condition. Provide pain management as appropriate. Euthanasia of the severely affected weaners may be advised.

Rectal prolapse ▶ VIDEO 23
Definition/aetiology
Prolapse of the rectum is quite common. Immediately prior to and during defecation the rectum will protrude through the anus, leading to prolapse.

Clinical signs
The rectum is visible external to the anus (**Figures 4.138, 4.139**).

Fig. 4.138
Rectal prolapse
in the finishing
pig.

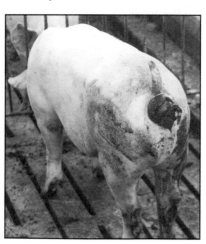

Fig. 4.139
Rectal prolapse
in the sow.

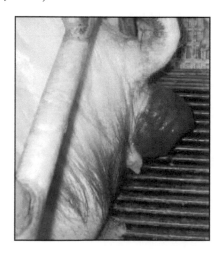

Causes

There are numerous events that can lead to a rectal prolapse, causing a protruding rectum to remain outside the body after defecation has finished. In pigs, rectal prolapses appear to be associated with:

- Increase in abdominal pressure:
  - Coughing: increases abdominal pressure – prolapse more likely to occur and then be bitten.
  - Piling: chilling draughts result in pigs standing on each other's abdomens causing increased abdominal pressure. Check for draughts and temperature variations over 24-hour periods.
  - Stocking density: too many pigs in the pen increases risk of piling.
  - Fat sows and large litters: appear to be associated with increased incidence of rectal prolapse in sows
- Increase in rectal straining:
  - Constipation: association with low water intake or low fibre levels in the feed.
- Increase in rectal irritation:
  - Feed ingredients: wheat-based diets and high starch diets. Hard wheat (varieties that produce sharp spicules) diets seem to be associated with more problems with rectal prolapses. This has been resolved by adding enzymes to the diet and rolling rather than hammer milling the wheat.
  - Mycotoxins: these can result in more straining and intestinal pain, especially with tannins.

- Salmonellae: there is an association with clinical salmonellosis on the farm and rectal prolapses and subsequent rectal strictures.
- Diarrhoea: other post-weaning diarrhoea problems including colitis. Is this a problem and is there a relationship between those pigs with severe diarrhoea and subsequent rectal prolapse? Straining with diarrhoea increases abdominal pressure and more prolapses being likely.
- Water: water quantity, quality and constipation. If the pig has to push harder to get the faeces out, there is an increased tendency to create a rectal prolapse.
- Decrease in anal muscle tone:
  - Angle of the floor: especially in sows in the farrowing house.
  - Tail length: has been stated to be associated with rectal prolapses but no association has been documented.
- Reproductive state:
  - In sows there appears to be an association with oestrus.

Management

In individual pigs, if you are going to replace a rectal prolapse, review the method described in Chapter 2.

Rectal stricture VIDEO 23

The grow/finish pig abdomen enlarges because the pig has a problem passing faeces. There is a scar in the rectum, which can often be palpated about 2 cm proximal to the anus (**Figures 4.140–4.143**). As the pig grows the rectal scar does not. Eventually, the pig cannot pass all the required faeces per day, which starts to back up

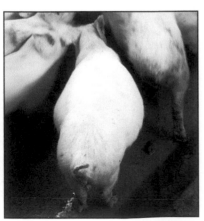

Fig. 4.140 **Appearance of a rectal stricture in a grow/finish pig.**

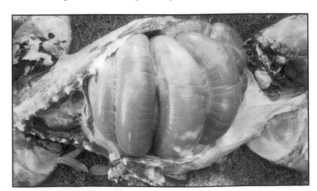

Fig. 4.141 **Gross view of the abdomen showing a grossly dilated colon.**

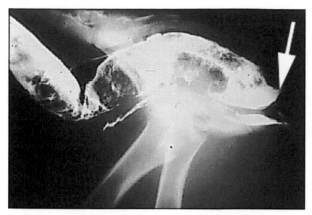

Fig. 4.142 Radiograph of a rectal stricture (arrow). The pig was given a barium meal to highlight the outline of the intestinal tract. Note there is some leakage into the vagina of the barium either from some anal leaked faeces or from the development of a fistula from the rectum.

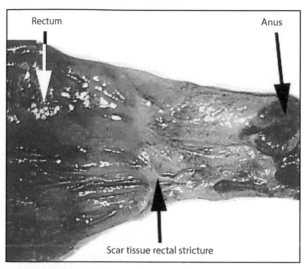

Fig. 4.143 Post-mortem internal view of the rectum. The scarred rectum is indicated by the black arrow.

in the colon. Progressively, the pig continues to eat but cannot adequately defecate and consequently the abdomen swells. The pig loses weight as it increasingly becomes toxic from the breakdown products being released from the stored faeces in the colon.

Possible causes of rectal stricture include trauma of the rectum during defecation (bitten by another pig), the end-stage of rectal prolapse, chronic salmonellosis and association with mycotoxins.

There is no effective treatment for rectal strictures. Once recognised, euthanasia is the only option. To control the problem, review the causes of rectal prolapse. Review *Salmonella* and feed management. Certain cereal grains may break into sharp spicules, increasing large bowl irritation. This may be reduced by the use of in-feed enzymes. Change from grinding to rolling as part of the investigation process.

Rotavirus infection

Definition/aetiology

Rotaviruses are double-stranded RNA non-enveloped viruses. There are five types (A–E) known in pigs. Type A is the most common, but there are many strains, making commercial vaccination difficult. The virus is ubiquitous. It is extremely resistant to temperature, chemicals and disinfectant, and pH changes. The virus will survive 3 months or more in the environment. Transmission is by the oral–faecal route. Sows may excrete the virus at the time of farrowing.

Clinical presentation

Piglets from parity 1 sows at 5–14 days of age have a sudden watery diarrhoea, which may start with a degree of vomiting (**Figures 4.144**, **4.145**). The diarrhoea is generally watery, yellow and white with flecks of tissue.

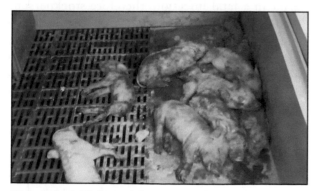

Fig. 4.144 Piglets with rotavirus diarrhoea.

Fig. 4.145 Diarrhoea. Piglets may also vomit.

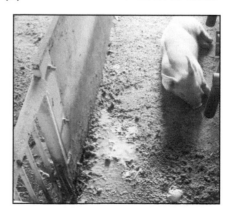

Diarrhoea continues for 3–5 days and mortality may reach 100%, but normally it is lower at 10–20%. In many cases rotavirus is combined with other problems including *E. coli*, which may increase the morbidity and mortality.

Differential diagnosis

Coronavirus diarrhoea of pigs including PEDV, TGEV and porcine delta coronavirus. Rotavirus infection plays a common role in other piglet diarrhoeas such as *E. coli* and coccidiosis.

Diagnosis

Definitive diagnosis can be difficult as the organism is common and antibodies are normal.

Recovery may occur within 72 hours and post-mortem findings can be very difficult to see in gross examinations. Even in acute cases, without secondary infections there may be few post-mortem findings. Post-mortem lesions include very watery diarrhoea and dilated small intestines. Histological examination will show the small intestinal villi to be shorter, possibly 10% of normal length (**Figure 4.146**). The pH of the intestinal contents is acidic (c.f. *E. coli* is normally alkaline).

Management

Treatment of individuals and litters: There is no specific treatment. Provide supportive therapy with electrolytes. Provide pain management as appropriate. Treat secondary infections.

Control: The problem is normally associated with a lack of colostral immunity and for this reason parity

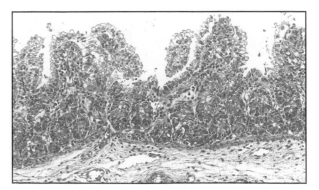

Fig. 4.146 Shortened villi with rotavirus infection. Compare these short villi with Figure 4.130.

1 litters have a higher prevalence. It is essential to ensure that the gilt is provided with experience of the farm's rotavirus population before farrowing, so she can pass this immunity on to her piglets. During the outbreak, aggressively carry out a natural planned exposure through feedback to all sows 6–3 weeks pre-farrowing during the outbreak.

Review colostrum availability and especially examine fostering protocols. Improving AIAO, batch farrowing and good hygiene between groups will help reduce clinical signs. Particularly note cross-contamination between batches through processing equipment and carts.

Vaccines are available in some countries but may not be effective due to the number of different strains and the frequency of mutation or genetic drift.

Zoonotic implications

Rotavirus infection is a common virus of mammals including man, but direct transmission between pigs and man has not been demonstrated.

Salmonellosis   ▶ VIDEO 24

Salmonella spp. can be associated with a range of different disorders in the pig. *Salmonella* belong to the Enterobacteriae and are a non-lactose fermenter, unlike *E. coli* which is a lactose fermenter. There are thousands of serotypes of *Salmonella* spp. *Salmonella* organisms are hardy and ubiquitous. They can persist for weeks or even years in the right environment. However, they are readily destroyed by heat, desiccation and many common disinfectants. Salmonellae live inside cells and thus cannot be reached by many antimicrobial agents. They can infect humans and may result in a fatal infection, therefore stockpersons handling sick pigs should wear gloves and take appropriate precautions. The classic salmonella infections of pigs are *Salmonella enterica* serotype *choleraesuis* var *kunzendorf* (septicaemic salmonellosis) and *Salmonella enterica* serotype *typhimurium* (salmonella enterocolitis).

Septicaemic salmonellosis

Definition/aetiology

Septicaemic salmonellosis is often associated with *S. enterica* serotype *choleraesuis* var *kunzendorf*, which is rare in Europe but common in North America. It is spread through contact with infected pigs and their faeces and through contaminated water supplies. *S. enterica* serotype *choleraesuis* is only rarely found in feed.

A disease outbreak is more likely to occur in animals that are stressed or have other diseases/disorders.

Clinical presentation

The incubation period is 24–48 hours. The condition is generally seen in pigs 3 weeks to 5 months of age (6–100 kg) and it is rare in suckling pigs, probably due to their intestinal lactobacilli predominance.

The disease presents as a group of weaners that are reluctant to move, are anorexic and have a high temperature (40.5–41.6°C). The pigs may have a shallow cough. Despite the high body temperature the pigs act as if they are chilled and are generally huddled. A few pigs may be found dead with purple (cyanotic) extremities indicating septicaemia. After a couple of days the pigs may develop yellow (golden) soft faeces/diarrhoea. *S. enterica* serotype *choleraesuis* is a pathogen that can cause pneumonia and diarrhoea in the same pig, which are highly suspicious clinical signs (**Figures 4.147, 4.148**). The mortality of infected pigs may be high.

Differential diagnosis

Aujeszky's disease (note similar liver changes with spots), porcine pleuropneumonia, erysipelas, classical and African swine fever.

Diagnosis

Diagnosis is based on clinical signs and isolation of the organism. Post-mortem examination reveals cyanosis of the ears, feet, tail and abdomen. The spleen is generally enlarged. The lungs are congested, possibly with interlobular oedema. Jaundice is not uncommon. There may be miliary white foci of necrosis in the liver. If pigs survive the initial stages they may also present with a necrotic enterocolitis.

Management

In many countries, all cases and isolates of *Salmonella* have to be reported to the local authorities.

Treatment of individual batches of pigs: Salmonellae live inside cells and thus cannot be reached by many antimicrobial agents. Treatment can therefore be difficult and unrewarding. Provide water and electrolytes as the main component of the treatment regimen. Consider using probiotics to restore gut microflora. Provide pain management as appropriate.

Control: Apply AIAO batching principles to minimise bacterial spread. Colour code batch equipment. Scrupulously adhere to cleaning regimens. Restrict staff and utensil movements. Note that one diarrhoetic pig will massively infect the environment. Remove all sick pigs and materials and isolate the pigs. Reduce stress factors where possible. Pay particular attention to water supplies. Reduce the pH of water and feed to less than 4. Salmonellae are not commonly found in liquid feed systems due to their acidic pH.

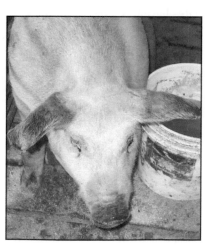

Fig. 4.147
Septicaemic pig associated with *Salmonella enterica* serotype *choleraesuis*.

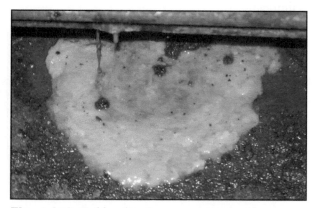

Fig. 4.148 **Golden diarrhoea associated with *Salmonella enterica* serotype *choleraesuis*.**

Salmonella enterica serotype *choleraesuis* vaccination is particularly useful and is unusual, as it can be used to good effect in the face of an outbreak.

Zoonotic implications
Salmonella enterica serotype *choleraesuis* does not cause human disease.

Salmonella enterocolitis   VIDEO 24
Definition/aetiology
Salmonella enterocolitis of pigs is generally associated with *S. enterica* serotype *typhimurium*, a very common *Salmonella* sp. found in rodents (especially mice) and the environment. It is common throughout the world. Infection is spread through contact with infected pigs and their faeces and through contaminated water supplies. A salmonella enterocolitis outbreak is more likely to occur in animals that are stressed or have other disorders. There is a carrier status for *S. enterica* serotype *typhimurium*, which may last for 5 months. *Salmonella enterica* serotype *typhimurium* can be found in feed, therefore this needs to be monitored.

The salmonellae found in pork may be contracted during the short time spent in the slaughterhouse lairage and may have nothing to do with the farm conditions. Salmonellae may be found in intestinal lymph nodes within 30 minutes of oral ingestion of the salmonella. The salmonella monitoring programmes around the world have done little to reduce the incidence in meat products. However, it should be remembered that pork is a rare cause of human salmonellosis.

Clinical presentation
Any age group can be infected but clinical signs are often seen in newly weaned pigs. The pigs present with a watery, yellow diarrhoea, initially without blood or mucus. The diarrhoea may reoccur in the same pig over the period of a couple weeks. Mortality is low, mainly associated with dehydration and potassium loss. A few pigs may remain unthrifty and some may develop rectal strictures. Clinical signs of enterocolitis may only be mild wasting and diarrhoea (**Figures 4.149, 4.150**). Many pigs infected with *S. typhimurium* have no clinical signs; the organism is merely present in their intestinal tract.

Differential diagnosis
Classical and African swine fever, swine dysentery, ileitis, coccidiosis, clostridial enteritis and other causes of diarrhoea.

Diagnosis
Isolation of the organism. There is a focal or diffuse necrotic colitis and typhlitis (infected colon and caecum) (**Figure 4.151**). This may also extend into the small intestine (ileum). Necrotic lesions may also be seen as adherent grey, yellow debris on the red roughened mucosal surface of an oedematous spiral colon and caecum. These may be well demarcated into button ulcers. The mesenteric lymph nodes are often greatly enlarged (**Figures 4.152, 4.153**).

Management
In many countries salmonella enterocolitis is a reportable condition and all infected cases and isolates have to be reported to the local authorities.

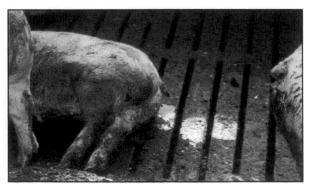
Fig. 4.149 Clinical salmonellosis in growing pigs.

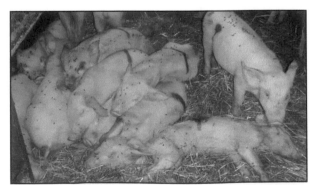
Fig. 4.150 Clinical salmonellosis in weaned pigs. Note the presence of flies on the extremely sick weaners.

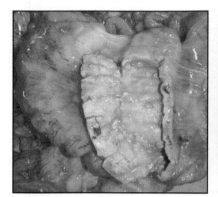

Fig. 4.151 Salmonella necrotic enteritis.

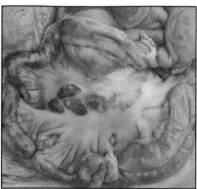

Fig. 4.152 Swollen lymph nodes associated with *S. enterica* serotype *typhimurium.*

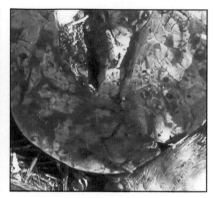

Fig. 4.153 Lung changes may include patchy consolidation.

Treatment of individual batches of pigs: Aminoglycosides such as gentamicin or apramycin have been useful on occasions. Provide water and electrolytes as the main component of the treatment regimen. Consider using probiotics to restore gut microflora. Provide pain management as appropriate.

Control: See septicaemic salmonellosis above. Vaccination against *S. enterica* serotype *typhimurium* is generally ineffective.

Zoonotic implications
Salmonella enterica serotype *typhimurium* can infect humans and may result in a fatal infection, so stockpersons handling sick pigs should wear gloves and take appropriate precautions.

Strongyle worms
There are two important strongyle worms in the pig: *Hyostrongylus rubidus*, the red stomach worm, and *Oesophagostomum dentatum*, which lives in the large intestine. Neither of these worms migrates through the body, but they live in the wall and lumen of

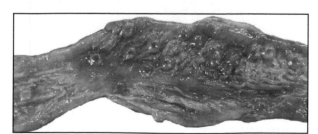

Fig. 4.154 *Oesophagostomum dentatum* nodules in the wall of the colon.

the intestines causing local damage (**Figure 4.154**) resulting in poor food conversion and growth. They both contribute to the 'thin sow syndrome' and while controlled in housed sows, may become an increasing problem with loose housing. The level of infestation is calculated via a worm egg count per g of faeces (see **Figure 4.41**).

Swine dysentery
Definition/aetiology
The presence of blood in the faeces is called dysentery. Swine dysentery is a classic condition associated with the presence of *Brachyspira* organisms. The condition is also called blood dysentery and bloody scours. The classic causal agent is *B. hyodysenteriae* but there are at least 12 serotypes known. *Brachyspira hampsonii* and *B. sunatina* may also cause similar clinical signs. However, even supposedly non-pathogenic strains such as *B. innocens* may be associated with clinical dysentery.

The condition typically affects pigs from 15 to 70 kg (6–18 weeks of age) but all age groups can present with clinical signs in an initial outbreak. The incubation period is 10–14 days. Pigs may transmit the bacteria for 90 days and mice for 180 days. These features are very important when designing eradication programmes. *B. hyodysenteriae* survives in:

- Mice: can shed for over 180 days.
- Faeces: can survive for 61 days at 5°C.
- Soil: can survive for 18 days at 4°C.
- Flies: can survive for 4 hours.
- Cats and dogs: can carry for 13 days.

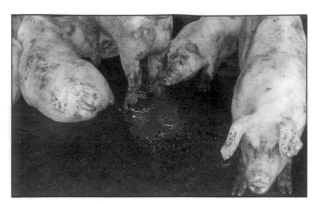

Fig. 4.155 Pig clinically affected with swine dysentery.

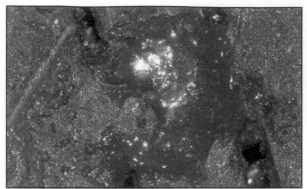

Fig. 4.156 Dysentery diarrhoea seen during a routine visit.

Clinical presentation

In an acute outbreak the first clinical signs might be death of one or two pigs before other pigs show any signs. A careful search of the pen normally reveals the presence of blood and mucus in some places (**Figures 4.155, 4.156**).

Over the following 2 weeks pigs present with diarrhoea with or without blood, and the severity is very variable. Infected pigs can have diarrhoea with large amounts of mucus in the faeces and afterwards with flecks of blood. With affected pigs there is a rapid loss of condition in some and pigs look hairy. Clinically affected pigs in a group can reach 50%. This loss of condition and wasting increases FCR by 0.6 and an extension of the finishing period by 20 days.

As the disease becomes established, finishing pigs present with dehydration and a painful abdomen and some pigs are weak and uncoordinated. The clinical signs often appear to be cyclic and reappear as outbreaks at 3–4-week intervals.

Differential diagnosis

Colitis (*Brachyspira* and non-specific), salmonellosis, ileitis, especially the haemorrhagic form. Other *Brachyspira* spp. can cause very similar signs, including mortality.

Diagnosis

The pathology is confined to the large bowel – caecum, colon and rectum – because *B. hyodysenteriae* is an anaerobe.

Typical changes in the acute phase include hyperaemia and oedema of the walls of the large intestine. Colonic submucosal glands may be more prominent and appear white. The mucosa is usually covered by mucus and fibrin with flecks of blood, and the colonic contents are soft to watery and contain exudate.

Confirmation of the diagnosis is through isolation of *B. hyodysenteriae* in the faeces. There are a number of other spirochaetes that are normal in the large bowel of pigs and may be associated with colitis.

PCR is available and may be used on faecal samples while IHC can be useful on tissue samples. Silver staining in the classic histological stain (**Figure 4.157**).

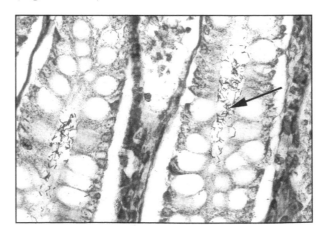

Fig. 4.157 Silver staining of the distal ileum revealing the S-shaped bacteria *Brachyspira hyodysenteriae* (arrow).

Management

Antibiotics used in treatment include tiamulin, lincomycin and tylan. If Carbodox™ is legal, it is highly effective but has a long withdrawal time. If metronidazole is legal in your area, it can be an extremely effective treatment. Unfortunately, *B. hyodysenteriae* has become resistant to many of the commonly used antimicrobials, making treatment difficult and elimination nearly impossible.

Treatment of individual groups – acute outbreak: Treatment via the water supply is essential for acute cases of swine dysentery, as affected pigs will not eat, and this should be extended to all animals in drainage contact. Follow treatment with in-feed medication once the pigs start to eat again (affected pigs and all animals in drainage/faecal contact). Very sick and weak pigs respond better using injectable medication. If treatment is unsuccessful, euthanasia may be warranted. Provide pain management as appropriate. The water supply should be supplemented using electrolytes.

Control: Pulse medicate with a suitable antimicrobial. Many *B. hyodysenteriae* serotypes are multidrug resistant, making treatment and control difficult, and elimination from the herd is the only practical control measure. The most effective on an isolated farm is to depopulate and repopulate with dysentery-negative stock.

Herd elimination: Several medication and intensive sanitation programmes have been effective in eliminating *B. hyodysenteriae*. Partial depopulation with medication is possible if the *B. hyodysenteriae* serotype is sensitive to a suitable antimicrobial agent:

- Have an effective rodent control programme.
- Drain all slurry pits.
- All buildings not containing pigs should be cleaned, disinfected and fumigated.
- Medicate all remaining pigs as prescribed.
- After 1 week of medication all equipment used for handling pigs, feed and manure should be cleaned and disinfected.
- Clean and disinfect floor as often as possible.
- Treat all farm cats and dogs as prescribed.

Note: It is fairly easy to spread swine dysentery: faeces, boots, clothing, truck wheels, rats, mice, cats and dogs.

Tapeworms

Taenia solium (*Cysticercus cellulosae*) is a tapeworm that affects pigs and man and is still a significant risk in Africa and parts of Asia. Effective slaughterhouse monitoring has eliminated the organism in many parts of the world. Separating human faeces from access to pigs by the use of properly constructed latrines is the first stage to control.

The significant issue with *Taenia* is that the adult worm develops in the human gut. It is also possible that people inadvertently eat the tapeworm eggs and cysts (*Cysticercus cellulosae*) then develop in the brain. This can cause headaches but, because the cysts occupy space in the brain, they can be life threatening. There are no clinical signs in infected pigs or humans with adult tapeworms in the gut. Normally, there is only one tapeworm in the adult human gut (**Figure 4.158**).

Treat the pigs with anthelmintics such as fenbendazole and similar products. Note that these products do not kill the eggs.

Teeth issues

Pigs can develop a range of dental problems but these are generally only recognised in pet pigs (**Figures 4.159, 4.160**). Teeth impaction and abscessation may be a significant cause of pleurisy and pulmonary abscessation. Many sows have pain and difficulty eating or reduced eating, which is associated with unrecognised dental issues. These result in ill thrift and ultimately culling.

Transmissible gastroenteritis

Definition/aetiology

TGE is caused by a virus belonging to the subfamily Coronavirinae (family Coronaviridae). These are RNA enveloped viruses. Several related viruses are found in pigs:

- PRCV, which is a mutant of TGEV.
- PED viruses (PEDV) I and II (see Porcine epidemic diarrhoea).
- Porcine delta coronavirus.
- Porcine haemagglutinating encephalomyelitis virus, which has worldwide incidence.

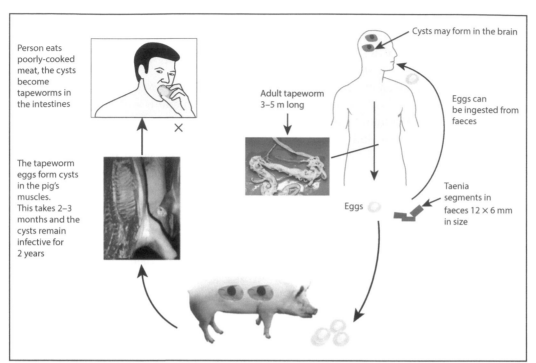

Person eats poorly-cooked meat, the cysts become tapeworms in the intestines

The tapeworm eggs form cysts in the pig's muscles. This takes 2–3 months and the cysts remain infective for 2 years

Cysts may form in the brain

Adult tapeworm 3–5 m long

Eggs can be ingested from faeces

Eggs

Taenia segments in faeces 12 × 6 mm in size

Fig. 4.158
Life cycle of
Taenia solium.

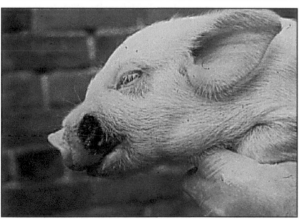

Fig. 4.159 Nasal necrosis following teeth clipping.

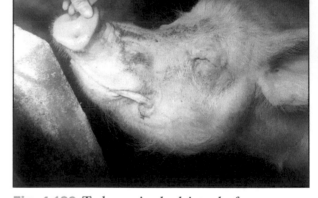

Fig. 4.160 Tusk growing back into the face.

Coronaviruses are relatively fragile and susceptible to disinfectants and drying. However, they can survive a few days in the cold, hence the disease is more severe in the winter/rainy season.

The emergence of PRCV in 1986 effectively vaccinated the European herd against TGEV. In America PRCV only appeared to reduce the clinical signs of TGE.

The pathogen spreads directly or indirectly through contact with infected faeces. With TGE, birds, particularly passerine birds such as starlings, are implicated in the spread of the virus. The incubation period for TGE varies from 18 hours to 3 days.

Clinical presentation

Pigs present with a watery diarrhoea (foul smelling, yellowish-green, often containing flecks of undigested milk particles in the piglet); vomiting and loss of appetite occur in pigs of all ages (**Figure 4.161**). The disease spreads rapidly around the farm. Piglets infected at less than 10 days of age generally die. Weaners become sick and recovery is difficult, and the recovered pigs appear unthrifty. Growers, finishers and adults are generally mildly affected and will survive if their water supplies are adequate. Outbreaks in smaller herds generally only last 3 weeks.

Fig. 4.161
Piglets clinically sick with TGE.

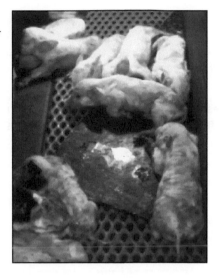

In large herds the disease can persist for some time, even becoming endemic, and this can contribute to post-weaning diarrhoea.

Differential diagnosis
PED, rotavirus, salmonellosis and ileitis in the growing herd.

Diagnosis
Clinical signs and the speed of infection spread around the farm is indicative of a viral diarrhoea. At post-mortem, the stomach will be empty and the intestines fluid filled and thin walled, indicating villus atrophy. Histological lesions are seen mainly in the jejunum and ileum. The duodenum is less affected. The lesions are villus atrophy (**Figure 4.162**) and placing a short section of jejunum in a water-filled test tube is frequently all that is

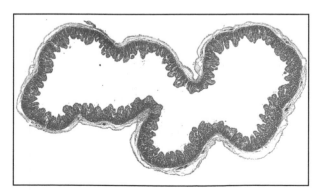

Fig. 4.162 Villus atrophy with TGE. Compare with the normal ileum shown in Figure 4.129.

necessary to visualise the villus atrophy. The pH of the intestine changes to acidic.

The virus is distinct from PEDV and PRCV. IHC of the infected intestines is very helpful. Antibody tests are useful, but virus and antibodies may be present without clinical signs. Pig-side lateral flow devices (see **Figure 4.132**) can be very helpful in the diagnosis (see Porcine epidemic diarrhea).

Management
Treatment: There is no specific treatment. Nursing and enhanced management of the piglets may reduce losses. Provide warmth, extra bedding and fluids (electrolytes). Provide pain management as appropriate. If sows develop hypogalactia provide milk replacer/creep to piglets.

Cross-suckle affected piglets onto recovered sows. On day 1 provide parity 1 piglets with colostrum from sows. Early wean into warm dry flat decks or similar accommodation. Use antibiotics to control secondary infections.

Practice a natural planned exposure (feedback) programme to ensure that all non-pregnant and pregnant (up to 3 weeks pre-farrowing) sows are exposed to the TGEV (intestines and faeces of affected piglets).

Sows about to farrow must not be exposed or they will infect their offspring and have inadequate colostral antibodies to provide adequate cover.

Control: Vaccines are generally disappointing. Critically assess general hygiene and disease control measures, including avoidance of unwanted visitors. Provide specific loading/unloading areas for pigs and keep them clean. Utilise adequate isolation facilities for introduced animals. Bird proof pig units where practical. Avoid spillage of feed around hoppers and where food is spilt clean it up. In yarding systems, cover all feed hoppers.

Whipworms
Trichuris suis is the pig whipworm. It lives in the large bowel and causes local damage to the intestinal wall. These worms do not migrate around the body. They may play a marginal role in the 'thin sow syndrome'. They are readily recognised with a worm egg examination because of their bipolar egg morphology (see **Figure 4.42**).

CLINICAL QUIZ

4.1 Look at the clinical signs illustrated in **Figures 4.16a–4.16j** (see pp. 158 and 159). What conditions may be associated with the different colours of the faeces?

4.2 Look at the gross pathology illustrated in **Figures 4.17–4.26** (see pp. 159 and 160). What are the classic conditions for each of the pathology states described; do not just look at the figure.

4.3 What do you see in **Figure 4.59** (see p. 166) that could affect pre-weaning diarrhoea control measures?

The answers to these questions can be found on page 473.

CLINICAL GROSS ANATOMY OF THE LOCOMOTOR SYSTEM

The domestic pig (*Sus scrofa*) is an artiodactyl (even-toed mammal) that has lost the 1st digit on all four feet. Apart from this adaptation, the skeleton is basically complete. Note that the rostral bone is an unusual mammalian feature.

Skeletal anatomy

The pig has six cervical vertebrae, 14 thoracic vertebrae (some Landrace breeds may have 15), six lumbar vertebrae, a sacrum and the coccygeal vertebrae forming the tail (**Figure 5.1**).

Detail of the limbs

From a clinical point of view, the clinician needs to appreciate the anatomy of the fore- and hindlimbs in a little more detail (**Figures 5.2–5.8**). An understanding of the anatomy of the limbs is essential to be able to pass professional judgement on the conformation of a pig or when reviewing a radiograph. Lameness is a common problem in the pig. The farm health team must spend more time and effort in maintaining the health of the limbs and especially the foot of the adult. Understanding the basics and being able to describe the structure of the lower limb is essential. It may be necessary to undertake a post-mortem examination of a foot.

Fig. 5.1 **General skeletal anatomy of the pig. Note the anatomy of the talus (astragalus) bone as the signature bone characteristic of all the artiodactyls.**

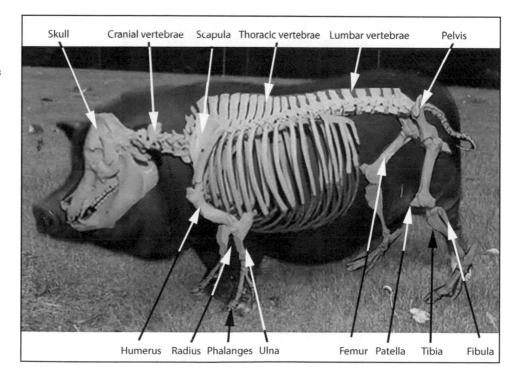

Skull   Cranial vertebrae   Scapula   Thoracic vertebrae   Lumbar vertebrae   Pelvis

Humerus   Radius   Phalanges   Ulna   Femur   Patella   Tibia   Fibula

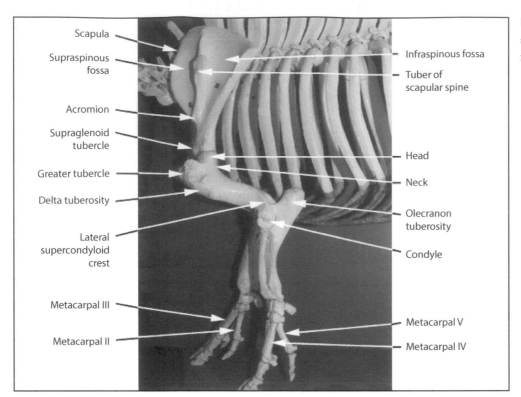

Scapula

Supraspinous fossa

Acromion

Supraglenoid tubercle

Greater tubercle

Delta tuberosity

Lateral supercondyloid crest

Metacarpal III

Metacarpal II

Infraspinous fossa

Tuber of scapular spine

Head

Neck

Olecranon tuberosity

Condyle

Metacarpal V

Metacarpal IV

Fig. 5.2 The anatomy of the forelimb.

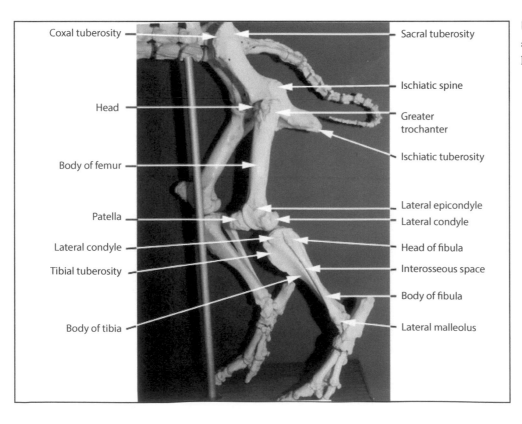

Coxal tuberosity

Head

Body of femur

Patella

Lateral condyle

Tibial tuberosity

Body of tibia

Sacral tuberosity

Ischiatic spine

Greater trochanter

Ischiatic tuberosity

Lateral epicondyle

Lateral condyle

Head of fibula

Interosseous space

Body of fibula

Lateral malleolus

Fig. 5.3 The anatomy of the hindlimb.

Fig. 5.4
Radiograph
of the leg.
(See Clinical
Quiz 5.1 on
page 226.)

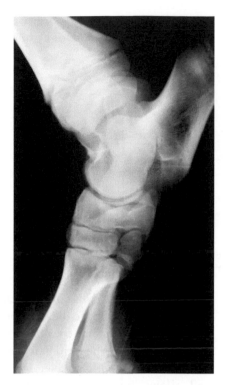

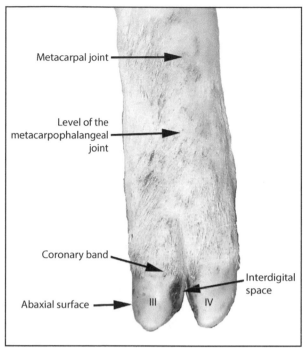

Metacarpal joint

Level of the
metacarpophalangeal
joint

Coronary band

Interdigital
space

Abaxial surface   III   IV

Fig. 5.5 Dorsal view of the distal front foot.

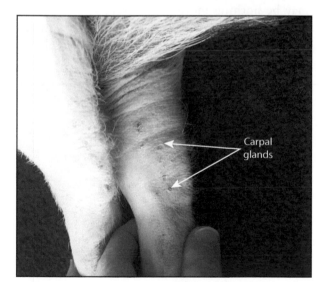

Carpal
glands

**Fig. 5.6 Lateral view of the distal front foot
illustrating the carpal glands.**

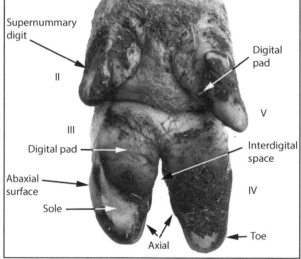

Supernummary
digit

Digital
pad

II

V

III

Digital pad

Interdigital
space

Abaxial
surface

IV

Sole

Toe

Axial

**Fig. 5.7 Plantar (front) or palmar (hind) view of the
foot.**

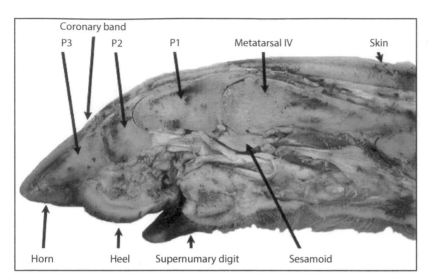

Fig. 5.8 Sagittal section through a digit (digit IV hind foot).

Surface musculature of the pig

It is beyond the scope of this book to detail all of the musculature of the pig, but the drawing below (**Figure 5.9**) will allow the reader to appeciate the major muscle masses once the skin is reflected during a post-mortem examination.

The clinician needs to appreciate that commercial pigs are assessed on their various breed characteristics and as the clinician becomes more interested in pigs, the difference between the different breeds and genetic lines can be fascinating and complex. Extreme conformities, for example double muscling, have been promoted by some genetic companies, but they may result in locomotor problems that the clinician should be aware of. It is vital that the pig's skeletal anatomy is normal and allows for normal function. Even in the pet pig industry, the development of micro pigs may be nothing more than severe starvation and enforced dwarfism. Mule feet (where the digits are fused) is a genetic disorder that should be selected against.

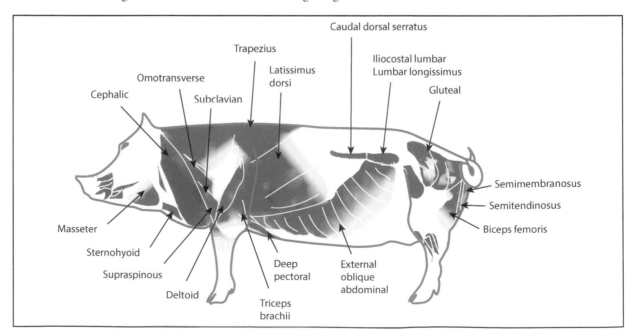

Fig. 5.9 The major superficial muscle masses in the pig with the skin reflected.

BACTERIOLOGY OF THE LOCOMOTOR SYSTEM

Locomotor conditions may be associated with bacteria. A swab should be taken carefully from the joint surface and the species of bacteria grown and identified. This is combined with an antibiogram to assist treatment programmes. *Table 5.1* describes the basic identification and characteristics of the major bacteria that may be isolated from joint disorders.

Table 5.1 **Basic swine bacteriology.**

ORGANISM	GRAM STAIN	GROWTH		SUGARS AND REACTIONS											
		ANAEROBE ONLY	HAEMOLYTIC BLOOD AGAR	MACCONKEY	TERGITOL	CATALYSE	OXIDASE	DEXTROSE BROTH	KLIGLER'S	KLIGLER'S IRON	LACTOSE	LYSINE	SIMMS	SIMMS CITRATE	UREASE
Actinobacillus suis	–B		β	–	–	+	V	+			+			P	+
Erysipelothrix rhusiopathiae	+B		N	–	–	–	–			+					
Haemophilus parasuis	–CB		N	–	–	+	–								–
Streptococcus spp.	+C		α/β	–	–	–	–								
Trueperella pyogenes	+B		N	–	–	–	–								

+ and green = positive; – and red = negative.
Gram stain: B = bacillus/coccobacillus; C = coccoid.
Sugars and reactions: G = gas.
Haemolytic: types α or β if yes; N = no.

Actinobacillus suis
See **Figures 5.10–5.13**.

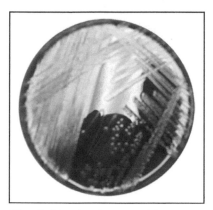

Fig. 5.10 Blood agar. Wide zone of β haemolysis.

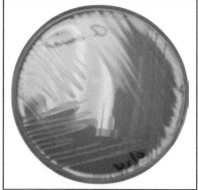

Fig. 5.11 MacConkey's. No growth. Sometimes very small.

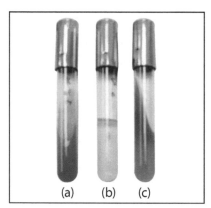

(a) (b) (c)

Fig. 5.12 Tests. No growth on MacConkey's is an important differential from *E. coli*. (a) Kligler's – lactose positive, dextrose negative, red; (b) Simm's – difficult, little reaction; (c) urease positive – red.

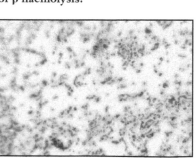

Fig. 5.13 Gram-negative rod.

Erysipelothrix rhusiopathiae

See **Figures 5.14–5.17**.

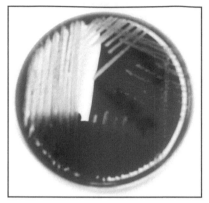

Fig. 5.14 Blood agar. Small colonies.

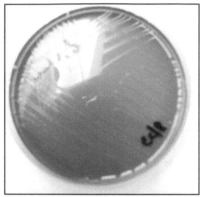

Fig. 5.15 MacConkey's. No growth.

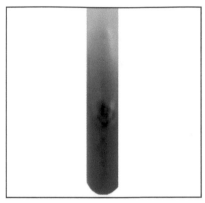

Fig. 5.16 Tests. Produces hydrogen sulfide (black streak) along stab line in Kligler's iron agar.

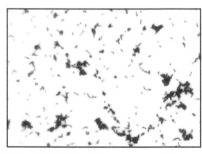

Fig. 5.17 Slender gram-positive rod of *E. rhusiopathiae*.

Haemophilus parasuis

See **Figures 5.18–5.21**.

Fig. 5.18 Blood agar. Very small colonies around the *Staphylococcus* streak. Chocolate agar may also be considered.

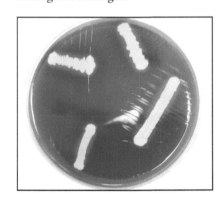

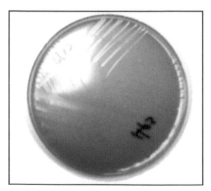

Fig. 5.19 MacConkey's. No growth.

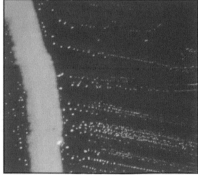

Fig. 5.20 Can be difficult to grow as requires NAD. Reputedly, grows best under CO_2 on chocolate agar. It is urease negative (yellow). Useful to distinguish from *Actinobacillus pleuropneumoniae* (urease positive; blue).

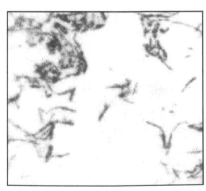

Fig. 5.21 Gram-negative coccobacillus.

Streptococcus suis
See **Figures 5.22–5.25**.

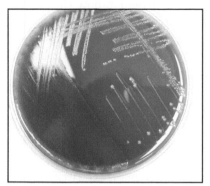

Fig. 5.22 Blood agar.

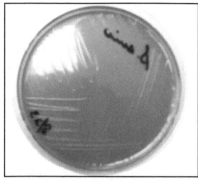

Fig. 5.23 MacConkey's. No growth.

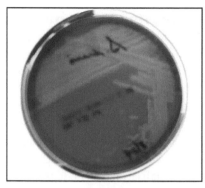

Fig. 5.24 Note the type of haemolysis. α haemolysis, green; β haemolysis, clearing. Catalase negative.

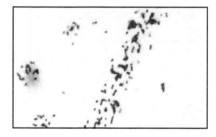

Fig. 5.25 Gram-positive small cocci; in chains or pairs.

Trueperella pyogenes
See **Figures 5.26–5.28**.

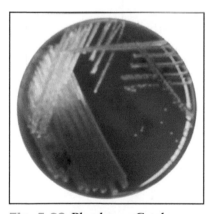

Fig. 5.26 Blood agar. Catalase negative.

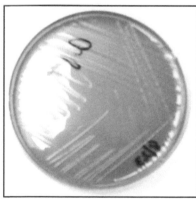

Fig. 5.27 MacConkey's. No growth.

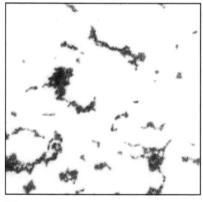

Fig. 5.28 Gram-positive pleomorphic rods; 'Chinese letters'.

Mycoplasma hyosynoviae

Mycoplasmas require special media. *Mycoplasma hyosynoviae* requires a long incubation period and a specialised laboratory to grow the organism. Polymerase chain reaction (PCR) is a possible alternative technique to demonstrate the presence of this organism.

INVESTIGATION INTO LOCOMOTOR DISORDERS

- Animal selection.
- Observe and record the locomotion of selected animals.
- Euthanase pig with typical signs.

- Submit a freshly dead pig, if available.
- Examine the brain and the spinal cord, if possible.

Assessing the conformation of a pig

The ideal animal provides good cushioning and flexion to all the joints. These animals will have an easier time getting up and down and are less likely to suffer from leg injuries and complaints and thus are more likely to be retained in the herd (**Figure 5.29**). When examining conformation on breeding farms, having a pit for the examiner to stand in and be below the animals walking in front, allows for better visualisation of the legs and underline of the pig being selected (**Figure 5.30**).

Dipped shoulders

To start examining the conformation of the pig, look at its general shape. In particular, note the position of the shoulder in relationship to the whole back. An example that can be seen from a distance are 'dipped shoulders', which may indicate a general weakness of the pig's back (**Figure 5.31**).

Examine the toes

When assessing the conformation, start with the toes. These are the foundation block on which the pig walks. Many pigs have poor feet. Toes should be big, even and well-spaced to take the weight of the animal (**Figures 5.32, 5.33**).

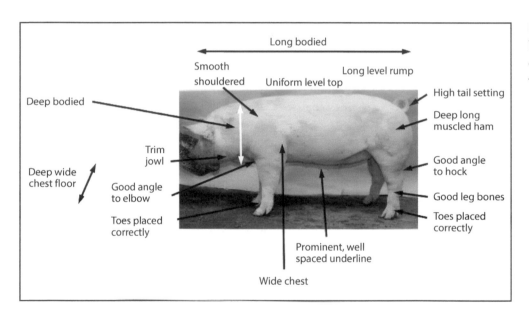

Fig. 5.29 The basics of pig conformation – what to look for.

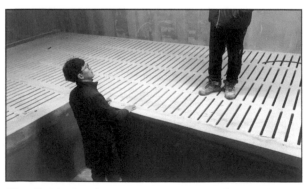

Fig. 5.30 Conformation pit within a selection house.

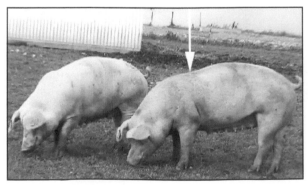

Fig. 5.31 Replacement gilt with a dipped shoulder (arrow).

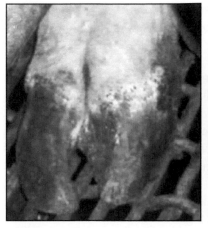

Fig. 5.32 Toes too close together.

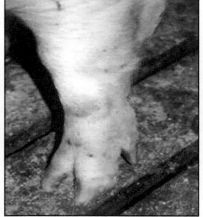

Fig. 5.33 Big well-spaced toes.

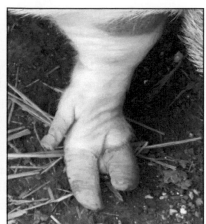

Fig. 5.34 Poor foot conformation in pet pigs can be a particular problem.

Ideally, the dew claws should be just off the floor. Reject animals whose toes are different by 1 cm or more (adult animal) (**Figure 5.34**). The toes should have no visible cracks, swellings or injuries. This should include the palmar (front) and plantar (hind) surfaces of the feet.

General examination of the conformation of the pig

Records should be kept of all selected and incoming young adults on the farm. Examples of a typical format that may be useful are provided in **Figure 5.35**.

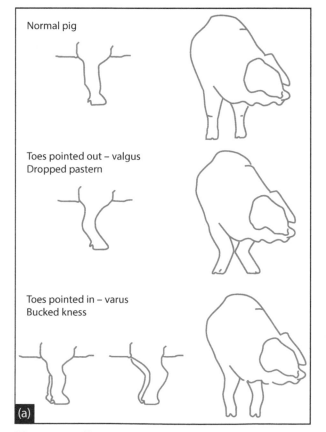

Normal pig

Toes pointed out – valgus
Dropped pastern

Toes pointed in – varus
Bucked kness

(a)

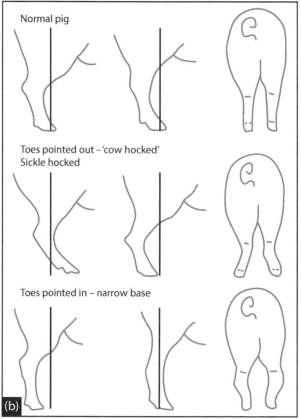

Normal pig

Toes pointed out – 'cow hocked'
Sickle hocked

Toes pointed in – narrow base

(b)

Fig. 5.35 Illustration of the conformation of legs. (a) Examination of the forelimbs. (b) Examination of the hindlimbs (the vertical line indicates the centre of gravity down the leg).

CLINICAL EXAMINATION OF THE LOCOMOTOR SYSTEM

Clinical examination of the locomotor system cannot be carried out in isolation and in particular, disorders of the neurological system (see Chapter 6) should be carefully considered in any differential diagnosis. Pigs do not like having their feet touched and examination can be difficult unless the pig is heavily sedated or anaesthetised. However, if the history indicates a lameness problem, take the advantages that are presented. For example, slowly and carefully examine the feet if the pig is lying down. Taking photographs can help further examination later.

Examination of the feet

See Chapter 1 for an overview of the clinical examination of a pig.

Treatment of the feet ▶ VIDEO 25

If the pig is small enough, place it in a sitting position (**Figure 5.36**) and the pig can then be easily restrained. If the pig is difficult, heavy sedation (not just azaperone) or anaesthesia is recommended (**Figure 5.37**). At this point the pig's feet can be easily and accurately trimmed.

Prevention and long-term treatment of feet problems of pet pigs

It is essential to provide pigs with a hard abrasive surface to allow for the foot to wear down normally. Pigs live in a variety of environments (**Figures 5.38–5.41**). The forest floor can be extremely hard.

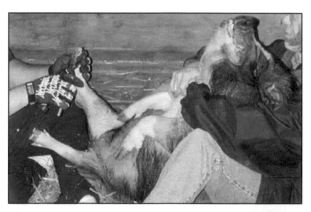

Fig. 5.36 Trimming the feet with the pig conscious.

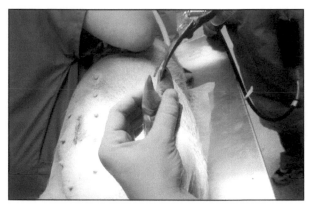

Fig. 5.37 Trimming under anaesthesia.

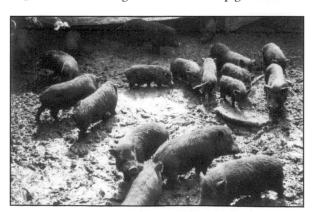

Fig. 5.38 Muddy paddocks make for soft feet.

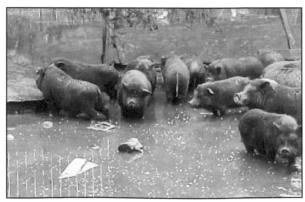

Fig. 5.39 Poor welfare conditions are often related to poor foot care.

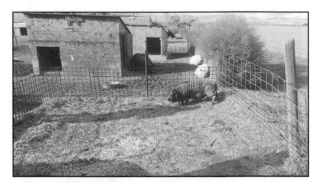

Fig. 5.40 Straw can be very clean but is non-wearing.

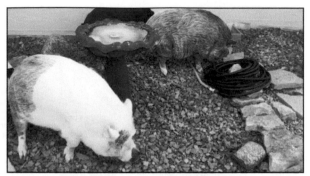

Fig. 5.41 An area of screenings will allow the pig's feet to wear more normally.

DISORDERS OF THE LOCOMOTOR SYSTEM ▶ VIDEO 16

Arthritis is a common problem in pigs, especially overweight pet pigs. It causes severe welfare issues and can be extremely difficult to treat. In commercial pigs it is generally a terminal condition as there are no economically viable solutions.

Non-specific arthritis

Arthritis is commonly seen in the slaughterhouse in otherwise clinically normal animals (**Figure 5.42**). If seen in the finishing herd the condition is often severe, with locomotor difficulties and structural deformities being observed. Less severe changes are often missed by stockpersons. Pain relief should be offered and if possible the pig should be sent to the slaughterhouse as soon as possible, but the pig has to be able to walk unaided.

Post-mortem examination of the affected limb will reveal the extent of the lesions, which may be outside the joint (tenosynovitis) (**Figure 5.43**).

Pet pigs

Pet pigs often present with structural issues and obesity resulting in excess strain and wear on the joint surfaces.

The pig presents with a variety of lameness problems (**Figure 5.44**). In the younger pig the lameness, even if severe, will generally resolve in 6–12 months. Medicate and provide pain relief. Take radiographs (under anaesthesia) to provide base line studies (**Figure 5.45**).

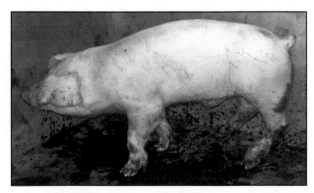

Fig. 5.42 Growing pig with severe arthritis and deformities of the legs.

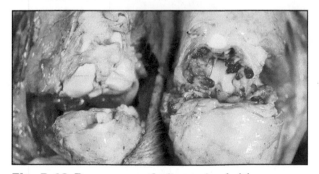

Fig. 5.43 Post-mortem findings of arthritis.

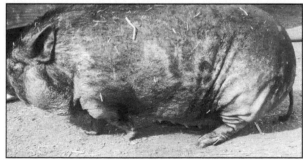

Fig. 5.44 Ten-year-old arthritic pet pig.

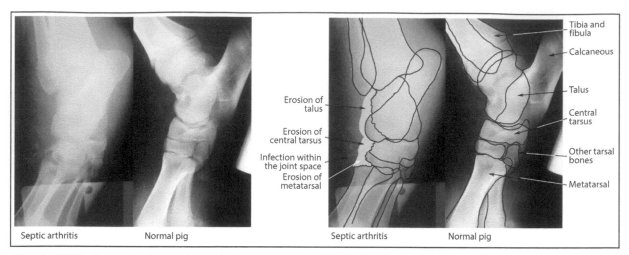

Fig. 5.45 Radiograph of an arthritic limb with and without labels.

Manage the pig's weight. Feed outside and spread the food in a wide arc and make the pig look and walk for its food. Do not use bowls. Make the pig work for its food.

However, as the pig ages the arthritis and lameness will return and require more pain management to provide an acceptable welfare outcome for the pig. Life expectancy will be reduced on welfare grounds.

Specific arthritis
Erysipelas
Erysipelas, caused by *Erysipelothrix rhusiopathiae*, is discussed in detail in Chapter 9. It is a major cause of chronic arthritis in the sow and boar. Proving the arthritis is associated with *E. rhusiopathiae* is difficult as it is associated with a hypersensitivity reaction and so the lesion may be sterile. Unfortunately, vaccines do not cover the problem. Treatment is difficult and unrewarding. Relief may be provided through painkillers given by mouth (hide the tablet in an apple, banana or chocolate). Erysipelas or chronic *Mycoplasma hyosynoviae* arthritis may be particularly important in breeding boars or boars on an AI stud as a cause of premature culling.

Mycoplasma arthritis ▸ VIDEO 26
Definition/aetiology: Mycoplasma arthritis is associated with *Mycoplasma hyosynoviae*. Because the condition is associated with a mycoplasmal organism, the clinical signs will not respond to penicillins because mycoplasma do not have a cell wall. The organism is very common on pig farms generally without any clinical signs. The problem is also complicated with injury to the joints, therefore environmental management needs to be considered.

Clinical presentation: The condition affects growers to young adults, generally newly introduced breeding stock that present with a sudden lameness. One hindlimb is often more severely lame, although lesions may be found throughout the pig, including the back. There may be swollen joints but quite often there are few outward signs on the leg apart from lameness. Typically, the condition is seen in a new group of gilts/boars 10–14 days post arrival onto the farm. There is no particular rise in rectal temperature (**Figure 5.46**).

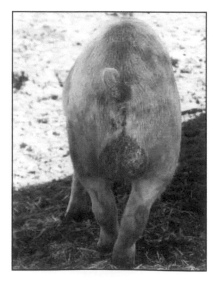

Fig. 5.46 Lame boar recently introduced to an outdoor unit.

Differential diagnosis: There are many reasons for a grow/finish pig to be lame. Taking a detailed history is a vital part of the clinical diagnosis. The condition is normally in a group that is newly arrived to the farm or buildings.

Diagnosis: Gross locomotion and absence of elevated rectal temperature. Pathology: in acute cases, affected joints present with a non-purulent synovitis (**Figure 5.47**). Antibody is present in synovial fluid. Note that the serum is normally positive in most pigs, both clinically affected and unaffected. Aspiration of the joint with confirmation by PCR.

Management: The environment, in particular poor quality floor surfaces, plays a role in the clinical expression of mycoplasma arthritis.

Treatment of the individual: Treatment is with mycoplasma active antimicrobials (e.g. tiamulin or lincomycin). Provide pain management as appropriate.

Control: Control can be difficult when the condition affects incoming gilts. Ensure that there is a sufficient introduction period for the gilts to recover fully from their lameness before breeding. A number of grow/finish pigs are diagnosed with mycoplasma arthritis but are actually sprains from chasing and bullying and therefore heal spontaneously. Review the pen layout, size of steps and floor condition.

Broken legs

Broken legs occur on farms (**Figure 5.48**) and, on occasion, they are associated with poor building design or failure due to wear and tear, for example due to holes appearing in the floor. Sows sleeping in a stall area may be trampled on by other sows and breakages occur. Miss-sizing boars and young sows can also lead to catastrophic breakage of the humerus (**Figure 5.49**). It is unlikely that nutritional imbalances are the cause of leg breakages, but it must be investigated when breakages become a herd issue. Gilts may have weakened bones with osteoporosis at weaning. Check lactation feed intakes and calcium and phosphorous concentrations in the feed. Broken legs and back can occur in the farrowing area when a sow stands on one of her piglets. Euthanasia is the only viable option.

Diagnosis of a break may be difficult, but auscultation at one end and tapping the other end of the bone may confirm the break in the live animal. However, this does not work for epiphysiolysis.

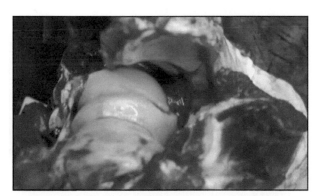

Fig. 5.47 Inflamed synovia in the elbow joint.

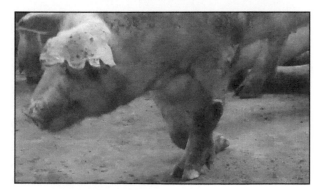

Fig. 5.48 Broken elbow in a finishing pig.

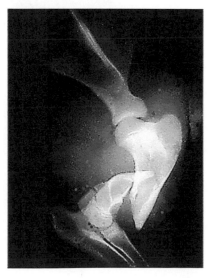

Fig. 5.49 Radiograph confirming a break in the humerus of a gilt mated with too large a boar.

Bursae

Bursae are liquid-filled protective swellings over joint surfaces. The body responds to chronic injury by covering the area with thickened skin with underlying liquids, generally from the tenosynovial surfaces. This can lead to unsightly swellings and may result in rejection of selected breeding animals (**Figures 5.50, 5.51**). Bursae can occur on the sternum from chronic chest trauma from the floor surfaces (**Figure 5.52**).

Bush foot   VIDEO 27

Bacterial infection can enter the foot through a number of routes:

- Puncture.
- Trauma wound to the lower leg.
- Toes can become trapped and torn in slats.
- Open wounds are not uncommon following abrasion from rough floors.

Bacterial infection can spread from the coronary band into the foot, resulting in severe necrosis of the internal tissues, including osteomyelitis (**Figures 5.53, 5.54**). The infection passes into the tendon sheaths, resulting in a spreading tenosynovitis. Once the infection has penetrated the internal tissues, treatment is generally hopeless. In the early stages, remove to a bedded hospital area and treat vigorously. Review flooring, particularly slat quality.

Treatment must be prompt as failure to respond quickly usually leads to euthanasia. Move the pig to a separate pen with good footing, ideally straw based.

Ensure the pig is encouraged to rise several times a day and make adequate provision for food and water. Provide pain management as appropriate.

Septic arthritis (joint ill)   VIDEO 28
Piglets and weaners

The organism generally associated with joint ill is *Streptococcus suis* serotype I. Many other species of

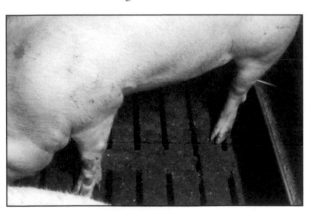

Fig. 5.50 Bursae on the fore- and hindlimbs of a 'selected' gilt, which was then removed from the breeding pool.

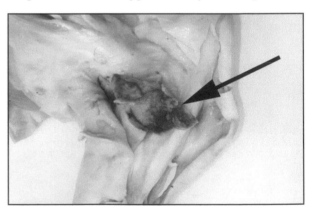

Fig. 5.51 Dissection of a bursa (arrow).

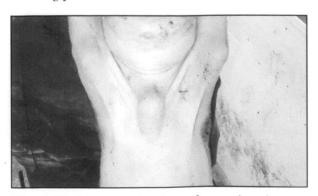

Fig. 5.52 A bursa on the chest of a growing pig.

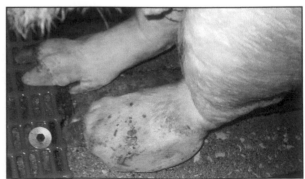

Fig. 5.53 Bush foot in a sow.

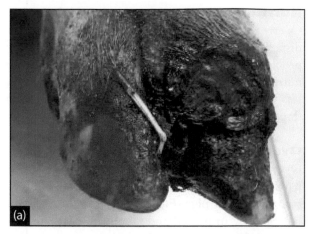

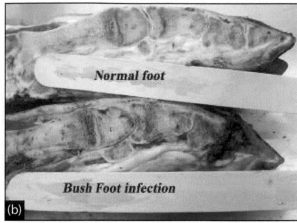

Fig. 5.54 Severe bush foot associated with flooring injuries in finishing pigs: (a) external view; (b) cross-section through the infected toe showing the osteolytic lesion of phalange 3.

streptococci can also be involved, as can *Trueperella pyogenes*. This may be confirmed by joint aspirate and culture. However, many chronic abscesses may be sterile. Pigs present with an acute swelling of one or more of the joints and may be acutely lame (**Figure 5.55**). Treatment should be vigorous with amoxicillin and pain relief. Commonly, corticosteroids are combined to provide effective treatments. If multiple joints are affected, euthanasia is advised. If the pig survives, with time the joint swellings resolve. At post-mortem a purulent tenosynovitis may be seen, which can be very severe (**Figure 5.56**). Always examine the umbilicus, as omphalitis is often seen. This may be the original nidus of infection.

Management: Review floor consistency. Rough floors are a major cause of stress. In the farrowing house consider lime washing to reduce the roughness of the floors. Check teeth clipping and tail docking equipment.

On many farms these pieces of equipment are dirty and infect the piglet during processing. Stopping teeth clipping has stopped the condition on a number of farms.

In adults and growing pigs, trauma to the legs can result in infection into the tissues around the joints and muscles. When the infection is severe enough to cause gross lameness and collapse, the response to treatment is generally poor and euthanasia is advised.

Osteochondritis dissecans

Osteochondritis dissecans (OCD) may be seen in young, growing and adult pigs. Some OCD lesions are common (**Figure 5.57**) but are only painful when:

- the lesion is severe enough to remove the joint cartilage, revealing the underlying bone within the joint;
- synovial tissue becomes trapped within the joint;
- when significant numbers of joint mice (pieces of cartilage or bone) are present.

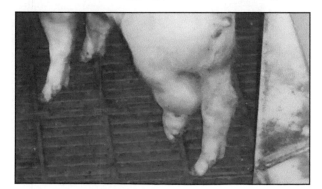

Fig. 5 55 Large infected hock joint in a weaner pig.

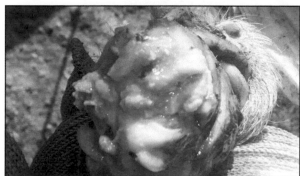

Fig. 5.56 Dissection of a joint with an abscess.

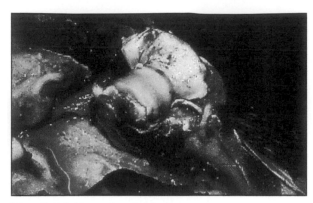

Fig. 5.57 Osteochondritis dissecans.

A small cartilaginous erosion in a pig is likely to be an incidental finding. Provide pain management as appropriate.

Femoral head separation (epiphysiolysis) ▶ VIDEO 29

Epiphysiolysis is a specific form of osteochondrosis affecting the neck of the femur. The lesion is seen following trauma, resulting in separation of the head of the femur from the shaft at the growth plate. The cause of the trauma may be:

- bullying;
- pushing through a narrow doorway;
- a mating injury.

Clinically, the young sow/gilt presents with sudden unilateral hindlimb lameness with collapse of her gluteal (hip) muscles, mainly on one side (**Figures 5.58, 5.59**). Fast growing pigs are a predisposing factor. There is no effective treatment.

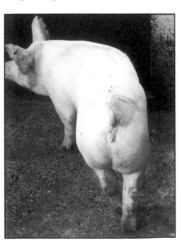

Fig. 5.58 A gilt with clinical epiphysiolysis. Note the hanging appearance of the affected left hindlimb.

Nutritional impacts on growth

Overly rapid growth of potential replacements predisposes them to early culling due to locomotor problems. May also be involved in poor lactation nutrition, because if their feet are sore, pigs may be less willing to stand to feed. Nutrition has a major impact on OCD.

Overgrown feet

Overgrown feet are not uncommon on pig farms, particularly in certain lines of pigs, and they are very common in pet pigs (**Figure 5.60**). Pig feet should be regularly inspected and trimmed, ideally immediately after farrowing. Sows do not like having their feet trimmed. They can be very hard and may be difficult to trim. Using a small grinder can be very effective. A bolt cutter during lactation can be very effective on overgrown supernumerary digits. Overgrown feet contribute to pre-weaning mortalities by making the sow clumsy.

Feet are a more serious consideration in the management of commercial pigs. It is possible to place the sow into a specific crate and then turn the crate, putting the sow on her back (**Figure 5.61**). Her feet can then be easily visualised and trimmed. While the sow may vocalise, the method is safe for both pig and stockperson. On release, the sow walks away and re-joins the rest of her group.

Porcine stress syndrome

If pigs become overstressed they can develop a hyperthermia, called porcine stress syndrome (PSS). The pig will present initially with incoordination and then rapidly collapse. The pig may just be found dead.

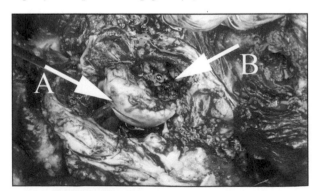

Fig. 5.59 Post-mortem view of the hip with the detached head of the femur demonstrated. A, the femoral head; B, the femoral neck.

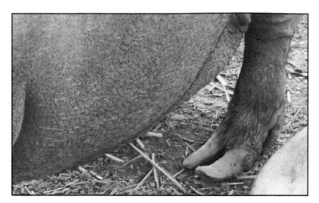

Fig. 5.60 Overgrown feet.

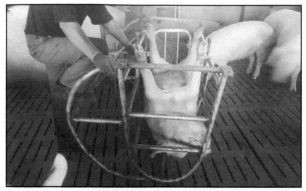

Fig. 5.61 A turnabout crate to allow foot trimming to be safely and easily carried out in gestating sows.

Body temperatures of 46°C may occur. Post-mortem examination of the back muscles reveal that they are very pale and may look like cooked pork. One form of this is specifically associated with a genetic abnormality. This gene is interesting as it was closely related to a gene for lean and also one for halothane sensitivity, where exposure to halothane resulted in PSS. This gene can be easily identified in a blood sample. Analysis of breeding company stock has removed or located this 'stress gene' in the breeding population.

However, if the pig is overstressed prior to slaughter there are two syndromes that may become apparent:

1 If the pH of the meat falls below 5.4, the meat becomes pale, soft and with high drip loss.
2 The alternative is the pH remains high, resulting in a dry, dark and firm meat, unsuitable for human consumption.

Spinal abscess

The grow/finish pig presents suddenly with hindlimb paresis (**Figure 5.62**). Both legs are on the same side of the pig. The abscess will normally be found on post-mortem examination at the thoracic/lumbar junction of the spinal cord. There is no treatment and euthanasia is the only option. If tail docking occurs on the farm, review the procedures.

Splayleg ▶ VIDEOS 30 and 31
Definition/aetiology

The piglet shortly after birth has splayed hindlimbs, sometimes called 'spraddlers' (**Figure 5.63**). The condition may rarely also affect the forelimbs and these pigs are referred to as 'starpigs' (**Figure 5.64**). There is no specific causal agent. The condition appears to be a problem associated primarily with the environment/management. Piglets staying wet and cold for too long and low birth weight piglets are

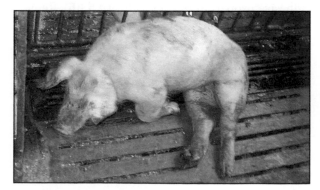

Fig. 5.62 Spinal abscess.

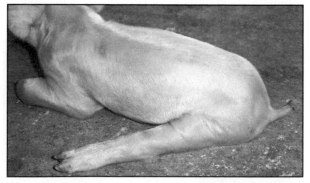

Fig. 5.63 Splayleg affecting the hindlimbs. (Note: This piglet should not have been tail docked until the splayleg had been resolved.)

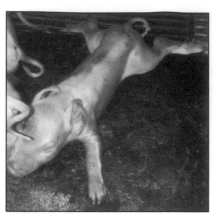

Fig. 5.64 Starpig with both the hindlimbs and the forelimbs affected. Euthanasia is the most humane action for this pig.

Diagnosis

The clinical signs are characteristic. Post-mortem examination is generally unrewarding. There may be some myofibrillar hypoplasia of the muscles of the back, the longissimus dorsi and the biceps femoris muscles. If the condition is primarily environmental there will be no anatomical issues in the newborn piglets. Failure to stand properly for 3 days may affect the anatomy of piglets at post-mortem when they are subsequently euthanased and submitted for histology.

Management

Treatment of individuals: If all four legs are affected, euthanase the piglets. If hindlimbs only are affected, tape legs together (**Figure 5.65**). Massage the hip area of the affected piglet. Provide support for the hindlimbs using tape and bands. Do not apply these bands too tight and cause circulation constriction. Remove the bands as soon as possible (after 48–72 hours). Whatever treatment is pursued, it is essential to provide adequate colostrum within 6 hours of birth.

Control: Adopt a split suckling routine where all piglets are placed in a warm box with a paper floor (to enhance grip) for 30 minutes prior to being released to get colostrum. Place mats or feedbags behind the sow during farrow. Provide shredded paper to the sow 24 hours prior to farrowing. Repair or replace the farrowing house floor, in particular behind and to the sides of the sow. Paint floor with lime wash to increase adhesive properties of floor (**Figure 5.66**). Remove mycotoxins and/or provide binders in the feed.

more prone. Stressed sows are more likely to deliver splayleg piglets. Zearalenone (F2) mycotoxin may be associated with increased incidence

There is probably a genetic component as Landrace piglets are more commonly affected than Large White piglets. The condition generally affects one or two pigs in the litter but can be seen in the whole litter. Males are more commonly affected than females. It is probable that splayleg of the forelimbs is a different syndrome.

Clinical presentation

Clinical signs are seen in piglets within hours of birth. Being splayleg seriously affects the piglet's ability to dry, suckle and get out of the way of the sow, thus increasing pre-weaning mortality. It may rarely appear in multiple litters and appears to be 'infectious' in nature.

Differential diagnosis

Spinal injury in the newborn piglet after being trodden on by sow. Other causes of weakness in neonatal pigs.

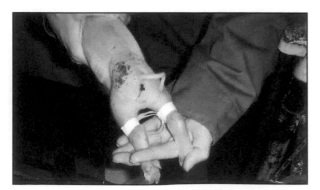

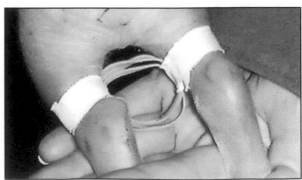

Fig. 5.65 Doubled elastic band held between the hindlimbs. Tape over the back may help stabilise the back as well.

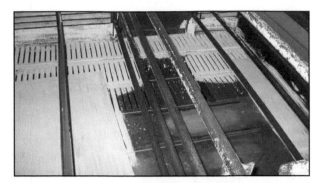

Fig. 5.66 Limewashing the farrowing area improves the grip on the floor.

Review gestation feeding. Increase feed intake from day 85 to day 110 of gestation. Birth weights need to be greater than 1.2 kg. Reduce gestation stress. Place sows into the farrowing house at least 5 days before farrowing. Ensure sow housing is adequate; length of sides, floor no draughts, etc. Do not breed from splayleg gilts or boars. While the animal recovers permanent damage may have been incurred.

Split hips

If a sow falls or does the splits, she can tear the pelvic muscles resulting in an inability to rise (**Figure 5.67**). There is generally no economic recovery and at the most, the sow should be euthanased 7 days after onset of the injury if no improvement is noted. Control the problem by reviewing the flooring and the lying patterns of the sows.

Trichinella spiralis

This is an important parasite of the pig, but is rare in developed countries. The worm is important as humans may become infected, resulting in severe muscular pains and swelling of the face.

The adult worm lives in the intestine of pigs, but no eggs are laid. The larvae develop within the female worm. The larvae are released from the female and migrate through the intestinal wall, moving through the body and eventually localising in muscle tissues (**Figure 5.68**). Here they wait (for up to 24 years) until the muscle in eaten by another pig, a rat or a person, when the live cycle starts again.

Diagnosis of *T. spiralis* infection is through examination of muscle tissues, especially the diaphragm.

Tumours affecting locomotion

As pet pigs age, tumours affecting a number of organs are recognised. If the lesion is a space-occupying lesion in the spinal cord, hindlimb paresis may be apparent (**Figure 5.69**).

Ulcerated granuloma

A large granuloma develops on the leg of the sow (**Figure 5.70**). The lesion looks more severe than the behaviour of the animal would indicate. There is no effective treatment. Lesion size can be controlled by housing on straw. Culling may be beneficial. The slaughterhouse veterinarian may become very concerned about the lesion, therefore telephone and discuss any welfare or transportation issues before sending in the animal. On occasion, *Borrelia suis* (*suilla*) or *Treponema pedis* may be a specific cause.

Other conditions

Foot and mouth disease is discussed in Chapter 9. Neurological conditions that may resemble locomotor

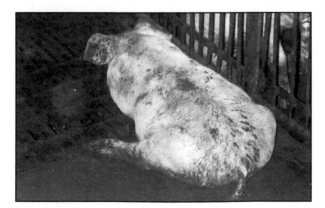

Fig. 5.67 Sow with split hips.

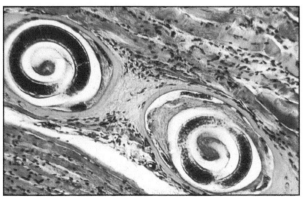

Fig. 5.68 *Trichinella spiralis* in a section of muscle.

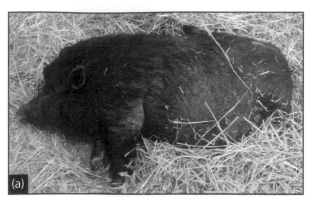

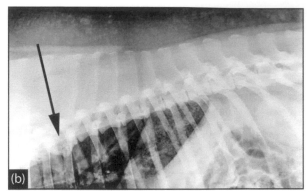

Fig. 5.69 (a) Paralysis of the hindlimbs. (b) Radiograph showing that in this case the paralysis is because of an invasive lymphoma growing adjacent to the spinal column (arrow).

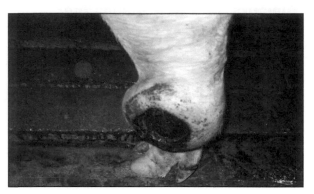

Fig. 5.70 Large ulcerated granuloma on the leg.

problems are discussed in Chapter 6. Many conditions, for example cystitis and pyelonephritis (see Chapter 7), can present as a locomotor problem associated with the back pain due to infected kidneys. This is a form of referred pain.

Many other systemic conditions can present initially as a lameness or locomotor problem, including swine influenza, classical swine fever and African swine fever.

CLINICAL QUIZ

5.1 Identify the anatomical structures in **Figure 5.4** (see p. 209).

5.2 Why does auscultation at one end and tapping the other end of the bone not work for diagnosing epiphysiolysis?

The answers to these questions can be found on page 474.

CLINICAL GROSS ANATOMY OF THE NERVOUS SYSTEM

See **Figures 6.1–6.4**.

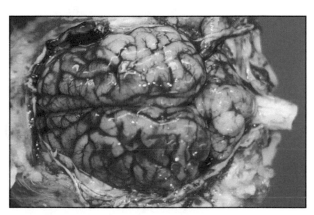

Fig. 6.1 The brain, dorsal view. (See question at end of chapter.)

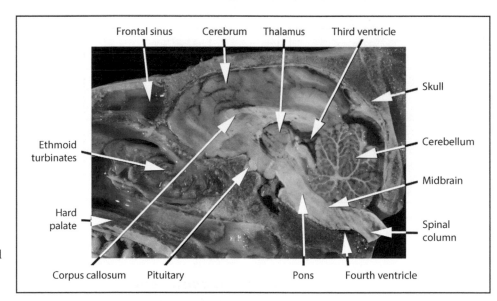

Frontal sinus   Cerebrum   Thalamus   Third ventricle

Skull

Cerebellum

Midbrain

Spinal column

Ethmoid turbinates

Hard palate

Corpus callosum   Pituitary   Pons   Fourth ventricle

Fig. 6.2 Longitudinal section of the cranial vault.

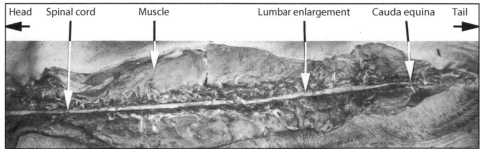

Head   Spinal cord   Muscle   Lumbar enlargement   Cauda equina   Tail

Fig. 6.3 Spinal column.

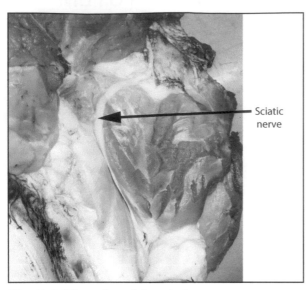

Fig. 6.4 Dissection of the sciatic nerve.

INVESTIGATION INTO NEUROLOGICAL DISORDERS

- Animal selection.
- Euthanase pig with representative signs.
- Observe and record with a video the behaviour of the selected animal.
- Submit a freshly dead pig, if available.

BACTERIOLOGY OF DISORDERS OF THE NERVOUS SYSTEM

The major bacteria of the nervous system are *Streptococcus suis*, *Haemophilus parasuis* (Glässer's disease; see Chapter 3) and *Escherichia coli* F18 (oedema disease/bowel oedema; see Chapter 4). Note that *E. coli* will not be found in the brain in cases of oedema disease as it is a toxaemia.

Escherichia coli
See **Figures 6.5–6.8**.

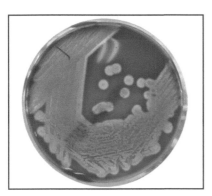

Fig. 6.5 Blood agar. Most pathogenic strains will be β haemolytic or smooth and mucoid.

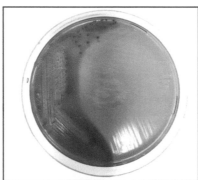

Fig. 6.6 MacConkey's. Pink colonies; lactose fermenter.

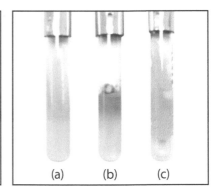

Fig. 6.7 Tests. (a) urease negative – yellow; (b) Simm's positive – red colour; (c) Kligler's positive with gas.

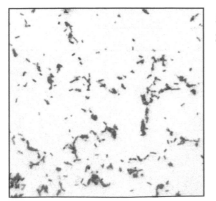

Fig. 6.8 Gram-negative rod; *E. coli*.

Streptococcus suis
See **Figures 6.9–6.12**.

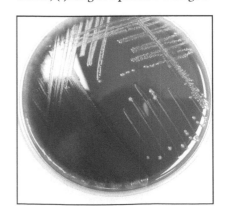

Fig. 6.9 Blood agar.

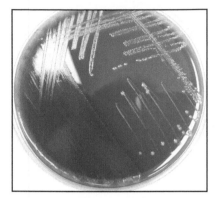

Fig. 6.10 Haemolytic. Note the type of haemolysis: α haemolysis, green; β haemolysis, clearing. Catalase negative.

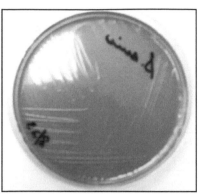

Fig. 6.11 MacConkey's. No growth.

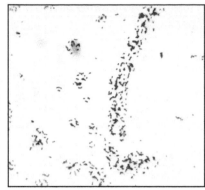

Fig. 6.12 Gram-positive small cocci; in chains or pairs.

Haemophilus parasuis

See **Figures 6.12–6.16** and *Table 6.1*.

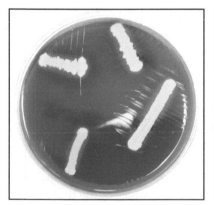

Fig. 6.13 Blood agar. Very small colonies around the *Staphylococcus* streak.

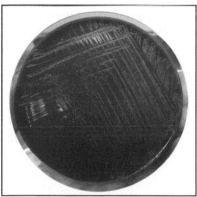

Fig. 6.14 Can be difficult to grow; requires NAD. Reportedly grows best under CO_2 on chocolate agar, shown above. Urease negative; yellow. Use to distinguish from *Actinobacillus pleuropneumoniae* (urease positive; blue). (See also Fig. 3.33.)

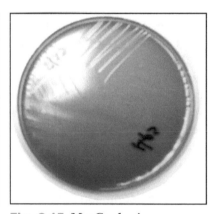

Fig. 6.15 MacConkey's. No growth.

Fig. 6.16 Gram-negative coccobacillus.

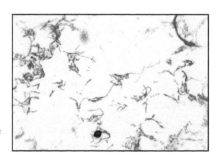

Table 6.1 **Basic swine bacteriology.**

ORGANISM	GRAM STAIN	GROWTH		SUGARS AND REACTIONS											
		ANAEROBE ONLY	HAEMOLYTIC BLOOD AGAR	MACCONKEY	TERGITOL	CATALYSE	OXIDASE	DEXTROSE BROTH	KLIGLER'S	KLIGLER'S IRON	LACTOSE	LYSINE	SIMMS	SIMMS CITRATE	UREASE
Escherichia coli	–B		N+β	+L	+L	+	–		+G		+		+		–
Haemophilus parasuis	–CB		N	–	–	+	–								–
Streptococcus spp.	+C		α/β	–	–	–	–								

+ and green = positive; – and red = negative.
Gram stain: B = bacillus/coccobacillus; C = coccoid
Sugars and reactions: G = gas.
Haemolytic: Type α or β; N = no.

DISORDERS OF THE NERVOUS SYSTEM

Bowel oedema/oedema disease

Definition/aetiology

Oedema disease is caused by *Escherichia coli* with the Shiga toxin (STx2e). Normally, the bacteria have the F18 (rarely F4) fimbriae attachment. The *E. coli* is β haemolytic. *Escherichia coli* is transmitted from pig to pig via the faecal–oral route. The Stx2e toxin is a vasotoxin that causes microangiopathy, which results in leakage from the capillary vessels and subsequent oedema. Venous pressure increases to 20 mmHg, resulting in oedema of the brain and thus neurological signs.

Clinical presentation

Pigs about 2 weeks post weaning present with a variety of clinical signs including sudden death and other neurological signs, including leg paralysis, splaying, staggering, circling and severe ataxia. Some pigs may also have a diarrhoea. Examination of the pig may reveal swollen eyelids associated with oedema (**Figure 6.17**).

Differential diagnosis

Meningitis associated with streptococci or *Haemophilus parasuis*.

Diagnosis

Post-mortem examination will reveal oedema of the mesocolon, stomach, eyelids and forehead (**Figures 6.18–6.20**).

Definitive diagnosis is by isolation of the F18 antigen and the STx2e toxin from intestinal contents. When submitting samples of the brain ensure that the medulla and midbrain are submitted intact in formalin. Bilateral, symmetric polioencephalomalacia of the brainstem, when present, constitutes a

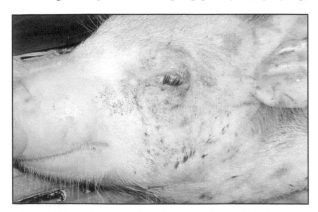

Fig. 6.17 Collapse and oedema of the eyelids in a pig with oedema disease.

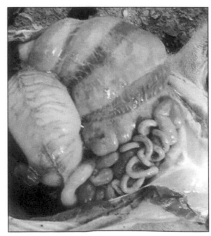

Fig. 6.18 Oedema in the loops of the spiral colon.

Fig. 6.19
Cobblestone appearance of the stomach mucosa.

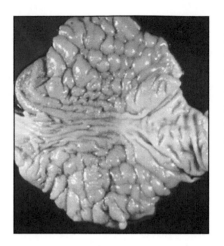

Fig. 6.20
Incision over the forehead without oedema. The normal skin is closely applied to the skull.

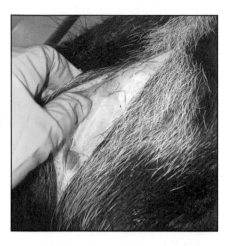

definitive diagnosis. Note that there is no meningitis in oedema disease cases.

Management

Treatment of affected litters: Acidify the water supply with 22 g citric acid per litre drinking water for the first 21 days post weaning. Add zinc oxide (ZnO) at 2,500 g/tonne. Ensure dosage is accurate. Review feed specifications and discuss with nutritional advisor. Consider increasing fibre and decreasing protein concentrations.

Antibiotics are very useful following culture and an antibiogram. Provide pain management as appropriate as neurological conditions can be extremely painful. Ensure water is plentiful and can be easily obtained by the compromised pigs.

Control: This can be difficult. Cleaning and AIAO should be practiced, but this does not eliminate the risk of an oedema disease problem.

Vaccination: Vaccinate with non-toxigenic F18 *E. coli*.

Prevention: Intensive sanitation is important. Removal with cleaning and disinfection of the nipple waterers and cups to remove *E. coli* contamination from the previous group has been shown to be helpful. The rooms must be properly cleaned with hot water and detergent, disinfected, dried and ideally lime washed before a new group enters. Diet changes may have to be gradual, with blending of two diets during the transition, or provide a diet containing a higher concentration of fibre.

ZnO should be included in the feed at a concentration of 3.1 kg per tonne to provide 2,500 mg/tonne of active ingredient. If phytase is used, the concentration of ZnO can be reduced.

Genetic control: In order to produce the clinical signs the pig needs to have suitable F18 attachment sites. Therefore, oedema disease cannot occur if the farm uses pigs that do not have the attachment site. The attachment is a recessive gene. Changing the boar line and possibly the sow line will provide excellent control. Discuss with the genetic supplier of your client's pigs.

Congenital tremor ▶ VIDEO 30
Definition/aetiology

Piglets are born with a tremor – thus the term congenital tremor (CT). There are a variety of events, diseases, toxins and genetics that can result in CT.

The most common cause, CT type A-II (CTAII) virus, is associated with a specific pestivirus. This is unrelated to other pestiviruses of pigs such as classical swine fever (CSF) and Bungowannah (porcine myocarditis) virus.

There are also a number of genetic causes (e.g. Landrace trembles and Saddleback tremors) but these will naturally be associated specifically with these breeds. CT type A-V is associated with organophosphate.

There are also other specific agents, notably CSF virus (CSFV), that can result in piglets with CT associated with a hypocerebellum (**Figure 6.21**) or hypomyelinogenesis. (See also Chapter 9.)

The rest of this section will deal with CTAII virus as a specific entity.

The agent would appear to be very infective. However, on modern farms pathogen transmission can be slow and it is possible for the pathogen to die out on a farm. All materials are infective – faeces, placenta, nasal droplets, macerated piglets/fetus and semen.

Pathogenesis of CTAII

Naïve sow becomes infected while pregnant. It would appear that becoming infected at any time during gestation will result in the production of trembling piglets. Once the female is immune/positive, subsequent litters will not demonstrate clinical signs.

Clinical presentation of CTAII

Classically, the problem occurs in parity 1 litters from newly introduced stock or homebred parity 1 sows. Piglets are born trembling in all the muscles. They may be unable to walk and often are unable to suckle efficiently. Once attached to the teat by the stockperson the piglet will suckle vigorously, but once it is let go by the stockperson the piglet will often shake itself away from the teat. Excluding sporadic cases, it is normal that there will be an increase in pre-weaning mortality and disorders, in particularly overlaids, increased lameness from trauma and outbreaks of scour. A trembling piglet that has problems suckling will clearly have problems ingesting sufficient colostrum. Mortality rates of 75–100% are common. Sometimes the trembling will be noticeably reduced when the piglet is asleep.

In the piglets that survive, the clinical signs subside with age. However, the tremble is often noticeable if the animal is watched over time and then relaxes, when mild muscle trembles will be evident over the ears and muscles on the back.

Start-up herds: In start-up herds the problem can be very severe and potentially disastrous, with almost 100% of litters presenting with CT piglets. In these cases it may also be seen in multiparity sows in subsequent years.

All other age groups: There are no clinical signs in weaners, growers or adults who become infected for the first time. The disease only affects the fetus.

Differential diagnosis

There are a variety of events, diseases, toxins etc that can cause a piglet to present with CT. There are also a number of genetic causes – Landrace and Saddleback breeds may also demonstrate CT as an inherited disorder. Other specific pathogens such as CSFV may result in CT.

Diagnosis

Congenital tremor virus may be revealed by PCR but it is extremely common. Diagnosis is achieved by clinical signs alone. There are no gross post-mortem findings.

In cases of CSF a reduction in the size of the cerebellum may be noted (hypocerebellum) (**Figure 6.21**).

Management of CTAII

Piglets with trembles: There is no specific treatment. The stockperson can only provide help and assistance to piglets with trembles. For example:

- Helping them to obtain colostrum, even by stomach tubing.
- Keeping the piglets warm.
- If necessary, euthanase the piglets and use the sow as a nurse sow.
- Do not breed from infected piglets, as it is possible they will produce trembling piglets themselves.

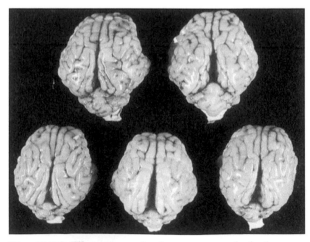

Fig. 6.21 The top two brains are normal, the lower three are affected with hypocerebellum associated with CSFV infection.

Control of CTAII: Adequate introduction programmes for the newly arrived gilt. A minimum of 6 weeks between arrival and first service. Ensure the gilts are adequately 'immunised' to the farm's pathogens using faeces, placenta and macerated fetuses and dead piglets. It is essential to 'infect' all naïve gilts before they become pregnant. On start-up units, obtain feedback material from the AI source and feed to gilts prior to first mating (e.g. dead semen) (see Chapter 11).

Do not cull unnecessarily the sow that had the trembling piglets as they should not produce affected piglets again.

If there are any signs of CSF, in many countries this is a notifiable disease. In enzootic countries check the vaccination programme.

If hereditary congenital tremor is believed to be the cause, avoid mating the sow and boar or siblings in subsequent matings.

Meningitis – bacterial   ▷ VIDEO 32
Definition/aetiology
The classical cause of meningitis in piglets, weaners and growers is *Streptococcus suis* 2. However, other types of *S. suis* may also be associated with meningitis in the pig. In addition, several other bacteria can cause meningitis, namely *Haemophilus parasuis*. *Haemophilus parasuis* in naïve finishing and adult pigs can cause a devastating acute fatal meningitis in any age group, but more commonly in adults introduced into a new herd. *Streptococcus* spp. are transmitted from the mother at birth through vaginal contact and later by nose to nose contact.

Clinical presentation
Meningitis can affect any age group, but it classically occurs between 2 and 15 weeks of age.

Most pigs infected with *S. suis* present without any clinical signs. The organism lives on the tonsils and upper respiratory tract of the normal healthy pig.

A few pigs may suddenly present with acute clinical signs, starting with swelling of the limbs. The pig becomes incoordinated often with uncontrolled eye movements (**Figure 6.22**). Rectal temperature is increased to 40–41°C. As the condition progresses the pig will fall over and thrash with all four legs on the floor (**Figure 6.23**). The pig may traumatise itself during these thrashing movements, especially around the head. Death can occur quickly, especially if the pig is stressed. In the farrowing house the condition can then be misdiagnosed as an overlaid pig. There may be a change in the voice of the pig associated with laryngeal oedema and the pain associated with the meningitis.

If death does not occur, a neurologically damaged pig may result.

Differential diagnosis
Haemophilus parasuis and septicaemic *E. coli*, intoxication with brewer products, water deprivation, porcine stress syndrome, trauma to the head, Aujeszky's disease, encephalomyocarditis, Japanese encephalitis virus, toxaemia, oedema disease and the terminal stage of many disorders may result in central incoordination.

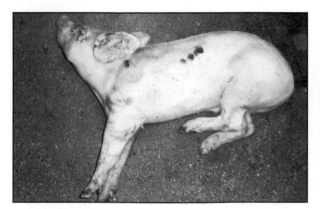

Fig. 6.22 A weaner pig in the middle of a meningitis fit. Note the opisthotonos.

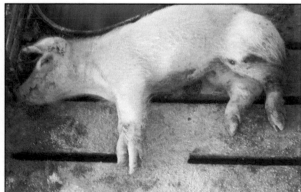

Fig. 6.23 A weaner pig with meningitis. Note the characteristic circular movement of food or bedding caused by the legs of the sick pig.

Diagnosis

There may be no particularly obvious post-mortem lesion. Meningeal congestion and tags are suspicious. Veterinarians should routinely open the skull to examine the brain and meninges (**Figure 6.24**).

If a diagnosis is absolutely required, culture of *S. suis* from cerebrospinal fluid obtained before starting the post-mortem examination is diagnostic. *Streptococcus suis* is so common, finding the organism in samples taken once the examination is underway may be due to contamination.

To obtain a cerebrospinal fluid sample, use a 40 mm 1.1 mm needle. Place the pig in a dorsal position. Flex the head over the edge of the post-mortem table. Feel for the atlas occipital junction. Swab the skin with surgical spirit. Insert the needle and 'walk' it down the back of the cranium towards the occipital joint. Attach a sterile 2 mL syringe; 1 mL of clear cerebrospinal fluid should be fairly easy to extract.

Histological examination of the meninges should include a Gram stain. This will allow differentiation between *Streptococcus* spp. and *H. parasuis*. (**Note:** DNA detection techniques (PCR) are difficult to interpret as the causal agents are ubiquitous.)

Management

Treatment of affected pigs: The pig is dying so treatment must be rapid and vigorous. Meningitis is extremely painful. Providing pain management is essential to the pig's possible survival. Antibiotics should be given using antimicrobials from the penicillin family. Isolate the pig in a darkened room so that it is not bullied. If seizures are extreme, administer a sedative as necessary. Provide water by mouth from a syringe if necessary. A pig drinks 1 litre per 10 kg per day so a few 'syringe fulls' is not sufficient.

Control: Most pigs carry *S. suis* on their tonsils and upper respiratory tracts. The causal factor that results in clinical signs is that the pig is subjected to too much stress or other disease. Wet and cold environments appear to predispose the pigs to meningitis. In outdoor situations the use of damp mouldy straw often

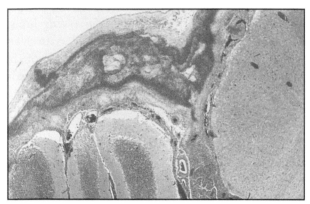

Fig. 6.24 Histology of the brain revealing a severe meningitis associated with *Streptococcus suis* (H&E).

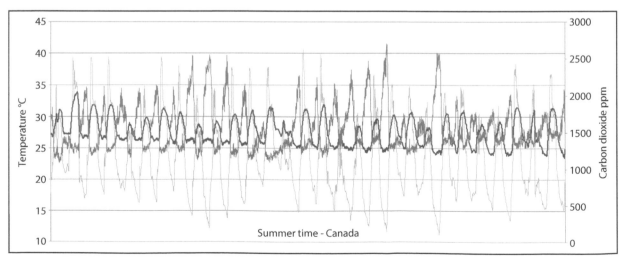

Fig. 6.25 Carbon dioxide concentrations on a farm with a streptococcal meningitis problem. The green line is the outside temperature, the red line the inside temperature and the blue line is the carbon dioxide concentration. Above 1,500 ppm is unsuitable for pig production.

precipitates a meningitis 'outbreak', as will excessive change in the temperature in the pigs sleeping area or pigs being moved and mixed, resulting in a disturbed social hierarchy. Poisonous gas concentrations have been associated with outbreaks; in particular monitor CO_2 concentrations over 2,000 ppm (**Figure 6.25**). Be aware also of carbon monoxide (CO) poisoning from gas heaters. Examine the environment carefully for draughts, particularly in the nursery.

Check colostrum management when meningitis occurs in piglets in the farrowing house. Review the rope feedback programme (see Chapter 11).

Zoonotic implications

Streptococcus suis can rarely cause a fatal meningitis in man following infection into a cut from the pig's skin, typically following cutting a finger following injection of a pig. It is a considered an occupational hazard. Outbreaks of human streptococcal meningitis have occurred following eating of poorly cooked previously sick weaners.

Check list

A check list for *S. suis* meningitis in weaners is shown below (*Table 6.2*).

Table 6.2 *Streptococcus suis* **meningitis in weaners – check list.**

FARM:	DATE:	
		CHECK
Undisturbed group of pigs	Examine and record lying pattern of undisturbed pigs – picture/video	
	Behaviour of pigs around the water supply – picture/video	
	Behaviour of pigs around the feeders – picture/video	
Stock	Clinically affected pigs respond to ceftiofur or penicillin	
Check for PRRSV	Blood results – note 21-day antibody delay	
PCV2-SD	Ensure that the pigs are correctly vaccinated against PCV2	
	Check vaccine purchases correspond to weaning numbers	
	Check medicine storage is 2–8°C	
Post-mortem	Ensure diagnosis is correct – picture/video	
Sick pigs	Treatment of sick pigs	
	Movement of recovered pigs	
	Collect true mortality and morbidity figures	
Check weaning age and weight	Age at weaning	
	Weight at weaning	
Immunology	Feedback programme	
Pig flow	Collect true weaning/farrowing/breeding and gilt numbers by batch	
AIAO	Ensure all the environment is thoroughly cleaned between batches	
Medicines	Ensure needles and syringes are not used between different groups	
Water in the nursery	Flow – 700 mL	
	Height – 13–30 cm	
	Number of drinkers	
	Cleaning programme between batches	
Floor	Nursery pigs need 0.3 m² per pig (to 30 kg liveweight)	
	Cleaning programme between batches	

(Continued)

Table 6.2 *(Continued)* **Streptococcus suis meningitis in weaners – check list.**

		CHECK
Air	The room temperature is 30°C on entry	
	Temperature cooling curve appropriate	
	Cooling 1°C per week to 24°C	
	Relative humidity (50–75% RH)	
	Gas heating – check colour of flame and CO concentration	
	Many farms with a meningitis problem have staff with 'headaches'	
	High dust and endotoxin issues	
	Note level of slurry under slats – air flow from underneath slats?	
	Draughts in the 'proposed sleeping area'	
	Examine defecation pattern of pigs	
	Smoke buildings and record air movement patterns – picture/video	
	Cleaning programme between batches	
Feed	Feed space (50 mm per 30 kg pig) and feeder management	
	What is the vitamin E concentration in the feed? Ideally 250 mg/kg	
	Gruel feeding regime 3–4 days post weaning	
	Problem coincides with a change in diet/feed type and feed size	
	Cleaning programme between batches	
Other problems	Eliminate any additional stressors at weaning – weighing, tagging, bleeding	

Middle ear disease   VIDEO 33

This condition is characterised by the pig walking with a pronounced head tilt (**Figure 6.26**). Many cases are associated with pyogenic bacteria; for example, streptococci. There is some evidence that *Mycoplasma hyorhinis* may play a role. Culture at post-mortem tends to reveal a mixed bacterial population.

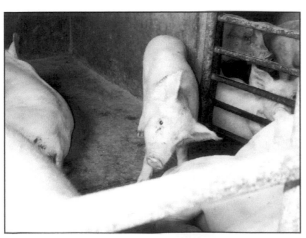

Fig. 6.26 The clinical signs of middle ear disease. The pig is circling towards the affected middle ear.

The condition is more common in weaners who develop sneezing 10–20 days post weaning. The problem tends to be sporadic.

Treatment of individuals may be unrewarding. Injections of ampicillin have been effective; these would not control *M. hyorhinis* but can be helpful in cases associated with *S. suis*. If there are a number of cases, ensure that the farm avoids chilling draughts.

If the problem occurs in pet pigs, radiological examination may reveal an abscess and occlusion of the middle ear on the side of the tilt (**Figure 6.27**).

In sows the condition may occur due to misplacement of drip cooling systems, which drip into the sow's ear.

Sciatic nerve damage

The pig will present with knuckling of the lower leg (**Figure 6.28**). Generally this is seen post weaning.

The cause is associated with damage to the sciatic nerve. This can be because of an injection, an abscess post injection or rough handling where the sciatic nerve is stretched and bruised.

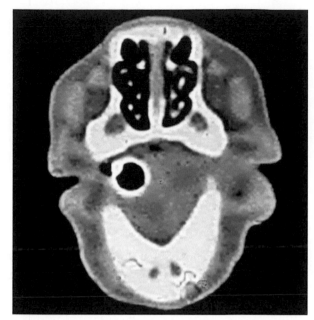

Fig. 6.27 **Computed tomography scan of a middle ear case demonstrating occlusion of the right middle ear – left is normal as indicated by the black circular hole.**

Treatment and control involves training the staff in injection and handling techniques.

Spinal abscess

The pig presents with both hindlimbs on the same side. This is discussed in more detail in Chapter 5.

Water deprivation/salt poisoning

Definition/aetiology

Pigs are found dead with neurological signs. There may be marks on the ground indicating that the pig paddled before death. Examination of the environment demonstrates a problem with the water supply. In rare cases, this may be associated with salt poisoning

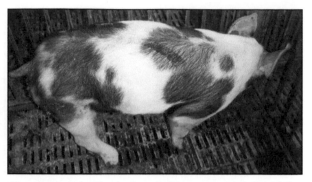

Fig. 6.28 **Damage to the sciatic nerve associated with an injection into the ham muscles (gluteals) has resulted in loss of sensation to the dorsum of the hind foot.**

if the salt concentration of the water supply is in excess of 7,000 ppm. If there is excess salt in the feed, the pigs will normally not eat the feed rather than present with salt poisoning. Pigs may be unable to reach the water supply, for example because of meningitis.

Clinical presentation

Initially a couple of dead pigs may be found. Live pigs may dog sit and stare into space. They will often twitch, which develops into a seizure every 5 minutes. Pigs may walk aimlessly and frequently fall over. Pigs appear blind and may head press. They may be very dirty, especially if the building is very hot.

Examination of the environment will generally reveal that the water supply is either turned off or at least inadequate (**Figures 6.29, 6.30**).

Once the water source is restored the clinical signs may become more pronounced. Pigs crowd around the drinkers (**Figure 6.31**) and drinking can be excessive. Pigs suddenly fall over, tremor and fit, associated with cerebral oedema. This may result in the mortality of several pigs.

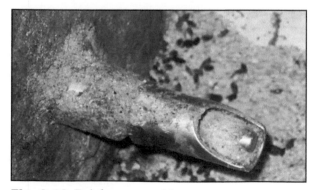

Fig. 6.29 **Drinker not working.**

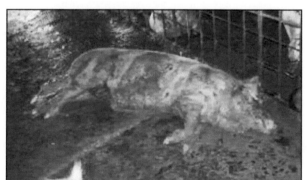

Fig. 6.30 **Dead pig in a pen without water.**

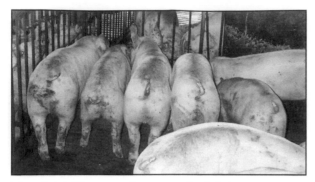

Fig. 6.31 Pigs crowding around a drinker.

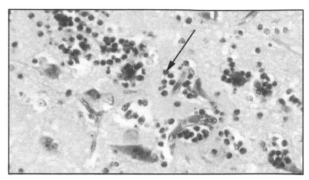

Fig. 6.32 Round eosinophils (arrow) in the brain specific to eosinophilic meningoencephalitis.

Differential diagnosis

Meningitis, Glässer's disease, Aujeszky's disease, CSF, oedema disease, teschovirus, blue eye disease and other viral infections, other poisons.

Diagnosis

No gross lesions may be seen at post-mortem examination. However, histological examination of the brain demonstrates the specific eosinophilic meningoencephalitis (**Figure 6.32**) and laminar cortical necrosis. Examination of salt concentrations in wet brains may reveal a level in excess of 1,800 ppm.

Management

Restore the water supply – but slowly. Corticosteroids may help to reduce brain swelling. Provide pain management.

Other important pathogens that can result in neurological signs

Aujeszky's disease virus (pseudorabies) (see Chapter 2) and Nipah virus (see Chapter 8).

CLINICAL QUIZ

6.1 Identify the structures in **Figure 6.1** (see p. 227)?

The answer to this question can be found on page 474.

URINARY DISORDERS

DIAGNOSIS OF URINARY TRACT DISORDERS

Suspicion

Male and female pigs may strain to urinate, which may be confused with spinal lameness. At urination there is blood or other abnormality noted. Observe the external genitalia for crystals or stones. Small stones may be seen adherent to the preputial hairs of the male. A white deposit may be seen on the floor behind the sow (crystalluria). A vulval discharge may be suspected by the presence of straw adherent to the vulva in the female.

Collection

Both males and females will urinate shortly after standing in the morning (**Figure 7.1**). This requires the stockperson to be ready or the veterinarian to be up early. Boars trained for semen collection may be encouraged to urinate when taken to the dummy sow as part of their libido behaviour.

Examination of the urine

Urine will have a range of colours from colourless to dark brown (**Figure 7.2**). Blood should not be present in the urine, but in recently bred females blood may be present because of trauma. In the male, preputial diverticulitis is common and this may result in blood in the urine.

Normal urine will not foam, but it will in the presence of protein. However, in the male this may be semen. The normal characteristics of urine are shown in *Table 7.1*.

The pH of free-catch boar urine may be quite alkaline, up to pH 11. This is associated with the action of urease from *Actinobaculum suis*, which is part of the normal microflora of the boar's prepuce.

Table 7.1 **Normal characteristics of urine.**

Volume (l/day) – depends on age	2–6
Specific gravity	1.000–1.040
pH	6–8
Bilirubin	None
Blood	None
Glucose	None
Protein	None

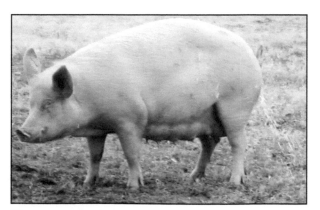

Fig. 7.1 Urinating sow.

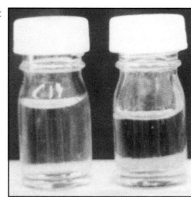

Fig. 7.2 Different normal urine colours.

Renal function

Renal function is ascertained by analysis of serum. Collect a blood sample for biochemistry analysis and note the serum concentrations of blood urea nitrogen, creatinine, GGT and protein (*Table 7.2*). For dead pigs, aqueous humour can be analysed.

Table 7.2 **Normal biochemistry in different aged pigs compared with a case of pyelonephritis.**

	UNIT	WEANER (10–30 kg)	FINISHER (30–110 kg)	ADULT	PYELONEPHRITIS*
γGT	IU/L			41–86	80
A/G	g/g	0.5–2.2	0.4–1.5	0.6–1.3	1
Albumin	g/L	19–39	19–42	31–43	**72**
ALP	IU/L	142–891	180–813	36–272	200
ALT	IU/L	8–46	15–46	19–76	37
Amylase	IU/L	528–2,616	913–4,626	432–2,170	
Anion gap	mmol/L			7.5–36	
AST	IU/L	21–94	16–67	36–272	200
Bicarbonate	mmol/L			8–31	29
Bilirubin	µmol/L	0.9–3.4	0–3.4	0–3.4	3
Calcium	mmol/L	2.02–3.21	2.16–2.92	1.98–2.87	3.0
Chloride	mmol/L			96 – 111	100
Cholesterol	mmol/L	1.06–3.32	1.37–3.18	1.24–2.74	2
CK	IU/L	81–1,586	61–1251	120–10,990	6,000
Conjugated bilirubin	µmol/L	0.9–3.4	0–1.7	0–1.7	1.2
Creatinine	µmol/L	67–172	77–165	110–260	**516**
Fibrinogen	g/L			1.60–3.80	**397**
Free bilirubin	µmol/L	0–3.4	0–3.4	0–3.4	3
Glucose	mmol/L	3.5–7.4	4.0–8.1	2.9–5.9	6
GSHPx	IU/gHb	30–137	40–141	48–135	110
IgG piglet blood at 7 days	mg/mL	25–35			
Iron	µmol/L	3–38	39–43	9–34	27
LDH	mmol/L			0–11	10
Magnesium	mmo/L			0.5–1.2	**1.7**
Osmolarity	mOsmol/kg			282–300	
Pepsinogen	ng/mL	149–313	230–570		400
Phosphorus	mmol/L	1.46–3.45	2.25–3.44	1.49–2.76	2.2
Potassium	mmol/L			3.5–4.8	**7**
Sodium	mmol/L			132–170	**121**
Testosterone	ng/mL			Male entire 2–130	n/a
Total protein	g/L	44–74	52–83	65–90	**143**
Triglyceride	mmol/L			0.2–0.5	0.4
UIBC	mmol/L	43–96	48–101	54–99	
Urea nitrogen	mmol/L	2.90–8.89	2.57–8.57	2.10–8.50	**29**

GSH-Px, selenium concentration and glutathione peroxidase; UIBC, unsaturated iron binding capacity.
* In cases of bacteriuria or cystitis there are no serum biochemistry changes. Figures in bold indicate abnormal.
See Appendix: Conversion factors (p. 469) to convert SI units to old/conventional units.

POST-MORTEM EXAMINATION OF THE URINARY TRACT

Split the pelvis to allow examination and extraction of the entire urinary tract from kidney to external os (**Figure 7.3**). The kidneys are opened on their lateral aspect (**Figure 7.4**). Examine the cortex, medulla and pelvis (**Figure 7.5**). Note the different papillae (**Figures 7.6, 7.7**). The proximal ureter can be easily found on the medial aspect of the renal pelvis. The ureter can be opened with scissors. Open the bladder from the ventral cranial aspect (**Figure 7.8**). Exteriorise the serosal surface to reveal the opening of the urethra. Examine the ureterovesical junction (**Figure 7.9**). Open and examine the urethra. Examine the vagina in the female and the prepuce in the male.

Fig. 7.3 General view of the urinary tract of the pig. The ureter and bladder are dissected and laid on paper for clarity.

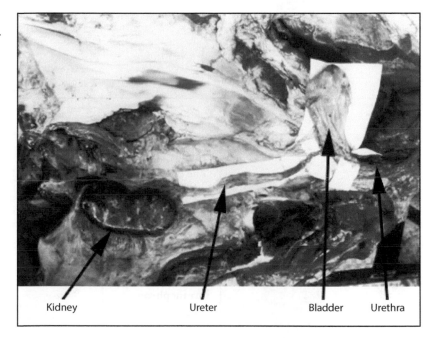

Kidney   Ureter   Bladder   Urethra

Fig. 7.4 Ventral surface of the kidney.

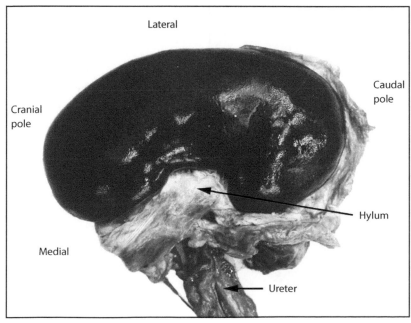

Lateral

Cranial pole

Caudal pole

Medial

Hylum

Ureter

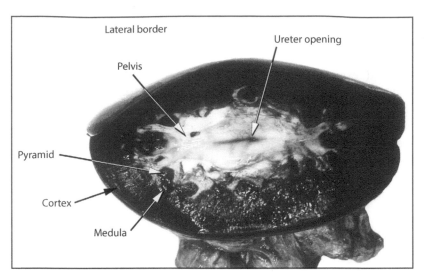

Fig. 7.5 Renal pelvis opened on the lateral border.

Lateral border

Ureter opening

Pelvis

Pyramid

Cortex

Medula

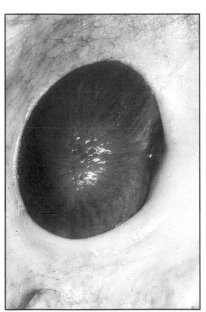

Fig. 7.6 Simple papillae. The entrance to the simple papillary ducts (formerly ducts of Bellini) are small and thus resist intranephron reflux.

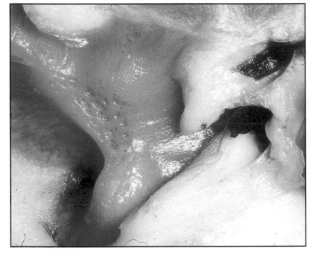

Fig. 7.7 Compound papillae, formed from the fusion of simple papillae, allow intranephron reflux through the open/larger ducts.

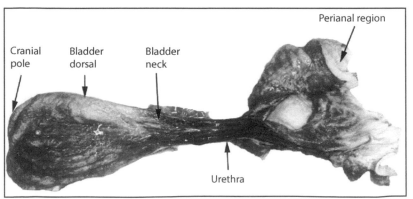

Fig. 7.8 The bladder and urethra in the sow.

Cranial pole

Bladder dorsal

Bladder neck

Perianal region

Urethra

Fig. 7.9 The ureterovesical junction in the pig.

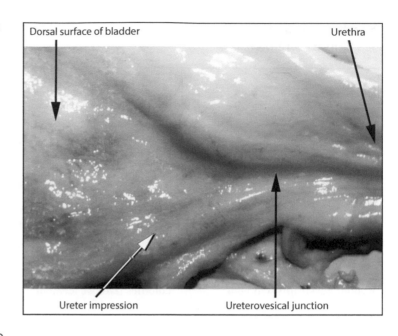

Dorsal surface of bladder | Urethra

Ureter impression | Ureterovesical junction

BACTERIOLOGY OF DISORDERS OF THE URINARY TRACT

The major bacteria of the urinary system are *Actinobaculum suis*, *Escherichia coli* and *Streptococcus suis*. See also *Table 7.3*.

Table 7.3 **Basic swine bacteriology – summary.**

ORGANISM	GRAM STAIN	GROWTH				SUGARS AND REACTIONS									
		ANAEROBE ONLY	HAEMOLYTIC BLOOD AGAR	MACCONKEY		CATALYSE	OXIDASE	DEXTROSE BROTH	KLIGLER'S	KLIGLER'S IRON	LACTOSE	LYSINE	SIMMS	SIMMS CITRATE	UREASE
Actinobaculum suis	+B	+	N	–	–	–	–								+
Escherichia coli	–B		N+β	+L	+L	+	–		+G		+		+		–
Streptococcus spp.	+C		α/β	–	–	–	–								

\+ and green = positive; – and red = negative.
Gram stain: B = bacillus/coccobacillus; C = coccoid.
Sugars and reactions: G = gas.
Haemolytic: type α or β if yes; N = no.

Actinobaculum suis

Actinobaculum suis are gram-positive, urease-positive, pleomorphic rods. See **Figures 7.10, 7.11**.

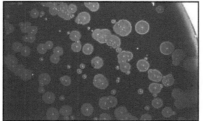

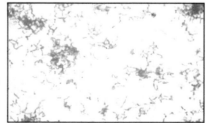

Fig. 7.10 Blood agar plates require anaerobic culture. Flat colonies, fried egg shaped.

Fig. 7.11 Pleomorphic rods (Gram stain).

Escherichia coli
See **Figures 7.12–7.15**.

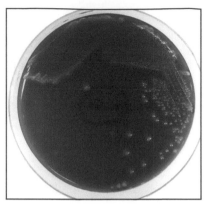

Fig. 7.12 Blood agar. Most pathogenic strains will be β haemolytic or smooth and mucoid.

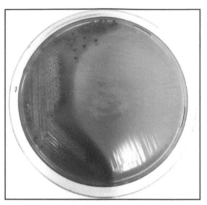

Fig. 7.13 MacConkey's. Pink colonies (lactose fermenter).

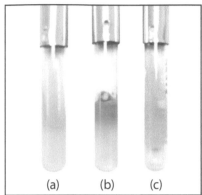

Fig. 7.14 Tests. (a) urease negative, yellow; (b) Simm's positive, red colour; (c) Kligler's positive with gas.

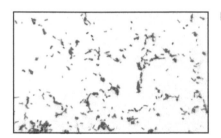

Fig. 7.15 Gram-negative rod.

Streptococcus suis
See **Figures 7.16–7.18**.

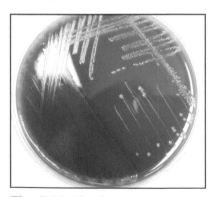

Fig. 7.16 Blood agar.

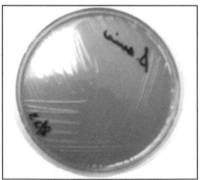

Fig. 7.17 MacConkey's. No growth.

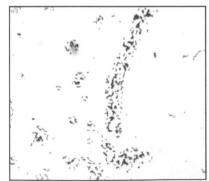

Fig. 7.18 Gram-positive small cocci; in chains or pairs.

INVESTIGATION INTO URINARY TRACT DISORDERS

- Animal selection – observe and record urination if possible.
- Euthanase pigs with typical signs.
- Submit a freshly dead pig, if available.
- Must collect a urine sample, serum, unclotted blood and a smear for haematology and biochemistry.

DISORDERS OF THE URINARY TRACT

Amaranthus reflexus intoxication

In the late summer/autumn pigs may present with acute kidney injury following ingestion of *Amaranthus reflexus* (redroot pigweed; **Figure 7.19**). The toxin results in calcium oxalate being deposited in the tubules. Clinical signs occur about a week after ingestion. Pigs present with weakness and trembling with incoordination.

Post-mortem findings are characterised by perirenal oedema (**Figure 7.20**). If the pig survives, the damage to the kidney may become chronic, resulting in chronic kidney disease. Serum biochemistry is useful in the diagnosis.

Differential diagnosis

Perirenal oedema may be seen associated with porcine circovirus 2 (PCV2) infection and other poisonings associated with oxalates (e.g. ethylene glycol).

Crystalluria

Definition/aetiology

Crystalluria is the presence of visible urinary crystal deposits in the bladder and on the vulva lips.

Clinical presentation

Sow presents with a white discharge closely adherent to the vulva lips. White stain may be seen on the slats behind the sow (**Figure 7.21**). The material can be 'putty like' and feel gritty to the touch.

Differential diagnosis

Purulent vulval discharges from uterine infections.

Diagnosis

Make a thin smear of the white material on a glass slide. Stain with a quick stain system to reveal the calcium apatite (calcium phosphate) and struvite (magnesium ammonium phosphate hexahydrate) crystals (**Figure 7.22**). A purulent discharge will demonstrate neutrophils.

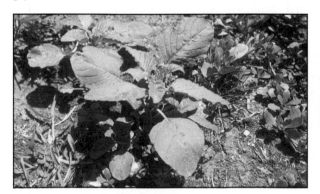

Fig. 7.19 *Amaranthus reflexus* plant.

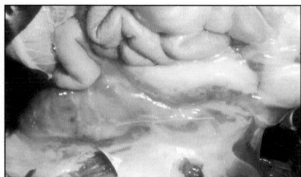

Fig. 7.20 Perirenal oedema.

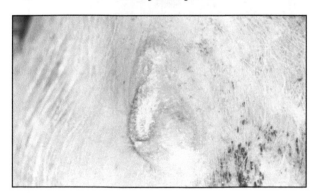

Fig. 7.21 White crystals on the vulva. This may also be seen on the floor.

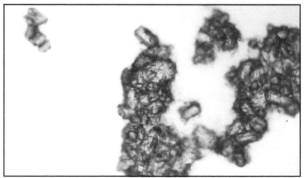

Fig. 7.22 Crystal violet stain of the white sediment quickly differentiates crystalluria from an inflammatory response.

Management

Ensure that the sow has plenty of water and exercise during pregnancy. It rarely causes mortality but large amounts of crystals (0.5 kg or more) may be found in the bladder at necropsy. May be used as a welfare indicator of inadequate water supplies.

Cystitis

Definition/aetiology

Inflammation of the urinary bladder. Many environmental and gut bacteria may be associated with cystitis, including *Actinobaculum suis*, *Escherichia coli*, *Proteus* spp., *Streptococcus* spp. and *Staphylococcus* spp.

Clinical presentation

May be asymptomatic to the stockperson. Urine may be seen to be darker or blood tinged. Sow may strain during urination. Around 70% of sows may be recognised as having a clinical cystitis in studies. Rare in the male without other problems such as prostatitis.

Differential diagnosis

Ascending pyelonephritis, which is life threatening. Other causes of vulval discharge.

Diagnosis

Examination of the urine. Post-mortem examination of the bladder (**Figure 7.23**). Histological examination is recommended. Note that post-mortem changes in the bladder are rapid. The transitional layer quickly becomes detached and may result in a purulent looking discharge. The exposed serosal surface can appear congested.

Management

The quality of the water supply for the pigs must be acceptable. Providing feed once a day in the afternoon to gestating sows enhances urinary health by encouraging urination in the afternoon and water intake. Drinking and urination are essential after mating. Reducing the number of natural matings and moving towards artificial insemination reduces the risk of introduction of potential pathogens. Improve the hygiene of the sow perineal region. The sow must not sleep in her faeces. This is particularly true for sows 3 days before and after farrowing. Enhance the hygiene of the sow and any interventions at farrowing.

Leptospirosis

Leptospirosis is the best known cause of interstitial nephritis, which may be particularly severe when associated with the *Leptospira pomona* serovar. However, leptospiruria is not unusual and is generally asymptomatic (**Figure 7.24**).

For further details on leptospirosis see Chapter 2.

Nephroblastoma

Nephroblastoma is a relatively common congenital embryonal tumour of the kidney. Normally only one kidney is affected. The kidney is extremely large.

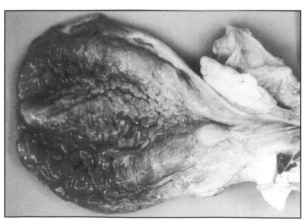

Fig. 7.23 Cystitis revealed as an incidental finding at post-mortem associated with *Escherichia coli* infection.

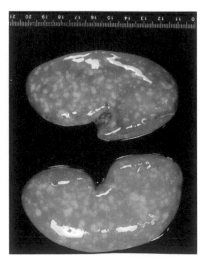

Fig. 7.24 Interstitial nephritis.

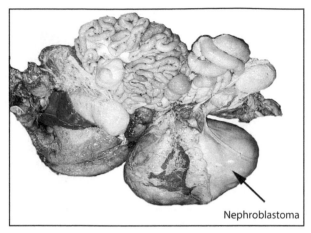

Fig. 7.25 Nephroblastoma. (See question at end of chapter.)

The other kidney is generally normal. Metastasis is unusual. The pig is asymptomatic. Nephroblastoma is found as an incidental finding at post-mortem or slaughter (**Figure 7.25**).

Porcine dermatitis and nephropathy syndrome

Porcine dermatitis and nephropathy syndrome is associated with urinary changes. The condition is discussed in more detail in Chapter 9.

In summary, the renal change is an enlargement of the kidneys (**Figure 7.26**), which often appear grey with multiple small red spots visible on the surface. Histological changes are characterised by fibrino-necrotising glomerulitis and interstitial nephritis (**Figure 7.27**).

Pyelonephritis and cystitis
Definition/aetiology
Actinobaculum suis is the classic organism associated with pyelonephritis and cystitis. However, other organisms may also be isolated (e.g. *Escherichia coli* and *Streptococcus* spp.). With *Streptococcus* there may be a purulent pyelonephritis.

A. suis is an anaerobic bacterium whose normal habitat is the prepuce of the boar. It should not normally be isolated from the sow or gilt. It has a powerful urease enzyme converting urea to ammonia, which raises the urine pH to ≥9.

Clinical presentation
In sows there are two major clinical presentations:

- **Acute pyelonephritis** in adult sows normally over third parity within a couple of weeks of breeding. Sows present off food, in collapse and urinating frank blood (**Figures 7.28, 7.29**). The sow may be found dead.
- **Chronic pyelonephritis** can occur at any time with the sow presenting with a variety of cystitis signs. Urinating smoky urine to frank blood. As the pig goes into renal injury her breathing rate increases. The sow goes off her food, presents with hindlimb weakness, eventually with collapse and eventually death. Many sows are misdiagnosed as clostridial hepatopathy if post-mortem examination is not carried out or is delayed by 12 hours.

Fig. 7.26
Grossly enlarged kidney in a case of porcine dermatitis and nephropathy syndrome (upper kidney) compared with a normal kidney (lower kidney).

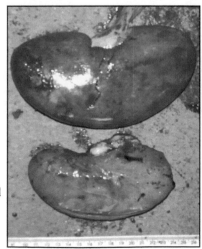

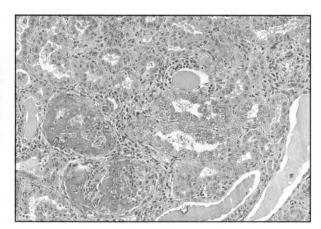

Fig. 7.27 Fibrino glomerulitis and interstitial nephritis.

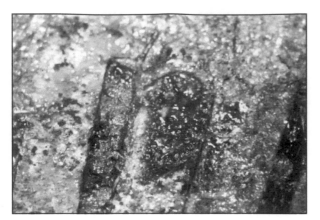

Fig. 7.28 Blood on the floor behind the sow after urination.

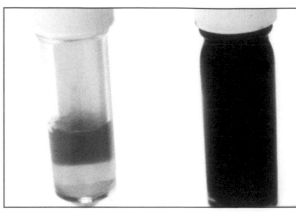

Fig. 7.29 Normal (left) and bloody urine (right) from a case of acute pyelonephritis.

Diagnosis

- **Live animal**. Urine sample revealing frank blood with renal casts. Urinary pH >8. Bacteriology demonstrates *A. suis*. Biochemistry examination of serum sample with elevated blood urea, creatinine and GGT concentrations. The potassium concentration rises precipitately as the pig progresses into renal failure.
- **Dead animal**. Post-mortem examination reveals pyelonephritis and severe catarrhal cystitis.

There are changes to the ureterovesical junction allowing for ureteric reflux. The extremely alkaline urine then causes ureteritis and necrosis of the renal papillae, resulting in massive blood loss. With the compound papillae (at the renal poles and middle) the alkaline and infected urine enters the renal nephron, leading to ascending pyelonephritis. A chronic end-stage kidney may be discovered as an incidental finding at post-mortem.

Post-mortem findings

Acute pyelonephritis: See **Figures 7.30–7.32**.

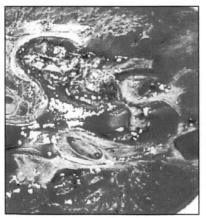

Fig. 7.30 Acute necrosis of the pyramids of the pelvis.

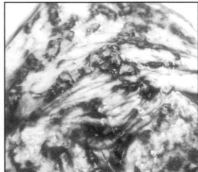

Fig. 7.31 Acute cystitis of the bladder wall.

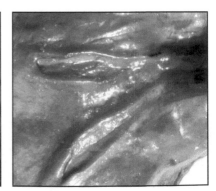

Fig. 7.32 Acute necrosis and damage of the ureterovesical junction. The damage allows for reflux of urine back to the kidney.

Chronic active pyelonephritis: See **Figures 7.33–36**.

Fig. 7.33
Gross
appearance
of the kidney
and ureter
in a case of
pyelonephritis
and ureteritis.

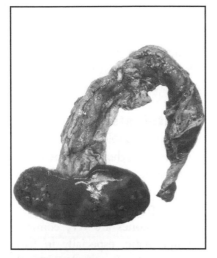

Fig. 7.34 Detail of
the chronic active
pyelonephritis common
over the pole of the
kidney.

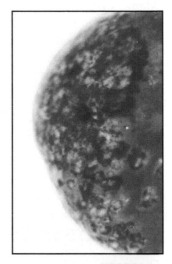

Fig. 7.35
Chronic
shortening
and thickening
of the
ureterovesical
junction.
This allows
occasional
ureteric reflux.

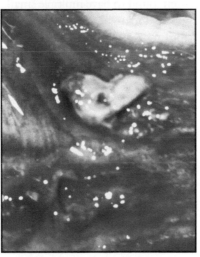

Fig. 7.36 Pyelonephritis
and hydroureteter
associated with
Streptococus suis.

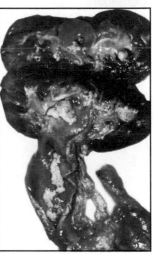

Differential diagnosis

Other causes of sudden death in the sow. Cystitis without pyelonephritis. Other causes of vulva discharge. Hindlimb weakness.

Management

Ensure that water management is excellent, especially in the breeding area (see Chapter 10).

A sow with cystitis becomes infected at breeding, especially with natural breeding. However, if the sow does not have cystitis, the *A. suis* organisms will be washed out at the next urination. Feed non-lactating sows once a day in the afternoon to encourage more urination and water intake.

Enhance management of hygiene of the farrowing and lactating sow.

Review breeding techniques and change to clean AI breeding management.

In chronic cases, lincomycin combined with tetracycline has proven effective, but note that chronic cystitis may be difficult to resolve. Acute cases often die within 2–3 days and can only be saved with fluid therapy and intensive care.

Stephanurus dentatus

Definition/aetiology

Stephanurus dentatus is the kidney worm. It is a strongyle worm most prevalent in warm climates, including the southern USA.

Clinical presentation

Many cases are asymptomatic and the problem is only revealed at post-mortem or slaughter. Condemnations in the abattoir are the most significant economic effect. If cases are seen, the pigs may have retarded growth and decreased food conversion. Larvae spend several months in the liver and during this time cause the majority of the pathological damage (**Figure 7.37**). The larvae leave the liver and migrate around the body. Adults develop in the perirenal tissues (**Figure 7.38**).

Differential diagnosis

In the liver *Ascaris suum*, although the chronic hepatitis changes are more severe with kidney worm infestation.

Diagnosis

Post-mortem examination of the liver and perirenal tissue. Demonstration of the eggs in the urine (**Figure 7.39**).

Management

The problem does not occur in countries with harsh winters. Avoid pasture-raised pigs. Avermectins are effective treatment options. Because of the long prepatent period, using once bred gilt management programmes (gilts are slaughtered after weaning their first litter) helps to break the worm life-cycle.

Urolithiasis

Definition/aetiology

Urolithiasis is the development of mineral stones within the urinary system, which may result in obstruction.

Clinical presentation

Urinary stones are very common and generally are asymptomatic, especially in female pigs. Boars are often found to have multiple small stones (calcium carbonate) looking like grit in the bladder at post-mortem (**Figure 7.40**). Obstruction of the urinary tract associated with urolithiasis is an acute presentation. The animal is often found dead with a distended abdomen.

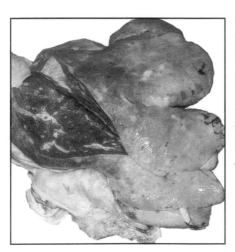

Fig. 7.37 Liver of a boar with chronic hepatitis associated with *Stephanurus dentatus*.

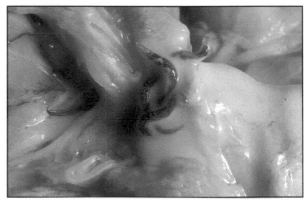

Fig. 7.38 Adult worms in the perirenal tissues.

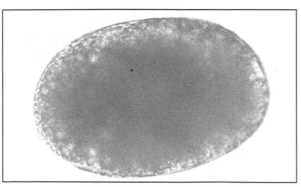

Fig. 7.39 An embryonated egg in the urine.

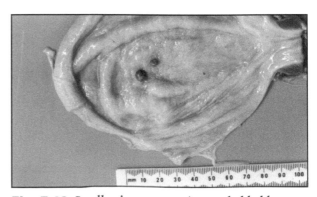

Fig. 7.40 Small urinary stones in a male bladder.

Differential diagnosis

Hindlimb weakness. Perceived sudden death.

Diagnosis

Stillborn piglets may present with urinary injury associated with heavy uric acid and urate uroliths present in the renal pelvis (**Figure 7.41**). This is characterised by an orange colour to the pelvis and pyramids. This may also be seen in dehydrated neonates.

In any age group, particularly males, if there is urinary blockage the bladder can be very large and fills the abdomen (**Figure 7.42**). Since the urinary bladder is significantly distended, it is easy to be punctured or ruptured when doing the necropsy. This releases the urine into the abdomen possibly together with the blockage stones. The clinician may think that the bladder ruptured, but this is extremely rare. Careful dissection of the whole urinary tract may reveal the stones.

If the pig is found live, it will have a distended abdomen and may look in distress. Generally, the pig is found dead with few gross lesions.

Management

Individual pigs may be difficult to manage. Urolithiasis is revealed as an incidental finding. If there is a problem with urinary blockage in growing pigs, review the food mineral concentrations and water supply. Review the type of urolith and modify the urinary pH as required.

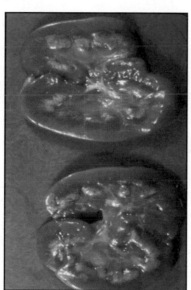

Fig. 7.41 **Orange urate stones/ deposit in a kidney from a stillborn piglet.**

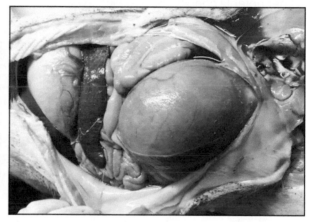

Fig. 7.42 **Male weaner mortality associated with urolithiasis. Note: This bladder would be easy to rupture if the post-mortem examination is performed too quickly.**

Other urinary necropsy findings

Congenital urinary tract conditions
See **Figures 7.43–7.48**.

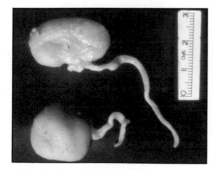

Fig. 7.43 **Congenital hypoplastic kidney.**

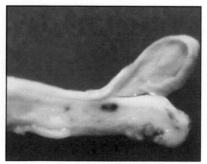

Fig. 7.44 **Ureteric diverticulum.**

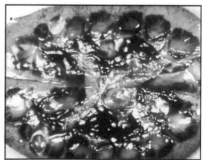

Fig. 7.45 **Congenital porphyria.**

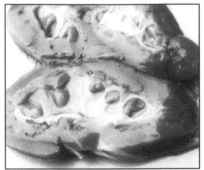

Fig. 7.46 Hydronephrosis.

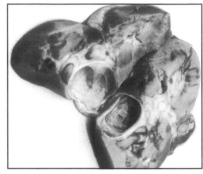

Fig. 7.47 Single large renal cyst.

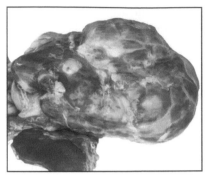

Fig. 7.48 Polycystic kidney (top). Note the otherwise normal kidney (bottom).

Other notable conditions of the kidneys
See **Figures 7.49–7.55**.

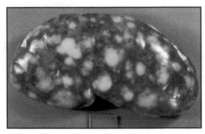

Fig. 7.49 Leukaemia affecting a kidney.

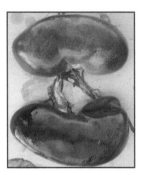

Fig. 7.50 Melanosis of the kidneys.

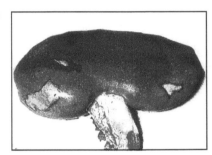

Fig. 7.51 Renal infarct.

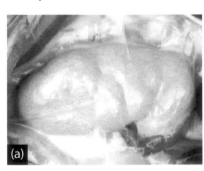
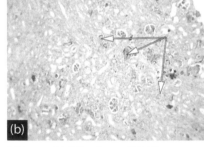

Fig. 7.52 (a) Melamine deposits in a kidney. (b) Histology (H&E) showing the melamine crystals (arrowed).

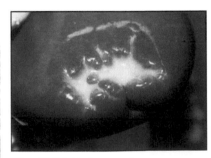

Fig. 7.53 Polar renal scar.

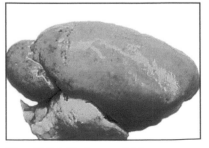

Fig. 7.54 End-stage kidney.

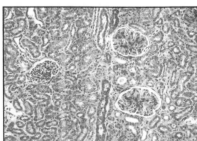

Fig. 7.55 Disseminated intravascular coagulation with the characteristic glomerulae cuffing often associated with salmonellosis (methylene blue stain).

CLINICAL QUIZ

7.1 Identify the major organs and the tumour shown in **Figure 7.25** (see p. 247).

7.2 Identify the major structures shown in **Figure 7.27** (see p. 247).

The answers to these questions can be found on page 475.

Acknowledgement
Figures 7.43, 7.49 and **7.51** reproduced, with permission, from Crown Publishing, originally published in *Pathology of the Pig: A Diagnostic Guide*. Eds. LD Sims, JRW Glastonbury. The Pig Research and Development Corporation Australia and Agriculture Victoria, 1977.

CHAPTER 8

IMMUNE SYSTEM DISORDERS

CLINICAL ANATOMY OF THE IMMUNE SYSTEM

Disorders and diseases affecting the immune system usually have significant impact on pig production. Immune responses are mediated by cells mainly present in lymphoid tissues, but not exclusively. Immune cells are present in virtually all body tissues and their response can occur at a regional or systemic level, depending on the triggering stimulus. Five major organised tissues represent the pig lymphoid system: lymph nodes (**Figure 8.1**), lymphoid follicles or aggregates, tonsils, thymus and spleen.

Porcine lymph nodes (and those of the hippopotamus) have the peculiarity of being histologically inverted compared with the rest of the mammals, with B-cell germinal centres located internally and cortical and paracortical areas dominated by T cells (**Figures 8.2, 8.3**).

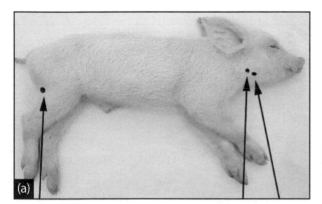

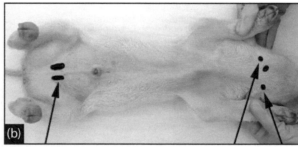

Fig. 8.1 (a, b) Superficial lymph nodes in the pig. (See Clinical quiz 8.1 on page 275.)

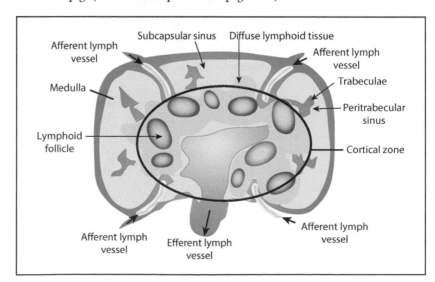

Fig. 8.2 Schematic representation of a pig lymph node.

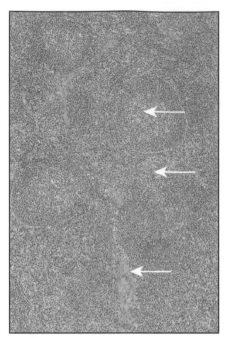

Fig. 8.3 The normal histological appearance of a pig lymph node. (See Clinical quiz 8.2 on page 275.)

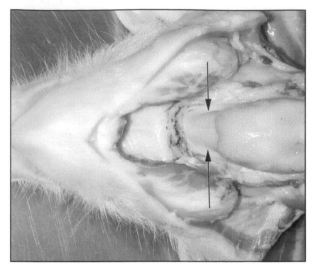

Fig. 8.4 Tonsils are located in the soft palate (arrows). Their identification is facilitated by the existence of tonsillar crypts, visible as small (<1 mm) dots on the surface of the soft palate.

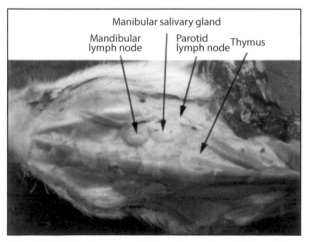

Fig. 8.5 The thymus and lymph nodes of the neck.

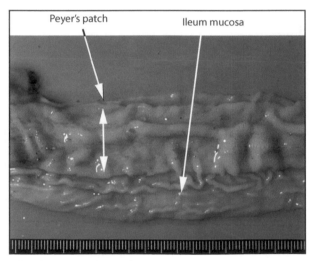

Fig. 8.6 Peyer's patches.

Lymphoid aggregates are mainly located in mucosal areas. They are usually designated as mucosa-associated lymphoid tissue (e.g. Peyer's patches in the digestive tract) and bronchus-associated lymphoid tissue in the respiratory tract.

The tonsils include those located in the soft palate (**Figure 8.4**), which are very big and easily identifiable grossly, but there are also tonsils in the pharynx, tongue and caecum. The tonsils are the most important entry site of pathogens to the immune system

due to their direct contact with the environment (see Chapter 3).

The thymus is identifiable in the ventral neck of young pigs and is the primary lymphoid organ for the development of T cells in the prenatal and neonatal pig (**Figure 8.5**). Identification of the thymus is complicated in chronically diseased animals, as it become atrophic.

The Peyer's patches in pigs are visible macroscopically (both from the serosal as well the

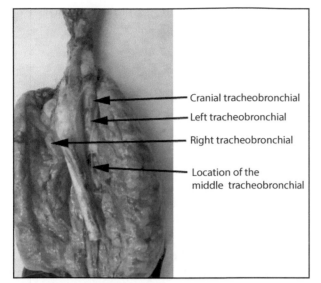

Fig. 8.7 The major lymph nodes of the respiratory tract – dorsal view.

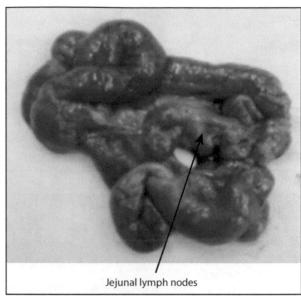

Fig. 8.8 The jejunal lymph nodes.

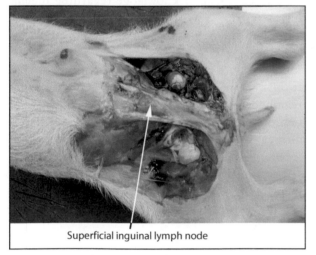

Fig. 8.9 Superficial inguinal lymph nodes. Normal size in a 25 kg pig: average length 38 mm, width 19 mm and weight 4.2 g.

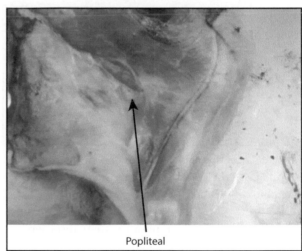

Fig. 8.10 The superficial popliteal lymph node.

mucosal surfaces). In the pig, Peyer's patches are mainly located in the ileum. They are large and protrude from the mucosal surface (**Figure 8.6**). They can be observed through the ileal serosa. Other lymph nodes are illustrated in **Figures 8.7–8.10**.

The spleen is the biggest lymphoid organ, playing a major role in immune responses against septicaemias (**Figures 8.11, 8.12**) (see Chapter 4).

The skin, one of the largest immune organs, is rich is antigen presenting cells, such as dentritic cells, and this feature can be used to great effect with needle free injections.

Besides specific lesions affecting tissues of the lymphoid system, there are a myriad of factors or elements including pathogens, vaccines, toxins, chemicals, nutrients and environmental and psychological (stress) factors that may up- or downregulate the immune responses. Such immunomodulation may affect the outcome of innate and/or acquired immune responses.

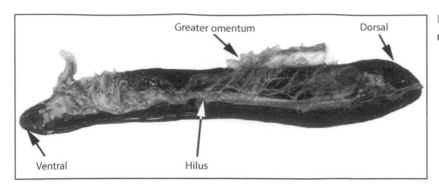

Fig. 8.11 **The visceral surface of the spleen.**

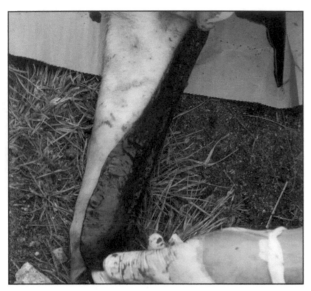

Fig. 8.12 **Is this spleen enlarged? A normal spleen should be of the approximate length as the elbow to the point of the toe!**

The majority of lymphoid system disorders are caused by infectious agents (alone or in combination), but environmental factors and management practices play a significant predisposing role. Moreover, although of no epidemiological significance, lymphoid tumours (lymphoma or lymphosarcoma) are the most frequent neoplasia in pigs.

Apart from tumours, infectious agents may cause local or systemic disease and lymphoid lesions. Pathogens causing lymphoid lesions, as part of a systemic infection, also cause lesions in other organs or systems.

An important cause of immunodeficiency in neonatal pigs is the failure of adequate colostrum intake. Due to the epitheliochorial placentation of the sow, pigs are born with an almost complete lack of serum antibodies and primed lymphoid cells.

Absorption of colostrum IgG antibodies and cells is normally limited to the first few hours of life.

Table 8.1 shows the main infectious and non-infectious causes of lymphoid system disorders and/or secondary immunodeficiency in pigs. The infectious causes are the most studied; there is still a significant lack of knowledge regarding mechanisms on how physical and physiological stress, nutrition and toxic products affect the immune system.

There are a number of infectious agents or their toxins that may affect the function of macrophages, lymphocytes or neutrophils by means of direct or indirect mechanisms. For example, porcine parvovirus, swine influenza virus, *Actinobacillus pleuropneumoniae*, *Mycoplasma hyopneumoniae*, *Salmonella enterica* serotype *choleraesuis* are pathogens that arc able to increase susceptibility to other agents, although they are not primarily affecting the lymphoid system themselves.

CLINICAL SIGNS AND DIAGNOSIS OF IMMUNE SYSTEM DISORDERS

The most important clinical signs associated with lymphoid system disorders and/or immunodeficiency associated with infectious and non-infectious origins are listed in *Table 8.1*. The majority of the infectious agents mentioned are not lymphoid system-specific. In consequence, observed clinical signs of diseases affecting the immune system may have a very variable outcome. This is specifically because the immunosuppressive status favours an outcome caused by the dominant infectious or non-infectious agents present in the farm and not necessarily a particular, unequivocal

Table 8.1 **Most frequent infectious and non-infectious causes of lymphoid system disorders in pigs and/or secondary immunodeficiencies, and their most frequently associated clinical signs.**

GENERIC CAUSES	AGENT/SPECIFIC CAUSE (DISEASE)	CLINICAL SIGNS
Physical and physiological distress	Thermal stress	Excess cold usually causes piling of animals, rough hair and trembling Excess heat usually causes a scattered resting of pigs, polydipsia and dyspnoea
	Crowding and mixing	Very variable; acute stress is difficult to assess clinically, unless it is displayed as fighting
	Weaning	Fighting due to hierarchy establishment
	Limit-feeding	Fighting due to restricted feeding and drinking areas
	Restraint	Screaming
Infectious agents	Porcine circovirus type 2	Growth retardation, rough hair, respiratory distress, death; susceptibility to concomitant infections; occasionally, diarrhoea and jaundice
	Porcine reproductive and respiratory syndrome virus	Growth retardation, rough hair, respiratory distress; susceptibility to concomitant infections; reproductive problems in pregnant sows
	Aujeszky's disease virus/ pseudorabies virus	Fever, central nervous clinical signs, depression, respiratory distress, death; susceptibility to concomitant infections; reproductive problems in pregnant sows
	Classical swine fever virus	Fever, central nervous clinical signs, depression, respiratory distress, diarrhoea, skin haemorrhages, growth retardation, death; susceptibility to concomitant infections; reproductive problems in pregnant sows
	African swine fever virus	Fever, haemorrhages of the skin, epistaxis, depression, bloody diarrhoea, death
	Nipah virus	Fever, central nervous clinical signs, depression, respiratory distress, non-productive cough, death; susceptibility to concomitant infections
	Mycobacterium avium complex, *M. bovis*, *M. tuberculosis* (tuberculosis)	Subclinical in most cases
Inadequate nutrition	Malnutrition	Growth retardation, death
	Overfeeding	Obesity
	Vitamin and/or trace mineral imbalances*	Very variable depending on the exact cause
Immunotoxic substances	Heavy metals	Very variable depending on the exact cause; some mycotoxins affect the immune system by predisposing to concomitant infections
	Industrial chemicals and pesticides	
	Mycotoxins	

*Key vitamins and minerals for optimal immune function are vitamins A, C, E and those from the B complex, and copper, zinc, magnesium, manganese, iron and selenium. It is very likely that the dietary requirements for optimal immune function are different from those to avoid deficiencies and their associated clinical signs.

clinical picture. In fact, immunosuppression or immunodeficiency can be clinically suspected in the following scenarios:

- Sickness due to pathogens with usual low pathogenicity or from an attenuated live vaccine.
- Recurrent sickness episodes that are usually not difficult to control.
- Failure to respond properly to vaccination.

- Unexplained neonatal sickness and/or death affecting more than one animal in a litter.
- A variety of disease syndromes occurring concurrently in a herd.

The aetiological clarification of lymphoid system disorders requires proper clinical, epidemiological and post-mortem investigations, but laboratory tests are obligatory in order to certify the specific cause of them.

A global diagnostic approach is recommended, including proper historical, clinical (*Table 8.1*) and epidemiological assessments at the herd level, as well as pathological examination of affected pigs and laboratory confirmation. Post-mortem examination of the lymphoid system is usually poorly informative, although in some particular cases the macroscopic diagnosis can be very suggestive.

The most frequent finding in the lymphoid system is regional or systemic lymphadenopathy. This terminology merely reflects an increase in size of one or most of the lymph nodes of the animal but does not give any clue regarding the specific cause. In fact, viral systemic infections, such as those caused by porcine circovirus type 2 (PCV2) and porcine reproductive and respiratory syndrome virus (PRRSV), as well as septicaemia caused by bacteria, are frequent causes of systemic lymphadenopathy. Regional lymphadenopathy is usually linked to the reaction of the drainage lymph node in respect of a lesion affecting the particular affected area (e.g. increase in size of mediastinal lymph nodes associated with catarrhal–purulent bronchopneumonia). It is important to provide an actual size in mm of a lymphadenopathy, not just record it as 'enlarged'. Other postmortem findings include: abscesses, granulomas or necrosis in lymph nodes, tonsil or spleen (usually associated with bacterial regional or systemic infections; rarely due to fungi); splenomegaly (frequent in septicaemia due to bacterial and systemic viral infections; the most striking one is that caused by African swine fever or erysipelas [see Chapter 9]; splenic infarcts (due to vasculitis or thrombosis); lymph node haemorrhages (usual finding in diseases causing haemorrhagic diathesis); and thymic atrophy (typical in all conditions causing a chronic catabolic state). Very rarely, lymphoma or lymphosarcoma can be diagnosed in slaughter-aged pigs due to the presence of malignant lymphoid proliferation in lymphoid tissues as well as non-lymphoid tissues. Many of these conditions are illustrated later in this chapter. Confirmation of most of these conditions requires histopathological examination.

Diagnosis of the specific cause of lymphoid system disorders will depend on the clinical assessment (if caused by physical and physiological alterations) or laboratory analyses (in cases of infectious diseases, nutritional deficiencies and immunotoxic substances). Determination of mycotoxins, heavy metals, chemicals and nutrients are done with different techniques and require specialised laboratories. For example, heavy metals and chemicals detection is mostly based on spectrometry techniques. Different analytical methods allow detection and quantification of mycotoxins and nutrients, such as high performance liquid chromatography, gas chromatography, capillary electrophoresis and ELISA techniques. For all these type of samples, feed is the most usual sample to be submitted, but in some cases it can be raw feed material, animal tissues or serum.

When the objective is to confirm or rule out the potential involvement of infectious agents (see *Table 8.1*), several laboratory techniques are available to determine the presence of particular lesions (histopathology), pathogens in lesions (immunohistochemistry [IHC], immunofluorescence, in situ hybridisation [ISH]), presence of an infectious agent (bacteriology or virus isolation), antimicrobial susceptibility of a bacterial agent (antibiogram), genome of the pathogen (PCR, RT-PCR, including real-time PCR) and antibodies against an infectious agent (ELISA and PCR tests). *Table 8.2* summarises the sample to be submitted for the potential diagnosis of a lymphoid disorder attributed to a pathogen.

MANAGEMENT OF IMMUNE SYSTEM DISORDERS

The management of a clinical condition primarily affecting the lymphoid system depends on the specific cause or causes that triggered it. Therefore, proper therapeutics or prevention of such problems must focus first on diagnosis. Once this is achieved (e.g. clinical, pathological), the nature of the intervention measure will adjust to the following actions:

- **Immediate actions:**
  - Antibiotic treatment in case of bacterial systemic infections; eventual use of anti-inflammatory drugs.
  - Urgent vaccination in case of certain viral infections (e.g. Aujeszky's disease [AD]/ pseudorabies).
  - Removal of feed or water in case of immunotoxic substances or nutritional imbalances.
- **Short-term actions:**
  - Change from immediate actions based on laboratory results if needed.

- Revision of the vaccine planning and strategic medications.
- Correction of the feeding management in case of malnutrition or overfeeding.

- **Mid-/long-term actions:**
  - Improve herd factors depending on structural or building issues.
  - Genetic background changes (significant effect on some systemic diseases affecting the immune system).
  - Enhance vitamin E concentration in the feed. In weaners this may require concentrations of 250 ppm. Vitamin C is generally not required by the pig as it is able to synthesise its own vitamin C.

The most frequently implemented actions against systemic disease outbreaks resemble the actions against respiratory problems, including the use of antibiotics and, eventually, non-steroidal anti-inflammatory medicines.

Most interventions are directed at preventing disease. Management of nutrition, raw feed materials and environment is the first control step. For a number of pathogens, vaccination is available and effective against a number of systemic diseases affecting the immune system (*Table 8.3*).

For notifiable diseases such African swine fever (ASF) and infection by Nipah virus, eradication applies in different parts of the world. Therefore, the main task of a veterinarian is early diagnosis of the

Table 8.2 **Samples to be selected depending on the laboratory technique.**

LABORATORY TECHNIQUE	SAMPLE TYPE	PURPOSE
Histopathology	Lymphoid tissue pieces (section of spleen, ileum and thymus, but complete lymph nodes – except mesenteric); fixation in formalin	Detection of microscopic lesions; usually very suggestive on the nature of the lesion
IHC/ISH	Same as for histopathology	Detection of a pathogen in the site of the lesion; detects antigen (IHC) or genome (ISH) of a pathogen
Bacteriology/virology	Complete lymphoid tissue, serum in some cases; refrigeration*	Isolation of bacteria or viruses; can be done for monitoring purposes
Antibiogram	Same as for bacteriology	Antimicrobial susceptibility of isolated bacteria
PCR/RT-PCR/qPCR	Complete lymphoid tissue, serum in some cases; can be refrigerated or frozen	Detection of pathogen genome; can be done for monitoring purposes
Antibody detection (ELISA)	Serum	Detection of antibodies against a pathogen; usually done for monitoring purposes

*Frozen samples are not a problem for virological tests.

Table 8.3 **Most common infectious agents causing systemic disorders that affect the immune system and their vaccine (and schedule) availability.**

INFECTIOUS AGENT	TYPE OF VACCINE	VACCINATION SCHEDULE
Porcine reproductive and respiratory syndrome virus	Modified live vaccines most often used; killed vaccines available	Piglet at weaning or later; gilt during acclimatisation; sows per cycle or in blanket coverage
Porcine circovirus type 2	Killed vaccines; genetically modified killed vaccine; subunit vaccines	Piglet at weaning or later; gilt during acclimatisation; sows pre-farrowing or pre-mating
Aujeszky's disease virus (pseudorabies virus)	Modified live DIVA* vaccines most often used; killed vaccines available	Piglet (two doses) at the end of nursery and during growing; gilts during acclimatization; sows in blanket coverage
Classical swine fever virus	Modified live vaccines ('chinese' or 'lapinised' strain) most often used; some are DIVA* vaccines (based on E2 protein).	Pigs (two doses) at 5 days of age onwards if coming from non-vaccinated sows, or around 35 days of age onwards if coming from vaccinated sows – second dose after 3–4 weeks; sows in blanket coverage or 3–6 weeks before farrowing

*DIVA, differentiation of infected from vaccinated animals.

condition and immediate notification to the appropriate authority. For other OIE (World Organisation for Animal Health [Office International des Epizooties]) pathogens such as classical swine fever virus (CSFV), however, there are different commercial vaccines available that can be applied in different geographical areas. Note that these vaccines may also result in injury to the immune system.

DISORDERS OF THE LYMPHATIC SYSTEM

Aujeszky's disease (pseudorabies)

A major early signs of a naïve farm breaking with AD is abortion. AD is discussed in more detail in Chapter 2.

Colostrum and innate immunodeficiency ▶ VIDEO 2

Because of the structure of the epitheliochorial placentation, which isolates the fetus in the uterus, piglets are born effectively immunodeficient. However, the fetus does start to activate its immune system at around 70 days of gestation. The pig is probably not fully immunocompetent until 70 days of life (about 30 kg in commercial pigs). This has significant impacts on the development of pig production system. (See Chapter 3

Table 8.4 Some factors affecting colostrum function/availability.

Mother	Udder oedema	Nervousness
	Insufficient teats	Constipation
	Damaged teats	Vaccination programme
	Mastitis	Too much Ca/PO$_4$ in feed: requires <1%
Piglet	Draughts	Competition
	Chilling	Litter size
	Hypothermia	First to last born birth order
	Fostering	Splayleg
		Congenital tremor

for the normal nursing pattern and disorders of the mammary gland.)

What can affect the availability of colostrum

Some factors affecting colostrum function and availability are listed in *Table 8.4*.

The clinician needs to pay attention to the behaviour of the sow and her reaction to her newborn piglets (**Figure 8.13**). Any sow that is reluctant to allow her piglets to suckle needs to receive additional attention and stockpersonship (**Figure 8.14**). This can involve the use of a sedative.

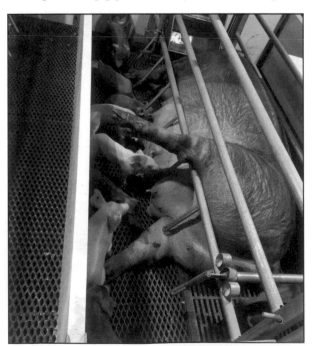

Fig. 8.13 Sow allowing her piglet to suckle.

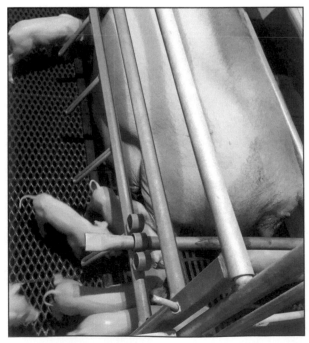

Fig. 8.14 Sow reluctant to allow suckling. The sow is 'protecting' her udder.

It is essential that newborn piglets have access to colostrum within 6 hours of the first suckle. Cellular immunity will only be transferred between mother and her own piglets. This is important in viral and mycoplasmal immunology.

A piglet can consume 250 g of colostrum in the first day, drinking 12 mL every hour. Once the production of milk stabilises at day 3, the milk is released for about 8 seconds every 45 minutes to 2 hours (more at the beginning of lactation and progressively less as lactation progresses).

What is colostrum?

Colostrum provides food and bioactive compounds and, vitally important, a source of warmth (*Table 8.5*).

Table 8.5 **Colostrum specifications.**

NUTRIENT COMPOSITION PER 100 ML	COLOSTRUM	MILK	BIOACTIVE COMPOUNDS PER 100 ML*	COLOSTRUM	MILK
Total dry matter (g)	24.8	18.7	Serum albumin (g)	1.46	0.45
Total protein (g)	15.1	5.5	IgG (g)	8.9	0.1
Casein (g)	1.3	2.6	IgA (g)	2.0	0.6
Whey (g)	13.7	2.9	IgM (g)	0.85	0.15
Lactose (g)	3.4	5.3	Lactoferrin (mg)	120	40
Total fat (g)	5.9	7.6	ECF (µg)	157	19
Palmitic acid (g)	2.0	2.8	IGF-I (µg)	40	1
Palmitoleic acid (g)	0.3	0.6	IGF-II (µg)	29	2
Stearic acid (g)	0.4	0.5	Insulin (µg)	1.5	0.2
Oleic acid (g)	2.2	2.5	TGF-β1 (µg)	4.3	0.2
Linoleic acid (g)	0.7	0.8	TGF-β2 (µg)	2.0	0.4
Vitamin A (µg)	170	100	Neutrophils	+++	
Vitamin D (µg)	1.5	0.9	Lymphocytes (memory T)	+++	
Vitamin E (µg)	380	260	Lysozyme	+++	
Vitamin K (µg)	9.5	9.2			
Vitamin C (µg)	7.2	4.7			
Total ash (g)	0.7	0.9			
Calcium (mg)	71	184			
Phosphorous (mg)	105	139			
Potassium (mg)	113	82			
Magnesium (mg)	8	10			
Sodium (mg)	71	43			

Note: Values highlighted in red indicate the major differences between colostrum and normal milk.

*Immunogloblins provide the piglet with an immediate source of antibodies to fight a variety of pathogens. IgG is for the blood stream, while IgA covers the surface membranes. Normal milk still contains a concentration of IgA. Lactoferrin is bactericidal through competition for iron, an important nutrient for enteric bacteria. TGF-β2 plays a role in controlling the intestines response to antigens. Memory T cells play a major role in passing on immunity to the piglet. Lactomorphine helps piglets sleep.

The cellular component in colostrum is also vital to providing the piglet with a degree of immunocompetence. However, the cellular component is only functional between the birth mother and her piglets. If the colostrum is from a surrogate mother, the immunolglobulins and other chemicals will be valuable, but the cellular function will be impaired.

Serum concentration of IgG in piglets

Piglets who have received sufficient colostrum will have a serum immunoglobulin concentration of >10 mg/mL (normal 25–35 mg/mL). If total protein is used (via a refractometer), a total protein <40 mg/mL implies insufficient intake. The movement of antibodies and maternal cells is maximal for the first 6 hours after the first suckle, not from the moment of birth. The provision of sow colostrum to gilt piglets reduces their mortality in the finishing unit and increases their growth rate. Colostrum also initiates a 30% increase in intestinal weight.

Enhancing colostrum intake by piglets: split suckling

Colostrum intake is vital to the survival of piglets. Each piglet needs a minimum of at least 200 mL of colostrum. Ideally, within the first 24 hours the newborn piglet should drink approximately 250 mL of colostrum. A system needs to be used that ensures all the piglets receive adequate colostrum (**Figures 8.15–8.19**).

Preparing the farrowing room helps ensure that the proper environment to ensure colostral uptake is maintained. The ambient room temperature for the sow should be about 20°C and for piglets it should be 37°C and draught free (less than 0.2 m/s air movement). Heat mats or creep lights need to be placed both behind the sow and in the creep area, which should be already dry and warm at +30°C.

Retention of maternal antibodies by the piglet

Table 8.6 details when maternal antibodies for various infectious agents are lost.

Iron and discoloured lymph nodes

Lymph nodes filter materials from the lymph draining an area of the body. This can be classically revealed following an iron injection into the hindlimb of a piglet. While it is preferable to inject iron into the neck, it is still common for 200 mg of iron gluconate to be injected into the muscles of the hindlimb. This iron is then distributed throughout the body. The iron present in lymph drains through the local lymph node, which will become black in colour (**Figure 8.20**).

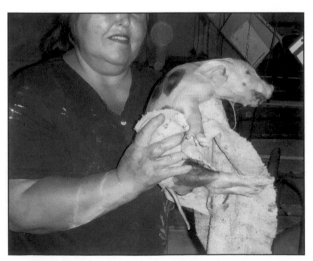

Fig. 8.15 Be there to collect and dry piglets as they are being born. This is very time-consuming.

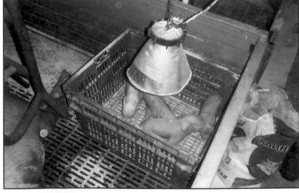

Fig. 8.16 Place newborn piglets into a basket under a heat lamp with the ambient air in the basket at 32–37°C. As soon as the first four or more piglets are dry and warm, place them on the sow to stimulate oxytocin release, which facilitates continuation of the birth process.

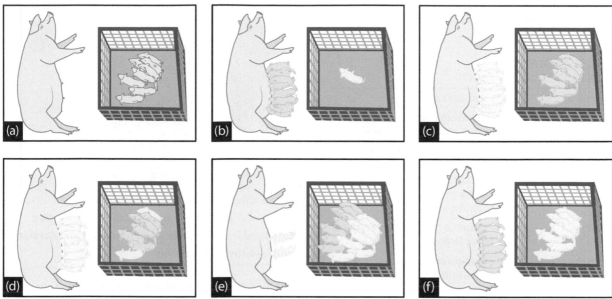

Fig. 8.17 Drawings illustrating piglet movements with split suckling. (a) Collect the piglets as they are born, dry and place them in a basket under a heat lamp. (b) After 1 hour, mark the piglets and release the warm and dried piglets onto the sow to suckle (group 1, blue piglets). Collect all the next group of newly born piglets, dry and place them into the basket under a heat lamp. (c) After 2 hours collect all the piglets that have been suckling. Release the second batch of piglets onto the sow to suckle (group 2, green). Place the group 1 (blue) piglets into the warming basket. (d) As new piglets are born continue to dry and place them in a warming basket (group 3 piglets, yellow). Mark with a different colour to the group 1 piglets (blue). (e) As new piglets are born continue to dry and place in warming basket – group 3 piglets (yellow). Mark with a different colour to the group 1 piglets (blue). (f) Release the group 1 piglets onto the sow for 30 minutes. Ensure all piglets have drunk colostrum. Collect and place in warming basket. Release the group 2 and group 3 piglets onto the sow for 30 minutes. Ensure all the piglets have drunk and release them as a group. By 4 hours farrowing should normally have been completed. With fostering, the split suckling may need to continue for a couple of hours more.

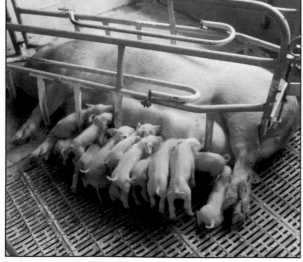

Fig. 8.18 Fostering and sorting can be completed after 24–48 hours.

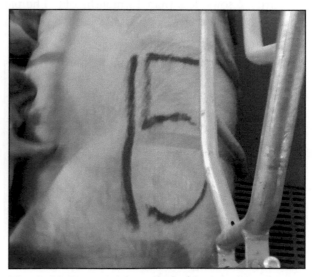

Fig. 8.19 Record the number of functioning teats on the rear of the sow pre-farrowing.

Table 8.6 **Retention of maternal antibodies by the piglet.**	
WEEK WHEN MOST ANTIBODY LOST	**AGENT**
Week 1	*Escherichia coli*
Week 2	Transmissible gastroenteritis virus Porcine epidemic diarrhoea virus
Week 3	*Actinobacillus pleuropneumoniae* *Brachyspira hyodysenteriae* *Haemophilus parasuis* Porcine reproductive and respiratory syndrome virus
Week 4	*Pasteurella multocida* and *Bordetella bronchiseptica*
Weeks 6–9	Aujeszky's disease (pseudorabies) Teschovirus *Mycoplasma hyopneumoniae* Porcine circovirus Porcine respiratory coronavirus Respiratory syncytial virus Swine influenza virus
Week 10	African swine fever virus Classical swine fever virus
Week 12	*Erysipelothrix rhusiopathiae*
Week 24	Parvovirus

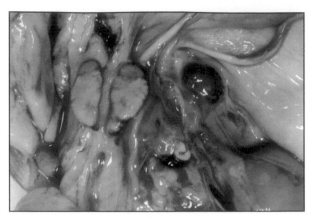

Fig. 8.20 Inguinal lymph nodes demonstrating unilateral iron discolouration following an injection of iron into the ham muscles.

Occasionally, an enlarged lymph node (e.g. a leukaemic node) may block local drainage and result in unilateral localised swellings (e.g. in one scrotum). There is no treatment and early euthanasia is recommended.

Two main forms of lymphosarcoma are recognised: lymphosarcoma of T cells originates in the thymus and develops in the cranial mediastinum; lymphosarcoma of B cells is multicentric occurring, for example, in the spleen and kidneys (**Figures 8.23, 8.24**).

Lymphosarcoma

Lymphosarcoma is a relatively common cause of wasting and ill thrift in young adult pigs (**Figures 8.21, 8.22**). It is therefore most commonly seen in gilts to parity 2 sows, less than 18 months old. The pig presents with a progressive loss of weight despite an appetite and no pyrexia.

Mycotoxicosis ▶ VIDEO 11

The clinical response to mycotoxins (some sources of mycotoxins are shown in **Figures 8.25–8.28**) can be variable, from acute to chronic. In most cases, the response is subacute to chronic and associated clinical signs are not specific enough. They can

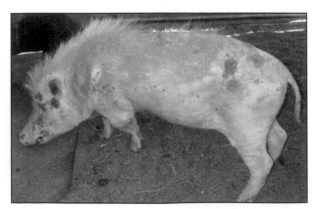

Fig. 8.21 A young sow that has become progressively emaciated associated with lymphosarcoma.

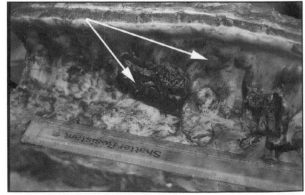

Fig. 8.22 Lymphosarcoma spread over the rib cage of a gilt (arrows).

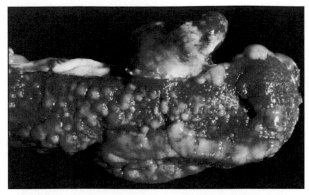

Fig. 8.23 Generalised distribution of malignant lymphoid proliferations of different sizes all over the splenic serosa (splenic lymphosarcoma).

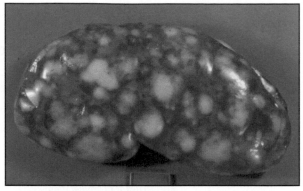

Fig. 8.24 Generalised distribution of malignant lymphoid proliferations of different sizes all over the kidney cortex (renal lymphosarcoma).

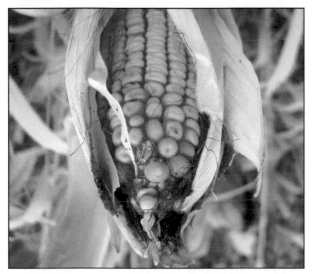

Fig. 8.25 Fungi growing on damaged corn (*Zea mays*).

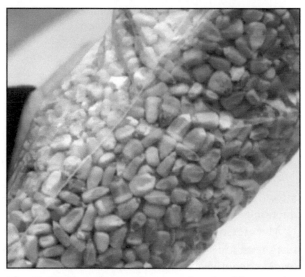

Fig. 8.26 Fusarium on harvested maize (*Zea mays*), in this case resulting in a zearalenone concentration of 10 ppm.

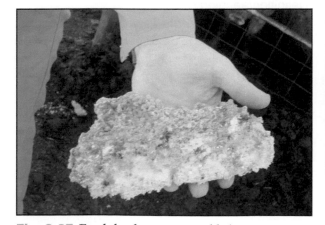

Fig. 8.27 Food that has gone mouldy in storage.

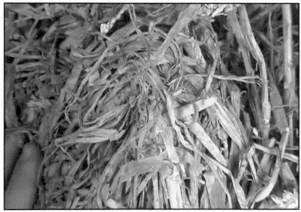

Fig. 8.28 Mould on bedding.

Table 8.7 **Mycotoxins.**

MYCOTOXIN	SOURCE	FIELD OR STORE	TOXIC CONCENTRATION	EFFECT
Aflatoxin	*Aspergillus flavus, Aspergillus parasiticus*	S	>0.2 ppm	Hepatitis; reduced growth; reduced feed intake; immunosuppression
Deoxynivalenol (vomitoxin)	*Fusarium spp.*	F	>0.5 ppm	Reduced feed consumption
Ergot	*Claviceps purpurea*	F	>1,000 ppm	Reduced feed intake; agalactia; gangrene
Fumonisins	*Fusarium moniliforme, Fusarium proliferatum*	F	>25 ppm	Liver dysfunction; pulmonary oedema
Ochratoxin, citrinin	*Aspergillus ochraceus, Penicillium viridicatum, Penicillium citrinum*	S	>0.2 ppm	Renal lesions; immunosuppression
Trichothecenes (T-2 toxin and diacetoxyscripenol)	*Fusarium* spp.	F	>3 ppm	Decreased feed intake; immunosuppression
Zearalenone	*Fusarium graminearum*	F	>1 ppm	Oestrogenic; pseudopregnancy; enlarged vulva in weaners
Plant toxins. There are numerous possibilities for poisoning from plants				
Gossypol	Cottonseed plant (*Gossypium* sp.)		>200 ppm	Reduced feed intake

S, mycotoxins that may increase in storage; F, mycotoxins that come from the field and do not increase in storage; 1 ppm = 1 mg/kg.

affect feed intake, feed efficiency, growth and reproduction and cause immunosuppression (*Table 8.7*).

Mycotoxins able to cause alteration of immune responses are aflatoxins (with values >0.2 ppm in feed), trichothecenes (>3 ppm) and deoxynivalenol (>0.5 ppm). If very high values of mycotoxins are found in the raw materials, feed refusal is the most frequent outcome.

Diagnosis of mycotoxicoses is difficult because other concomitant conditions might be present and the exact role of these toxins is still not completely defined. Moreover, the potential additive effect of multiple toxins below the limits of causing overt clinical signs is virtually unknown. Diagnosis is established by means of detection of mycotoxins in the feed by chemical methods; ELISA tests are available to detect aflatoxins. In face of a suspicion or occurrence of mycotoxicosis, interventions include a change of feed source and cleaning of equipment and feed storage places.

Mould inhibitors (often clays) are widely used, especially when moisture in feed storage places is observed; however, these products do not remove existing toxins. Dilution of contaminated grain is also common practice, but care should be considered to avoid introduction of new fungi or other mycotoxins.

Increasing methionine in the diet may be useful to combat mycotoxins in the feed. It assists with the detoxification of mycotoxins (vomitoxin [deoxynivalenol] and aflatoxin) in the liver.

Nipah virus infection

Definition/aetiology

Nipah virus belongs to the Paramyxoviridae family. It was initially detected in the Malaysian village Nipah. It has subsequently been found in other South-East Asian countries. The major concern for this infection is its zoonotic threat and cause of significant human mortality. Cats and dogs may also die following infection. It is believed that pteroid bats are the reservoir of this virus.

Clinical presentation

Clinical signs can vary significantly, since pigs may develop outcomes from subclinical to fatal. Nipah virus infection may result in acute fever accompanied by respiratory (from dyspnoea to paroxysmal, 'barking' cough) and/or neurological signs (muscle fasciculation, hindlimb weakness and inco-ordination). Mortality is especially high in suckling and early nursery pigs, but low (<5%) in grow/finish and adult pigs. Epistaxis is often seen in sudden death animals. Abortion may also be seen in sows. It is considered that the high mortality in young animals is probably associated with concurrent bacterial infections.

Differential diagnosis

Nipah virus infection should be differentiated from AD, CSF and ASF, PRRS and PCV2-SD. There are no characteristic gross or microscopic lesions that can be used to differentiate Nipah virus infection from other diseases. The existence of human mortality may be an unfortunate indicator that the pathogen is present. The zoonotic component of this infection is the major differential trait with other diseases causing neurological and respiratory disease in pigs.

Diagnosis

If Nipah virus infection is suspected, immediately contact the local government officials. A severe cough together with neurological signs in the geographical areas where Nipah virus has been described might suggest the condition. Histopathology may be of help since besides interstitial pneumonia and non-suppurative meningoencephalitis, lymphocyte depletion and vasculitis can be seen. Definitive diagnosis is usually established through detection of viral RNA by RT-PCR. Since Nipah virus is a high-risk zoonotic agent, samples should be taken with appropriate protective equipment and most of the diagnostic work should be performed in high biocontainment laboratory units. Indeed, methods that replicate the virus (cell culture) are not indicated in order to minimise the handling of potential infectious material. Viral antigen can also be demonstrated by IHC in formalin-fixed, paraffin-embedded tissues. Recommended samples to test are lungs, meninges, brain (olfactory bulb), trigeminal ganglion, lymph nodes and kidney. Screening for antibodies is mainly performed by an ELISA test.

Management

There is no treatment for Nipah virus infection, and when an outbreak has been established an eradication policy is applied. Prevention should include avoiding contact between pigs and virus reservoirs (pteroid bats) and strict biosecurity and quarantine to avoid entrance of infected pigs. The major focus is to prevent infection of humans.

Porcine circovirus diseases ▶ VIDEO 34
Definition/aetiology
PCV2 is the essential infectious agent causing the so-called porcine circovirus diseases. This group of diseases includes different clinical pictures, namely PCV2-systemic disease (PCV2-SD, formerly known as post-weaning multisystemic wasting syndrome), PCV2-reproductive disease (PCV2-RD), porcine dermatitis and nephropathy syndrome (PDNS), and PCV2-subclinical infection. Importantly, PDNS is an immune-complex disease and PCV2 is the suspected antigen associated with it; however, many cases are found with minimal involvement of PCV2. From 2007 onwards, the first PCV2 vaccines became available and the clinical picture was widely controlled.

Several different genotypes of PCV2 are recognised with PCV2b being the most prevalent genotype followed by PCV2d. Cross-reactivity and cross-protection have been shown between genotypes PCV2a, PCV2b and PCV2d.

Clinical presentation
The most well-known clinical expression of PCV2-SD is wasting or growth retardation (**Figures 8.29, 8.30**), which may be accompanied by different degrees of skin paleness, respiratory distress, diarrhoea, icterus and increased mortality. In early disease phases, an increase in the size of lymph nodes can be seen. The inguinal superficial lymph nodes may appear to increase in size, but most of this is associated with cachexia and loss of fat covering, making the lymph nodes more apparent.

Chronically affected pigs, surviving the acute phase, tend to develop cachexia. Since PCV2-SD affected pigs are immunosuppressed, they are very likely to suffer from concomitant diseases; additional clinical signs caused by these concurrent conditions can confuse the overall picture. The use of a PCV2 vaccine may improve the growth of the pigs by 20 g/day.

PDNS is recognised by red-to-black erythema, haemorrhage and necrosis of the skin, usually with circular to irregular shapes, mainly located in the hindlimbs and perineal area. In some cases, such skin lesions are generalised. The role of PCV2 in

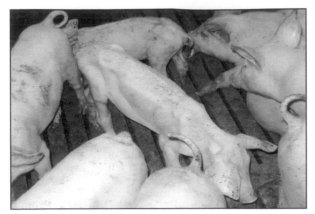

Fig. 8.29 Severe case of PCV2-SD illustrating post-weaning multisystemic wasting syndrome with no vaccination.

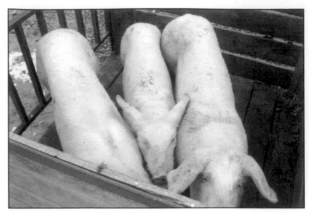

Fig. 8.30 The pig in the middle showing growth retardation was diagnosed as a PCV2-SD case.

cases of PDNS has not been determined, although on farms with PCV2-SD, cases of PDNS are more common (see Chapter 9).

PCV2 may also act as a SMEDI (stillborn, mummified, embryonic death and infertility) virus with some late-term abortions and premature farrowings being observed. This may be associated with fetal myocarditis. The severe form tends to occur in newly established herds with poor herd immunity programmes (see Chapter 2). On most farms the impact of PCV2 on the reproductive performance will be negligible.

Differential diagnosis

PCV2-SD differential diagnoses must be established with all causes of growth retardation, the most important being PRRS and ileitis. However, chronic respiratory and enteric diseases must also be included as potential diagnoses. Importantly, the differential list does not preclude other pathogens that might be found concomitantly together with the systemic disease. In fact, and in the absence of vaccination, co-infections of PCV2 and PRRSV or other pathogens are very frequent.

PCV2 reproductive disease must be differentiated from cases of late abortion and premature farrowing, including mainly PRRSV. When mummified fetuses are found, the most likely differential is porcine parvovirus.

PDNS is a rather characteristic condition; therefore, it is not easy to confuse it with other diseases. However, CSF, ASF and erysipelas must be included

in the differential diagnosis list. PDNS may occur without any apparent association with PCV2 (see Chapter 9).

Diagnosis

A herd diagnosis of PCV2-SD disease can be established based on two major criteria: significant increases in the percentage of wasted pigs and mortality compared with previous records and fulfilment of individual diagnostic criteria in at least one out of five necropsied pigs (some post-mortem findings are shown in **Figures 8.31–8.37**). Individual diagnostic criteria include three facets:

1 Clinical signs compatible with the condition.
2 Histopathological confirmation of moderate to severe lymphocyte depletion and granulomatous inflammation of lymphoid tissues.

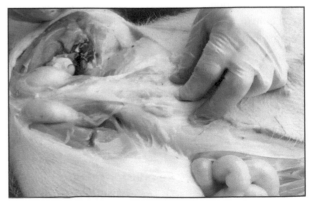

Fig. 8.31 Prominent lymph nodes.

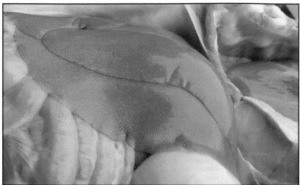

Fig. 8.32 Pale liver.

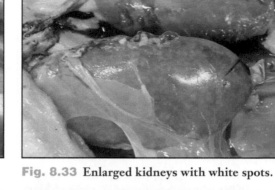

Fig. 8.33 Enlarged kidneys with white spots.

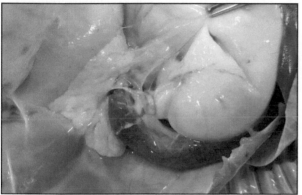

Fig. 8.34 Enlarged gastrohepatic lymph node.

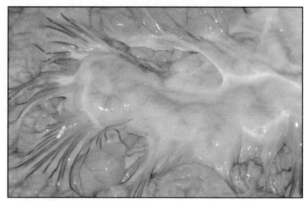

Fig. 8.35 Marked enlargement of the mesenteric lymph nodes.

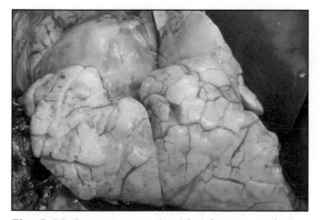

Fig. 8.36 Severe pneumonia with pulmonary oedema.

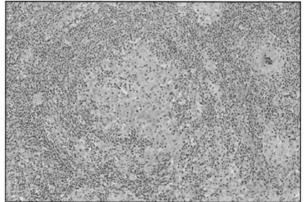

Fig. 8.37 Lymphoid depletion in the lymph node.

3 Moderate or high amount of PCV2 genome or antigen in these lymphoid lesions (**Figure 8.38**).

Note: Any draining lymph node from an infectious nidus is going to be enlarged. In cases of PCV2-SD the problem is systemic not local.

Detection of antibodies
Detection of antibodies against the virus does not constitute a diagnosis of the systemic disease, but it helps monitor the infection when cross-sectional studies are carried out.

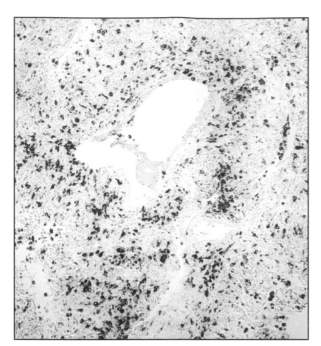

Fig. 8.38 Immunohistochemistry for porcine circovirus.

PCV2-subclinical infection does not have diagnostic usefulness since PCV2 is a ubiquitous virus. However, monitoring of PCV2 infection is interesting in the context of vaccination. This is mainly performed by antibody detection by ELISA methods or PCR detection of the virus, using serum or oral fluids as the most usual matrices.

PCV2-SD histological score

A PCV2-SD score can be made by histological examination (**Figures 8.39–8.41**). The score assesses lymph nodes or other lymphoid tissues. The tissues are examined for two characteristics:

- The degree of lymphoid depletion on a 0–3 scale.
- The degree of histiocytic granuloma formation on a 0–3 scale.

Immunohistochemistry scoring

The degree of PCV2 in the tissues, as assessed using IHC, can be determined on a 0–3 scale based on the degree of staining and the percentage of follicles with positive staining (**Figure 8.42**). Positive is indicated by the brown stained areas. A score of 1 = 10% or less of the follicles have PCV2 present; a score of 2 = 10–50% of the follicles have PCV2 present; a score of 3 = more than 50% of the follicles have PCV2 present. This may even be visible with the naked eye.

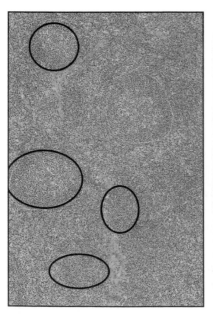

Fig. 8.39 Normal lymph node (some of the follicles are circled).

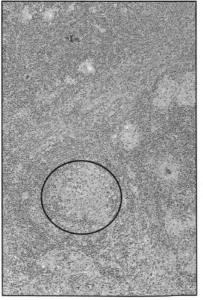

Fig. 8.40 Lymph node with lymphoid depletion – lack of cells and the follicular picture is lost (circled).

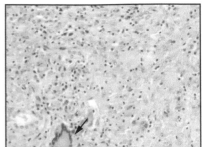

Fig. 8.41 A granuloma (multinucleated cell) (arrow) in a lymph node.

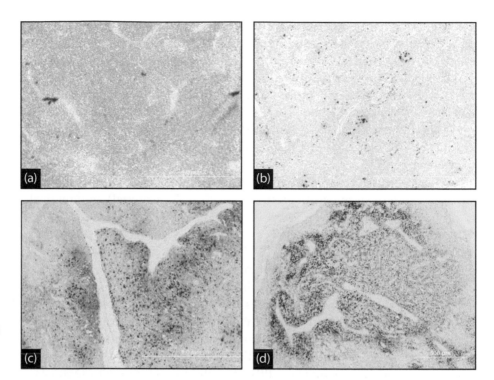

Fig. 8.42 Examples of PCV2 IHC scores. (a) IHC score 0; (b) IHC score 1; (c) IHC score 2; (d) IHC score 3.

Add the score for each of the criteria together and divide by 3. If multiple tissues are examined – ideally five lymph nodes – the tissues are added together and divided by the number of tissues. Samples should be taken of tonsil, spleen and superficial inguinal, bronchial and mesenteric lymph nodes.

Polymerase chain reaction

The use of quantitative PCR (qPCR) in serum or tissues can orientate clinicians towards the disease, especially if these values are high. However, individual variation and timing of sample collection during the course of infection makes establishment of the diagnosis difficult. It is recommended to take samples from affected pigs in the first week of clinical signs (both for pathological and molecular biological analyses).

Quantitative PCR cycle time interpretation and viral load: The initial viral load can be determined approximately by the PCR cycle time (*Table 8.8*).

This scale can be used for a number of other viruses and gives the clinician an indication of the prevalence of one virus versus another.

Table 8.8 PCR cycle time and approximate viral load.

CYCLE TIME	APPROXIMATE VIRAL LOAD
8	6×10^{13}
13	6×10^{11}
16	6×10^{10}
18	6×10^{9}
20	6×10^{8}
22	6×10^{7}
30	6×10^{6}
34	6×10^{5}
35	6×10^{4}
37	6×10^{3}

Management

PCV2-SD is considered a multifactorial disease in which management, concurrent infections, host genetics, nutrition and PCV2 infection timing play major roles. Therefore, intervention is recommended to ameliorate the impact of the disease. However, the most effective current prevention system is by means of vaccination. Piglet vaccination around weaning is the most common practice, but sow and gilt vaccination is an increasingly used in order to homogenise the immunological status of the herd as well as to protect against potential reproductive problems. The generalised use of PCV2 vaccines demonstrated the subclinical effects of the infection.

While the role of PCV2 in cases of PDNS is difficult to ascribe, the rise of PDNS cases in PCV2 vaccinated herds may be used as a valuable sign of improper or failed vaccination and this should be discussed with the farm health team.

Porcine reproductive and respiratory syndrome ▷ VIDEO 19

PRRS is a serious, economically significant pig infectious disease worldwide. It is caused by a porcine arterivirus. The most important features of PRRS are described in Chapter 2. Although the clinical signs are mainly of a reproductive and respiratory nature, PRRSV causes a systemic disease with important implications for immune function. PRRSV is able to replicate in macrophages and is considered to cause modulation of the immune system, especially affecting the innate antiviral responses. From a clinical point of view, such an effect on the immune system is recognised by means of concomitant infections with other pathogens. In some farms, such a scenario is the basis of enzootic pneumonia or porcine respiratory disease complex. Lesions in lymphoid tissues are usually absent. However, enlargement of lymph nodes has been described and, histopathologically, there is early lymphocyte depletion with necrosis followed by lymphoid follicle hyperplasia. These microscopic lesions are relatively mild and can affect the thymus, spleen, tonsils and Peyer's patches. As PRRSV is associated with respiratory symptoms, it is discussed further in Chapter 3.

Swine fever

CSF and ASF cause classic haemorrhagic lymph node lesions (**Figure 8.43**) and are discussed further in Chapter 9.

Tuberculosis

Definition/aetiology

Pigs are susceptible to several species of the genus *Mycobacterium*, including *M. avium* complex (MAC),

M. tuberculosis and *M. bovis*. There are also a number of other fortuitous species isolated. In many instances different isolates can be isolated from different cases within the same 'outbreak'. MAC isolates are the most frequent ones causing lesions in domestic pigs. Statistics indicate that the prevalence of tuberculosis in pigs has been decreasing over time worldwide, but sporadic cases still occur, mainly when there is backyard production and, rarely (because of feeding with contaminated material), in intensively reared pigs.

Clinical presentation

Tuberculous lesions in pigs are usually limited to foci in a few lymph nodes of the digestive tract, without observation of clinical signs. If there are extensive lesions, loss of body condition can be seen, but not specific enough to suspect tuberculosis. Most cases are detected at slaughter.

Differential diagnosis

Since most of the cases are subclinical, it is virtually impossible to establish a differential diagnosis. At slaughter, observed lesions might be confused with abscesses or granulomas of bacterial or parasitic origin.

Diagnosis

Post-mortem findings include granulomatous lymphadenitis and differentiation between causal *Mycobacterium* spp. (**Figures 8.44, 8.45**) is virtually impossible (although it has been noted that

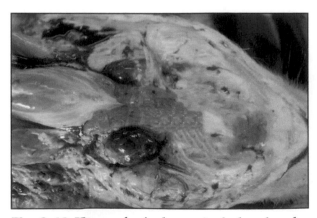

Fig. 8.43 Haemorrhagic changes in the lymph nodes in a case of African swine fever.

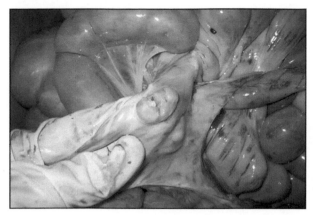

Fig. 8.44 Tuberculous lesion in a mesenteric lymph node.

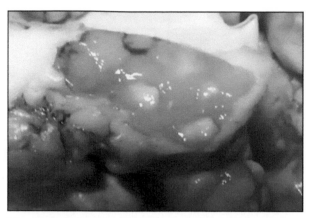

Fig. 8.45 Granulomatous lesions in a bronchial lymph node.

mineralisation is rare in MAC cases but frequent in *M. bovis* and *M. tuberculosis* infection). Generalised tuberculosis is rare in swine. Histopathology of granulomatous lesions and detection of acid-fast bacilli are characteristic of tuberculosis. Confirmation of the condition is made by *Mycobacterium* spp. detection through PCR and bacterial isolation (slow and tedious). The best samples to test are from those tissues showing granulomatous lesions. Although not frequently used, the intradermal skin test (in ear or vulva) with tuberculin can help in the diagnosis.

Management

Prevention of the condition is based on avoiding the source of infection, which can be variable (wood shavings, sawdust, peat, coal, feed and water). Once infection is within a farm, the most common approach is test (with the intradermal skin test) and removal. If affected animals are just nursery pigs and growers, slaughtering and controlling the source of infection should be enough. Adequate measures should be coupled with disinfectants. The most effective intervention is total depopulation if infection has been shown persistently in a herd.

CLINICAL QUIZ

8.1 Identify the superficial lymph nodes arrowed in **Figures 8.1a, b** (see p. 255).

8.2 Identify the structures shown in the histological section of a porcine lymph node in **Figure 8.3** (see p. 256).

The answers to these questions can be found on page 476.

DISORDERS OF THE SKIN

INTRODUCTION

Conditions affecting the skin are usually very evident to the observer. It is, therefore, important that the clinician is able to recognise the major disorders of the skin and advise appropriate treatment plans. As a few of the disorders of the skin are self-limiting, it is also an opportunity for the clinician to demonstrate that antimicrobial treatment is not required.

To examine the skin of the pig requires the same systematic approach demonstrated in the other organ systems. In describing the lesions it is important to be able to describe your orientation around the pig (**Figure 9.1**).

The position of the lesion on the pig can be very important in the differential diagnosis of disorders of the skin and a simple examination chart can be very revealing (**Figure 9.2**). The drawings can be customised for different breeds and even species. **Figure 9.3** shows the outlines for the skin examination of a wart hog.

Once the clinician has described the position of the lesion, its appearance should be described (see Chapter 1).

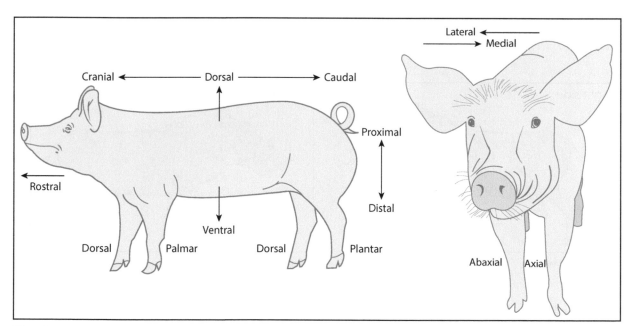

Fig. 9.1 **Orientation of the pig.**

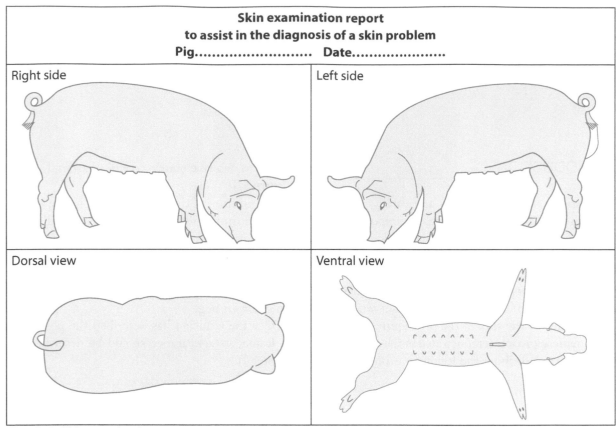

Fig. 9.2 Skin examination report.

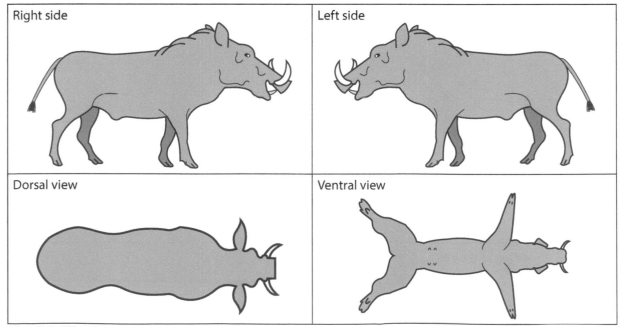

Fig. 9.3 Wart hog outlines.

Wattles

Many breeds of pigs have an appendage 5–7 cm in length hanging from the neck. Wattles, warts and protuberances are a classic Suidae characteristic (**Figures 9.4–9.7**).

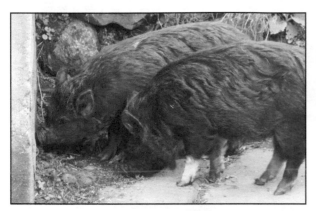

Fig. 9.4 **Wattles in a Kunekune pig.**

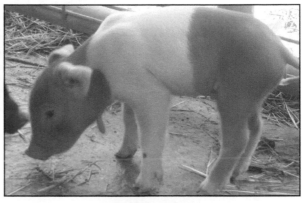

Fig. 9.5 **Wattles in a red wattle pig.**

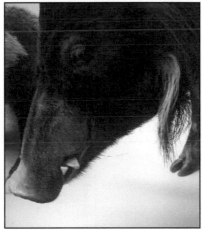

Fig. 9.6
**Tassels in a
Philippine pig
(*Sus philippensis*).**

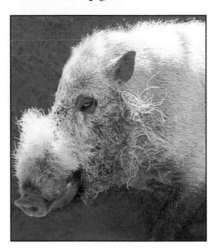

Fig. 9.7
**A bearded pig
(*Sus barbatus*).**

Describing skin lesions in specific terms

- Macule – localised change in skin colour and reveals no change in colour with palpation.
- Papule – well-circumscribed raised area of skin. Papules may coalesce into a plaque.
- Vesicle – raised area containing serosal fluid. Large vesicles (>3 cm) are called bullae.
- Pustules – raised area containing purulent material.
- Nodules – solid, palpable lumps.

BACTERIOLOGY OF SKIN DISORDERS

Several skin conditions are associated with bacteria and a swab can be taken, the species identified and an antibiogram created to assist treatment programmes. Many of the bacteria identified are also commensals or opportunistic pathogens of the skin. The skin naturally should have a healthy microbiota, which acts as a major component of the defence mechanisms. *Table 9.1* shows the basic identification and characteristics of the major bacteria that may be isolated from skin lesions.

Table 9.1 **Basic bacteriology of the skin.**

ORGANISM	GRAM STAIN	ANAEROBE ONLY	HAEMOLYTIC BLOOD AGAR	MACCONKEY	TERGITOL	CATALASE	OXIDASE	DEXTROSE BROTH	KLIGLERS	KLIGLERS IRON	LACTOSE	LYSINE	SIMMS	SIMMS CITRATE	UREASE
						SUGARS AND REACTIONS									
Erysipelothrix rhusiopathiae	+B		N	–	–	–	–			+					
Staphylococcus spp.	+C			–	–	+	–								
Streptococcus spp.	+C		α/β	–	–	–	–								
Trueperella pyogenes	+B		N	–	–	–	–								

Gram stain: B = bacillus/coccobacillus; C = coccoid.
Haemolytic: if yes, type α or β; N = no.

Erysipelothrix rhusiopathiae

See **Figures 9.8–9.11**.

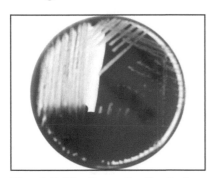

Fig. 9.8 Blood agar. Small colonies.

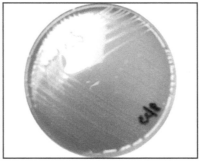

Fig. 9.9 MacConkey's. No growth.

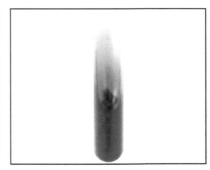

Fig. 9.10 Kligler's black streak.

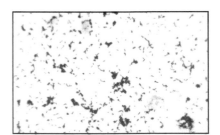

Fig. 9.11 Slender gram-positive rod.

Staphylococcus spp.

Staphylococcus hyicus is shown as an example in **Figures 9.12–9.14**.

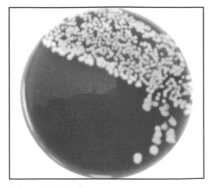

Fig. 9.12 Blood agar.

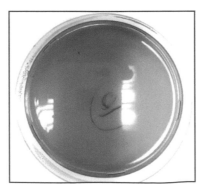

Fig. 9.13 MacConkey's. No growth.

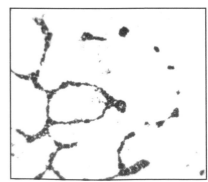

Fig. 9.14 Gram positive.

Streptococcus suis
See **Figures 9.15–9.17**.

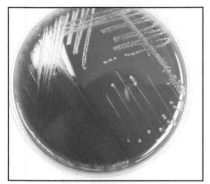

Fig. 9.15 Blood agar.

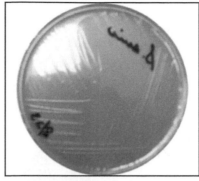

Fig. 9.16 MacConkey's. No growth.

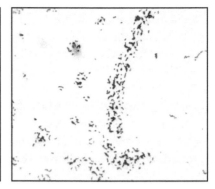

Fig. 9.17 Gram-positive cocci in chains.

Trueperella pyogenes
See **Figures 9.18–9.20**.

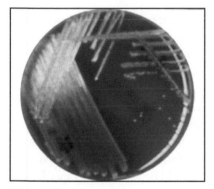

Fig. 9.18 Blood agar.

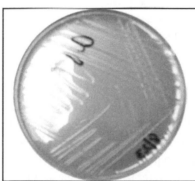

Fig. 9.19 MacConkey's. No growth.

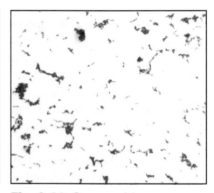

Fig. 9.20 Gram-positive pleomorphic rods: 'Chinese letters'.

Note: When examining ear swabs, *Malassezia* organisms (yeast) are common in the external ear canal of pigs and may be identified.

EXAMINATION OF AN EAR WAX SAMPLE

Take a sample of ear wax/scrape from the inner pinna and external ear canal using a speculum. The scrape should include some of the surface tissue, ideally with a hint of blood in the scrape. Place a small piece on a microscope slide. There are two techniques that may then be utilised: potassium hydroxide, or liquid paraffin oil with the slide warmed. Place another glass slide over the sample and 'crush' it between the two slides. Examine the specimen with a microscope under low-power magnification.

Interpretation

The potassium hydroxide will 'clear' the specimen making the parasitic mites easier to see. With a warmed slide and paraffin oil the mites will be actively moving. The eye is trained to notice movement and mites will be easier to identify from the debris (see Mange).

INVESTIGATION INTO SKIN DISORDERS

- Animal selection.
- Euthanased pig with typical signs.
- Observe and carefully record the animal in the various visible planes.
- Submit a freshly dead pig, if available.

- Pieces of skin should include normal skin about 2 cm square. Take photographs before removing the skin sample. Submit the sample for histological examination.
- A skin scrape can be useful. Collect an ear wax scrape from the inner pinna for examination for mange.

Radiographic investigation

It may be necessary to investigate a draining route of an abscess, especially in pet pig medicine. The use of radiography may be indicated (**Figure 9.21**).

DISORDERS OF THE SKIN OF PIGS

Abscessation ⏵VIDEO 35

Pigs are prone to abscesses (**Figure 9.22**). Subcutaneous abscesses can be very large and may contain over 6 litres of purulent material. The presence of an abscess can be confirmed by inserting a long clean needle into the softest part of the 'lump' and drawing back with a 10 mL syringe to reveal a yellow creamy liquid. If the abscess contents are fluid, release the purulent material using a cross-cut at the bottom of the abscess, not at the point (top). It is essential that the skin wound does not heal too fast as the abscess will reappear, hence the use of a cross-cut. The cut at the bottom allows adequate drainage; no pockets of abscess should be left. Flush with running water using a hose 2–3 times daily. Provide pain management.

In the early stages of an abscess, before the contents become liquid, it may be possible to clear the

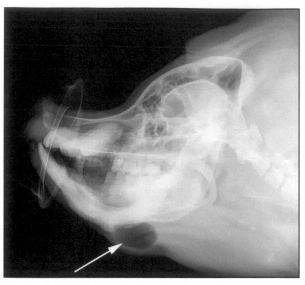

Fig. 9.21 Radiograph of a pig's head illustrating a tooth root abscess (arrow).

infection using antibiotics such as lincomycin HCl. If abscessation becomes a group problem, review the causes of fighting amongst the pigs to try and eliminate the inciting cause of the abscess. However, pigs will fight when housed together and abscessation is an inevitable consequence.

A granuloma (not necessarily an abscess) may appear in the neck following oil-based vaccination; there is no specific treatment, but the injection technique and hygiene should be critically reviewed. Note that abscesses can occur in any organ, not just the skin. The source of the abscessation may be skin wounds such as tail biting, foot lesions or even from infected

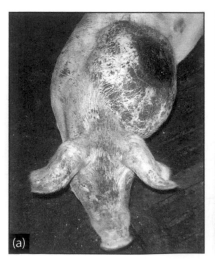

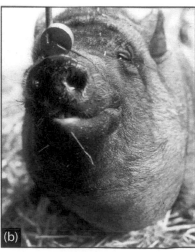

Fig. 9.22 (a, b) Abscessation is very common in pigs. The large shoulder abscess in the sow on the left was associated with *Trueperella pyogenes* and the neck abscess in the pet pig (a) with *Actinobacillus suis*.

teeth, which may occur following poor piglet processing technique. Pulmonary abscesses and endocarditis lesions can seed bacteria to the rest of the body via the blood stream. The causal organisms associated with abscessation are typically *Streptococcus* spp., *Actinobacillus suis* and *Trueperella pyogenes*. By the time the abscess is presented for treatment the lesion may be sterile.

Allergic/atopic response

Pigs can become allergic to compounds. This is generally an issue with pet pigs. Investigate the cause of the allergic response in a similar manner to an investigation into atopy. Chemical dyes in bedding are quite often the cause in pet pigs (**Figure 9.23**). However, food allergies and pollen allergies have all been observed.

Alopecia

It is normal that pigs will lose their hair seasonally and grow quite a long coat in the winter months.

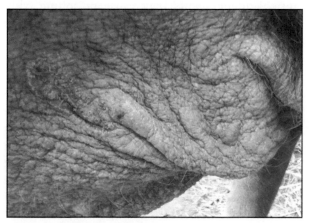

Fig. 9.23 **Allergic reaction to colour dye in bedding material in a pet pig.**

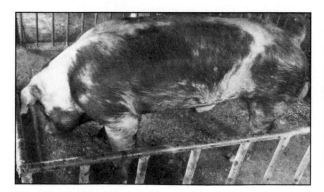

Fig. 9.24 **Alopecia in a Duroc boar.**

However, some individual pigs seem to be particularly susceptible to alopecia (**Figure 9.24**). This can be quite alarming to the client. Investigate for mange or other parasites and treat systematically. Increasing essential oils in the feed may help. In many cases there may be little that can be done if the pig appears unconcerned.

Anaemia

Anaemic pigs present whiter/paler than normal and are sometimes called ghost pigs. This can be quite difficult to appreciate in white pigs and with poor lighting. There are three ways in which pigs can become anaemic:

1 Loss of blood through haemorrhage such as following a bleeding gastric ulcer.
2 Loss of haemoglobin due to dietary insufficiencies such as inadequate iron. This is classically seen in older piglets and weaners.
3 Reduced number of red blood cells due to disease, infection or toxaemia of the bone marrow or erythrocytes.

The pig will be pale with, perhaps, a yellow (jaundice) tinge. The pig's breathing may be laboured. Anaemic pigs have more diarrhoea, especially post weaning. In piglets, iron deficiency anaemia occurs because milk is low in iron and if the pigs are housed indoors there will be no access to external iron sources such as the soil (**Figure 9.25**). Therefore, it is advised that indoor piglets should receive 100–200 mg iron dextran by injection on days 3–5 of age.

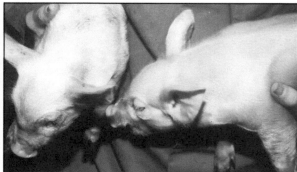

Fig. 9.25 **Iron anaemia in weaned piglets: right (white and hairier), anaemic; left, normal. Can be subtle in white breeds.**

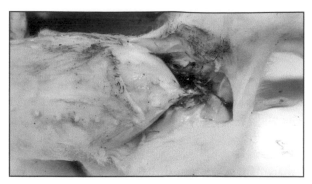

Fig. 9.26 Pale pig with watery blood associated with anaemia due to a gastric ulcer.

At post-mortem examination the muscles are pale and the blood may not clot and appears watery (**Figure 9.26**).

Anthrax

If you suspect anthrax as a diagnosis, take great care as anthrax is zoonotic. Anthrax is caused by the bacterium *Bacillus anthracis*. The source of *B. anthracis* is normally through contaminated feed; outdoor sows may contract spores through the soil or contact with carcases. When this bacterium infects a pig there may be very few clinical signs, but occasionally the bacterium causes an acute illness, fever, respiratory distress and sudden death. Anthrax should be suspected in any pig found suddenly dead with a swollen neck, with copious blood tinged mucus and large haemorrhagic lymph nodes. When suspicious, make an incision into the swollen neck region and take some of the lymph fluid. Do not fix the slide with

heat; allow to air dry. *B. anthracis* does not form the characteristic capsule readily in pigs and the capsule that does form is broken down with heat (**Figure 9.27**). If the suspicions are confirmed, stop the post-mortem examination and inform a government veterinarian.

Antimicrobial and iatrogenic intoxication

Skin reactions have been recorded three to four days after the administration of an antimicrobial agent. These reactions can range from only a mild rash and blushing to a very severe ulceration. If the offending medication is removed, recovery is generally rapid unless other organ failure is involved.

Cases of tiamulin and florfenicol toxicity are reported. However, in many cases the causal agent is not determined. Note that warfarin and other anticoagulent agents may cause poisoning, skin haemorrhages (**Figure 9.28**), bruising and even death.

Aural haematoma   VIDEOS 15 and 36

Acute aural haematoma is characterised by swelling of the pinna (ear) (**Figure 9.29**). The condition is associated with head shaking, therefore fighting and mange are important predisposing factors. The head shaking results in blood leaking under the skin of the ear. When handling an acute haematoma, the swelling is soft and fluctuating. If a needle is inserted into the swelling, gelatinous blood can be revealed.

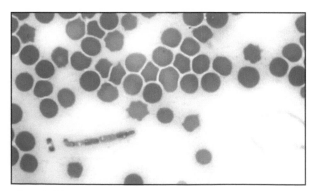

Fig. 9.27 *Bacillus anthracis* in a blood smear stained by MacFadyen's methylene blue.

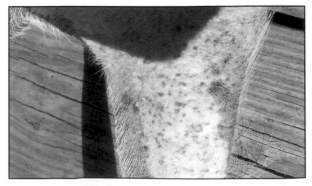

Fig. 9.28 A pig that ate some rodent bait containing an anticoagulant agent.

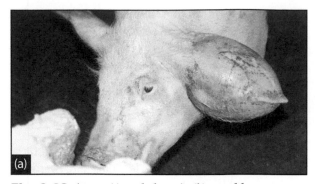

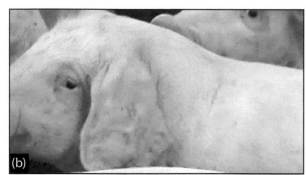

Fig. 9.29 Acute (a) and chronic (b) aural haematoma.

Treatment

Do nothing as the lesion resolves with time, but the ears can be very heavy and they may become infected. Provide pain management as required.

Surgical opening of the aural haematoma is sometimes performed, but there is a risk of the pig bleeding to death if the internal bleeding has not stopped. Further, even if initially successful, a subsequent seroma with associated swelling is likely. So, if drainage is advised, such as is possible with pet pigs, it is best to wait for 2 weeks. Chronic pain management must be practiced in this case.

Bites from insects

See **Figures 9.30**.

Chronic aural haematomas are regularly seen in grow/finish pigs as a crumpled ear where the original haematoma has become organised. While this can look disfiguring it has no consequence for the welfare of the pig.

Control and prevention

If aural haematomas are common within a group, test for mange and, if evident, eliminate it. Examine the reasons for aggression and fighting among the pigs. For example, check water and feed availability.

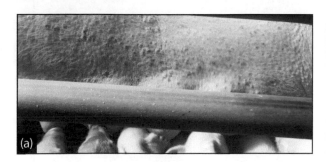

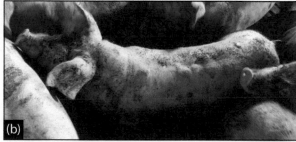

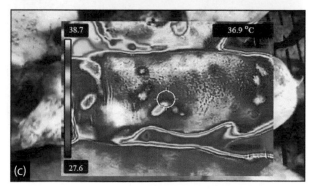

Fig. 9.30 (a) Multiple insect bites (mosquito) on a sow in lactation. (b) Hypersensitivity reaction to stable fly (*Stomoxy calcitrans*) bites. Note the raised lumps similar to erysipelas. Single pig is not pyrexic and shows no behavioural abnormality. (c) Same pig, infrared. Note that the lumps are cooler than the surrounding skin temperature. (Red/white hotter to blue/black colder.)

Burns

Occasionally, pigs can be involved in a farm fire and become burnt. They require local treatment to the skin. If the burn is severe, euthanasia may be the only option. If young piglets touch the heat lamp they may blister their nose, resembling a foot and mouth lesion.

Chemical burn

Chemicals are often added to the floor and surfaces as part of the terminal cleaning and disinfection routines on pig farms. Lime (CaCO₃) is a cheap and common disinfectant. However, if these chemicals are not allowed to dry adequately and pigs are then exposed to the wet surfaces, the chemicals can burn the skin. The lesions are concentrated on the hind quarters and ventral surfaces, especially the face and rump (**Figure 9.31**). The tongue may also be burnt.

The pigs will normally recover within a week but pain management is advised.

Unusual skin conditions can also become apparent associated with chemical poisoning. These must be investigated in detail as they become apparent. Note antibiotic intoxication as a differential.

Cyanosis and blue ears

A bluing and blushing of the ears. This may result in severe circulatory collapse to the pinna and, over time, gangrene and loss of the tips of the ear (**Figure 9.32**).

Causes

Bacterial causes include: *Haemophilus parasuis*, *Actinobacillus pleuropneumoniae*, *Escherichia coli*, *Erysipelothrix rhusiopathiae*, *Salmonella* spp., *Streptococcus* spp. or infection by *Pasteurella multocida* (**Figures 9.33, 9.34**). Viral causes include

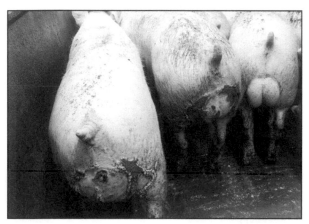

Fig. 9.31 Lime burn. Note the location on the ventral surface and the rump.

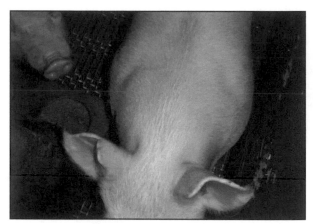

Fig. 9.32 Gangrene of the ear resulting in loss of the tips of the ear.

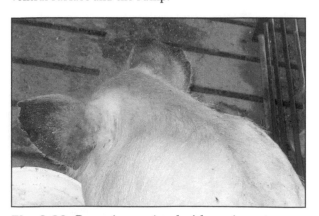

Fig. 9.33 Cyanosis associated with septicaemic salmonellosis.

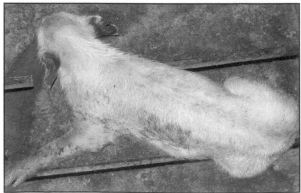

Fig. 9.34 Cyanosis with pericarditis.

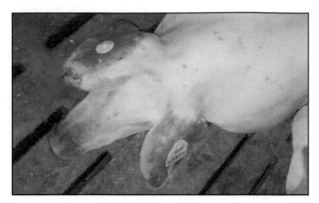

Fig. 9.35 Blue ears and nose in a pig with ASF.

porcine reproductive and respiratory syndrome virus (PRRSV) (**Figure 9.35**), classical swine fever virus (CSFV) and African swine fever virus (ASFV).

Other causes include poisons (carbamate, organophosphates), deficiencies (thiamine), accidents (electrocution) and under some natural conditions (at farrowing and associated with a stressful circumstance).

'Dippity pig'

This condition presents as an acutely affected pig with a necrotising cellulitis of the skin, normally along the back (**Figure 9.36**). The pig is usually young, 3–10 months of age. There is no specific treatment for 'dippity pig'. However, giving the pig a good bath with a medicated antiseptic shampoo, combined with topical treatment with anaesthetic gel smeared liberally over the affected area, will provide temporary relief. An injection of lincomycin HCl followed by 3 days of lincomycin HCl tablet medication will assist skin healing.

However, the condition will self-heal within 2–3 days without any medication. This condition can be seen in outdoor commercial pigs associated with acute sunburn.

Epitheliogenesis imperfecta

In this condition pigs are born with a portion of their skin missing (**Figure 9.37**). Assuming the lesion is not too extensive, treat with skin disinfectants and the lesion will progressively heal. Pigs generally heal with only a scar area visible by the time of slaughter.

Erysipelas ▷ VIDEO 37
Definition/aetiology

Erysipelas of pigs is caused by the bacterium *Erysipelothrix rhusiopathiae*, which is common in soil samples and, therefore, can enter the farm through the feed or water supply; when grain is harvested, 1–2% of the weight is soil. The organism also lives in fish, and fish meal can be a source of infection. The organism can cause problems in turkeys and sheep, which can then cross-infect pigs on farms with birds, sheep and pig being farmed together. In addition, 20% of the pigs on the farm may carry the organism on their tonsils without any clinical signs.

There are over 25 serotypes but types 1 and 2 are the most common and commercial vaccines only cover types 1 and 2. The disease is recognised around the world and is also called diamond skin disease, or measles, by farmers. Erysipelas is one of the major diseases of the pig and its clinical signs need to be recognised by all clinicians.

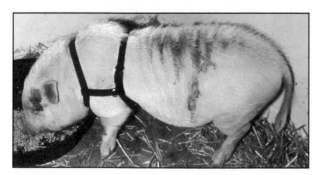

Fig. 9.36 'Dippity pig' in a pet pig.

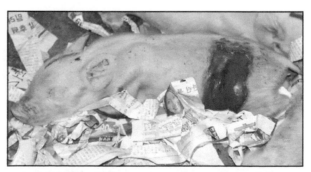

Fig. 9.37 Epitheliogenesis imperfecta in a new born piglet. This lesion will heal given time. Note the shredded paper, which is commonly used as bedding in the farrowing area.

Clinical presentation

Erysipelas can affect any age group. However, most weaners below 12 weeks of age are protected by colostral antibodies passed on from their mother and, therefore, clinical signs are rare in piglets and weaners. Stressed pigs are more likely to show clinical signs, such as sudden changes in diet, or changes in temperature or introduction of other disease such as swine influenza. Six phases of the disease are recognised clinically.

Peracute: With peracute erysipelas the pig is found dead with no clinical signs. This may occur in one or two pigs in a pen. There are many reasons for pigs to die. One reason is lack of observation, but if the death is unexplained, erysipelas must be considered as part of the differential diagnosis. Run your hand over the skin of the pig before post-mortem examination and the diamond lesions may be felt, even if not seen. There may be few lesions at post-mortem, but a very large spleen is suggestive (see **Figure 9.39**).

Acute: The disease appears to start with a sudden onset. However, it takes 2–3 days post infection for the pigs to demonstrate the classic diamond lesions of erysipelas (**Figure 9.38**). The 'diamond' lesions may be felt before they are seen. Affected animals present with a high temperature (40–42°C) and infected pigs often separate from the rest of the group and may appear chilled and cold (typical of a high fever). When the group of pigs is examined, the affected pig will generally be found lying down and when encouraged to rise, will walk stiffly, appear to have a sore abdomen and may be tucked up.

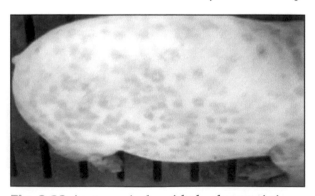

Fig. 9.38 Acute erysipelas with the characteristic diamond lesions on the skin.

The affected pig will then attempt to find an area to lie down again. The pig generally appears very dejected. Affected pigs are often off their feed and may be constipated (although young animals may have diarrhoea). As the condition develops the 'diamond' lesions will change from a pink to dark purple lesions. The skin lesions may progress to a necrotic centre and slough leaving a scar, which can be permanent.

Associated with the pyrexia (high body temperature), sows may abort and boars may become infertile, which may be permanent or last 6 weeks. Therefore, erysipelas can also be considered to be a reproductive disease and can have a significant impact on the pig flow of the farm. Acute pigs left untreated may die or start to recover in 4–7 days.

Subacute: The pig presents with diamond lesions but with only a few other clinical signs, including no loss of appetite. The lesions self-heal in 1–2 weeks.

Chronic arthritis: Three weeks or more after infection, with or without clinical signs, some pigs may present with a chronic lameness in one or two joints. This can affect the vertebrae and thus the pig may have a sore back and difficult painful walking. In pet pigs, erysipelas arthritis is a major problem in geriatric pig care. Note that the vaccine does not prevent the arthritic form and arthritic lesions are generally lifelong.

Chronic endocarditis: After infection, the *E. rhusiopathiae* bacteria may adhere to the cardiac valves, resulting in a vegetative endocarditis. As the damage to the heart valves becomes more extensive, the pig develops clinical signs of chronic heart failure including breathlessness and poor circulation, especially after exertion. This can result in sudden death, especially after mating for instance. Associated with the poor circulation, the ears and tail of the pig may go purple and become necrotic and gangrenous.

Carrier status: Some 20–50% of pigs may carry the organism on their tonsils without any clinical signs being exhibited in their lifetime.

Pathogenesis

With regard to the clinical signs, examining the pathogenesis is useful. The organism can gain access to the pig by many routes. Classically, most infections are oral from contaminated feed and/or water. In acute cases the pathogen enters the blood stream via the pharynx, hence the widespread clinical signs. The diamond lesions are actually the consequence of microthrombi and bacterial emboli in dermal capillaries and venules, which may lead to circulatory stasis and necrosis, usually in pigs that have already been sick for 2–3 days before the lesions become large enough to be visible. In the chronic form, arthritis can take months to develop and therefore definitive diagnosis can be difficult as the lesions are sterile by the time the clinical signs are recognised.

Differential diagnosis

The peracute and acute forms of erysipelas need to be differentiated from other causes of sudden death, in particular swine fever (CSF and ASF), salmonellosis and anthrax. Diamond skin lesions are non-specific and will occur with a number of allergic conditions, notably on a herd basis to food stuffs, but most allergies are individual cases not group cases. For the chronic form of erysipelas with arthritis, *Mycoplasma hyosynoviae* would be the major differential. In cases of endocarditis, *Streptococcus* spp. may also be isolated from the lesions.

Diagnosis

Clinical signs: While diamond lesions are not definitive, they are very suggestive and the major visible and palpable clinical sign. Suspected pigs should be treated with penicillin immediately. If there is a significant improvement by 24 hours, this is very suggestive of erysipelas.

Post-mortem lesions: In peracute cases there may be very few lesions visible. Possibly, an enlarged spleen may be seen (**Figure 9.39**) and the diamond lesions may be felt (but not seen). In acute cases the skin lesions may be seen or felt. The spleen is generally greatly enlarged but few other gross changes will be recognised. In chronic cases, endocarditis will be evident and a vegetative (cauliflower) valvular lesion seen (**Figure 9.40**). Associated with the general poor circulation, the heart may be visible enlarged. Severe arthritis in one or more joints may be recognised in chronic erysipelas (**Figure 9.41**).

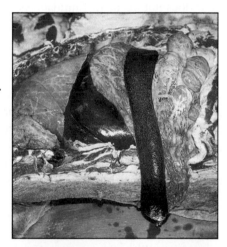

Fig. 9.39 Enlarged spleen in a peracute erysipelas case.

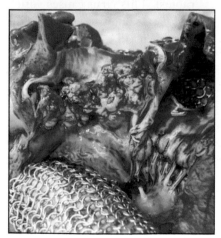

Fig. 9.40 Endocarditis of the atrio-ventricular valve.

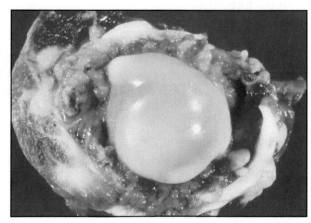

Fig. 9.41 Arthritis associated with erysipelas in a boar.

In acute and some peracute cases, bacterial culture of the blood can be performed but obtaining a blood sample may be difficult. Note that the organism can live on the skin so sample contamination is a risk. In chronic cases, the organism can be difficult to isolate and serology may be useful, although most pigs are vaccinated or the organism can be present in 20% of pigs without clinical signs.

Management
Treatment of individuals or a group
- **Acute/subacute erysipelas**. Penicillin and tylan phosphate-based medicines are very effective in the treatment of erysipelas. Acute cases should also be given analgesics.
- **Chronic erysipelas**. There is no practical treatment except analgesia in the arthritic form.

Prevention and control: Erysipelas is easily and effectively controlled by vaccination. Injectable and oral vaccination is possible. Vaccination protection lasts about 6 months, therefore the following programme is recommended:

- Pigs over 3 months are vaccinated once and again 3 weeks later. Selected breeding animals should be vaccinated.
- Sows are vaccinated either pre-farrowing or post farrowing or every 6 months. If a sow is vaccinated pre-farrowing, it will boost her erysipelas colostrum antibodies and further protect her offspring.
- Boars are vaccinated every 6 months (but are often forgotten).

Poor vaccination protocols may result in unvaccinated pigs that the health team believe to be immunised. The classic reason why vaccines are inactivated is because they are frozen in a poorly maintained refrigerator.

Zoonotic implications
Erysipelas can infect humans and usually results only in a skin infection; however, the condition can be more severe. Note that 'erysipelas' of humans is actually caused by a *Streptococcus* sp. infection.

Foot and mouth disease and other vesicular diseases
Definition/aetiology
Foot and mouth disease (FMD) is caused by an Aphthovirus (meaning virus causing vesicles) of the Picornoviridae family named FMD virus (FMDV). This pathogen is extremely common around the world, but pig industries are trying to eliminate the virus from their production systems. This has been very successful in Europe and North America. South America and selected parts of the Asia are progressively achieving negative status. The World Organisation for Animal Health (OIE) is particularly responsible for monitoring this virus around the world.

FMD affects all of the artiodactyl (even toed) mammal family, although individual viruses may affect more or fewer species. FMD occurs in pigs, cattle, sheep, goats, deer and camels, for example, but does not occur in Equidae. As with many other conditions, there are a number of other diseases that can clinically resemble FMD:

- Swine vesicular disease (SVD) caused by a calicivirus, another member of the Picornoviridae.
- Rarely seen is vesicular exanthema (VE) of swine and the San Miguel Seal Lion virus.
- Senecavirus A (SVA, formerly known as Seneca virus), another picornavirus, also produces mild clinical signs although elevated pre-weaning mortality may be evident.
- Vesicular stomatitis (VS) is unusual as the virus is a Rhabdovirus (same family as rabies). This virus causes vesicles in pigs and cattle but also equines, and occurs in Southern USA.

These viruses are important because they cause clinical signs that mimic the classic signs of FMD. Due to the severe trade restrictions imposed on the farm/area to control FMD, they can have a big impact. With the advent of PCR and DNA technologies, these other non-FMD viruses are becoming less important. It is still vital, however, that any case of suspected FMD is reported by the practicing veterinarian. The government veterinarians will then decide the outcome for the farm and its animals. Primarily, pigs are initially infected through the oral route, through contaminated feed, hence the regulations prohibiting the feeding of swill in many countries. Airborne spread is more commonly from cattle.

Clinical presentation

Pigs of all ages can be affected in the initial outbreak. In enzootic regions, lesions are unusual in piglets and weaners less than 3 months of age as the pig is protected via colostrum. In an outbreak, the clinical signs may not be seen for 1–5 days, but can take as long as 21 days. The major clinical sign is that several pigs are suddenly lame. When the animals are clinically examined, the skin around the snout (**Figure 9.42**), lips, tongue, inside the mouth, around the coronary band and the soft skin on the feet becomes whiter (blanched) (**Figure 9.43**). Then, within hours, vesicles (blisters) may develop. These may also be seen on the sows' teats. The vesicles are rarely seen as they rupture within 24 hours and secondary infection of the exposed skin occurs. Without secondary infection healing is rapid, especially around the mouth, making lesions difficult to observe. Over a few days, in a few pigs the hoof may become detached, revealing the painful raw tissues underneath. The hoof can regrow, but is often deformed and this can take months. The pigs may have a pyrexia of 40.5°C.

The disease affects nearly all susceptible animals, but few animals will die as a direct consequence of the disease. The clinical signs spread rapidly through the air, by animal contact and via vectors such as clothing, utensils and vehicles. The pathogen may be spread from farm to farm and country to country through meat and meat by-products, especially fast frozen feeds.

Semen from infected animals is contaminated and so artificial insemination is a potential means of spread. Pigs produce aerosols 3,000 times more concentrated with FMDV particles than cattle and therefore pigs are a major source of FMD spread to other animals, especially when combined with high humidity, cloud cover and moderate temperatures, which favour airborne spread (over 20 km). While a carrier status occurs in cattle this is not reported in pigs.

Differential diagnosis

Swine vesicular disease, VE, San Miguel Sea Lion virus, SVA, VS, trauma such as lime burn or contact with a heat lamp. If there in any doubt, report suspicions to the appropriate authority.

Diagnosis

In the field via clinical signs and perhaps at postmortem examination for vesicles, generally ruptured, in the mouth, nose and on the feet (coronary band). Final diagnosis will be made by government laboratories.

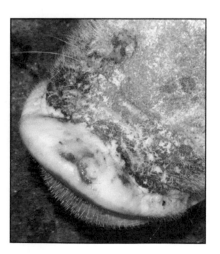

Fig. 9.42
FMD lesion on the nose of a pig.

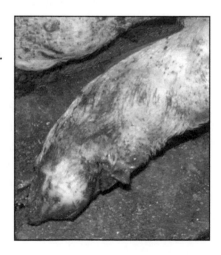

Fig. 9.43
FMD lesion on the foot of a pig.

Management

Treatment: If FMD is notifiable in your area, immediately report to your veterinary practice and government officials. If FMD is endemic, a vaccine is used. If the correct vaccine is used, field and vaccine strains can be differentiated. Note that the different strains of the virus need different vaccines and that official notification may still be required. The protection offered by the vaccines is not great and protection only lasts for 6 months. In vaccinated sows, colostrum will protect their piglets for about 3 months.

Control: Strict regulation of importation of animals and animal products infected with vesicular diseases.

Government controlled euthanasia and disposal of animals via burial, composting, rendering or burning. This may be within a 3 km zone of a suspected infected case.

Zoonotic implications

Human infection is claimed but it is extremely rare and usually without clinical signs. Children can get hand, foot and mouth disease (teschovirus), which many clients may confuse with FMD in an outbreak.

Procedure for dealing with a notifiable condition

Know the local notifiable and reportable conditions of pigs. The protocols to follow if you suspect a notifiable condition are shown in *Table 9.2*.

Table 9.2 **Suspected notifiable disease protocols.**

CLIENT SUSPECTS AN UNUSUAL OR POTENTIALLY NOTIFIABLE DISEASE

Request client seal the property

Place 'Keep out' notices at all public entrances

Request that all personnel remain at the property until the veterinarian arrives

VETERINARIAN'S RESPONSIBILITY

Wear disposable outer clothing and wear only farm boots

Take disinfectant in the car

Ensure you have a camera and mobile phone that works

Ensure you have a rectal thermometer

Upon arrival examine stock carefully. Photograph, video and catalogue any observed clinical signs

THE VETERINARIAN SUSPECTS AN UNUSUAL OR NOTIFIABLE DISEASE

Phone practice to inform partners. Email photographs of clinical signs

Phone appropriate authority; know their telephone number

Provide full name and address of the farm and GPS location if possible

Provide clear details of how to get to the location of animals/farm

Email photographs and or video and clinical details of the observed lesions

BEFORE THE GOVERNMENT VETERINARIAN ARRIVES (UNLESS OTHERWISE AUTHORISED)

Stop movement of all animals from and to the farm

Stop all movement of vehicles from the farm

Divert all vehicles that are to arrive at the farm such as feed trucks etc.

Ensure farm perimeter entry points prohibit vehicle movements; for example, place tractor across entrance, ensure signs are in place, if necessary place stockpersons at entrance

Proceed with a detailed clinical examination of all the other stock on the farm, including all species

(Continued)

Table 9.2 *(Continued)* **Suspected notifiable disease protocols.**

LEAVING THE FARM
Follow all advice given by the authorised veterinarian
Leave disposable overalls
Leave farm boots
Leave rectal thermometer
Do not remove any items contaminated with faeces or blood
If necessary, rewrite notes on clean paper or photograph
Provide counselling and support to the client with regard to consequences if the suspect disease is confirmed
Implement suitable additional biosecurity measures
Spray car wheels and wheel hubs with disinfectant
On the way home wash car in hot steam car wash
Double wash all clothing with detergent
Shower thoroughly (minimum 3 minutes) including watch and glasses
Clean and disinfect all equipment removed from the farm (phone, camera)
DURING A ROUTINE VISIT THE VETERINARIAN SUSPECTS A NOTIFIABLE OR UNUSUAL ANIMAL DISEASE
Proceed from veterinarian's responsibility, point 3
Do not take personal boots and overalls from the farm
Ensure you have a small supply of disinfectant in the car at all times

Frostbite

Pigs that are exposed to a very cold environment may suffer from frostbite, especially of their extremities: ears, toes and tail (**Figure 9.44**). The compromised circulation may result in death of the area, gangrene and loss of the area. The frostbite is often due to a combination of cold air and wind chill.

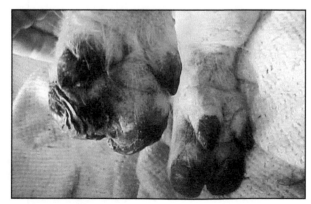

Fig. 9.44 **Pet pig with frostbite of its feet. The ears were also affected.**

Greasy pig disease/exudative epidermitis ▶ VIDEO 38

Definition/etiology

Greasy pig disease/exudative epidermitis is associated with *Staphylococcus hyicus* infection. This bacterium is normal on pig skin and is found in the vagina, and the piglet's skin is colonised at birth. The clinical disease is caused by this normal bacteria penetrating into the skin lesions from fighting. Therefore, to understand the problem the clinician needs to examine the farm for areas of aggression.

Clinical presentation

The major clinical signs are seen in piglets and weaners less than 8 weeks of age (pigs less than 20 kg body weight). There are three major clinical presentations.

Piglet: Facial necrosis is a form of greasy pig disease associated with litters with more piglets than functional teats or poor milk output, resulting in excessive fighting between the piglets and damage to the face. Note that *Treponema pedis* may also be isolated from cases of facial necrosis (see also Vices).

Older piglets and weaners: The newly weaned pig suddenly presents covered in patches of dirty brown greasy wet skin. The hair is matted and may become a grey colour (**Figure 9.45**). The condition extends rapidly, covering the whole body, and affected pigs stop eating and drinking and become very dehydrated. Without treatment, after 7–10 days affected pigs may be found dead.

Chronic in weaners: The pig presents with 3–5 cm patches of the above skin condition but the disease does not spread. The condition most commonly affects the upper neck and hindlimbs, areas where the pigs tend to direct their aggression (**Figure 9.46**). The condition will resolve spontaneously 5 days after the fighting stops. At any age, wounds that do not heal properly may have a localised region of *S. hyicus* infection.

Chronic in adults: A chronic black spotty appearance on the back and neck of sows is often associated with culture of *S. hyicus* from the lesions.

Differential diagnosis

In the more severe cases the visible signs are classic. The major differentials would be a moderate to severe pityriasis rosea. Pityriasis rosea occurs on the ventral surface predominately whereas greasy pig disease is initially on the neck and back. Mange may be considered but *Sarcopes scabiei* var *suis* is clinically unusual in the piglet immediately post weaning.

With a mineral deficiency, particularly zinc, the pig may present with a parakeratosis. Generally, this occurs on home mill and mixers because of a milling mistake, with the mineral mix being forgotten.

Diagnosis

Clinical signs and post-mortem lesions of a severe exudative epidermitis. In severe acute cases lymph nodes may be swollen and abscessed. Culture of the bacteria may be relatively meaningless as culture from normal skin is also positive, but it is very significant when isolated from subcutaneous lymph nodes. Isolation does allow for an antibiogram to be arranged.

Management

Treatment of an individual: Isolate and place in a separate 'compromised pig' pen. Inject with a staphylococcal active antimicrobial, which concentrates in the skin (e.g. lincomycin HCl). Wash the pig in a suitable disinfectant. Ideally, use lanolin in the wash to soothe the skin. Inject with multivitamins and provide pain management. Provide plentiful water through bowl drinkers and, if necessary, provide extra water by mouth. The animals will be quite dehydrated and additional water management will be an essential part of the treatment. A normal pig may drink 1 litre per 10 kg, therefore a couple of syringes full of water will not be significant. Provide heat from a light source. Ideally, place the pig in a hospital pen with dry clean straw as bedding. Unfortunately, this level of care can be difficult on large commercial farms.

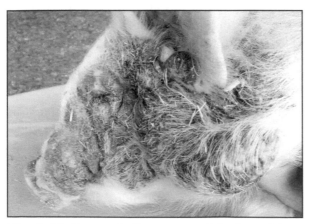

Fig. 9.45 Greasy pig disease around the face of the weaned pig.

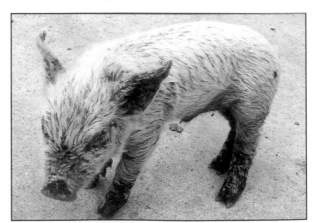

Fig. 9.46 Severe chronic greasy pig disease in a weaner.

Control

In the young piglet: The young piglet presents with facial necrosis. This is associated with fighting over the milk supply. Rather than advising teeth clipping, understand and resolve the reasons why the sows are providing inadequate milk supplies.

In the older suckling piglet: If the problem is seen in the older piglet, especially from gilt litters, ensure feedback programmes and colostrum management are adequate in gilts and parity 1 sows.

In the weaner: Greasy pig disease is the end result of fighting. Therefore, review all causes of fighting and increased aggression. Classic reasons are:

- Fighting over water.
- Inadequate space availability.
- Inadequate water; supply sufficient drinkers of appropriate flow rate.
- Draughts and piling; find and fix.
- Mixing and moving; minimise.

On rare occasions it has been necessary to change genetics to a more sociable pig. Check fly control; in particular look for biting flies such as *Stomoxys calcitrans*, which can transmit the bacteria and injure the skin in large numbers of pigs at the same time. In herd 'outbreaks' it is possible to control the problem by adding lincomycin HCl to the water supply together with a sweetener to encourage the pigs to drink. If present, control mange on the farm as this will reduce pigs traumatising their skin by scratching.

Herniation ▶ VIDEO 13

There are four common forms of herniation seen in the pig: umbilical; inguinal/scrotal; perineal; traumatic.

Umbilical hernia

An umbilical hernia is a congenital defect affecting around 1.5% of pigs. Clinically, it is generally seen in pigs over 30 kg, after which the hernia can reach a gigantic size (**Figure 9.47**). These can occur as a major problem on pig farms. The animal only has an economic future if the hernia diameter stays less than 30 cm and none of the skin is ulcerated. Once the hernia makes contact with the ground, euthanasia is advised. Large umbilical hernias may require the farm to inform the slaughterhouse before delivery. There is no economically viable treatment. There is some genetic basis to the condition but it is complex and does not follow simple Mendelian genetics. On rare occasions intestinal entrapment may occur in the hernia. If there is a group problem on the farm, check farrowing protocols, in particular that the umbilicus is not being pulled or traumatised during birth. Review navel management in the farrowing area.

Inguinal/scrotal hernia

These occur in the male when the inguinal canal does not close, and they can become very large (**Figure 9.48**). Strangulation of a portion of the intestines can occur through the hernia on rare occasions (**Figure 9.49**). Assuming the animal is not castrated, these animals will grow without problems to slaughter weight. If castration has to be performed, recognise the scrotal hernia before castration and then carry

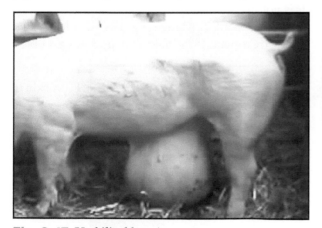

Fig. 9.47 Umbilical hernia.

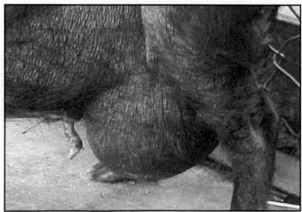

Fig. 9.48 Scrotal hernia – note the paraphimosis.

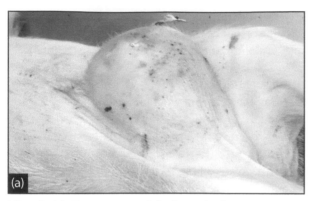
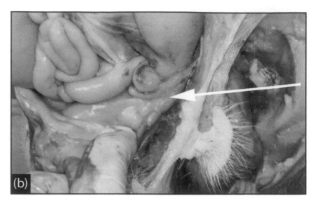

Fig. 9.49 Entrapment of the intestinal tract in a scrotal hernia. (a) Gross appearance. (b) Post-mortem appearance (arrow).

out a closed castration. If the scrotal hernia is not recognised, then prolapse of the intestine and death will occur rapidly after castration. Scrotal hernias appear more commonly in some breeds than others. Vietnamese Pot Bellied pigs are one example, making castration of pet pigs a little problematic at times.

Perineal hernia

In older sows, the whole of the perineal region can present in collapse with the rectum and vagina

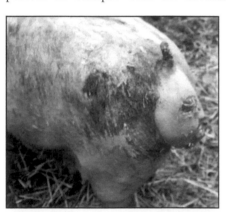

Fig. 9.50 Perineal hernia.

prolapsing into the hernia (**Figure 9.50**); there is no economic treatment. If the sow is close to farrowing, keep her until farrowing if the welfare of the animal can be maintained. However, manual removal of piglets or caesarean section are likely to be required. Provide the sow with a bran diet or add liquid paraffin/mineral oil from time to time to help with the passage of faeces until slaughter.

Traumatic hernia

Typically occurs due to sows biting the piglet, which may result in a hernia through the abdominal wall. Traumatic hernias are only of consequence if intestinal strangulation occurs (**Figure 9.51**). If the conformation is so badly disfigured that it may result in problems in the slaughterhouse, immediate euthanasia is advised.

Hyperkeratinisation/flaky skin

It is not unusual for adults to present with dry flaky skin (**Figure 9.52**). Mange as a cause should be ruled out by treatment. If the flaky skin presents a problem

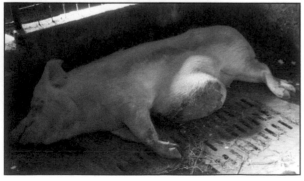

Fig. 9.51 Traumatic hernia.

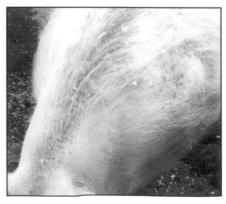

Fig. 9.52 Flaky skin in a boar.

for the owner more than the pig, wash the pig with a skin disinfectant. Add cooking oil/olive oil to the pig's diet to increase the fat content, which will be expressed on the skin. Several pet pig diets are quite basic in order to reduce calories, reduce pigs putting on too much weight and keep costs down, and therefore are short in essential oils.

Jaundice – icterus

Jaundice (icterus) is a yellow discolouration of the tissues that may be seen pre-mortem in the white of the eyes or the mucosal surface of the vulva, but is often diagnosed at post-mortem (**Figure 9.53**). It is caused by a build-up of bilirubin pigments in the tissues.

This build up can occur due to liver disease (hepatitis, *Leptospira icherohaemorrhagica* [see Chapter 2]) gallbladder disease or blockage (gallstones) or associated with an excessive haemolysis (*Mycoplasma suis*).

Differential diagnoses may include yellowing of the carcase associated with corn oils, diets high in carrots, tetracycline deposition. Note that the carcase and fat may also change colour in other conditions; for example, congenital porphyria (see Chapter 2) (carcase more brown than yellow), diets high in shrimp (pink colouration to the fat) or other oils and stains (e.g. blue fat in Uganda associated with soap being fed as a wormer).

Diagnosis is confirmed by finding a serum total bilirubin concentration >3.4 µmol/L.

Lice and ticks ▶ VIDEO 39

The pig biting louse is *Haematopinus suis*. These are the biggest lice known to man and are readily observed (**Figure 9.54**). The life cycle occurs on the body and takes 30 days to complete from egg to adult; however, the louse cannot live for more than 3 days away from the pig, making control technically easier than with mange, although in practice this has proven more difficult. It is possible that swine pox may be carried by lice. Lice are very sensitive to standard mange (*Sarcoptes scabiei*) treatment including avermectins.

A few ticks can be found on pigs, especially pet pigs or outdoor units. The major tick of concern in pig farming is the *Carios (Ornithodorus)* (soft body) tick, which acts as a host for ASF virus (ASFV).

Mange ▶ VIDEO 40
Definition/aetiology

Sarcoptic mange is a serious parasitic infection of the pig caused by *Sarcoptes scabiei* var. *suis*. This is a species adapted to the pig. Other sarcoptes mites may be found on pigs but they are of little significance. *Demodex phylloides*, which is the cause of demodectic mange, may also be found incidentally. *Sarcoptes scabiei* var. *suis* is common and should be assumed to be present unless an eradication programme has been undertaken. Most breeding companies are mange free.

The pathogen is spread through pig to pig contact and through pigs coming into contact with infested buildings. The mite is able to survive for 21 days off the host in ideal situations. The condition can have a high economic importance. The impact varies depending on infestation, but a growth rate loss of 10% is not unusual in moderate to severe infestations. Mange will weaken the pig and is an added stress, and the constant rubbing causes damage to buildings. It may appear to occur cyclically with the various degree of stress on the pigs.

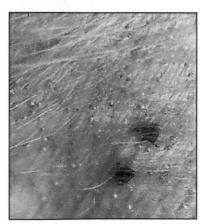

Fig. 9.54 *Haematopinus suis* visible on the skin.

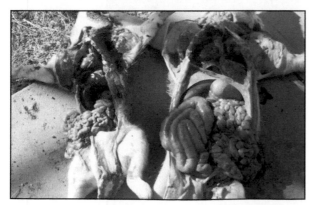

Fig. 9.53 **Normal pig (left); jaundiced pig (right).**

Life cycle of the mange mite: The female lays about 1–3 eggs a day in the skin and the adult female lives for about 1 month; therefore, some 30–40 eggs are laid per female. Most of the eggs are laid in the soft tissues of the inside of the ear. There may be as many as 18,000 mites per gram of ear skin. The eggs hatch out in about 5 days and the larvae moult to the nymph, which moult to the adult in 10–15 days. The life cycle remains on the pig at all times.

Sarcoptes scabiei var. *suis* can live off the pig for about 21 days. The warmer the conditions the shorter the survival time. This can be important information when designing an eradication programme. The pig mange mite does not survive in or on other hosts although it can 'live' for a few days on humans and in some cases cause a skin rash.

Clinical presentation

The major clinical presentation is scratching (pruritus) (**Figure 9.55**). Affected pigs appear uncomfortable and have intermittent body scratching.

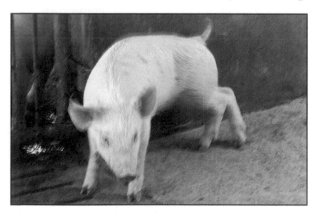

Fig. 9.55 **Clinical sign of pruritus.**

Following a recent infestation, the pigs demonstrate persistent itching and rubbing.

Ear wax increases, sometimes forming plaques. As the condition becomes chronic, hair will be rubbed off in places and the skin may become thickened (**Figures 9.56, 9.57**). Areas of the skin may become traumatised and this can result in a secondary greasy pig disease outbreak. Chronic skin lesions are more common behind the ear and tail head. Mange affects all age groups, although sows and growing pigs most often exhibit the characteristic clinical signs. The problem may be more apparent in the cooler months.

Differential diagnosis

Sows may scratch when exposed to cigarette smoke or perfumes including aftershaves. Forage mites in straw/bedding may cause irritation and scratching. Any other causes of skin hypersensitivity/allergy may cause scratching, and this is a problem in some pet pigs. The skin may be thickened with parakeratosis or dry and scaly with deficiencies of essential fatty acids or zinc, but these pigs are generally not itchy. *Malassezia* yeast infestations may increase the amount of ear wax.

Diagnosis

The skin itching and subsequent skin damage is a secondary hypersensitivity reaction to the mange mite. *Sarcoptes scabiei* mites may not be found in the damaged skin area so the clinician needs to examine the ear wax (**Figure 9.58**). Individuals need to be examined to find evidence of the mite to confirm the diagnosis. Absence is very difficult to ascertain.

An ELISA blood test is available, but false positives can occur. However, the test is

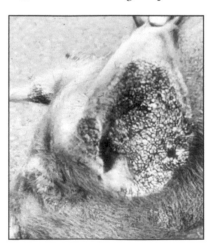

Fig. 9.56 **Chronic mange in the ear of a boar.**

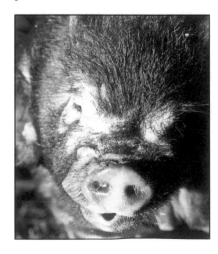

Fig. 9.57 **Mange lesions on the face of a pet pig.**

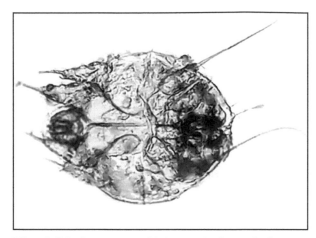

Fig. 9.58 *Sarcoptes scabiei* var *suis* through the microscope.

useful in breeding nucleus herds to demonstrate absence.

From a commercial point of view, visual inspection of the skin of finishing pigs in the slaughterhouse can be useful as part of the monitoring programme (**Figure 9.59**).

Management
Treatment: Avermectins can be used via various routes; injection and feed are common. Failure to adequately treat large boars is a common reason for failure to provide adequate control.

Control/eradication: Where possible, mange should be eradicated from units. Mange should be considered a welfare problem and with avermectins it can be eliminated from all units. Future breeding stock will need to be purchased from sarcoptic mange-free farms (see Chapter 11).

Methicillin resistant *Staphylococcus aureus*
Methicillin resistant *Staphylococcus aureus* (MRSA) is a significant human pathogen. It causes no clinical signs in pigs, but they may act as carriers to some porcine-adapted strains. This has the potential to be a zoonotic condition.

Mycoplasma suis
The organism *Mycoplasma suis* grows on the surface of erythrocytes. There are generally no or few clinical signs. Infection may be suspected in pigs that are anaemic without other obvious cause (**Figure 9.60**). In chronic cases a degree of jaundice may be visualised in affected pigs. Examine a blood smear and stain using Giemsa; the black small bodies may be seen associated with the erythrocytes (**Figure 9.61**). Treatment with tetracycline is generally effective.

Fig. 9.59 Skin lesions of mange. These lesions can be more prominent in the slaugtherhouse and even in the supermarket.

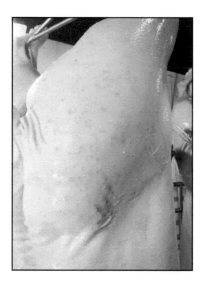

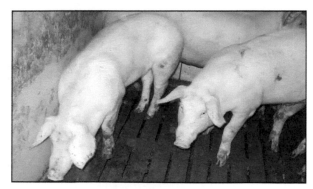

Fig. 9.60 Anaemic finishing pig.

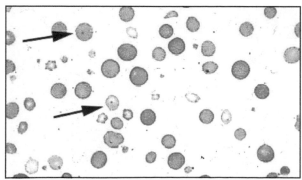

Fig. 9.61 *Mycoplasma suis* in erythrocytes (arrows) demonstrated by Giemsa staining.

Papilloma

Papilloma wart-like lesions on the skin may be seen on the forelimbs, sheath, scrotum and teats. Rarely, a congenital fibropapillomatosis may be seen with large patches of skin with cauliflower-like aspects (**Figure 9.62**). These may grow rapidly. Diagnosis is confirmed with a skin biopsy and histology. Other warty growths include squamous cell carcinomas, especially associated with the ears in white pigs in sunny climates.

Parakeratosis

Parakeratosis is generally seen in young weaned pigs (**Figure 9.63**). It is usually associated with zinc deficiency (occasionally high calcium reducing zinc availability). The lesions take 4–6 weeks to develop. The pig's skin becomes scaly, which may progress to covering the whole body in a thick encrustation. Exudative epidermitis is the major differential. Diagnosis is confirmed by a blood test showing low zinc levels (approximately 5 mmol/L; normal = 20 mmol/L).

Photosensitisation

Photosensitisation is associated with sloughing of the skin, generally in minimally pigmented areas of the body exposed to sunlight. The incident is normally triggered by exposure (ingestion) of a photodynamic agent (**Figure 9.64**). Ingestion of St John's wort (*Hypericum* sp.), a classic causal agent, is a good example. In many cases the photodynamic agent is not recognised. Treat the clinical signs, hydrate the pig, provide pain management and remove from sunlight.

Swine pox

Swine pox is caused by swine pox virus. The condition is seen clinically as small circular scabs 10–20 mm in size (**Figure 9.65**). Occasionally, small vesicles may be seen. The pathogen is thought to be widespread on most farms, although the problem can appear as a herd epidemic problem. Affected pigs recover in 10 days. Provide skin disinfectant washes to control secondary infections and improve basic pen hygiene. A congenital form can present with lesions seen on the newborn piglets (**Figure 9.66**).

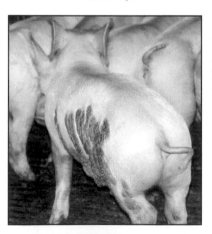

Fig. 9.62 Congenital giant fibro-papillomatosis tumour.

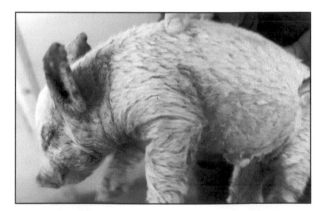

Fig. 9.63 Parakeratosis in a weaned pig.

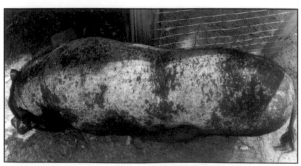

Fig. 9.64 Pet pig recovering from photosensitisation following the ingestion of parsnips.

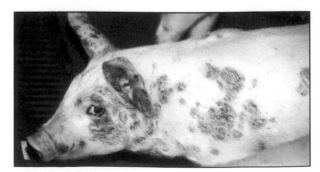

Fig. 9.65 Swine pox in a weaner pig.

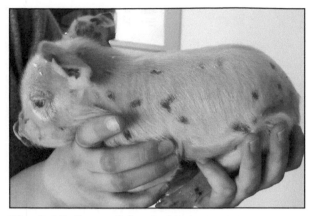

Fig. 9.66 **Congenital swine pox.**

Pityriasis rosea ▶ VIDEO 41

This is a genetic condition that suddenly appears in weaned and growing pigs 10–60 kg in weight (**Figure 9.67**). The pig presents with scabby lesions over its body, in particular the ventral abdomen. The lesions are often in rings with a red raised edge and a blanched centre. With time, the lesions may grow and coalesce. The pig is not ill and grows normally, although it looks quite alarming. No treatment is necessary. Rarely does the condition present by the time of slaughter. It is wise not to breed from afflicted animals.

Porcine dermatitis and nephropathy syndrome ▶ VIDEO 42
Definition/aetiology

Porcine dermatitis and nephropathy syndrome (PDNS) is a conditions of older growing pigs and occasionally adults. PDNS is considered an immunocomplex (type III hypersensitivity) disease and glomerular nephritis and a systemic necrotising

vasculitis are the most striking associated lesions. This is recognised on the skin as a purple lesion. The condition is non-specific, but there is an association with farms having a problem with PCV2-SD. The condition is also not infective. In all farms this can occur sporadically. An 'outbreak' of up to 10% of finishing pigs on a farm may point the clinician towards problems with PCV2-SD on the farm. Review the possible role of PCV3 on the farm.

Clinical presentation

The most obvious clinical sign is the presence of irregular red to purple patches (macules and papules) in the skin, particularly around the hindlimbs and perineal area. The lesions tend to merge with time and if the pig survives, scarring may occur. The pigs also show anorexia and depression and they lie down. They may have a stiffened gait and may have problems rising.

The problem classically affects pigs from 40–70 kg (12–16 weeks of age), although it has been seen occasionally in adults and can be associated with abortions. In grow/finish pigs it is generally fatal within a few days of the first clinical signs.

Differential diagnosis

The major differential diagnoses of PDNS are CSF and ASF. Therefore, in all cases of PDNS rule out the possibility of swine fever. Severe salmonellosis and erysipelas may also present with similar clinical signs.

Diagnosis

The striking skin changes are very suggestive (**Figure 9.68**). At post-mortem the lesions on the skin

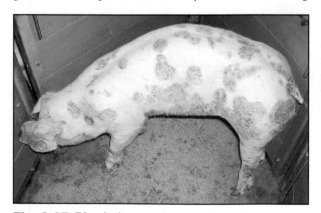

Fig. 9.67 **Pityriasis rosea in a growing pig.**

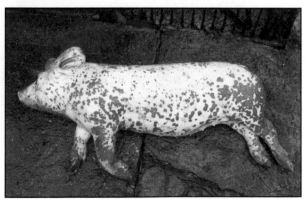

Fig. 9.68 **Dead pig with PDNS lesions.**

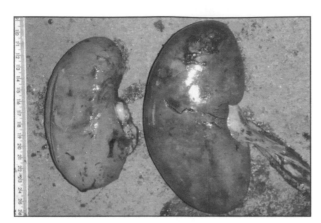

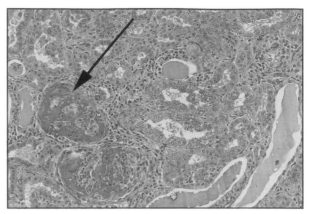

Fig. 9.69 The kidney on the left is a normal kidney from a 60 kg finishing pig. The kidney on the right is an enlarged kidney from a 60 kg pig with PDNS.

Fig. 9.70 Histological lesions of glomerular nephritis (affected glomerulus arrowed) in a case of PDNS.

are classic. The kidneys are bilaterally 2–3 times larger than normal and are paler than normal (**Figure 9.69**). There may be cortical petechiae visible on the surface of the kidney. The subinguinal lymph nodes draining the affected skin areas are grossly enlarged with a red, haemorrhagic appearance. Definitive diagnosis is only possible following renal histology demonstrating the glomerular nephritis (**Figure 9.70**).

Management

As yet there are few real clinical strategies that are effective. Control PCV2-SD by vaccination and ensure water supplies are excellent.

Ringworm

Affected pigs show characteristic round, light brown, gradually spreading circular lesions on

their bodies (**Figure 9.71**). Healing can take several weeks. They otherwise demonstrate no undue clinical signs. For treatment, it is necessary to wash the pigs with a skin disinfectant or, in a herd situation, consider the use of an antifungal agent such as griseofulvin.

Scrotal haemangioma

Haemangiomas arise from blood vessel endothelial cells and are common benign tumours on the scrotum of boars (**Figure 9.72**). They generally have no clinical significance.

Sunburn

A skin reaction is triggered by ultraviolet B rays with a maximum impact at 307 nm. The impact is worse in pigs with little or no pigmentation and

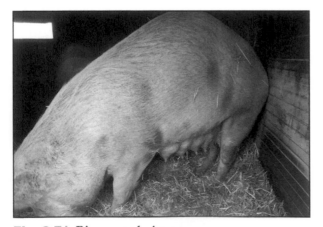

Fig. 9.71 Ringworm lesions on a sow.

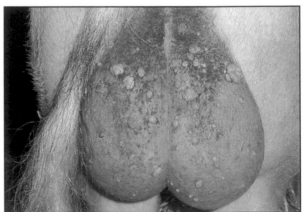

Fig. 9.72 Scrotal haemangiomas.

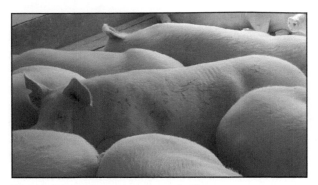

Fig. 9.73 Sunburn in selected gilts.

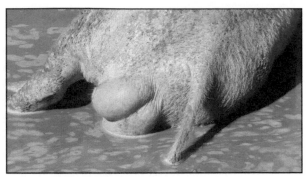

Fig. 9.74 Sunburn affecting the testes of a boar.

those exposed to sunlight (**Figure 9.73**). The animals can be severely affected, being ataxic and stiff, possibly becoming prostrate and then eventually die. In males this may affect the testes, often the dorsal aspect, with resulting infertility (**Figure 9.74**).

Provide adequate shade and wallows to outdoor pigs and monitor the impact of the sun in indoor housed pigs.

Swine fever(s)

The practicing clinician is not in the position to differentiate between CSF (hog cholera) and ASF. While there may be pathological differences, they are subtle. Following a clinical examination that indicates a suspicion of a swine fever, in countries where it is reportable, the practicing veterinarian needs to immediately report to the government authorities and their practice. In Asia, the correct diagnosis of a possible ASF outbreak is complicated by the natural presence of CSF. Likewise, in Africa, the correct diagnosis of a CSF outbreak can be complicated by the natural presence of ASF. Both swine fevers are caused by viruses resulting in a severe systemic viraemia with death and characteristic petechial haemorrhages in the skin. While presenting with very similar clinical signs, the two viruses are very different from each other.

Classical swine fever
Definition/aetiology
CSF, also known as hog cholera, is a highly contagious viral disease considered of worldwide importance and included in the notifiable disease list of the OIE. It is caused by CSFV, a pestivirus antigenically related to bovine viral diarrhoea virus (BVDV)

and border disease of sheep. CSFV is divided into three major genetic groups, each containing 3 or 4 subgroups. There are significant genetic differences among these groups, which are also translated into antigenic variability. Moreover, the virulence of CSFV isolates also differs, which explains the variation in clinical signs observed in infected animals. The major worldwide trend is to eradicate the infection with the aid of vaccines (with or without gene deleted characteristics), although the infection is still endemic in many countries in Asia and some in Central America.

Clinical presentation
CSFV infection can cause peracute, acute, chronic and pre-natal clinical signs, depending on the viral strain but also on pig age, health status and immunity. Highly virulent strains usually cause high fever, cyanosis, cutaneous haemorrhages (**Figure 9.75**) and

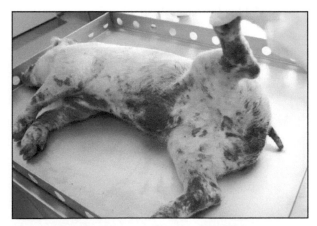

Fig. 9.75 Multiple cutaneous haemorrhages in a pig with a virulent CSFV infection.

high mortality rates. Depending on the strain, these signs can be milder and are difficult to differentiate from many other diseases. Piling is usual in pigs displaying fever. The effect of CSFV replication on the immune system (causing immunosuppression) facilitates concurrent infections and a variety of respiratory and/or enteric signs can be seen. On the reproductive side, CSFV infection can cause abortion and stillbirths. Immunotolerant pigs that show persistent viraemia have been described as a result of *in-utero* infection around 50–70 days of gestation; these pigs may look normal but may develop the so-called 'late-onset CSF', which represent chronically affected animals with rough hair, growth retardation and high susceptibility to concomitant infections. Importantly, these pigs are viral shedders and may play a significant epidemiological role in virus maintenance in the herd. CSFV may induce viral persistence on early post-natal infection.

Piglets may be born with congenital tremor.

Differential diagnosis

Cutaneous and internal organ haemorrhages caused by CSF must be differentiated from those of ASF, highly virulent PRRS, PDNS, septicaemic salmonellosis and erysipelas. In these cases, taking into account the notifiable nature of CSF, communication with the competent authority is compulsory. When less severe forms of CSF are observed, the differential diagnosis is more complicated since it can include general conditions causing fever and specific diseases such as PCV2-SD, PRRS, Aujeszky's disease and chronic respiratory/digestive problems. Congenital tremor is common on farms because of a variety of causes.

Diagnosis

Haemorrhagic diathesis is one of the hallmarks of peracute and acute CSF. These haemorrhages can be seen virtually everywhere, although those of the kidneys, larynx and lymph nodes are the most typical ones (**Figures 9.76–9.79**). Moreover, infarcts

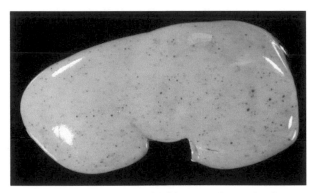

Fig. 9.76 Multiple petechial haemorrhages in the kidney of a pig infected with CSF.

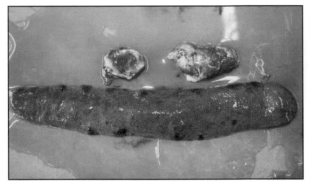

Fig. 9.77 Relatively normal sized spleen displaying infarcts in the margins of the organ in a pig experimentally infected with CSFV.

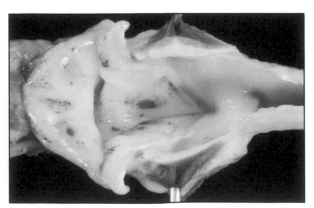

Fig. 9.78 Multiple petechiae in the larynx of a pig affected with CSF – laryngeal haemorrhages.

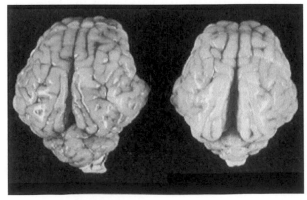

Fig. 9.79 The left brain is normal; the right demonstrates CSF hypocerebellosis.

in the margins of the spleen are fairly characteristic of CSF.

In the piglet, congenital tremor may be associated with a visible reduction in the size of cerebellum.

Diagnosis must be confirmed by laboratory tests and differentiated from other pestiviruses such as BVDV and congenital tremor virus. Most often, reverse transcription PCR methods are the preferred option to detect viral RNA due to their high sensitivity. The virus can also be isolated in cell culture and detected by an antigen-capture ELISA test. The best tissue samples to test include tonsils, spleen, kidney and ileocecal and retropharyngeal lymph nodes. Also, blood serum or buffy-coat can also be used from live pigs. The reference assay to detect antibodies is virus neutralisation, although ELISAs have also been developed. It is of paramount importance to detect the virus in the first instance; a scenario of positivity against antibodies and negativity against viral presence would imply detection was too late.

Management

For international trade purposes, CSF-free areas maintain a non-vaccination policy against CSF and eradication policies are in force. Therefore, in a suspicious case, the first step is communication with the competent authorities. In some of these CSF-free areas, however, there are eventual outbreaks due to the virus being endemic in wild boar populations. Therefore, wildlife represents a serious threat in these countries. For disease prevention, different CSF vaccines are available. These are live attenuated vaccines based on 'Chinese' C strain (the most commonly used), the Thiverval strain and recombinant

vaccines with the gene deleted concept (through the E2 protein). Although vaccines prevent clinical signs, they do not prevent transplacental infection and, therefore, persistent infections and a subsequent late-onset form of CSF. Oral vaccination of wild boar through baits has been tested, but adequate immunisation is difficult to guarantee due to possible difficulty in accessing the baits.

African swine fever
Definition/aetiology
ASFV is the only representative of the Asfarviridae family. It is one of the largest and most complex viruses and is able to cause a fatal disease of pigs of all breeds and ages. Moreover, ASF is also an OIE notifiable disease. The lack of vaccine availability and its current expansion into different parts of the world suggests it should be considered a global animal health priority. So far, 22 ASFV genotypes have been identified and cross-protection among them is considered poor. In addition, due to the fast clinical evolution of disease, immune responses are non-existent in many animals. In Africa, the virus transmission cycle is complex since it may involve domestic pigs, wild suid species (mainly wart hogs and bush pigs [**Figures 9.80, 9.81**], which are subclinically infected) and soft ticks (*Carios* spp. [**Figure 9.82**]). In Europe, the most common transmission route is by direct contact between sick and naïve pigs, as well as between domestic pigs and wild boar. Besides being currently endemic in some parts of Russia, Ukraine and some Eastern European Union countries, it has also been endemic on the island of Sardinia for many years. Traditional methods of rearing pigs in

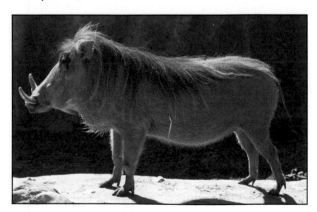

Fig. 9.80 Wart hog (*Phaeochoerus africanus*).

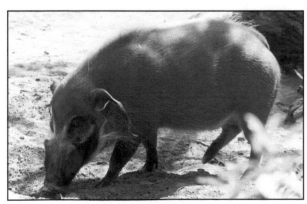

Fig. 9.81 Bush pig (*Potamochoerus porcus*).

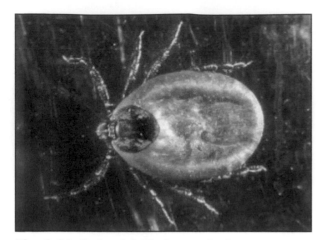

Fig. 9.82 Carios tick (*Carios erraticus*).

Sardinia facilitate the permanent transmission and maintenance of the virus.

Clinical presentation

Although wild African suids are resistant to the disease, domestic pigs and European wild boar can develop a number of clinical signs. Mortality is the usual outcome for highly virulent strains, although lower mortalities can be observed in moderately (20–80%) and low (10–30%) virulent strains (**Figures 9.83, 9.84**). Acutely affected animals develop a high fever with the pigs becoming very quiet and reluctant to move. Many pigs may vomit and present with dyspnoea (due to severe pulmonary oedema) besides the haemorrhagic lesions. Sows will abort and lactating sows stop milking. In most cases, a haemorrhagic diathesis develops, with potential cutaneous haemorrhages, epistaxis and bloody diarrhoea.

In subacute/chronic cases the clinical picture is similar, although the number of affected animals is lower and the course of the infection longer.

Differential diagnosis

Cutaneous and internal organ haemorrhages caused by ASF must be differentiated from those of CSF, highly virulent PRRS, PDNS, septicaemic salmonellosis and erysipelas. Splenomegaly can also be present in ASF and some of the above mentioned diseases. In these cases, taking into account the notifiable nature of ASF, communication with the competent authority is compulsory. Because of severe effects on the immune system, concurrent infections may appear; however, in acute cases there is usually not enough time for them to develop.

Diagnosis

Haemorrhagic diathesis is one of the hallmarks of ASF as well as splenomegaly (**Figures 9.85–9.88**). Haemorrhages can be seen virtually everywhere, although those from the kidneys, lung, heart, lymph nodes, urinary bladder and gallbladder are the most typical ones. Diagnosis must be confirmed by laboratory tests. Most often, PCR methods are the preferred option to detect viral DNA due to their high sensitivity, although direct immunofluorescence and haemadsorption tests have been traditionally used. The virus can also be isolated in cell culture but it is not practical from a rapid diagnosis point of view. The best samples to test include spleen, kidney, lymph nodes, lungs, blood and serum.

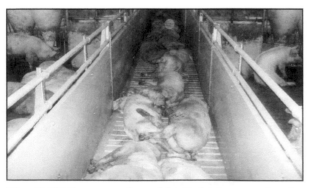

Fig. 9.83 Large number of dead pigs in an outbreak of ASF.

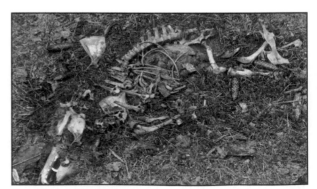

Fig. 9.84 Dead wild boar which died with ASF. The virus particles were still viable.

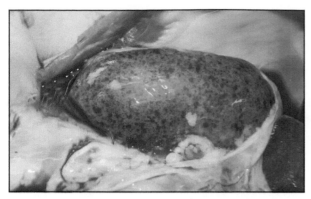

Fig. 9.85 Multiple petechial to diffuse haemorrhages in the kidney of a pig experimentally infected with ASF.

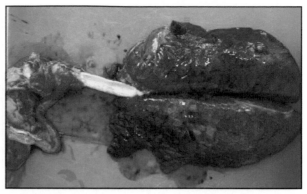

Fig. 9.86 Multiple haemorrhages in the lung parenchyma and marked pulmonary oedema with tracheal foam in a pig experimentally infected with ASF.

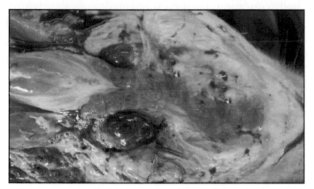

Fig. 9.87 Diffuse, severe haemorrhages in the submandibular lymph nodes of a pig experimentally infected with ASF.

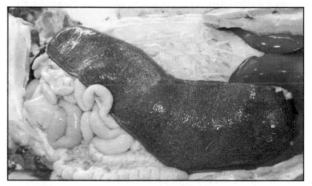

Fig. 9.88 Marked splenomegaly in a pig experimentally infected with ASF. The spleen can increase its size by 3–4 times; it is full of blood that can be observed when cutting the organ.

Management

No vaccination is available for ASF and eradication policies apply in ASF-free countries. As long as the disease is clinically suspected, communication with the competent authorities must be established and pig movements restricted, followed by performance of appropriate diagnostic studies.

Thrombocytopaenia purpura

This condition is seen only in young piglets from 3–10 days of age. The cause is antibodies to the piglet's platelets in the colostrum of multiparous sows. Piglets present dead and on close examination reveal small haemorrhages on the skin (**Figure 9.89**). Postmortem examination reveals small haemorrhages throughout the carcase; transfer surviving piglets to another sow. This condition is a differential for the swine fevers, but the age group is revealing.

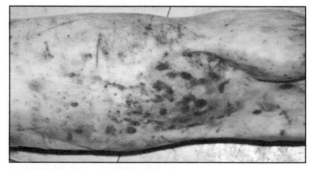

Fig. 9.89 Haematomas on the skin of a piglet with thrombocytopaenia purpura.

Trauma of the skin
Piglet

Abrasions to the carpus are very common in the piglet and weaner. They arise from the suckling motion/activity of the carpus on the floor of the

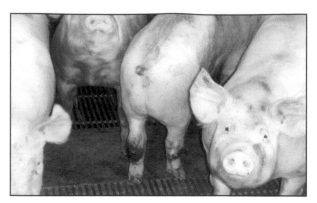

Fig. 9.90 Tuber ulcer/erosion.

farrowing pen (**Figure 9.90**). The lesion develops into a callus and presents few obvious health problems; however, it may progress to joint ill. Proper care and attention to farrowing floors is to be encouraged to reduce the severity of the problem as much as possible. Provide pain management as appropriate.

Grow/finish

Erosions are not uncommon on many pig farms and are generally associated with rough flooring or sharp contact surfaces. They are very common with new floors, which should always be checked for sharp points before entry of the pigs. Secondary infections are not uncommon if the animal remains in a dirty abrasive environment. Review the environmental conditions. Consider lime washing floors and walls to reduce sharp points. Provide pain management as appropriate. In individual cases that are severe, remove the animal to a compromised pig pen, ideally with bedding such as straw, and cover the exposed tissues with wound sprays.

Adults

Shoulder sores: Shoulder sores are classically seen in the later stages of lactation and generally associated with a thin sow (**Figures 9.91, 9.92**). Some of the modern lean sow genotypes may easily develop shoulder sores. The problem is ischaemia (no blood supply) with secondary infection by *Staphylococcus* spp. resulting in necrosis over the shoulder blade. Treatment is to keep the wound clean until weaning. Provide pain management as appropriate. After weaning, place the sow in a hospital pen with straw. Feed the sow to restore body condition. Healing is normally complete within a month. The sow, however, should be bred as normal after weaning. Occasionally the wound becomes cannibalised by piglets within the litter and this can create a very deep injury, which may even require euthanasia of the sow.

Injuries: Fighting among pigs is extremely common in both males and females and between the sexes (**Figures 9.93–9.99**). Occasionally injuries, sometimes life threatening, may occur.

Skin injuries through bites and the use of tusks can be very dramatic and may require sutures. However, also remember that the pig has evolved to be able to cope with these injuries and their healing powers are exceptional.

Ulceration may occur in other related species and require systematic care; for example, an ulcerated wound in a hippopotamus (*Hippopotamus amphibious*) (**Figure 9.100**).

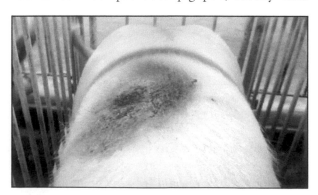

Fig. 9.91 Housing injury.

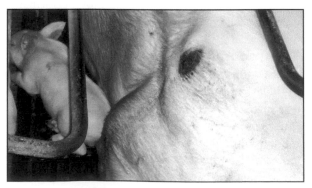

Fig. 9.92 Shoulder sore.

Fig. 9.93
General points of injury in the pig.

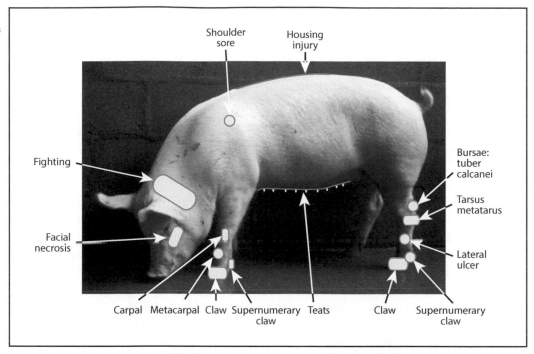

Shoulder sore

Housing injury

Fighting

Facial necrosis

Bursae: tuber calcanei

Tarsus metatarus

Lateral ulcer

Carpal   Metacarpal   Claw   Supernumerary claw   Teats   Claw   Supernumerary claw

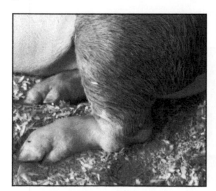

Fig. 9.94 Fighting – tusk injury gilts and boar.

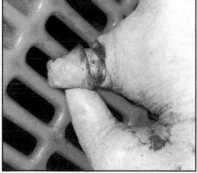

Fig. 9.95 Teat trauma.

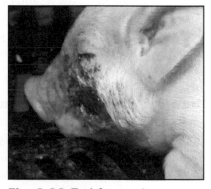

Fig. 9.96 Facial necrosis.

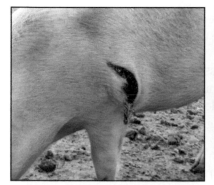

Fig. 9.97 Bursa.

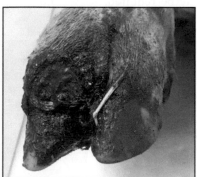

Fig. 9.98 Claw injury.

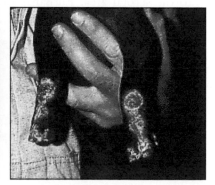

Fig. 9.99 Carpal injury.

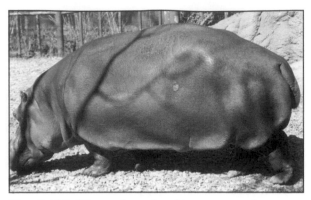

Fig. 9.100 Ulcerated area in a hippopotamus in a zoo.

Ulcerated granuloma

A large granuloma can develop on the leg of the sow, although the lesion looks more severe than the behaviour of the animal would indicate. There is no effective treatment but lesion size can be controlled by housing on straw. Culling may be beneficial. The slaughterhouse veterinarian may become very concerned about the lesion, therefore telephone and discuss any welfare or transportation issues before sending in the animal. On occasions *Borrelia suis* (*suilla*) may be a specific cause. Also look for *Treponema pedis* (see Chapter 5).

Ventral/preputial gangrene

A spreading dry gangrene of the prepuce is seen in finishing pigs and young adults (**Figure 9.101**). The lesions start as a small ulcer, which rapidly develops into a black necrotic zone on the ventral surface around the prepuce. This can spread and become quite extensive on the ventral surface and extend into the scrotal area. Euthanasia may be required.

Treatment needs to be aggressive with lincomycin HCl and using medicated washings of the area. Examine skin scrapes for spirochaetes. It may be possible to isolate *Treponema pedis* from these lesions.

Vices ▶ VIDEO 36 and 43

Definition/aetiology

A group of pigs in a stressed environment will readily demonstrate a tendency to bite, nibble and suck other pigs in the group:

- Facial necrosis in piglets; see also greasy pig disease/exudative epidermitis.
- Penile sucking in newly weaned pigs.
- Ear sucking/ear biting in nursery pigs.
- Tail biting in grow/finish pigs, rarely in adults.
- Flank biting in grow/finish, especially in tail docked pigs.
- Vulva biting in adult females when loose housed.
- Bar biting and other stereotypies.

The body area injured by the behaviour of other pigs is often age dependent.

Causes of stressed and deprived pigs

The clinician must ensure that the environment of the pig is suitable for farming. It is advisable to check for the following:

- Pig factors:
  - Check tail length, in particular variability.
  - Facial necrosis associated with lactation failure and consequent fighting between hungry pigs.

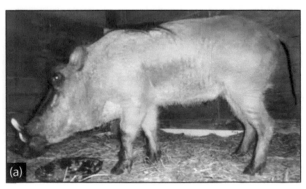
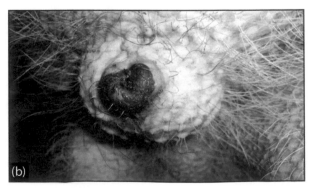

Fig. 9.101 (a, b) Ventral/preputial gangrene in a wart hog.

- Environmental factors:
  - Check for evidence of draughts at pig heights (draught air speed >0.2 m/sec). In about 9/10 cases, tail biting has been associated with a chilling draught.
  - Check air quality (target: NH_3 <20 ppm; H_2S <10 ppm; CO_2 <1,500 ppm).
  - Check 24-hour temperature fluctuations. Note weather changes and high pressure changes.
  - Check humidity (target between 50 and 75% RH).
  - Check light intensity.
  - Check water supplies.
  - Check stocking density.
  - Check feed particle size (target >500 μm).
  - Check salt (NaCl) concentration in feed.
  - Check feeder space availability.
  - Mycotoxin needs to be kept below toxic concentrations.
  - Examine mixing and moving protocols

Post-mortem findings

Following injury to the skin from vices, there are a number of internal sequelae to the subsequent bacteraemia. These include pulmonary miliary abscesses, vegetative endocarditis, spinal abscessation and single or multiple discrete abscesses throughout the body. Each of these may complicate the clinical findings in an individual pig.

Management

Treatment: Find the offending pig(s), which may be difficult. Look for the gaunt, smaller, middle order pig, often with chronic mild diarrhoea. Remove affected pigs to a hospital pen and treat with sprays/wound dressings. Provide pain management. Consider euthanasia if pigs are severely affected, lame or have other abscesses. Lesions may become secondarily infected with *Staphylococcus hyicus* and/or *Treponema pedis* externally, or with bacteria introduced into the body of the pig, which would include *Streptococcus* spp. and *Trueperella pyogenes*.

Control: Increase NaCl concentration in the feed to 0.9% and ensure the water supply is excellent. It may also be worth considering increasing the concentration of potassium chloride (KCl) in the feed. The addition of magnesium oxide (MgO) may also help to reduce the degree of vice in the group of pigs by modulating their behaviour.

- Review environmental factors and remove any adverse stressors.
- Review pig sleeping area provisions.
- Some genotypes may be more aggressive in some environments.
- Provide distractions through toys (e.g. chains).
- Improve pig flow to remove under- and overstocking ▶ VIDEO 5D
- Check tail docking principles as pigs do not like variable pig tail lengths

Areas of vice
See **Figures 9.102–9.109**.

One way to visualise to the client the impact of all these various problems on a pig farm is to image the iceberg effect of management and health issues (**Figure 9.110**). The small end result – tail biting – is associated with an array of errors in production.

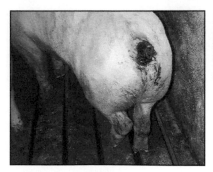

Fig. 9.102 Tail biting.

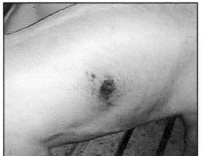

Fig. 9.103 Flank biting.

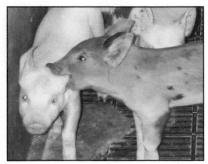

Fig. 9.104 Ear biting.

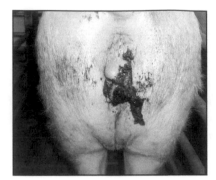

Fig. 9.105 Vulva biting.

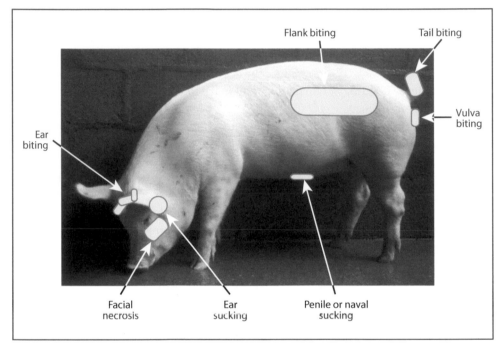

Fig. 9.106 Areas on the body where biting occurs.

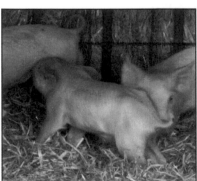

Fig. 9.107 Penile or naval sucking.

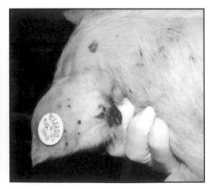

Fig. 9.108 Ear sucking.

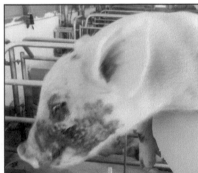

Fig. 9.109 Facial necrosis.

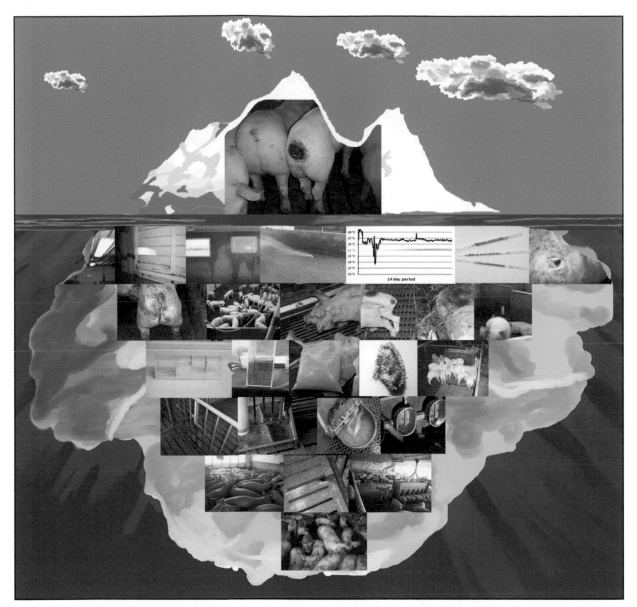

Fig. 9.110 The iceberg effect of different 'stress' factors resulting in tail biting in a group of finishing pigs.

CLINICAL QUIZ

9.1 Label the other structures shown in **Figure 9.21** (see p. 282).

The answer to this question can be found on page 477.

ENVIRONMENTAL MEDICINE

INTRODUCTION

Understanding population health maintenance is important in animal production. This chapter looks at the skills required to allow the veterinarian to examine the whole farm as a living organism. In order to do this, a systematic approach is recommended. There is little difference between the skill-set necessary to examine an individual animal, a group or a whole farm.

WATER SUPPLY MANAGEMENT

All stockpersons know water is essential for survival and production. While water can be demonstrated to be a limiting factor to pigs, the pigs will only rarely present with 'salt poisoning' (see Chapter 6) and many of the signs of water shortage are subtle and thus missed by the farm team.

Fresh water is a limited resource and should be treated as such and not squandered. All wasted water is an expense through increased slurry disposal. However, if the farm's slurry bills are high, do not restrict water availability. Instead, use better designed water systems. Remember, leaking drinkers, cooling systems, power-washing, general cleaning, rain run-off and poor drainage all contribute to the volume of slurry produced.

Water consumption

The water supply needs to provide at least 1 L per 10 kg body weight per day. A lactating sow may use as much as 80 L per day at peak lactation (around day 18 of lactation). **Note:** This is water used, not necessarily water consumed. Because of poor design, many water delivery systems waste 20–50% of the water they supply.

Equipment useful for monitoring the water management on the farm

See **Figures 10.1–10.8**.

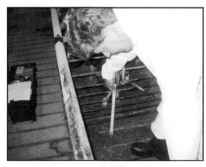

Fig. 10.1 Tape measure for height – check the available smart phone measuring apps.

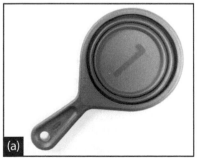

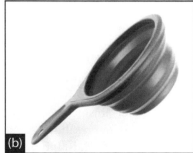

Fig. 10.2a, b Measuring cylinder – this is collapsible, reducing the space taken up by the equipment.

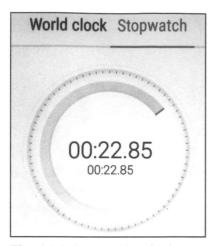

Fig. 10.3 Stop watch – check your smart phone apps.

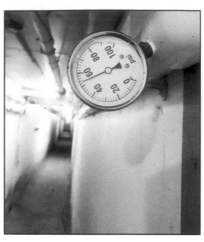

Fig. 10.4 Water pressure gauge.

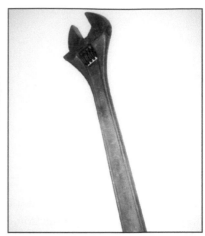

Fig. 10.5 Wrench to remove drinker.

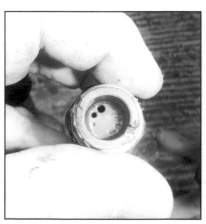

Fig. 10.6 Have sufficient tools to take drinker apart; a Swiss Army knife, for example. One of the three holes in the drinker is selected to adjust the flow of water through the drinker.

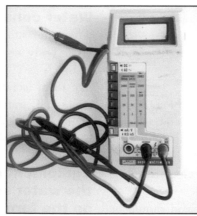

Fig. 10.7 Check for stray voltage with a volt meter.

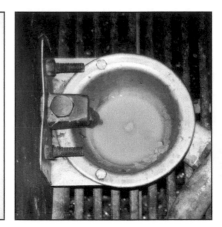

Fig. 10.8 Note the colour, smell and taste of the water. A total dissolved solids meter can be very helpful.

Water quality and source

Ensure the water quality is suitable for pigs (*Table 10.1*). Water from artesian bore holes may supply water unsuitable for pigs because of high salinity. Maximum salinity should be less than 1,000 mg/L dissolved solids. It is important to position the bore hole away from the slurry storage lagoon as the slurry may contaminate the ground water. However, even contaminated bore water may be adequate for power-washing and cleaning and thus significantly contribute to the farm's attempt to reduce the cost of production.

Clinical issues that may occur with contaminated water supplies
High sulphate

This has been associated with:

- Diarrhoea/scouring at >3,000 mg/kg.
- Poor weight gain and feed efficiency.
- Nervousness in various age groups.
- Increased water intake by growing pigs.
- Decreased water intake by lactating sows.
- Decreased feed intake.

Table 10.1 **Guidelines for water quality suitable for pigs to drink.**

ELEMENT	MAXIMUM mg/kg (ppm) OF WATER
Aluminum	5
Arsenic	0.5
Beryllium	0.1
Boron	5
Cadmium	0
Calcium	1,000
Chloride	400
Chromium	1
Copper	5
Fluoride	2
Hardness – calcium carbonate	<60 classified as soft 120–180 classified as hard >180 classified as very hard
Iron	0.5
Lead	0.1
Magnesium	400
Manganese	0.1
Mercury	0.003
Molybdenum	0.5
Nickel	1
Nitrites	10
Nitrates	50
Phosphorus	7.8
Potassium	3
Sodium	150
Selenium	0.05
Solids (dissolved)	1,000
Sulphate	1,000
Uranium	0.2
Vanadium	0.1
Zinc	40
Total viable bacterial counts per mL 37°C 22°C	Counts should be low and not vary between samples $<2 \times 10^2$ $<1 \times 10^4$
Coliforms/100 mL	Zero

As the water becomes more alkaline the laxative effect of sulphates is more pronounced, especially in young pigs.

Total dissolved solids

<1,000 mg/kg	No risk
1,000–3,000 mg/kg	Mild diarrhoea in pigs not adapted to the water
5,000+ mg/kg	Avoid in pregnant and lactating sows
7,000+ mg/kg	Avoid in any pig

Total dissolved solids can be removed, but this is generally expensive. It is more important when producing water for semen extension in artificial insemination (AI). This is achieved by use of filters, reversed osmosis and water softeners

High iron (Fe) content

Iron levels in excess of 0.3 mg/kg can stain clothes. At this concentration it may also support iron bacteria (part of the biofilm), which results in foul odours and plugging of water systems. Levels over 0.3 mg/kg may also result in reduced water intake.

High sodium (Na) content

Sodium sulphate is a well-known laxative. Water with over 400 mg/L sodium may warrant an adjustment to the sodium concentration in the diet, but ensure that chlorine deficiency does not result. At 800 mg/L, sodium can cause diarrhoea.

High coliform counts (e.g. *Escherichia coli*)

- Check for sources of animal faecal contamination.
- Shock chlorination (using sodium hypochlorite at 5.25% chlorine solution).
- High levels of organic matter will promote the conversion of chlorine into chloramines. This interferes with the ability of disinfectants to work.

Counts should be kept at no higher than 1 colony forming unit (cfu)/100 mL to ensure that diarrhoea does not ensue.

Algae

- Green algae – control growth by applying 1 mg/L copper sulphate to the water.
- Blue green algae – find a different water source as the water will poison the pigs.

Other pathogens that may be transmitted via the water supply

Erysipelothrix rhusiopathiae, *Salmonella* spp. and *Leptospira* spp. are examples. Other local farming operations may contaminate the water source (e.g. a local fish farm in cases of erysipelas).

Water filter

There should be few suspended solids, such as sand and mud, in the water supply. Dissolved solids and high mineral content can affect the palatability of the water and can form deposits in the pipe, reducing flow. If you filter the water, ensure the filters are cleaned and managed regularly (**Figure 10.9**).

Water delivery systems to and around the farm

In many countries it is illegal to take water straight from the municipal mains water supply. A non-return valve must be fitted within the pipeline. Check with the local water company to determine the legal situation.

If a storage tank is used, the height to the water surface determines the maximum pressure in the down pipe (*Table 10.2*). A low-pressure system runs

Table 10.2 Relationship between height of the header tank and water pressure.

HEIGHT (m)	PRESSURE (kpa)
0	0
1.5	14
3	28
6	62

between 0 and 100 kpa and a high-pressure system at 100–500 kpa (normally from the mains or pumped supply).

If a water header tank is used, the tank needs to fill quickly even when the farm water demands are high, for instance during power-washing or during hot weather. Ensure that the water tank has a tight fitting lid and is rodent proof. The tank needs to be checked regularly.

Length of pipes used

On farms using storage tanks, ensure that the drinkers are not too far from the tank. Check the flow in the first drinker and compare with the flow in the drinker farthest from the tank (**Figures 10.10, 10.11**). If there is a relatively large pressure reduction, it may be necessary to use more than one storage tank in the building. Consider the water availability when all the animals are trying to drink at once, such as after feeding. When washing rooms, water flow may become critical.

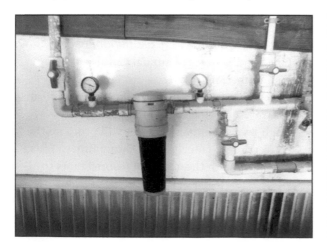

Fig. 10.9 Filter poorly maintained and full of sediment.

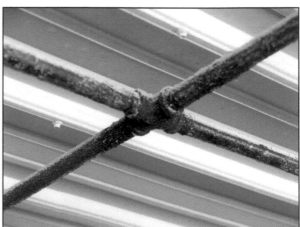

Fig. 10.10 Water is distributed along many long pipes thus constantly reducing the water pressure.

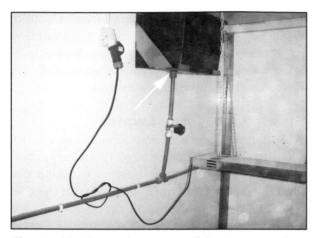

Fig. 10.11 The single pipe out of the storage tank (arrow) halves the pressure in the system compared with having two pipes out of the storage system to supply both sides of the house.

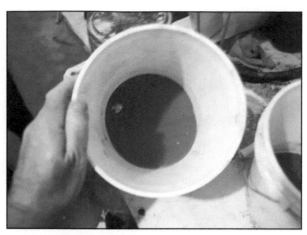

Fig. 10.12 Sediment in the water system released when a drinker was removed.

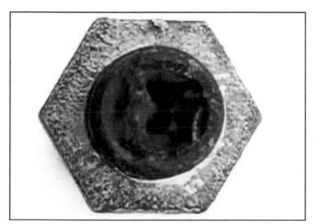

Fig. 10.13 A down pipe blocked with calcium carbonate deposit. This resulted in serious respiratory problems in the finishing pigs, associated with problems with the mucociliary escalator.

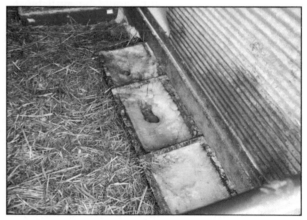

Fig. 10.14 Frozen water in the hospital pen. It is little surprise that the pigs in the hospital pen did not do well.

Sediment in the pipe work

A narrowing of the down pipe can be an insidious cause of reduced water availability. Some sediment can be dislodged with acids, which may ultimately improve water availability, but in the short term may also lead to blockage of drinkers as the sediments enter the pipelines (**Figures 10.12, 10.13**).

Freezing

The farm should have adequate provision to cope with adverse weather conditions, especially in the winter when water delivery systems may freeze (**Figure 10.14**). Does the farm have adequate provisions to easily transport water to all pigs if the need arises?

Water drinker to the pig

Ensure that the correct drinker type is used for every age group. Adult bite drinkers are totally inadequate for piglets. Regular checking will reveal any abnormal wear; an incorrect drinker will only create more wasted water.

Number of drinkers per pen

As many drinking systems are placed at the rear of pens they may not be checked on a daily basis.

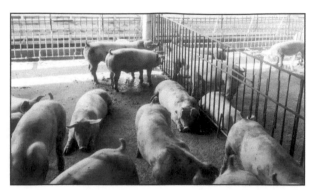

Fig. 10.15 Inadequate water supply is illustrated by the pigs crowding behaviour and subsequent poor performance.

Therefore, there should be two drinkers in each pen (in case one fails). Welfare codes recommend that one nipple drinking point should be available for each ten pigs; a water bowl normally provides water for 20 pigs; check your local regulations. A trough can supply 12 finishing pigs per 30 cm of water trough. Watch the behaviour of the pigs using the drinker (**Figure 10.15**).

Height and angle of the drinkers

Incorrect height for the age group is one of the commonest mistakes, resulting in pigs struggling for water. Follow the manufacturer's recommendations but as a general guide a nipple or bite drinker should be sited slightly above the shoulder. Are the drinkers properly re-set when the pigs enter the building? Reference heights are shown in *Table 10.3*.

Where the pen is designed for animals over a wide growth range, provide either a number of watering points at different heights or some means of adapting drinker height to current pig size. It is not sufficient to provide steps, which the pigs must climb to reach water, unless a bowl type drinker is used and the step is intended to limit soiling of the bowl.

Flow or pressure of water

This is probably the most common fault restricting water availability (*Table 10.4*). Initially, check for variability between drinkers in the same house. This should alert the farm health team that there is a water problem (**Figures 10.16, 10.17**):

* With low-pressure systems any blockage results in low flow rates.
* With high-pressure systems excessive water pressure results in the drinker spraying pigs in the next pen.

Some drinkers will not provide the required flow rates without creating a pressure problem; the manufacturer's recommendations must always be followed. If water enters the mouth at too high a pressure, the animal will gag and increased water waste will result. Another consideration is that the animals have evolved drinking from ground level and while a sow can consume 3 L in 45 seconds from a trough, water intake may be reduced when drinking with a raised head.

Purchasing a manufactured drinker, removing the filter and pressure regulator because of persistent blockage problems, and then drilling out the orifice to increase and stabilise the flow, is not an acceptable alternative to the purchase of a correct drinker in the first place.

Table 10.3 **Height of drinker for weight of pig.**

WEIGHT OF PIG (kg)	HEIGHT TO NIPPLE DRINKER (cm)
<10	10–13
10–30	13–30
31–60	30–60
61–110	60–76
>111 and adult	76–90

Table 10.4 **Suggested water flow rates.**

WEIGHT OF PIG (kg)	FLOW FROM A NIPPLE (L/min)
<10	0.3
10–30	0.7
31–60	1.0
61–110	1.5
Adult	1.5–2.0
Lactating sow	2.0

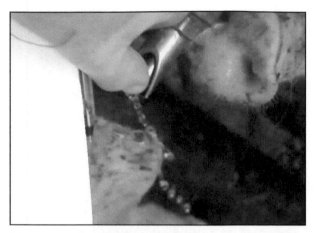

Fig. 10.16 Water flow too slow.
VIDEOS 44A and 44B

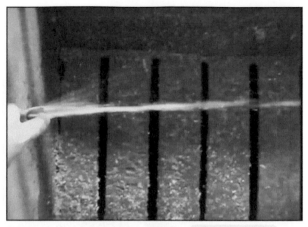

Fig. 10.17 Water flow too high. VIDEO 44C

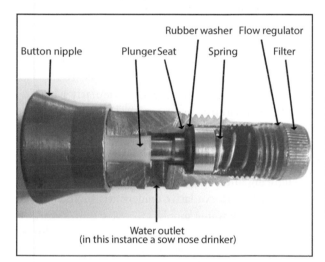

Fig. 10.18 Dissection of a nose or button drinker.

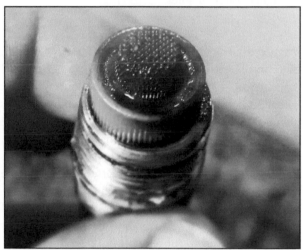

Fig. 10.19 Example of a filter and water pressure regulator.

Drinker design

It is a useful skill to be able to understand and repair the drinker types used on pig farms (**Figures 10.18, 10.19**).

Depth of water

The depth of water in a trough is very important. For instance, sows require a depth of 4 cm as pigs are not designed to lick up water. If the pig cannot bubble air through the water, check the depth. With water troughs in the gestation/dry sow area, check that there are no shallow areas (**Figures 10.20, 10.21**). On some farms the angle of slope in the trough is too great for a sufficient depth of water to build up. The slope must be decreased and more header tanks installed.

In outdoor systems the water trough may also be used as a wallow and fill up with soil, which reduces the water depth. Ideally, there should be a separate water supply and mud wallow.

Water through feed

Many finishing pigs receive the bulk of their water supply through wet feed systems. These can be a very efficient means of watering growing pigs. Ensure that the water and feed mix is correct; it is recommended

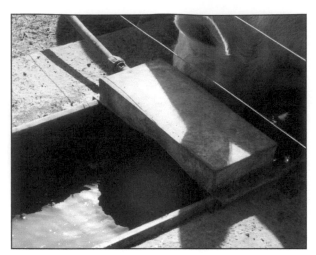

Fig. 10.20 Water depth is very important in troughed water supplies.

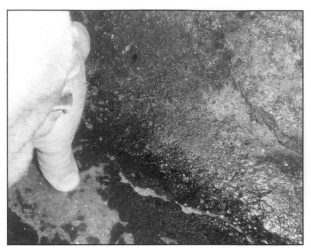

Fig. 10.21 Inadequate depth makes it very difficult for the pigs to drink as they cannot suck up the water.

that a dilution of 2.5:1 (water/feed ratio) is used. A ratio of 3 or even 3.5:1 may provide a better food conversion. There should always be additional water through a nipple or bite drinker, including farms using wet/dry single spaced feeders or liquid feeding systems. Not every pig will want to eat every day, but it is likely it will want a drink, particularly if it is sick. The demand for water greatly increases if the animals have pneumonia or diarrhoea.

In the farrowing house, wet/damp feeding of sows can greatly enhance dry matter intake plus water intake and so subsequent milk production, litter weaning weights and reduction in the wean to service interval.

Behaviour of pigs using the drinkers

Veterinarians (and stockpersons) should watch pigs manipulate the various aspects of the environment in order to gain valuable information on the adequacy of the system being observed:

- **Time spent drinking.** Weaners are reluctant to drink for more than 6 minutes a day whereas lactating sows are more willing to spend time drinking. However, lactating sows should spend time caring for their piglets rather than drinking for 2–3 hours a day.

- **Crowding around drinkers.** Stockpersons should be concerned when their pigs are crowding around drinkers, particularly when this behaviour is not associated with feeding times.

- **Increased aggression.** If the water supply becomes limited, this can lead to increased fighting and aggression in the pigs. Investigations into vice and exudative epidermitis should always include the water supply.

- **Bizarre behaviour patterns.** Sows that exhibit bizarre behaviour patterns, such as playing with the drinker all the time, or have an over full water/feed trough may have been desperate for a drink of clean water previously.

- **Is it just one pig's problem?** Water deprivation can be an individual pig's problem. After weaning, for instance, some weaners do not find the drinker and will rapidly lose weight and dehydrate. Such animals can be difficult to identify in the early stages when mixed within a larger group, and every effort should be made to ensure all the pigs know how to use the water supply. Making nipples leak for 48 hours, spreading water under the drinker or having a concrete dish placed below the drinkers prior to piglets entering the nursery may help this transition period.

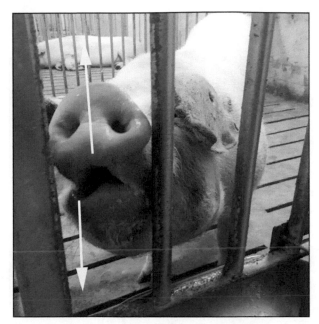

Fig. 10.22 Twisted snout associated with problems in using the water supply. Note the lower jaw does not align with the middle of the snout (arrows). The drinker was turned towards the wall for 6 months.

- **Off feed.** It will take 24–36 hours of water deprivation to make a noticeable difference to feed intake and even when present this simple observation is often missed. In *ad-libitum* feed systems, it can be very difficult to see when pigs are not eating properly.
- **Changes in anatomy.** Deformities of the head can be seen associated with difficulties in using the water supply (**Figure 10.22**). These may be dismissed as cases of atrophic rhinitis.

Position of drinkers

If drinkers are too close together, a dominant sow can stop others having access while she is drinking (*Table 10.5*). Check that the drinkers are accessible to the pig; this is particularly important in the farrowing house with nose drinkers installed in a feed/water trough too small for the sow's head. Drinkers can be made inaccessible if placed too close to feeders or walls.

Table 10.5 Recommended minimum distance between two drinkers.

AGE OF PIG	DISTANCE
Nursery	26 cm
Finisher	60 cm
Adult	1.8 m

Stray voltage

In areas where electrical grounding may be difficult, for instance farms on very sandy soil, it is always worth periodically checking for stray voltage and ensuring that all metal work is well grounded. This requires a qualified electrician.

Water as a therapeutic route

When using water medication ensure that the system is clean before addition of medications. If there is any problem, clean the system out with organic acids, hypochlorate or proprietary products. Ensure all the drinkers are free-flowing after treatment with medications. Various antibiotics can be inactivated by high calcium or iron concentration. Some medications use sugar as a carrier and this can encourage slime growth, whereas citrate carriers acidify the water, dislodging lime deposits which then block the drinkers. Water is an excellent route for medication but requires good management to maintain the system. Always check the drinkers regularly (twice daily) while medicating the pigs and, once finished, ensure the system is restored to full working capacity. When determining the therapeutic dose, a guide to daily water use is 1 L/10 kg bodyweight assuming the water supplies are adequate to start with.

Water is also used for cooling

This is further discussed under the management of the ventilation system.

Water: other uses

Water on the farm may also be used in the production of on-farm diluted semen for AI. Water also washes floors and flushes toilets.

Examples of poor water supply management
See **Figures 10.23–10.42**.

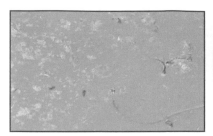

Fig. 10.23 The water source needs to be clean and regularly checked for bacterial contamination.

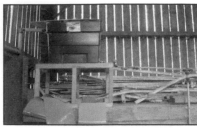

Fig. 10.24 Water may be stored on farm in header tanks, but these need to be secure.

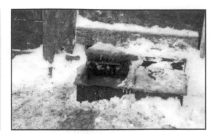

Fig. 10.25 If the water supply is liable to freezing, ensure suitable arrangements are made.

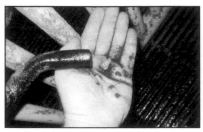

Fig. 10.26 Where the water is distributed through pipelines in the house, ensure the system is not blocked and is clean.

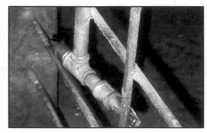

Fig. 10.27 Is the drinker accessible to the pigs? These drinkers have turned, causing limited access.

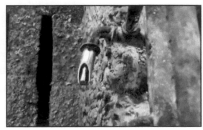

Fig. 10.28 This drinker has turned towards the wall, making it difficult to access.

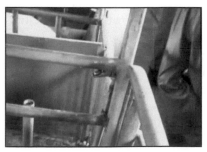

Fig. 10.29 This drinker is very difficult to access due to the design of the pen.

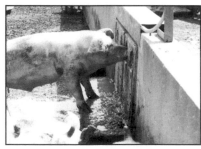

Fig. 10.30 Do not make pigs climb to reach the water supply.

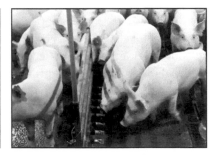

Fig. 10.31 These drinkers are too low for adequate access without spillage.

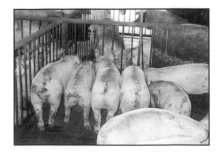

Fig. 10.32 There is an insufficient number of drinkers in this pen.

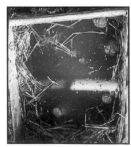

Fig. 10.33 This water was clearly contaminated with faecal materials.

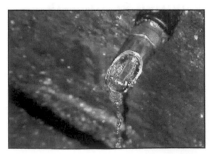

Fig. 10.34 This drinker is leaking water, a serious cause of waste.

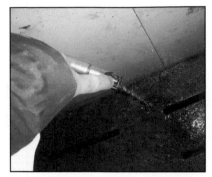

Fig. 10.35 Check the water flow. In this instance it is inadequate for the age of the pigs.

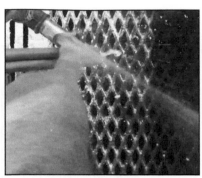

Fig. 10.36 This flow, from a high-pressure system, is excessive.

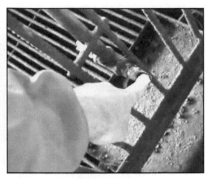

Fig. 10.37 There is no flow from these drinkers, which will result in the death of pigs.

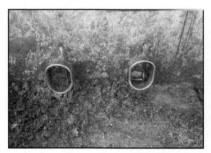

Fig. 10.38 Water flow problems can often be seen at a distance. Check for variation between drinkers.

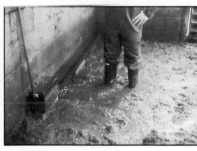

Fig. 10.39 Drinkers can overflow and lead to water wastage and potentially wet sleeping areas.

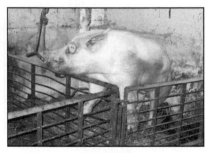

Fig. 10.40 Observe the behaviour of the pigs while drinking to see if the water supply is adequate.

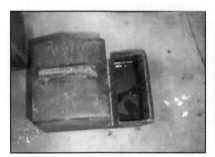

Fig. 10.41 Drinkers used for compromised pigs must be clean and readily accessible.

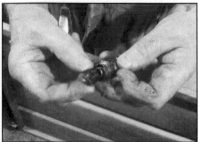

Fig. 10.42 A working knowledge of how drinkers work will help the investigation.

AIR MANAGEMENT

Equipment useful for monitoring the quality of the air supplied to the pigs
See **Figures 10.43–10.53**.

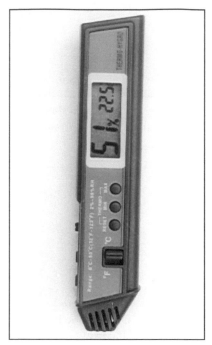

Fig. 10.43 Temperature and humidity pen.

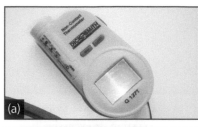

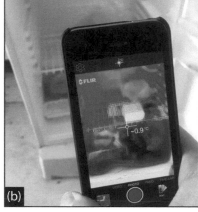

Fig. 10.44 Infrared thermometer (a) and, ideally, a camera (b).

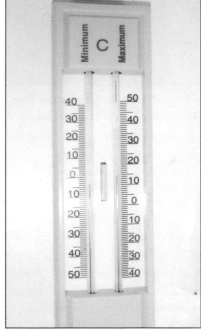

Fig. 10.45 Maximum and minimum thermometer.

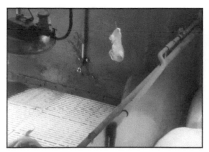

Fig. 10.46 Temperature loggers.

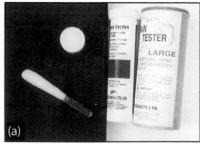

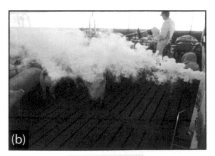

Fig. 10.47 (a, b) Smoke sticks in various sizes. ▶ VIDEO 45

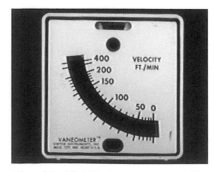

Fig. 10.48 Wind vane to quantify air speed.

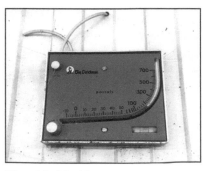

Fig. 10.49 Air pressure gauge.

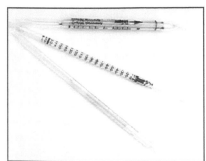

Fig. 10.50 Gas concentrations detectors: CO, CO_2, NH_4 and H_2S.

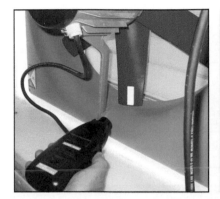

Fig. 10.51 Tachometer for fan speed.

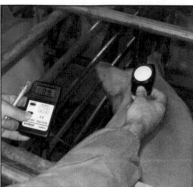

Fig. 10.52 Light meter – check smart phone apps.

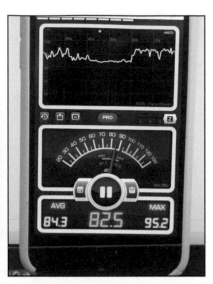

Fig. 10.53 Sound meter – check smart phone apps.

Note: Smart phones increasingly provide apps that may be useful to the population animal specialist – distance measurements, light and sound meters, for example.

Monitoring the air by observing at the pigs

Acute air patterns

Examine the pigs before you enter the room. This means that all rooms should have a window (which must be clean) from which the farm team can view the pigs (**Figure 10.54**). It may be useful to have a drawing of the room so the location of the pigs can be quickly noted.

Quietly enter the room and watch and observe the pigs. Count/note the number of coughs and sneezes that occur in a minute. Get to know the normal behaviour of the pigs pre- and post entry. If the group of pigs are clinically affected with swine influenza or porcine pleuropneumonia, they will tend to be very quiet, a different behaviour pattern from normal.

The various lying patterns of the pig should be noted and understood. If pigs are cold, they will lie on the floor with their legs tucked under their body to reduce floor contact and the whole group of pigs will huddle together (**Figures 10.55–10.58**). The group will often lie close to a wall, unless the wall is cold and wet. The pigs may shiver and, over a short

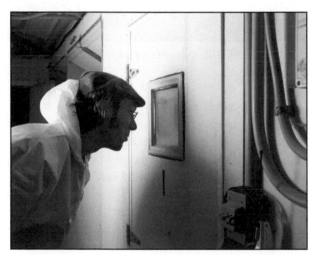

Fig. 10.54 Examining the pigs prior to entering the room.

time, may become hairy. Larger pigs seem unable to adopt this tucked position for very long and tend to lie semi-recumbent with their legs tucked into their body. The pig is trying to conserve heat.

It is also normal for pigs to sleep together so it is important to differentiate between cold pigs huddling and normal pigs sleeping in a pile.

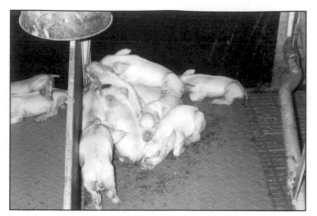

Fig. 10.55 Cold piglets. Note the legs tucked under the body and chest held off the floor.

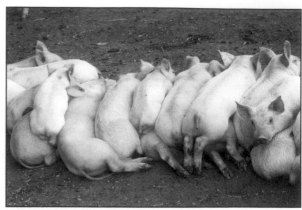

Fig. 10.56 Chilled weaners.

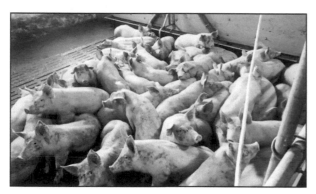

Fig. 10.57 Chilled growing pigs in a new building that is wet.

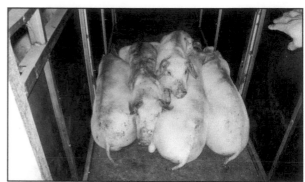

Fig. 10.58 Chilled and cold pigs in a hospital house that is not conducive to recovery.

If the pig is comfortable

Within a group of pigs there will be a selection of lying patterns (**Figures 10.59, 10.60**). The main group of pigs will sleep together in a pile; however, other pigs will be lying spread out but with maximum contact with the floor. These separated pigs will be the more dominant pigs. The lower order pigs will lie on the edge of the main group. Pigs sleep with their legs stretched out from the body.

If the pig is too hot

If the pigs are too hot they will generally be dirty and covered in faeces or soil. Individual pigs will lie away from other pigs, if possible, sometimes against a cold wall (**Figure 10.61**). The pigs will not pile. The pigs will lie in any water or cooler area, ideally a wallow. As the pigs get hotter they will start to dig into the earth, especially in bedded floors. This can cause considerable damage to the building. Hot pigs will choose to wallow in faeces and slurry to assist cooling. Sometimes this is unavoidable but its occurrence should be minimised. Once pigs become 'dirty' they can be extremely difficult to retrain, even when provided with an ideal environment (**Figure 10.62**).

Watch the pig's breathing; a hot pig will pant to loose heat through the mouth. Panting is breathing above 40 breaths per minute. If pigs continue to be too hot, they will start to die.

Chronic air patterns

Pigs are inherently clean animals and generally avoid lying in faeces. From a few days of age pigs will become toilet trained to defecate in a specific area. The defecation pattern of the pen provides a good long-term indicator of thermal comfort. The farm team can see the defecation area even after the pigs have left the building. Abnormal defecation patterns indicate a chronic reduction in optimal environment.

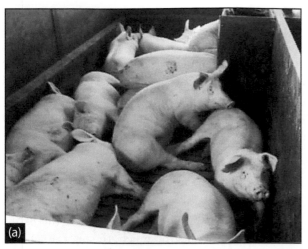
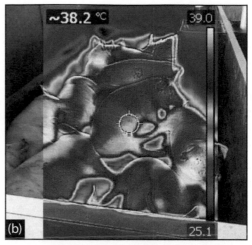

Fig. 10.59 Comfortable finishing pigs sleeping well (a) with the infrared image on the right (b). The temperature at the left top indicates the temperature at the indicator circle (an explanation of infrared images can be found at the end of this chapter).

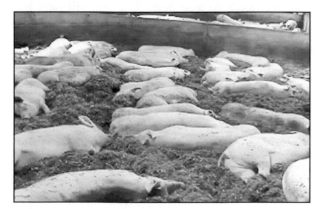

Fig. 10.60 Comfortable sows.

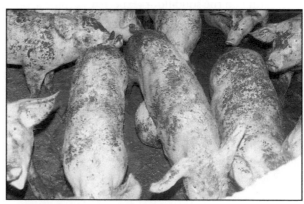

Fig. 10.61 Hot finishing pigs. Note that they are very dirty.

Fig. 10.62 The environment must be suitable for the intended pigs. The farrowing heat mat illustrated is too hot at 50°C. The piglets will not sleep on the heat mat and will choose to sleep by their mother, increasing their chance of being overlaid.

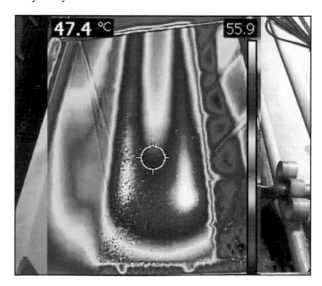

Monitor the defecation pattern (photograph or drawing) at the end of each batch.

The pig's defecation area (toilet) should be where these characteristics are present:

- The pen is coolest.
- The pen has a draught – the pigs will defecate under the cold dropping air.
- The pen is wettest.
- The pen is darkest.
- The pen is most private.

The other side of the defecation area is the sleeping area, which would normally not include any other features of the toilet. Do the defecation and sleeping patterns match the expected pig behaviour or are the pigs defecating and sleeping in the wrong place? For example, pigs sleeping on slats (expected toilet area) but defecating on the solid floor (expected sleeping area).

Thermal control: heat loss and conservation in a pig

Understanding how pigs gain and lose heat is an important consideration in designing pig barns. Pigs lose heat by four natural methods (**Figure 10.63**):

1 Conduction to the floor.
2 Convection to the air.
3 Radiation to other surfaces.
4 Latent heat (or moisture) mainly by respiration.

Thermal neutral zone

The thermal neutral zone is the external temperature zone where the pig is able to control its internal body temperature with minimal effort and expenditure of energy. Within the thermal neutral zone the pig is able to move its body position and/or control its blood flow to the periphery to maintain its internal body temperature. If the external temperature is below the thermal neutral zone (lower critical temperature [LCT]) the pig needs to use energy (food) to maintain its internal body temperature, thus the food conversion efficiency is poorer and the cost of production goes up. If the external temperature falls too much, the pig is unable to maintain its internal body temperature, resulting in hypothermia.

If the external temperature is above the thermal neutral zone (upper critical temperature [UCT]), the pig needs to lose heat. The pig will pant and attempt evaporative cooling. Pigs do not have the ability to sweat and lose heat. The pig will reduce its feed intake to reduce its metabolic heat production. This will then reduce growth rate and increase time to slaughter, thus increasing costs.

It is important to keep the pig within its thermal neutral zone. Unfortunately, the zone is not fixed and varies with age and the environment of the pig (*Table 10.6*). As the pig becomes bigger the zone becomes wider and the pig becomes more thermal tolerant.

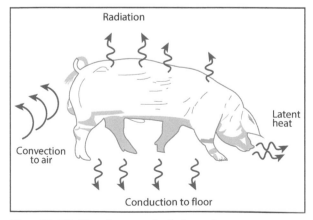

Fig. 10.63 Heat loss methods in a pig.

Table 10.6 **Guide to the thermal neutral zone.**

PIG WEIGHT (kg)	LCT (°C)	UCT (°C)
Gestating sows	10	21
Lactating sows	16	20
Piglets	30	34
4-week-old piglet	25	30
Weaned	24	34
20 kg	20	28
40 kg	16	26
100 kg	14	20

Temperature requirements of pigs

Using the thermal neutral zone information, a guide to the temperature requirements of pigs is shown in *Table 10.7*.

Table 10.7 **Guide to room temperature requirements of the pig.**

TYPE OF PIG	WEIGHT RANGE (kg)	DEGREES C		
		SAFE TEMP.		+/−
		IN	OUT	MAX
Suckling piglet	1–7	30	30	0
1st stage nursery	7–15	30	24	1
2nd stage nursery	15–25	24	21	1.5
Growing	25–50	18	20	2
Finishing	50–110	14	18	2.5
Lactating sows	180–250	16	20	1
Individual adults	180–250	14	18	2.5
Group housed	180–250	12	18	2.5

Table 10.8 **Review of factors that can influence thermal neutral zone.**

	DEGREE C CHANGE
Management that allows a reduced ambient temperature	
Straw bedding	4
Deep straw	6
Lids over pens	2
Management that increases the LCT	
Slight draught (>0.2 m/s)	5
Draught (>0.4 m/s)	10
Very cold and draughty	15
Pig housed on its own	8
Wet floor	4
Wet bedding	4
Fully slatted floor	2
Showers	4
Poor lying area	8
Restrict feeding	4

Factors that can affect the thermal neutral zone

A variety of management and environmental factors can influence the LCT and UCT (*Table 10.8*). Management can adjust these factors, making the pig more comfortable.

Daily liveweight gain decreases by 10 g/day/°C above UCT.

Using lower critical temperature and upper critical temperature in real time

The impact of LCT and the influence of management can be used in real time by the clinician to provide advice to the farm (**Figure 10.64**).

Take a pen of pigs with an average weight of 40 kg, housed on straw with a kennelled (enclosed) area. The pigs are restrict-fed. There is a small draught and there are only a few pigs in the pen because there were insufficient sows bred in the batch. Therefore, these pigs need a minimum temperature of 19°C to stay above their LCT.

Note: Even if providing a minimum temperature of 19°C for the group, the small pigs could still be chilled.

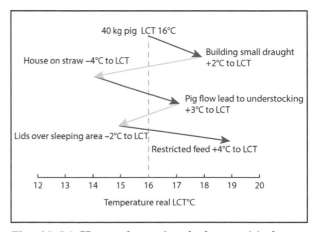

Fig. 10.64 How to determine the lower critical temperature in real time.

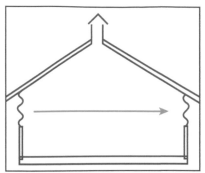

Fig. 10.65 Wind effect across building – cross flow.

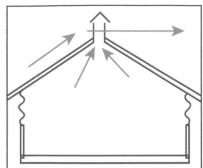

Fig. 10.66 Ridge effect creating a negative pressure.

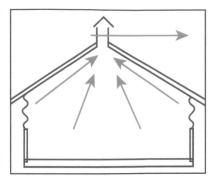

Fig. 10.67 Chimney effect creating a negative pressure in the house.

Basic design of pig ventilation systems

Over time many different building designs have been used to house pigs. Pig buildings can be broken down into the broad categories of natural or forced ventilation.

In addition to the building type, the farm team must be aware of the climate zone the building is situated in and realise that the climate zone may vary with the seasons. Thus, farms in mid-continental areas need to cope with dry and very cold winters and very hot and humid summers. If building designs that work well in one climate zone are used to house pigs in anther climate zone, the results could be a disaster.

Natural ventilation

Natural ventilation is controlled by curtain opening, wind direction, ridge (length of the building) and the chimney (local may be multiple) effect (**Figures 10.65–10.67**).

Mechanical ventilation systems

There are two primary mechanical ventilation systems: those that involve fans that pull air out of the building (negative-pressure building) and those that involve fans that push air into the building (positive-pressure building). Fans that merely recirculate air have no effect on the pressure in the building and so have no effect on air change.

To monitor the effect in the mechanically ventilated building a manometer is required to measure the pressure in the building (**Figure 10.68**). One simple way of examining the pressure is to observe the door. On entry to the room does the door close behind you because of the positive pressure in the building?

Reviewing the ventilation systems

The veterinarian is generally not a ventilation specialist. However, a basic review of the air flow pattern can be visualised using smoke. This can be very rewarding and produce great conversation concerning the ventilation system with the whole farm team.

Example of environmental impacts on a building ventilation system.

The effect of wind direction on naturally ventilated buildings can be useful to illustrate how the air patterns within a house can rapidly change. The illustrations below (**Figures 10.69–10.71**) demonstrate how even one factor can have a profound impact on the health of the pigs in individual pens. The air patterns expected in cross-flow ventilated houses with different wind directions are shown. The red areas indicate zones where the air quality will be seriously compromised.

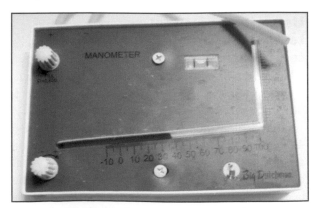

Fig. 10.68 Check the ventilation system by measuring the pressure in the system.

Fig. 10.69
Naturally ventilated building when the wind strikes 90 degrees to the curtains/openings – all pens equally ventilated.

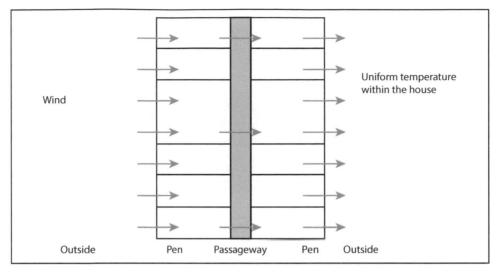

Uniform temperature within the house

Wind

Outside   Pen   Passageway   Pen   Outside

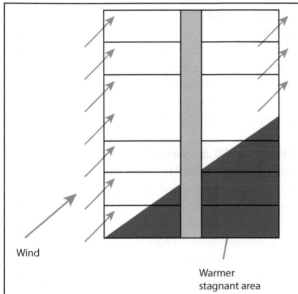

Wind

Warmer
stagnant area

Fig. 10.70 Naturally ventilated building when the wind strikes 45 degrees to the curtain. A diagonal or poor underventilated area exists in the house.

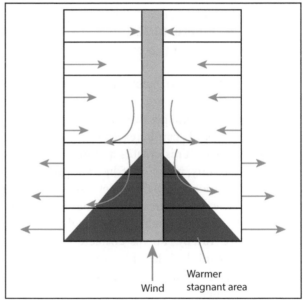

Wind   Warmer
stagnant area

Fig. 10.71 Naturally ventilated building when the wind strikes 0 degrees to the curtain. A triangle of underventilated area exists in the house.

Visualising air patterns using smoke ▶ VIDEO 45

The big issue with examination of the ventilation system is time. The clinician needs to realise that the results obtained are only valid during the time of the examination; the time of day, wind speed, external temperature, number of pigs and weight of the pigs in the room. A change in any of these, and other, features will change the ventilation system's capacity and the physical characteristics of air, heat and humidity movements. However, examination of the air flow pattern can still be very revealing.

Smoke can be used to visualise ideal air flow, excess or insufficient air flow, and may help to explain unexpected disturbance of the air flow.

Ideal ventilation

When the ventilation is ideal, the air will have a rotation pattern with the following properties: good mixing of the air, warming of the cold incoming air,

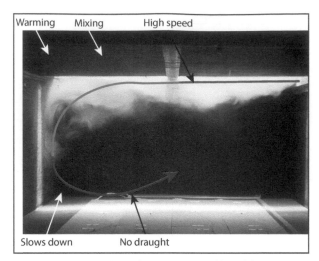

Warming   Mixing   High speed

Slows down   No draught

Fig. 10.72 Good air flow into a small building.

Table 10.9 **Suggested ventilation rates and air speed for pigs.**

PIG WEIGHT (kg)	VENTILATION RATE (L/s)	MAXIMUM AIR SPEED SUMMER (m/s)	OTHER (m/s)
25	1.5–17	0.25	0.25
30	1.8–20	0.30	0.25
40	2.0–25	0.36	0.25
60	2.2–30	0.41	0.25
80	2.5–35	0.46	0.25
100	3.0–40	0.51	0.28
115	3.5–45	0.61	0.30

reduction in speed and no draught, together with air exchange (**Figure 10.72**). Suggested ventilation rates and air speed for pigs are shown in *Table 10.9*.

The ventilation can be excessive – excessive operating pressures

If the operating static pressure is too high, the animal level air speeds can be excessive, especially for younger animals. This creates a draught as the air has no time to mix, warm or reduce its speed.

The ventilation can be too slow so air does not possess sufficient speed to allow mixing. The cold air (heavy) falls rapidly, resulting in draughts near the inlet (**Figure 10.73**). This is characterised by condensation around the inlet. The poor mixing results in poor air quality and the defecation pattern moves towards the inlet.

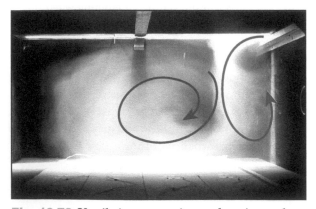

Fig. 10.73 Ventilation pattern in very low air speed: fresh air falls rapidly from the ceiling, causing a draught.

Unexpected air pattern due to an obstruction

Obstructions can interfere with air flows. Air patterns will move in one direction until they hit an obstruction, when they will change direction. If air hits a light or a beam, it will change direction and then may drop down onto the backs of the pigs, resulting in a stressful chilling draught (**Figure 10.74**).

Infrared to assess the temperature resources within a room

An infrared camera can be another resource for the veterinarian to help visualise the temperature sources within a room and to ensure that these sources are working adequately (**Figure 10.75**). Remember that the infrared temperature is different from the air temperature. When looking at a heater, the infrared camera gives a number that is generally warmer that the ambient air temperature, but conversely, when examining a pig, it will be colder than the body core temperature.

Temperature sources can be divided into three components:

1 Heat input – heat lamp, for example.
2 Cold sink – slatted floor, for example.
3 The pigs.

The feature that this often undervalues are the pigs themselves. Ventilation systems only work when healthy pigs of the correct size are in the room, thus providing a heat source. You cannot assess

Fig. 10.74 Air pattern after hitting a beam. The air pattern is indicated by the red arrows.

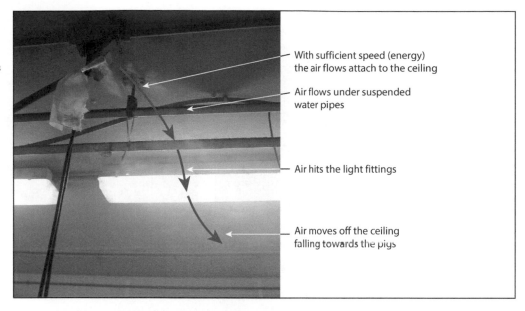

With sufficient speed (energy) the air flows attach to the ceiling

Air flows under suspended water pipes

Air hits the light fittings

Air moves off the ceiling falling towards the pigs

Fig. 10.75 The various heat sources within a nursery (a) are revealed by an infrared camera (b).

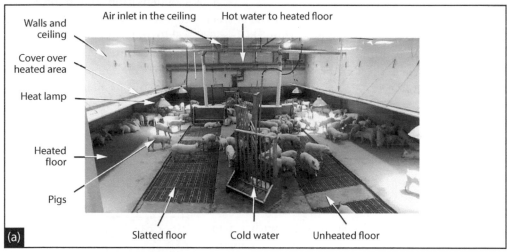

Walls and ceiling

Air inlet in the ceiling

Hot water to heated floor

Cover over heated area

Heat lamp

Heated floor

Pigs

Slatted floor

Cold water

Unheated floor

(a)

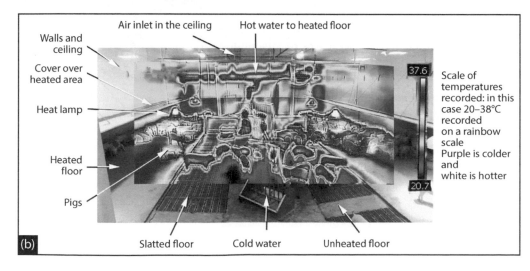

Walls and ceiling

Air inlet in the ceiling

Hot water to heated floor

Cover over heated area

Heat lamp

Heated floor

Pigs

Slatted floor

Cold water

Unheated floor

37.6

Scale of temperatures recorded: in this case 20–38°C recorded on a rainbow scale Purple is colder and white is hotter

20.7

(b)

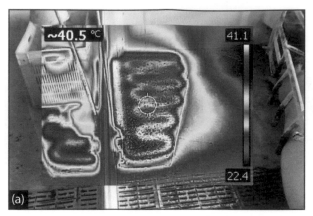
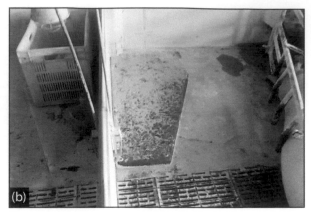

Fig. 10.76 An infrared picture of the farrowing house piglet heat mat illustrating the electric warming coils (a). Note the farm is practicing split suckling (see Chapter 8).

accurately the ventilation performance of an empty cold building.

The infrared camera can also reveal the correct workings of the heat resources within the room (**Figure 10.76**). A prime example is within the farrowing house where there are two clear environmental requirements:

1 The piglet – requiring an air temperature of about 30°C.
2 The sow – requiring an air temperature of about 18°C.

Humidity

Pigs, like humans, are able to cope with a wide range of humidity without ill effects. Normally, if the humidity is between 50 and 75% there will be few impacts on pig health. Low humidity (less than 50%) results in a reduced size of suspended particles and, therefore, more particles enter the lungs and these can carry pathogenic agents. Dry air may cause injury to the mucociliary apparatus. Relative humidity over 75% results in a damp environment, which may overwhelm the respiratory defenses. Only at 100% humidity is the air actually 'cleaned' by the large droplets falling out of the air (e.g. sweat box systems, which are illegal).

Condensation

Condensation and poor insulation will often go together. Water droplets will form where there are cold patches associated with poor insulation on a ceiling (**Figure 10.77**). These water droplets may become big enough to fall from the ceiling, wetting the pigs below. Condensation will also lead to increased ageing of the building through rust. Condensation may also raise the room's humidity levels above 75%, which can compromise pig health.

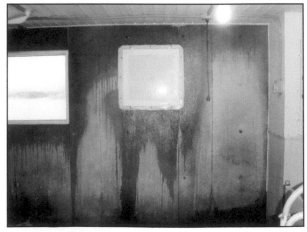

Fig. 10.77 Condenstation on the walls indicating areas of poor insulation.

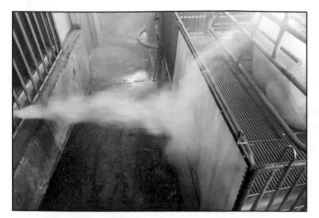

Fig. 10.78 Draughts from an evaporative inlet directed away from piglets using a simple screen to redirect the air flow pattern.

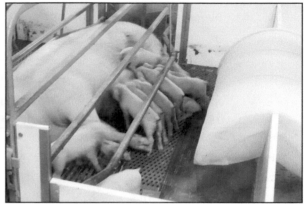

Fig. 10.79 Piglets in the farrowing house can be protected from chilling down draughts by mobile covers.

Draughts

A chilling draught is possibly the number one environmental factor that affects the pig's ability to fight disease (**Figures 10.78–10.80**). Chilling draughts are a serious stress factor affecting the animal's ability to sleep properly. It is vital that producers provide pigs with zones and, in particular, a draught-free sleeping area. A draught can be defined as any air movement in the sleeping area in excess of 0.2 m/sec. Make two chalk marks, 1 m apart (one stride), and measure whether smoke takes 5 sec or less to cross between the two marks. If it does, then the air is moving at more than 0.2 m/sec and so constitutes a draught. Holes in curtains or walls can result in unexpected draughts.

Draughts can be revealed using smoke sticks and an accurate anemometer for low wind speed evaluation.

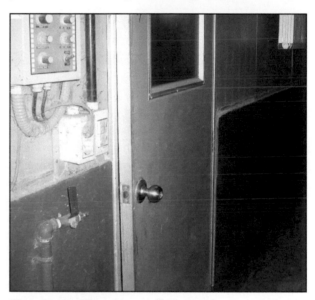

Fig. 10.80 Draughts can be caused by doors being left open.

Fan maintenance

Most farms have very poor fan maintenance programmes and a dirty fan can be 40% less efficient than a clean fan (**Figure 10.81**). This results in poor air quality and variable air patterns throughout the building. It also costs more money to run a dirty fan. A typical reduction of 25% on the electricity bill can be obtained simply by cleaning and painting the fans.

A tachometer is used to measure the speed of the fan. Note that fans can be dangerous and must be examined with caution.

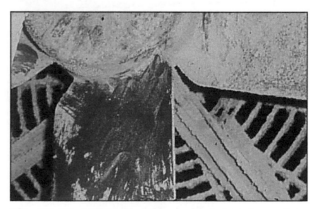

Fig. 10.81 A dirty fan with one blade starting to be cleaned.

Table 10.10 **Suggested air exchanges in different pig houses.**

| | | | | NO TUNNEL | | TUNNEL ONLY | | TUNNEL AND EVAPORATIVE | |
| | | | | | | HOT | | | |
	WEIGHT (kg)	COLD (m³/hr/pig)	MILD (m³/hr/pig)	(m³/hr/pig)	AIR CHANGE (sec)	VELOCITY (m/s)	AIR CHANGE (sec)	VELOCITY (m/s)	AIR CHANGE (sec)
Farrowing	181	34	136	1,100	30–40*			1	
Nursery	4–7	3–9	25	65	40–50			0.5	
Grow/finish	27–100	9–17	60–85	200	30–40	1.5–2.0	30–40	1.5–2.0	30–40
Wean/finish	4–100	3–17	60–85	200	30–40	1.5–2.0	30–40	1.5–2.0	30–40
Gestation	147	20	85	255	30–35	1.5–3.0	30–35	1.5–3.0	30–35
Boar	200	24	85	510	30–35	1.5–3.0	30–35	1.5–3.0	30–35

* Farrowing with evaporative cooling using 45 sec air change.

Suggested air exchanges for different pig houses are shown in *Table 10.10*.

Inlets
Curtains
Used properly, curtains can provide good air patterns through cross-flow ventilation. However, it is important to ensure the curtains do not result in draughts. Regularly raise the curtain completely to remove any mice nests. Mice can eat through the curtain, resulting in a hole allowing a draught onto the pigs (**Figure 10.82**). Curtain band settings need to be checked so that the curtain is not always moving when trying to correct the temperature. A 2°C band setting is normal.

In the summer, curtains can contain water pools that promote mosquito breeding and may lead to a biosecurity risk to the pigs inside the building (**Figure 10.83**).

Mechanical inlets
The inlet should be centrally controlled and slaved to the outlet, but this is usually not the case. Inlets are often too open and the lower air speed reduces the mixing of cold and warm air in the house. However, the most common mistakes that the clinician can identify are inlets that are:

- Broken (**Figure 10.84**).
- Different from other inlets.

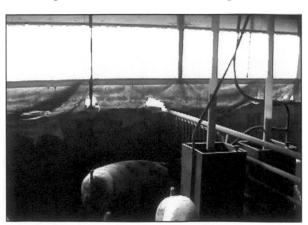

Fig. 10.82 Holes in the curtain, which were resulting in draughts in the winter months.

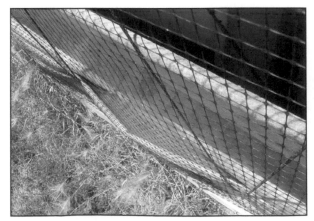

Fig. 10.83 Pooling of water in curtains can be a serious mosquito breeding area.

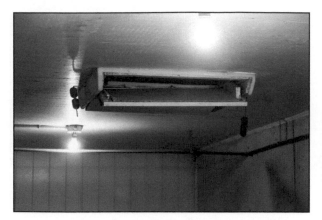

Fig. 10.84 Inlet broken, allowing air to fall off the inlet onto the pigs.

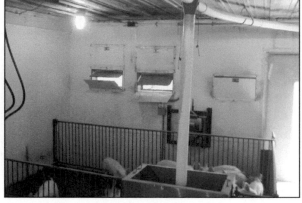

Fig. 10.85 Inlet miss-set. The right one is causing a draught into the building.

- Miss-set, which often occurs during the cleaning process (**Figure 10.85**).
- Missing.
- Open.

When there appears to be a problem with an inlet, note and discuss this with the farm team.

Evaporative cool cells

Many farms will utilise evaporative cool cells to reduce room temperature. Warm air is pulled through a cool wet surface and the evaporative cooling of the air reduces air temperature by about 5°C from the outside temperature.

The clinician needs to ensure that the evaporative cool cell is working optimally. This can be gauged by observing the moisture patterns (c.g. are there wet and dry areas on the cool cell?). Reasons for evaporative cool cell failure include poor maintenance with blocked water nozzles (**Figure 10.86**). Air may also bypass evaporative cool cells because of poor sealing (**Figure 10.87**).

Non-controlled inlets and outlets

In some naturally ventilated buildings the inlet and the outlet may be the same structure and act as an inlet or outlet depending on weather conditions; for example, buildings that utilise Yorkshire

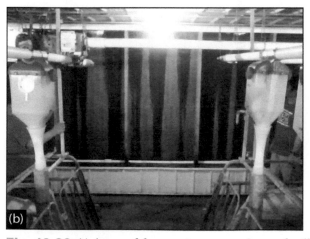

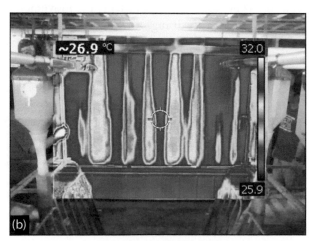

Fig. 10.86 (a) Areas of dryness in evaporative cool cells are areas where the water is not running. The external air then passes uncooled into the building. (b) This is demonstrated by the infrared camera picture.

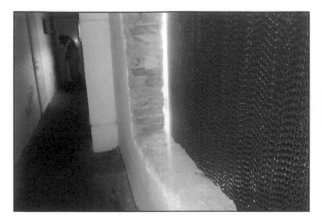

Fig. 10.87 Poor sealing around the evaporative cool cell.

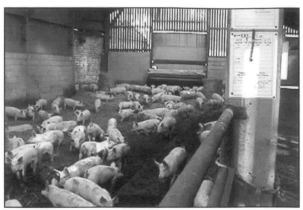

Fig. 10.88 Pigs in a yard with temperature control through Yorkshire boarding and straw bedding.

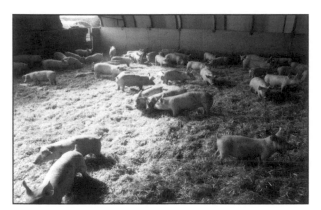

Fig. 10.89 A hoop structure utilising straw bedding.

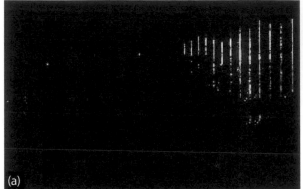

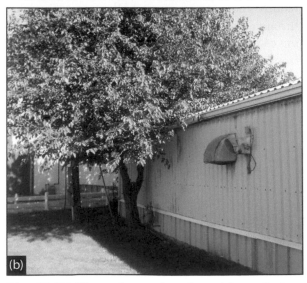

boarding, or other netting, to reduce the air speed (**Figure 10.88**). Being non-controlled it can be very difficult to control air movements and thus prevent draughts. This lack of control results in an increased LCT; however, this can be compensated for by the use of bedding (**Figure 10.89**).

Physical blockage of the ventilation system

Vegetation growing up the edge of buildings poses a serious vermin risk as it provides rodents with protection prior to entering the buildings (**Figure 10.90**). On many farms, vegetation even enters the ventilation system, disturbing the inlet or outlet. Rubbish/old equipment being discarded along the side of buildings can pose a similar risk and increases the risk of rodent infestation.

Fig. 10.90 Vegetation can interfere with ventilation systems. (a) This Yorkshire boarding ventilation system was completed blocked by ivy and the pigs had severe pneumonia. (b) Trees around buildings can interfere with the ventilation systems.

Trees surrounding the buildings can progressively affect the air patterns around and into buildings.

Insulation

Many pigs living in old buildings suffer severe temperature variations associated with insufficient or damaged insulation panels. Insulation is important both to maintain the temperature in the winter and keep the building cool in the summer. The major problem with insulation is that it can be destroyed by rodents.

An infrared camera can be useful to illustrate areas where insulation is inadequate. This may indicate areas of rodent infestation or where contractors failed to install adequate insulation when constructing the building (**Figure 10.91**).

Cooling

In many parts of the world cooling is more important than heating (**Figures 10.92–10.97**).

In outdoor systems, pigs should be provided with a wallow to allow them to utilise evaporative cooling (**Figure 10.98**).

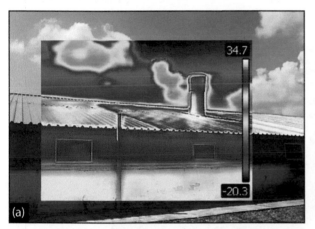
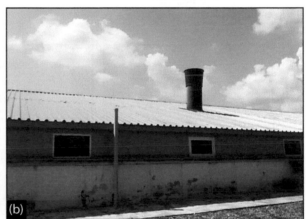

Fig. 10.91 (a) Infrared image of the roof of a building revealing a significant difference in heat over the roof where the insulation was missed during construction. (b) On close examination this area can be seen as a premature rusting of the roof metal panels in the visible light picture.

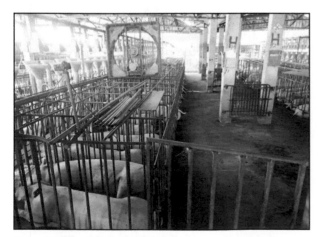

Fig. 10.92 Cooling the whole room. Cooling fans re-circulating air in a breeding area.

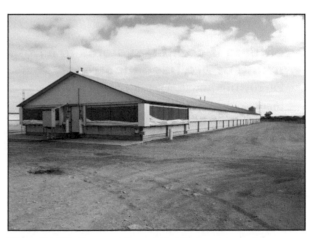

Fig. 10.93 Evaporative cool cells in a tunnel ventilated building.

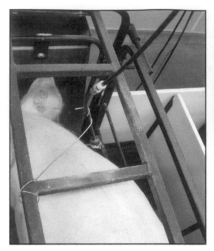

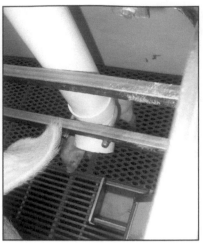

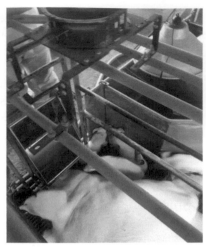

Fig. 10.94 Cooling the sow directly. Drip cooling in lactating sows.

Fig. 10.95 Snout cooler.

Fig. 10.96 Fan coolers above the sow's head.

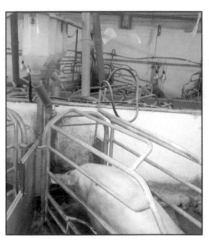

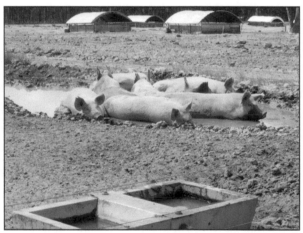

Fig. 10.97 Directed air to cool the sow.

Fig. 10.98 Wallows used in outdoor pig production.

Problems if cooling systems are not working or are used incorrectly

- **Farrowing house**. Wet farrowing pen floors increase diarrhoea problems in piglets. Sows may slip on damp floors.
- **Boar/gestation**. Floors may become slippery if pigs remain wet. At breeding, animals can be injured if they slip on the wet floor. Sows can over cool, chill and abort.
- **Grow/finish**. Wet pigs may be over cooled and, particularly with high ventilation rates, this may lead to increased stress and disease risk as well as reducing growth.

- **Spray not directed properly**. If spray-cooling system sprays into the feeders, this can result in bridging that blocks feeders. If they spray onto the walls it can damage insulation. If the spray/drip cooler drips into the ear, it can lead to mental behavioural problems in stalled sows being cooled.
- **Spray system not working, not being maintained**. The animals supposed to be cooled will be too hot. It is common in farrowing areas for drip cooling systems to be poorly maintained and the outcome is poor feed intakes. The consequences of poor nutrient intakes during

lactation include increased wean-to-service intervals (reduction in farrowing rate and litter size) and reduced pig weaning weights (increased days to market and reduced finishing rate, and more pigs die).

- **Water storage tank**. Note warm/hot water does not provide adequate cooling so ensure main storage tanks are properly placed and not subjected to direct sunlight.
- **Humidity**. High humidity can interfere with evaporative cooling.

Gases

Ammonia has an effect by increasing mucus viscosity and so slowing the mucociliary escalator. This reduces the pig's ability to clear its airways. The effect of ammonia on lacrimal flow in humans is shown in *Table 10.11*. The management of the slurry system can have significant impact on the gases in the room. Many ventilation systems fail by allowing air to move from the slurry pit back into the room;

remember that the pig's nose is closer to the floor than the stockpersons.

Target air–gas concentrations are shown in *Table 10.12*.

Veterinarians do not need expensive detectors for ammonia concentration. With practice and observation, an educated guess as to the ammonia concentration can be made.

Diurnal carbon dioxide variations are shown in **Figure 10.99**.

Where do these gases come from?

- Body excretions: ammonia.
- Respiration: carbon dioxide.
- Slurry system: ammonia, hydrogen sulphide, carbon dioxide, methane.
- Heating systems: carbon monoxide, carbon dioxide.

Dust

Dust in a pig house is made up of 30% feed powder, 30% skin dander and 40% faecal dust. Air should contain less than 10 mg/m^3 of inhaled dust.

There are three aspects to dust. The majority of dust falls in the particle size greater than 3.6 μm. Assuming the respiratory tract is not damaged, these particles are removed before entering the alveoli. Particles less than 1.6 μm will not settle in the alveoli and will move in and out of the respiratory tract. Only particles between 3 and 1.6 μm will enter and settle in the lung alveolar tissues. This is important

Table 10.11 Effect of ammonia on lacrimal flow in humans.

CONCENTRATION NH$_3$	TYPICAL HUMAN EFFECTS
Below 5 ppm	No effect
5–10 ppm	Detect its smell
10–15 ppm	Causes mild eye irritation
Above 15 ppm	Causes eye irritation and tear flow

Table 10.12 Target air gas concentrations.

GAS	CHEMICAL FORMULA	COSHH LONG-TERM LIMIT (ppm) (8 hours)	COSHH SHORT-TERM LIMIT (ppm) (10 min)	EFFECTS OF HIGH EXPOSURE
Ammonia	NH$_3$	25	35	200 ppm sneezing, salivation and appetite loss; 30 ppm some respiratory signs, reduces mucociliary escalator speed
Carbon monoxide	CO	50	300	Abortion in pregnant sows
Carbon dioxide	CO$_2$	5,000	15,000	Aim to keep the building under 1,500 ppm; 100,000 ppm narcotic used in slaughterhouses
Hydrogen sulphide	H$_2$S	10	15	20 ppm appetite low, fear of light and nervousness; sudden exposure to 400 ppm is lethal. Low concentrations smell of rotten eggs; high concentration no smell

COSHH, Control of Substances Hazardous to Health.

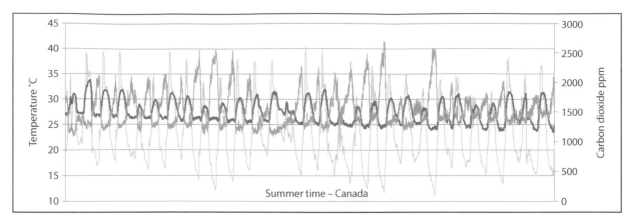

Fig. 10.99 Diurnal carbon dioxide variations. The carbon dioxide is illustrated in blue. The temperature in the finishing house is illustrated in red with the outside temperature in green. Note: CO_2 concentration is highest at night. Normal CO_2 concentrations are 400 ppm (2016) (and rising about 2 ppm/year). Note that the poor ventilation never reduced the CO_2 concentration to less than 1,000 ppm (about 2.5× outside) and during the night the CO_2 was often above 2,000 ppm. It is generally recommended not to have concentrations above 1,500 ppm. The room ventilation system, however, was able to stablise the outside temperature but it was still very hot for finishing pigs.

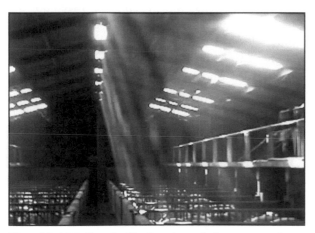

Fig. 10.100 Respirable dust in a pig house seen in the shafts of sunlight.

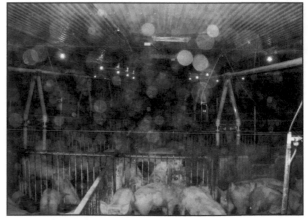

Fig. 10.101 Dust can be recognised in photographs as the dust particles reflect the flash light.

as it means viruses require a 'piggy back' to gain entry into the lungs (**Figures 10.100, 10.101**).

Endotoxin

When gram-negative bacteria die, their cell wall becomes a lipopolysaccharide toxin, also known as endotoxin. When this compound is released into the air it can have a significant effect on the respiratory tract, resulting in bronchial constriction and reduced lung function in any animal in the airspace, including the stockpersons.

Light

Pigs should be kept in light with an intensity of at least 40 lux for a minimum of 8 hours per day. The major area of the farm where light is required is in the gilt breeding area, where it is advisable to have a minimum of 300 lux for 16 hours on and 8 hours off to help stimulate gilts to cycle. Adequate light also facilitates accurate oestrus detection. While light is provided, the maintenance of lighting systems is generally poor and this can be a useful guide to the general level of building hygiene. One of the classic

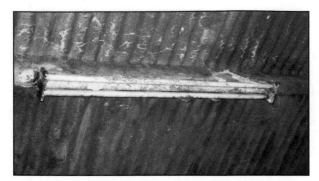

Fig. 10.102 **Poor light because of fly faeces on light fittings.** ▶ VIDEO 26

reasons for poor lighting in buildings is the build up of fly faeces on the light fittings (**Figure 10.102**). There are many light meters available for your smart phone.

Noise
National codes or legislation will vary but to comply with European Union (EU) legislation a sound limit of 85 dBA is required. This can be extremely difficult to achieve on a pig unit. Therefore, it is advisable that ear protection is used when feeding or bleeding pigs. Sound levels can be measured on a smart phone.

Ventilation maintenance programme
All farms should have a written SOP (standard operating procedure) for maintenance of the ventilation system on farm. An example is shown below.

DAILY CHECK
Observation of pigs – too hot, too cold, variable around the house
Check the room for smells – check for gases
Check the room is not too dusty
Check the area for evidence of condensation
Does the air feel too damp and heavy (over 75% or under 50% relative humidity)
Is there evidence of inadequate spray cooling
Repair leaking water supplies and dripping drinkers
Repair any other leaks (e.g. guttering)
Check the room for draughts or hot spots
Examine the creep lights – too bright, different types, pig lying patterns

Check room lights so that pigs can be seen
Ensure that the vents and fans are working as expected

WEEKLY
Clean fan blades and shutters
Check alarm systems and fail-safes
Clean heater cooling fins and filters
Check gas jets and safety shut-off valves
Check inlet baffles
Check feed coverings
Check thermostats: measure current conditions; inlet, outlet and piglet height
Check rodent control
Ensure AIAO effective in cleaning ventilation system

MONTHLY
Ensure shutters open and close freely
Check insulation panels including creep areas
Check recirculation air ducts for dust accumulation
Check curtains for rodents in the bottom of the curtains
Check that records are being used to maintain required air quality

3–6 MONTHLY
Ensure fans operate as expected
Clean fan motors and controls
Clean and repair chipped areas on fans or shutters
Check air inlets for debris, especially attic and soffits
Check fuel bills for deterioration in air quality
Check passive ventilation systems
Check for seasonal variations

Examples of poor ventilation management
Nearly all the examples are associated with poor maintenance and management of the ventilation system.

Obstructions on the outside
On many farms the air entering the building does so via the attic. However, if the air cannot access the attic, it cannot get into the room (**Figures 10.103–10.105**). It is imperative that daylight is clearly visible when you examine the entry areas. Likewise, inlets must be able to work as required.

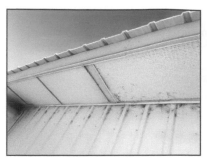

Fig. 10.103 Soffits blocked with dust and ice.

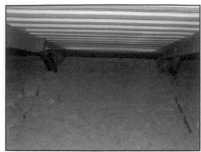

Fig. 10.104 Insulation blocking soffit.

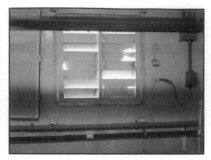

Fig. 10.105 Fan louvres broken and stuck with dirt.

Internal obstructions to air flow

Use smoke to illustrate the air movement patterns. See **Figures 10.106–10.108**.

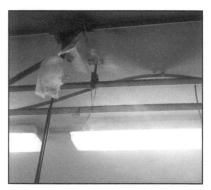

Fig. 10.106 Lights diverting air patterns. (See Figure 10.74 for air pattern arrows.)

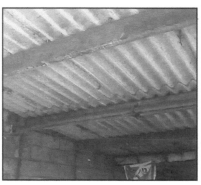

Fig. 10.107 Ceiling obstructions forcing the air off the ceiling.

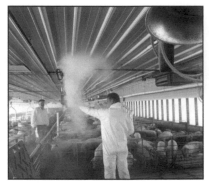

Fig. 10.108 Power board obstructing air flow.

Inadequate static pressure
See **Figures 10.109–10.111.**

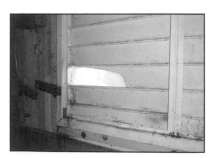

Fig. 10.109 Broken louvres.

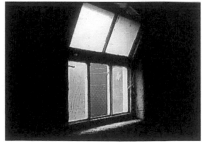

Fig. 10.110 Broken/open windows/doors.

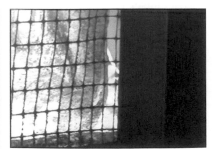

Fig. 10.111 Poor curtain maintenance.

Air has insufficient energy

See **Figures 10.112–10.114**.

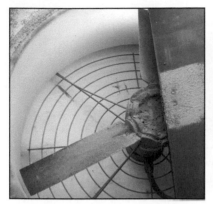

Fig. 10.112 Dirty fan blades.

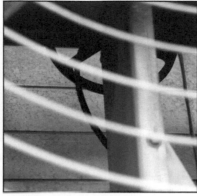

Fig. 10.113 Poor belt drive – fan off.

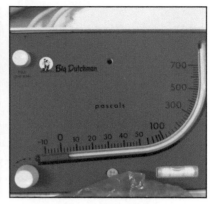

Fig. 10.114 Inadequate static pressure.

Pig behaviour

The behaviour of the pigs is the best indication that the ventilation system is working satisfactorily. Note that this requires undisturbed pigs. When you examine the pigs be quiet and ideally examine through a window. See **Figures 10.115–10.122**.

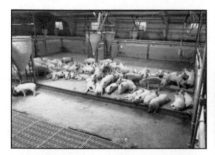

Fig. 10.115 Normal comfortable weaners. Pigs in all positions, some together as a social group and others on their side allowing heat loss to floor.

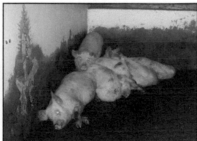

Fig. 10.116 Finishing pigs who are piling. The pigs were sleeping in a draught. Tail biting, pneumonia and colitis are common in chilled grow/finish pigs.

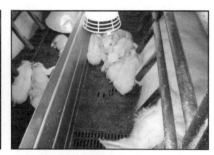

Fig. 10.117 Chilled piglets. These animals are very prone to pathogens, such as *E.coli* diarrhoea, and to overlay from their mother.

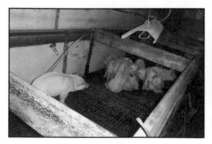

Fig. 10.118 Chilled weaners. These weaners are very prone to Glässer's disease, meningitis and diarrhoea problems.

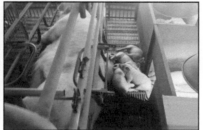

Fig. 10.119 Piglets that are too hot. The creep ambient air was at 48°C. The piglets are then forced to sleep outside their safe creep area.

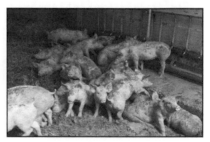

Fig. 10.120 These weaners are too hot. The animals were breathing very heavily. Pigs lose heat through evaporation.

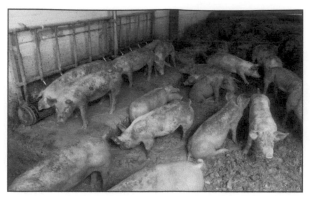

Fig. 10.121 As pigs get too hot they will start wallowing in their own manure to keep cool and thus look very dirty.

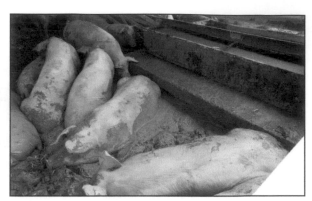

Fig. 10.122 Sows too hot. Lactating sows that are too hot are unable to milk properly.

Draughts

Draughts are the major factor in the onset of many diseases of the pig. It is essential to avoid draughts in the sleeping area. See **Figures 10.123–10.130**.

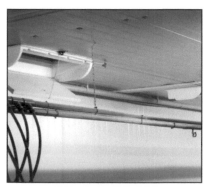

Fig. 10.123 Broken inlets leading to draughts.

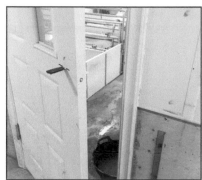

Fig. 10.124 Doors left open or do not shut properly result in draughts.

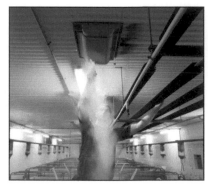

Fig. 10.125 Incorrect fitting of inlets.

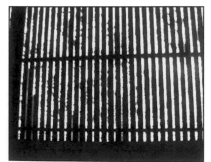

Fig. 10.126 Poor building design. This Yorkshire boarding is too wide, resulting in draughts.

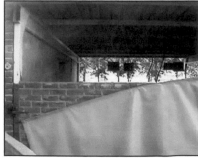

Fig. 10.127 Curtain not shutting properly.

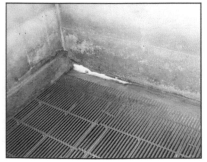

Fig. 10.128 Holes in the wall can lead to draughts.

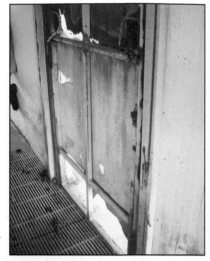

Fig. 10.129 Draught from a damaged/broken door.

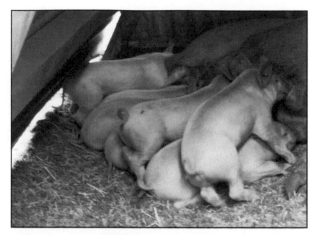

Fig. 10.130 Draughts are also common in outdoor pigs with poorly maintained arcs.

Dust particles and cooling
See **Figures 10.131, 10.132**.

Fig. 10.131 Dust. (a) Pig housing can produce a lot of dust. (b) The respirable dust is very hazardous to the health of the pigs and people.

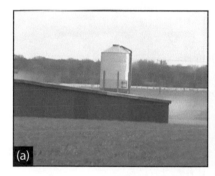

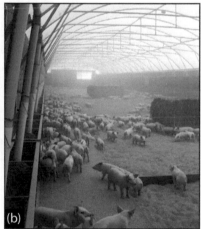

Fig. 10.132 Cooling. (a) It is essential to prevent pigs from getting too hot. If the relative humidity is low enough, they lose a lot of heat through evaporative cooling. Note that heat is lost by evaporation, not by the wetting. To be effective, sows must be allowed to dry. The spray cycle should be defined as x minutes on/y minutes off (the ventilation specialist should fill in details). (b) For outdoor pigs, provide shade.

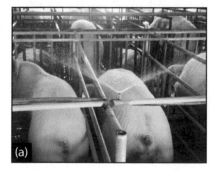

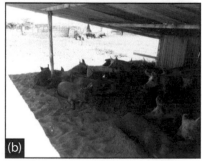

Management errors

Management errors are all too common on pig farms due to poor maintenance, failure to repair and lack of protocols (**Figures 10.133–10.150**).

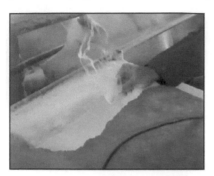

Fig. 10.133 Damaged creep lid resulting in excessive heat loss and chilling of the piglets.

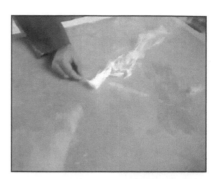

Fig. 10.134 A normal insulated creep lid with little air movement.

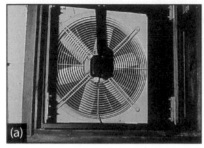

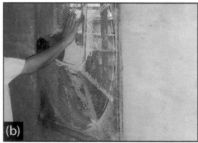

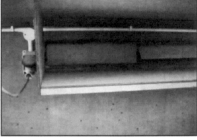

Fig. 10.135 (a, b) Fan maintenance is generally very poor with dirty fans causing poor ventilation and pneumonia. A dirty fan is 40% less efficient than a clean fan.

Fig. 10.136 Internal air vents. One is stuck shut thus reducing ventilation. The other was stuck open, resulting in draughts.

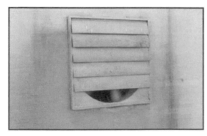

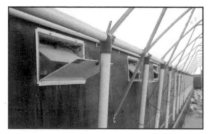

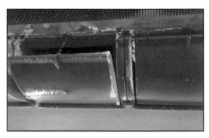

Fig. 10.137 Missing flap resulting in back pressure on the fan and reducing its efficiency.

Fig. 10.138 Inlet direction opening obstructed by feed down pipe.

Fig. 10.139 Inlets frozen closed.

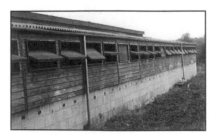

Fig. 10.140 Automatically controlled natural ventilation (ACNV) flaps, which are open variably due to damaged hydraulics. Variable ventilation patterns resulted.

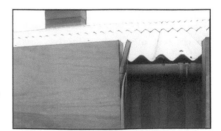

Fig. 10.141 Inlet direction cowling needing repair.

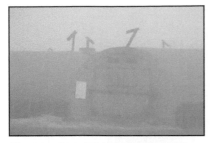

Fig. 10.142 This outside building has a wide variety of weather conditions to contend with on a daily basis (shown is a particularly foggy damp day).

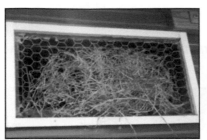

Fig. 10.143 Outlets blocked by a bird nest.

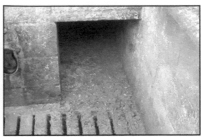

Fig. 10.144 Kennel systems require additional flaps in the winter time, and in the summer time may need removing.

Fig. 10.145 Thermostats that monitor the environment also need to be clean and in good working order.

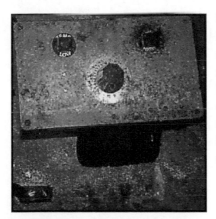

Fig. 10.146 Farm electrics are often very poorly maintained. This box became wet and shorted out a fan, resulting in severely heat stressed pigs.

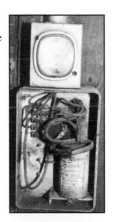

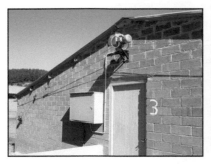

Fig. 10.147 Safety flaps and alarms have to be in good working order and regularly (weekly) checked to ensure they work.

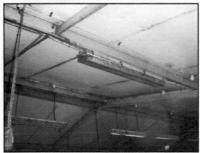

Fig. 10.148 Light is also part of the air. Light is part of the reproduction requirements (300+ lux) and is needed to see the pigs (>50 lux).

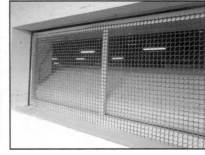

Fig. 10.149 Adequate bird proofing is required to reduce feed wastage and reduce risk of diseases (e.g. *Salmonella*).

Fig. 10.150 The siting of a building will affect the ventilation inside the building. These trees were a wind break but vortexed the air.

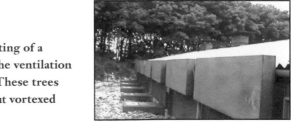

FEEDING SYSTEM MANAGEMENT

Equipment useful for monitoring feed management on the farm

See **Figures 10.151–10.155**.

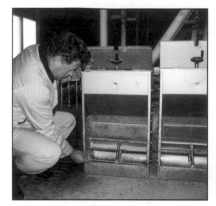

Fig. 10.151 Measure the dimensions of the feeder.

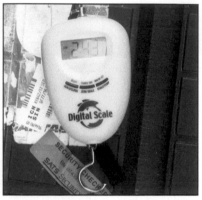

Fig. 10.152 Check weight of feed delivered against volume.

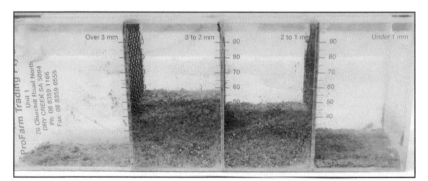

Fig. 10.153 Particle size calculator, which may also measure the amount of powdered feed.

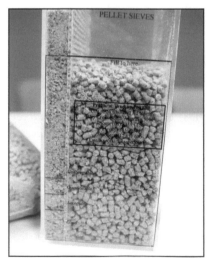

Fig. 10.154 Appearance of the feed, especially the quality of the pelleting.

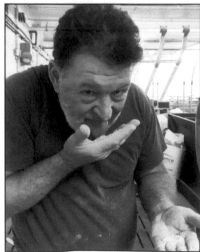

Fig. 10.155 Note the look, smell and taste of the feed.

Calculations that may be useful

Feeders and feed bins are generally based on circles. It is important, therefore, to be able to determine the volume of a feed bin (**Figure 10.156**). This can also be expressed as an equation: the area of a circle is πr^2; the volume of a cylinder is $\pi r^2 h$; the volume of a cone is $\frac{1}{3} \pi r^2 h$.

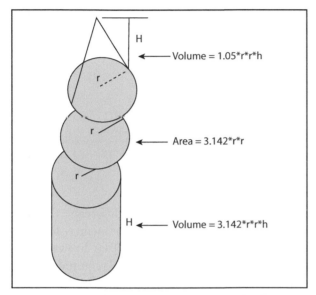

Fig. 10.156 Calculating surface, area and volume of a cylinder.

Nutritional requirements of the pig

The clinician needs to know the basic nutritional requirements of the different stages of pig growth (*Table 10.13*).

Energy

Net energy (NE) (MJ/kg feed) is recommended as the unit of dietary energy measurement. This estimates the energy actually available to the pig. The energy density requirement is high when the pig is young and decreases with age. With pigs at the end of finishing, their feed energy intakes are decreased to reduce back fat deposition.

In lactation, feed energy density is increased if feed intake is likely to be reduced (e.g. primiparous sows or during hotter times of the year). If increased dietary fat is included, it will also decrease feed intake. High energy intakes also help to reduce the wean-to-service interval.

Table 10.13 Basic nutrition requirements of the pig.

DIET	BODY WEIGHT	ENERGY NET ENERGY	PROTEIN CRUDE PROTEIN	TOTAL LYSINE	FIBRE CRUDE FIBRE
Units	kg	MJ/kg	%	%	%
1st creep	7–12	11	22	1.8	1
2nd creep	12–18	11	22	1.8	1.5
Weaner	18–30	10	21	1.4	2
Grower	30–65	9.9	19	1.3	3
Finisher	65–90	9.4	19	1	4
Finisher 2	90–120	9.2	17	0.9	3
Gilt rearer	60–130	9.4	14	0.8	5
Gestating sow		9.2	16	0.7	7
Lactating sow		10	18	1.0	4.5
Boar		9.2	14	0.7	7

Protein

Protein levels are described around the percentage of lysine, which in the pig is the first limiting amino acid. Other amino acids are described as their concentration in relationship to the lysine concentration. The dietary protein density is high in young animals and decreases with age. The lysine level reduces correspondingly. As the animal matures, protein deposition reduces.

In some countries feed additives such as ractopamine hydrochloride can be added to the final finishing ration to boost the growth potential and reduce feed conversion ratios while enhancing the protein deposition. This is particularly useful to the smaller pigs in the group.

In lactating sows, extra protein (and lysine) is required to enhance milk output and thus litter weaning weights. The dietary total lysine level for lactating sows needs to be above 1% to enhance piglet performance. During mid-gestation, feeding is designed to provide only a maintenance diet for adults.

Others

The gilt rearing diet is designed to allow the gilt to continue growing, build bone and leg strength and increase their fat reserves before farrowing, and often will have enhanced biotin, zinc, calcium and phosphorous concentrations.

There may be some ingredients that have a specific veterinary role and the clinician may request a modification of the diet to enhance health. For example:

- In the nursery the concentration of calcium may make the pig more prone to diarrhoea.
- Zinc oxide (ZnO) can be used to reduce the incidence of *Escherichia coli* diarrhoea. This use may be barred in some areas. Always check local requirements.
- Note the concentration of vitamin E may be different to maintain health versus the nutritional requirement for growth.
- Salt(s) (NaCl for example) concentration(s) may be manipulated to assist in the control of tail biting. Ensure there is plenty of water available in the pen.
- Magnesium oxide (MgO) may assist as a laxative and as a behavioural modulator.
- EDTA can be considered in control of *Brachyspira hyodysenteriae*.
- Betaine or bicarbonate may be included in the diet as they are heat sparing; very useful in lactation diets.

Feed intake and growth rate potentials of pigs

It is important to know the expected weight of pigs at each of the different stages of growth and to be able to estimate their weight. Accuracy can only be achieved through practice (**Figure 10.157**, *Table 10.14*). A graphical illustration of a growth curve for a Large White x Landrace finishing pig is shown in **Figure 10.158**.

Table 10.14 Expected liveweight and growth rates for Large White × Landrace finishing pigs.

AGE OF THE PIG		DAILY LIVEWEIGHT GAIN (g/day)	WEIGHT (kg)
WEEKS	DAYS		
4	28	215	7.0
6	42	395	12.5
8	56	630	21.3
10	70	660	30.5
12	84	715	40.5
14	98	800	51.5
16	112	965	65.0
18	126	1000	80.0
20	140	1100	95.0
22	154	1100	110.0

Different markets have different finishing weights. The Parma ham requirement is for a pig over 12 months of age and 170 kg liveweight, so different growth curves may be required for different clients. Potential breeding gilts should have their own growth curve and should not be treated as finishing pigs. Different genetics may also have genotype-specific requirements and targets. The genetic companies often produce excellent nutrition guidelines.

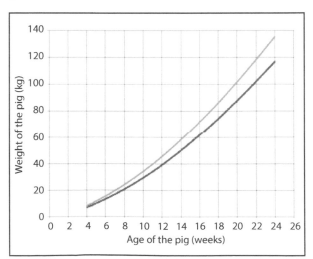

Fig. 10.158 Graph of expected growth rates in finishing pigs. The green line is optimistic growth whereas the red line is below expectations.

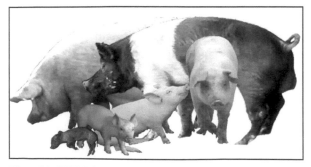

Fig. 10.157 Pigs change shape as they grow. With practice, this can provide the clinician with a useful guide to the likely weight of the pig.

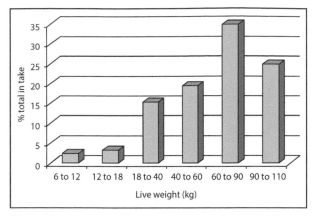

Fig. 10.159 Example of percentage of total feed usage on a farrow to finish farm. Pigs fed weaning to 110 kg liveweight.

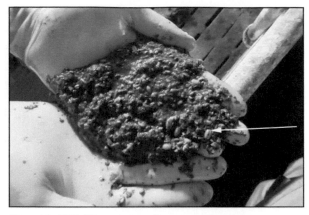

Fig. 10.160 Pigs cannot digest whole grain (arrowed), therefore grains that are not broken open are effectively wasted.

Using the right feed at the right time

It is essential that pigs progressively move to the cheaper diets as soon as possible while maximising their growth potential. Keeping pigs on expensive early diets for longer than warranted increases costs. Often, pigs are kept on expensive weaner diets too long to compensate for the poor feed intake and growth in the first week post weaning. Carry out regular feed budget audits to ensure that the farm is allowing for appropriate levels of feed intake (**Figure 10.159**).

Use correct feed

It is essential to provide a suitable diet. In times of high prices it is tempting to simplify and cheapen the feed, but growth and health could be affected. If the pigs' growth slows down, this cannot be allowed to affect pig flow and AIAO systems. Poorly formulated diets are more likely to result in diarrhoea, resulting in raw feed ingredients ending up on the floor and thus the slurry pit.

Feed preparation

Feed that is incorrectly prepared (i.e. whole grains, or poorly ground or rolled grains) are not digested by the pig and result in increased feed wastage (**Figure 10.160**).

Feed available when pigs enter a house

It is essential that pigs are fed the correct diet immediately they enter the barn. Requiring the

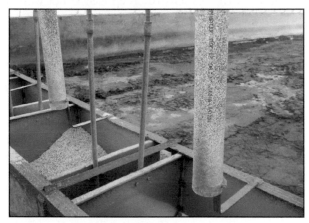

Fig. 10.161 Final finishing feed left to be eaten by the next group of 30 kg pigs.

pigs to eat up the last of the previous group's feed is not acceptable (**Figure 10.161**). Such feed may contain incorrect ingredients or medications (or lack of prescribed medications) or, if it has been left for more than a couple of days, has become spoiled with moulds or rodent/bird faeces and urine.

Feeding routines

Creep feeding in the farrowing house

If the farm practices 3-week weaning, it is unlikely that most of the pigs will consume sufficient creep feed to improve weaning weights and post-weaning feed intakes (**Figure 10.162**). With 4-week weaning, creep feeding can be beneficial. However, it must

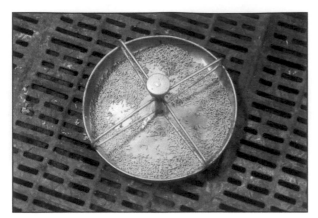

Fig. 10.162 Farrowing house creep feeder. Ensure that creep feed is not wasted.

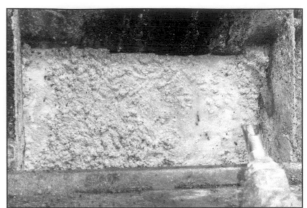

Fig. 10.163 Farrowing house feeder demonstrating poor management.

be done so that expensive creep feed is not wasted and soiled; creep feed should be fed at least three times daily (i.e. little and often).

Adult pig feeding

The feeding routines practiced in the farrowing, breeding and gestation areas can result in enormous feed wastage. In the farrowing area, attempting to get lactating sows to eat too much can result in loss of appetite. The sow then fails to clean out the feed trough, resulting in mould development and, in the worst cases, fly infestation of the feed (**Figure 10.163**). The feed problems can also impair water consumption, affecting milk supply to the piglets.

In the breeding area, when sows are in oestrus they often will not eat and this results in feed remaining in the feed troughs, souring and being wasted (**Figure 10.164**).

In gestation areas, feeding routines can be very careless, resulting in large amounts of feed being wasted on the floor. Combined with poor cleaning routines this feed becomes soiled. Overfeeding of the gestating sow is common on pig farms. This extra feed is wasted, does not benefit the growing fetuses and may reduce subsequent feed intake during lactation.

Calculations

Approximate daily feed intake wean-to-finishing: 4% of body weight; approximate daily adult gestation feed: 1% of body weight.

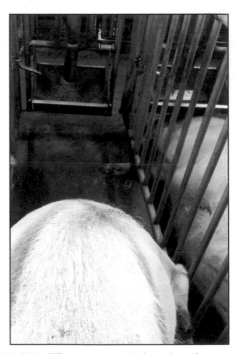

Fig. 10.164 The sow came in heat but she was still being fed.

Feeder set up VIDEO 46

Adequate feed space

To allow all the pigs to grow evenly it is essential to provide sufficient feeder space for all the pigs in the pen (*Table 10.15*). This is particularly important in the first 3 days after weaning.

Calculation

Restricted feeding space needed is 1.1 × shoulder width of the pig. Different genetics may have different

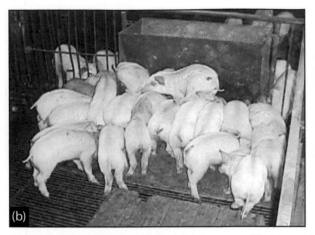

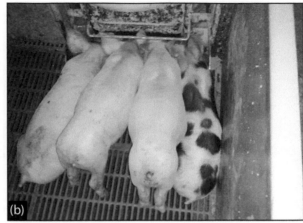

Fig. 10.165 (a, b) Insufficient feed space will change the behaviour of the pigs, resulting in fighting over feed space. ▶ VIDEO 4

Table 10.15 **Feed space availability in a trough feeder.**

WEIGHT OF PIG (kg)	TROUGH/HOPPER LENGTH (mm)/PIG	
	RESTRICTED FED	*AD-LIBITUM* FED
5	100	75
10	130	33
15	150	38
35	200	50
60	240	60
90	280	70
120	300	75
Sow	400	N/A

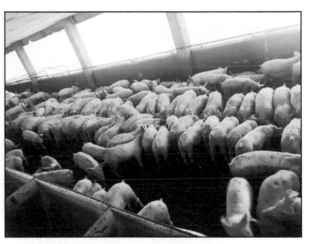

Fig. 10.166 The use of an additional narrow trough can enhance post-weaning feed intake for the first 3 days post weaning and allows for normal group behaviour to be exhibited.

shoulder widths and therefore may have different feed space requirements.

The newly weaned pig requires 3 × longer feed space than is required a week later. This is because newly weaned pigs feed as a group (restricted feeding) and do not understand the concept of *ad-libitum* feeding (**Figures 10.165, 10.166**).

Feed distribution

Ensure that the feed is distributed evenly along a feeder to minimise aggression at the feed space. This will also minimise uneven growth within a group of pigs. Do not place the feeder on a sloped floor.

Feeder in wrong position in the pen

When siting the feeder consider the ability of the pig to reach it. Feeders placed in cold corners will often become fouled with urine and faeces as the pigs use the area as a toilet. Feeders placed too close to a divider or other obstacle, a drinker for example, may have feed spaces that are inaccessible. Pigs should not have to jump up to gain access to the feeder. This is typically seen when young pigs have to cope with raised feeders.

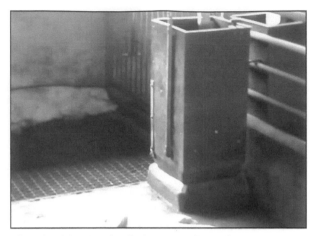

Fig. 10.167 Feeder facing away from the passageway making it difficult to visually monitor the feeder.

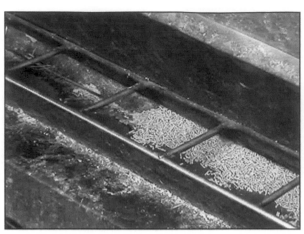

Fig. 10.168 Poor feed distribution. Ensure that the down pipe is properly placed.

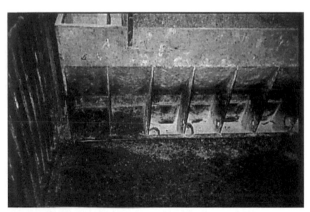

Fig. 10.169 Feeder in the wrong place in the pen and being used as a toilet area.

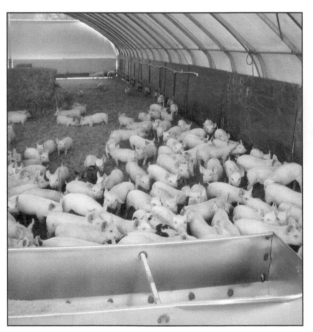

Fig. 10.170 Distance between the feeder and drinkers is too great, resulting in feed being spilt.

Feeders placed so that they cannot be easily examined

All feeders should be placed so that the stockperson can easily examine the feed pans for leakage, feed overflowing or soiling (**Figure 10.167**).

Feed and drinker position

Pigs like to drink shortly after feeding. If the drinkers are more than 2 m from the feeder, pigs will walk between the feeder and drinker and carry food in their mouths (**Figure 10.168**). This feed will be dropped (and wasted) on the floor and bedding. Ensure that the pigs do not have to cross the sleeping area to get from the feeder to the drinker (**Figures 10.169, 10.170**).

Covering feeders

Uncovered feeders contribute up to 30% of the dust in the air. The feeder is exposed to rodents and possibly birds, which can both eat the feed and soil the remaining feed. All feeders should be covered. If the stockperson needs to examine the feed level, ensure that the feeder has a see-through area where this can be assessed. (**Note:** many of the figures illustrate uncovered feeders.)

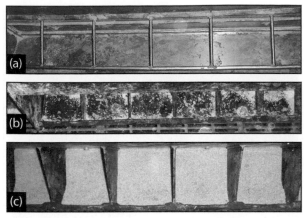

Fig. 10.171 All feeders on the farm should have information sheets clearly describing how the feeder should be running. (a) Too little feed. (b) Feeder working correctly. (c) Feeder overrunning.

Feed quantity available ▶ VIDEO 15

The adjustment of feeders should be done daily; this is one of the most important jobs for grow/finish stockpersons. It is not acceptable that feeders are allowed to overrun just to ensure pigs have 'sufficient' feed. Feed efficiency can be maximised when the pigs have to work for their feed. Placing less feed in the feeder by lowering the down pipe into the feeder pan will reduce feed wastage and the dust production, although the feed auger may need to run more often. All stockpersons should understand in detail how the feeder works and how to adjust the feed availability (**Figure 10.171**). A feeder that is overrunning will also tend to allow the feed to become powder (**Figures 10.172–10.175**). This can result in reduced feed intake, increased environmental dust and increased respiratory problems in the pigs.

It is essential to ensure that the pigs actually get to eat the feed in the desired form. It is important to realise that there are four types of feeds on the normal farm:

- The feed formulated by the nutritionist.
- The feed manufactured by the feed mill.
- The feed actually in the feeder for the pig.
- The food actually swallowed by the pig.

Unfortunately these are not always the same.

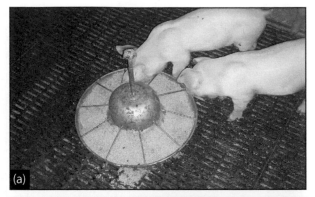

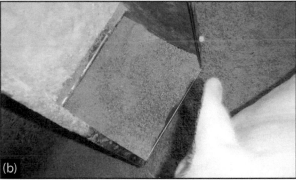

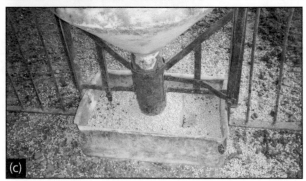

Fig. 10.172 (a–c) Three different feeder designs, all providing too much feed resulting in feed wastage.

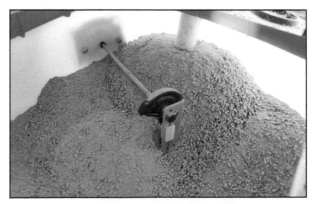

Fig. 10.173 Very powdery feed being fed.

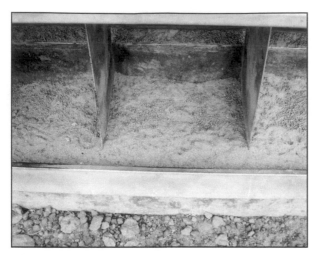

Fig. 10.174 Wasted dusty food inside feeder.

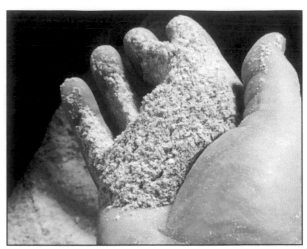

Fig. 10.175 Examination of the feed in the feeder – a lot of powder

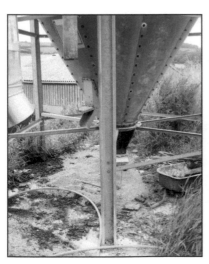

Fig. 10.176 Feed spillage under a feed bin.

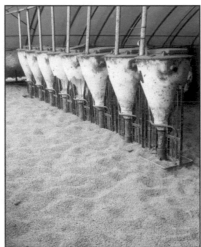

Fig. 10.177 Feed being spilt during delivery with a broken pipe.

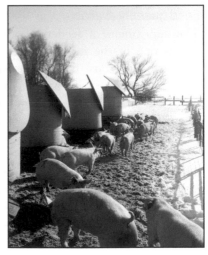

Fig. 10.178 These pigs ran out of feed. They then ate snow, resulting in gangrene of the stomach with *Clostridium septicum* infection (braxy).

Feed outage is the ultimate insult to the pig: Manage and understand feed movement within a feed bin and ensure that feed outages do not occur (**Figures 10.176, 10.177**). If a pig is without feed for 24 hours, a gastric ulcer may occur (**Figure 10.178**). This results in poor feed digestion and leakage of blood. It is relatively common for pigs to go without feed for more than 6 hours on pig farms and may even be considered a normal occurrence at least once in every batch of pigs produced. It is good management to have sufficient feed in the feeders for at least 24 hours. Then, if there is a problem with feed delivery from the bin to the feeder, it can be detected and corrected before a feed outage occurs. If the pigs have been transported a long distance, consider providing a high-fibre, large particle size formulation for the first week post arrival to enhance gastric health.

Feed spoiling

There are many ways in which the feed can be spoilt:

- **Feeder incorrectly placed.** As discussed previously, ensure the feeder does not look like a toilet area to the pig.
- **Effects of the weather and the feeder.** The feed must not be spoilt by the effect of the weather, in particular during rain storms (**Figure 10.179**). This includes feed barrows and bagged feed areas.
- **Floor feeding/feed as bedding.** Floor feeding of grow/finish pigs, for whatever reason, should be avoided (**Figure 10.180**). Feed is a very expensive bedding material. While it is not uncommon in the immediate post-weaning period to feed on a floor mat, the provision of a simple inexpensive trough will not only reduce waste but also provide the stockperson with details of feed consumption per pig rather than just usage per group. The number of farms where feed is spread on the floor merely to indicate to the pigs where their sleeping area is located is particularly surprising. Review pen layout and provide a draught free sleeping area for all pigs.
- **Mouldy feed.** The feed can become soiled by water running into a feeder (e.g. from a poorly managed drip cooling system) (**Figure 10.181**). This wet feed can rapidly become mouldy and fly infested. Feed bins that are not sealed after filling or are sited where condensation can occur in the bin, resulting in feed wastage through mould; feed bins placed directly in front of outlet fans are an example of this. Mould not only results in wastage but is a potential health risk when eaten by the pigs.
- **Farrowing and gestating sows.** Sow feed is at particular risk for spoiling through attempts to overfeed by stockpersons.
- **Rodent and vermin control.** Birds, mice and rats can consume vast quantities of pig feed and their faeces and urine contribute to the soiling of even more feed. Discourage vermin by immediately cleaning up any feed bin spills (**Figure 10.182**). Feeders should be covered to reduce access to vermin. Buildings should be bird-proof to reduce access and thereby improve *Salmonella* control (**Figure 10.183**). The food conversion rate (FCR) has been reduced by 0.3 (from 3.0 to 2.7 from 30–100 kg liveweight) in pigs merely by covering the feeder. In outdoor units, seagulls and other birds can swoop down and take several pellets at one time. An adult rat will eat 15 g/day; with a 1,000 rats on the farm this is nearly 5 tonnes per year. A seagull will eat 100 g/day; with 100 seagulls this is 3.7 tonnes per year.

Feed wastage

Feed is the largest single expense on a pig farm, accounting for 60–80% or more of the cost of production. It is essential that feed wastage is minimised. On the average farm it is estimated that 12% of feed delivered is wasted. On a 10-sow weekly batch farrowing farm, 12% feed wastage can be more than 250 tonnes

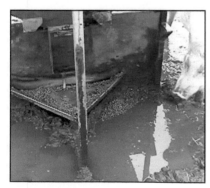

Fig. 10.179 Feed exposed to the weather.

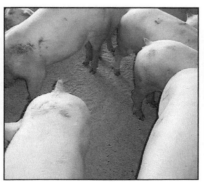

Fig. 10.180 Floor fed gilts; note the feed wastage.

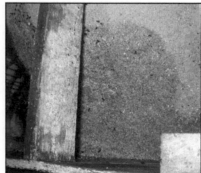

Fig. 10.181 Feed spoilt by a leaking water line.

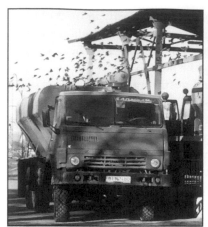

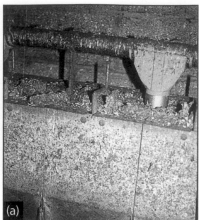

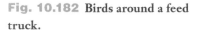

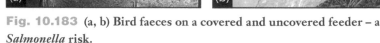

Fig. 10.182 Birds around a feed truck.

Fig. 10.183 (a, b) Bird faeces on a covered and uncovered feeder – a *Salmonella* risk.

of feed per year (whole farm – farrow to finish – feed consumption at 9 tonnes per sow per year). Feed is wasted along the entire feed line from field to rectum.

Health on a farm comprises about 3% of total costs. On the average farm, 12% of the feed used is wasted. If feed is 60–80% of total costs, this wastage is about 9% of the cost of production (i.e. three times the health farm costs).

Interaction between feed and air

Ensure that the pigs are kept within their thermal comfort zone. If pigs are housed too cold, feed will be consumed to help keep them warm. If the pigs are too hot, feed consumption will drop, and therefore growth slows. In addition, extra effort will be expended in panting to help the pig lose heat. In the farrowing area, feed only at the cooler times of the day.

Interaction between feed and water

If the pigs do not have sufficient water supplies, they will reduce their feed intake and ultimately stop eating. There is a very close correlation between water and feed intake. The distance from the feeders and the water supply will affect feed intakes.

Interaction between feed and floor

Poor placement of the feeders in the pen can have a dramatic impact on aggression over feed and thus impact on feed availability and growth rates or the reproductive performance in adults.

Examples of poor feed management
See **Figures 10.184–10.213**.

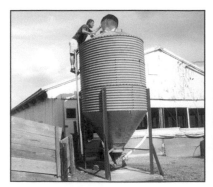

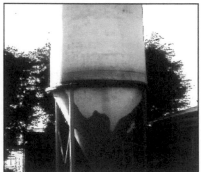

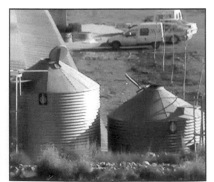

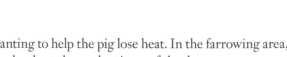

Fig. 10.184 It is essential to regularly check feed bins.

Fig. 10.185 A bin that can be seen through helps reduce the likelihood of mould being missed.

Fig. 10.186 Bins with their lids left open. The rain got in and spoilt 3 tonnes of feed.

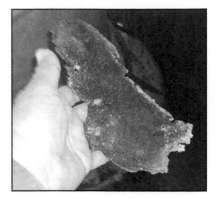

Fig. 10.187 Inadequate bin hygiene routines. Feed bins need regular cleaning.

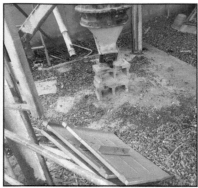

Fig. 10.188 Poor placement of the feed bin and cleaning up afterwards.

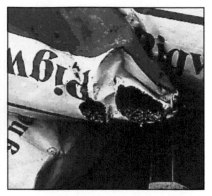

Fig. 10.189 Poor storage allowing rat infestation, waste and disease risk. Do not leave bags of feed outside to get wet.

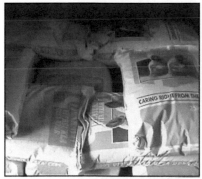

Fig. 10.190 Creep feed should only be stored on pallets.

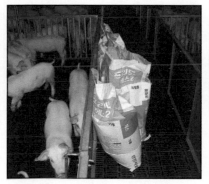

Fig. 10.191 Poor storage; the creep feed is too hot. Note that creep feed is basically milk.

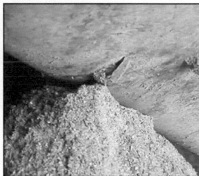

Fig. 10.192 Holes in the home miller and mix plant.

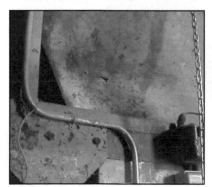

Fig. 10.193 Holes in the bin/auger piping lead to chronic feed loss.

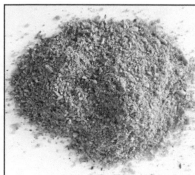

Fig. 10.194 Poor milling leading to feed being unusable. Pigs cannot digest whole or poorly milled grains.

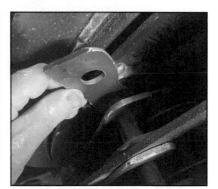

Fig. 10.195 The poor milling (see Figure 11.194) was associated with a blunt hammer in the mill.

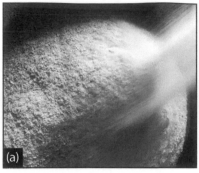
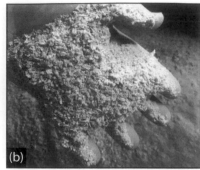
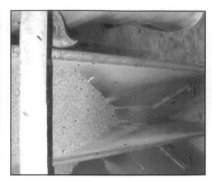

Fig. 10.196 (a) Dusty feed in the feed hopper. Detailed examination is not necessary. (b) Check the quality of feed at the top of the feeder and compare with what the pigs are actually trying to eat.

Fig. 10.197 Poor placement into feed hoppers can result in fighting over feed.

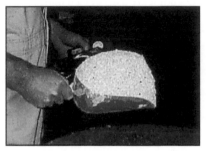
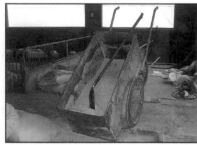

Fig. 10.200 Poor management of feeders as part of AIAO, resulting in wasted feed.

Fig. 10.198 Feed scoop management resulting in increased waste at delivery.

Fig. 10.199 Poor hygiene of feed barrow around farm. Maintain all trailers and tote bins.

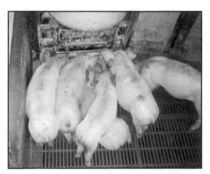
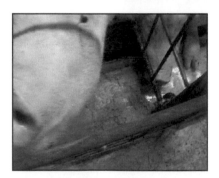

Fig. 10.201 Inadequate feeder space for all the pigs; variable growth is inevitable.

Fig. 10.202 A sow in heat may not eat. Ensure all uneaten food is distributed and not wasted.

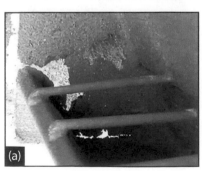
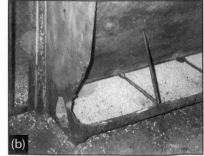
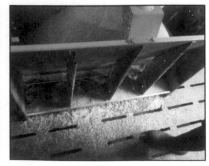

Fig. 10.203 (a, b) Holes in feed hopper, both large and small, result in waste. Poorly repaired feeders are the number one error on most pig farms.

Fig. 10.204 Design of feed hopper where pigs can throw food out of the hopper.

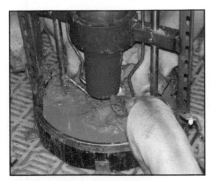

Fig. 10.205 Management of feeder with too much food presented.

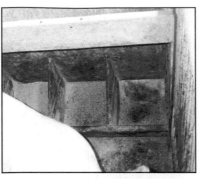

Fig. 10.206 Poor feeder slide adjustment resulting is variable feed availability and waste.

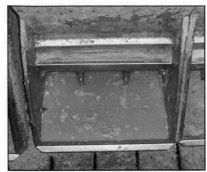

Fig. 10.207 Feeder blocked with water.

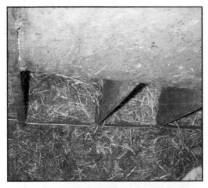

Fig. 10.208 Bedding management resulting in blocked feeders. Items such as straw or marker cans can block feeders.

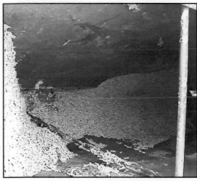

Fig. 10.209 Feeders that have allowed water to enter, thus spoiling the food.

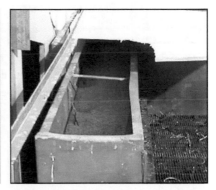

Fig. 10.210 Partially covered feeders. Birds and rodents spread the *Salmonella* organisms.

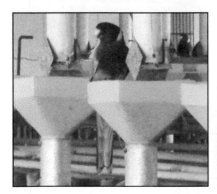

Fig. 10.211 Feeders with birds.

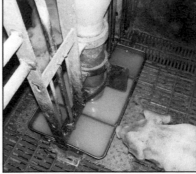

Fig. 10.212 Water overflowing into the feeder, thus limiting feed accessibility and resulting in increased wastage.

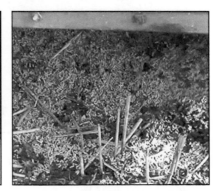

Fig. 10.213 Feed wastage under the feeder not only costs money but encourages rodents to the farm.

MANAGEMENT OF THE FLOOR

Equipment useful for monitoring the management of the farm floor
See **Figures 10.214–10.218**.

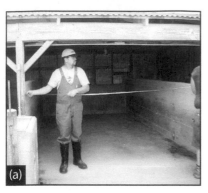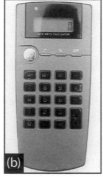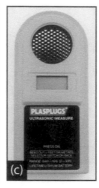
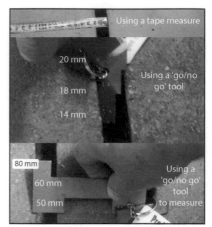

Fig. 10.214 (a–c) Stocking density measuring tape, calculator and ultrasound – area, volume, stocking density measures and actual distance measure apps. The ultrasound can be useful in dark pig buildings.

Fig. 10.215 Measure solid/void/step. Distance measurer. A simple template tool can be used to measure distance.

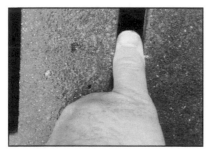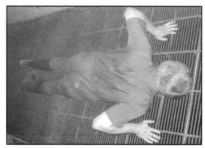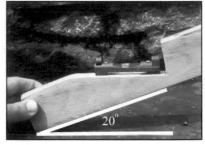

Fig. 10.216 Note rough edges using your hand. You can also estimate wet and dry area.

Fig. 10.217 Determine total floor comfort using your whole body.

Fig. 10.218 Slope of the floor; 20 degree measure shown. Check smart phone apps.

Calculations required
The calculations shown in **Figure 10.219** may also be useful when examining the floor space.

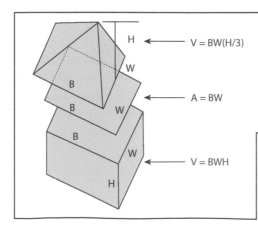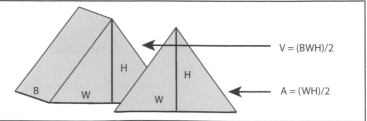

Fig. 10.219 Area and volume calculations for squares and triangles. Square: area = base × width; cube: volume = base × width × height; pyramid: volume = base × width × (height/3); triangle: area = (width × height)/2; isosceles triangular prism: volume = (base × width × height)/2 – this is useful for the roof space.

Stocking density ▶ VIDEO 16

Grow/finish stocking density

In many countries there is a legally required, or recommended, industry standard for stocking densities based on pig weights, and the whole farm team must understand these requirements.

Another aspect of stocking density requirements is to look at the floor space a 100 kg pig requires to ensure that it does not touch another pig. A 100 kg pig requires 0.93 m² in order not to touch another pig, which it needs when it is too hot. As the pig gets bigger so does its space requirement. In reality, not all the floor is used as within the thermal neutral zone, many pigs will pile, releasing 'their' floor space to other pigs.

There is also the reality that in most farms the heaviest pigs will be 'cherry picked' once they reach the selected slaughter weight and their floor space is released to the remaining pigs.

Example of legal requirements in the EU: See *Table 10.16.*

The major change in legal floor space requirements in the EU occurs when the average liveweight is more than 110 kg, when there is suddenly a requirement to have 30% more floor space. This is highly significant as the European industry aims to finish at a weight of 115 kg or more liveweight and thus all pigs require a minimum space of 1.0 m².

Example of moral (industry standard) requirements: See *Table 10.17.*

A minimum stocking density does not take into account the flooring type. In Canada, standards are made that take this in to account and also include protocols to take into account hot weather (*Table 10.18*).

Example based on mathematics: Stocking density based on mathematics is practiced in Australia where the stocking density is based on a factor of the total body mass.

Required: space (m²) = $0.3 \times$ (bodyweight kg)$^{0.67}$.

Therefore, a 110 kg pig requires 0.70 m².

Table 10.16 **The stocking density required for pigs under EU directives (UK interpretation).**

EU LEGISLATION 91/630

AVERAGE LIVE WEIGHT OF PIG (kg)*	MINIMUM SPACE REQUIREMENT (m²)
≤10	0.15
≤20	0.20
≤30	0.30
≤50	0.40
≤85	0.55
≤110	0.65
>110	1.00

* In the UK ≤ (less than or equal too) is used, whereas in the European directive it is only < (less than). Individual governments can make legislation harder than the directive but not less.

Table 10.17 **The stocking density recommended by the US pig industry. (Swine Care Manual, National Pork Board, 2001).**

WEIGHT OF PIG		SUGGESTED FLOOR SPACE	
lb	kg	ft²	m²
12–30	5.4–13.6	1.7–2.5	0.16–0.23
30–60	13.6–27	3–4	0.28–0.27
60–100	27–45	5	0.46
100–150	45–68	6	0.56
150–market	68 and more	8	0.65

Table 10.18 **The stocking density recommended by the Canadian industry and government bodies.**

PIG WEIGHT (kg)	MINIMUM SPACE REQUIRED (m² per pig)		
	FULLY SLATTED	PARTIALLY SLATTED	SOLID BEDDING
10	0.16	0.18	0.21
20	0.26	0.29	0.33
50	0.48	0.53	0.61
75	0.62	0.7	0.8
90	0.7	0.78	0.91
100	0.76	0.85	0.97
110	0.81	0.9	1.03

Note: This housing may need to be increased in hot weather by 10–15%.

Application of stocking rate requirements

The floor stocking rates described above need to be closely applied by the farm team. Over- and understocking is not conducive to good health. A small increase in stocking density will general improve performance, but chilling must be avoided. When the pen is overstocked the other resources such as water, food and air may also be compromised. All aspects of the pen must be reviewed before the veterinary surgeon believes that the health of the pigs is not being compromised. As a general rule, every 0.1 m² reduction from the 'ideal' space results in a 5% reduction in feed intake. However, from a production view, the more pigs per sq metre, generally, the lower the cost despite the production losses. From an ethical point of view, the differences around the world pose significant differences in production capabilities and production costs. *Table 10.19* illustrates the amount of pig that can be 'legally' produced around the world.

The more pigs that can be sold per batch the lower the cost of production. The EU industry is at a disadvantage compared with all the other production systems illustrated.

Unoccupied floor space

The various requirements indicate suitable floor space for pigs, but the environment of the pig is complex with feeder, drinkers, toys and walls also vying for space. Unoccupied floor space is the floor space minus all these other structures. In most pens, space is lost by the feeder. The floor space lost to the feeder can be minimised by using a circular feeder rather than a rectangle feeder. See *Table 10.15* for feed space required for different ages of pigs.

For example: 40 pigs at 60 kg require a feed space of 60 mm per pig. A rectangular feeder of 0.3 m wide would occupy a space of 0.04 m², whereas a circular feeder can provide this feed space but only occupy 0.005 m².

Pen layout

Finishing pens should not be less than 2.5 m wide. If pens are long and narrow, an increase in lameness will occur as the pigs will charge around. To create a tolerant social structure, the group should be more than 60 pigs per pen. If the pens are long and narrow, provide a chicane using partial walls to slow the pigs down.

Sleeping versus defecation areas

The two major different areas of a pen are: (1) the space where the pigs sleep; and (2) the space where the pigs defecate (*Table 10.20*).

It is possible to help pigs determine their defecation area by:

1 Preparing the house with the above considerations in mind (**Figures 10.220, 10.221**).
2 Marking the defecation area.

Table 10.19 **Cost of production implications of local stocking density rules. Based on a farm that has a batch space of 100 m² of finishing floor with pigs finishing at 120 kg liveweight.**

PART OF THE WORLD	KG OF LIVEWEIGHT FINISHED
Australia	16,080
Canada (fully slatted)	15,720
European Union	12,000
United States of America	18,360

Table 10.20 **Sleeping and defecation area definitions. Fill in the empty boxes. The answer can be found on p. 482.**

SLEEPING	DEFECATION

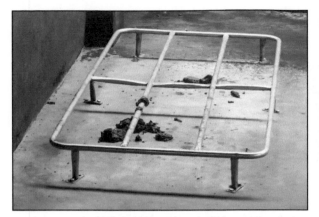

Fig. 10.220 Room preparation with faeces from the same group/batch placed in the defecation area.

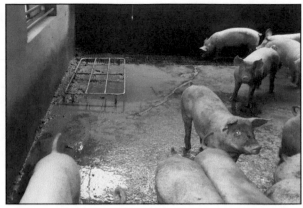

Fig. 10.221 The defecation area in use.

It is important to have sufficient sleeping area. Watch pigs sleeping; all pigs should have a suitable dry area to sleep. If pigs have to sleep in the dunging area, the sleeping area is too small (**Figure 10.222**).

Passageway – big pens versus small pens

A major loss of space in a finishing building is the passageway. The passageway is classically 15% of a building's total floor space. If the passageway is released to pigs, this can reduce the cost of production. Increasing numbers weaned from 10 to 12 per batch farrowing place increases output by 20% and much of this increase in output can be accommodated by the farm adopting big pen production methods and still allow the farm to remain within the legal or industry

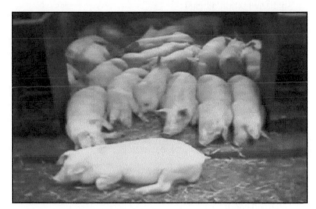

Fig. 10.222 The sleeping area is insufficient and some pigs have to sleep in the dunging area.

standards (**Figures 10.223, 10.224**). The pros and cons of big pen versus small pen production are listed in *Table 10.21*.

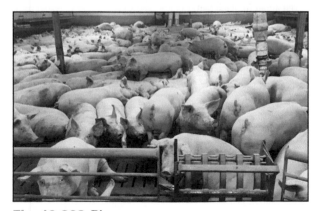

Fig. 10.223 Big pen.

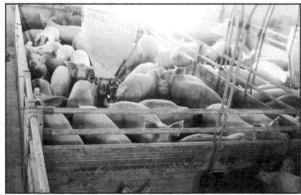

Fig. 10.224 Small pen.

Table 10.21 **Production comparison between big and small pens. Red indicates a negative aspect.**

BIG PEN	SMALL PEN
Pig effects	
Choice	No choice
Poor identification	Good checking individual pigs
Space to show clinical signs	Little space for clinical signs
Catching individual pigs	Injecting individual pigs
Less tail biting	More tail biting
Run away from bullies	Nowhere to run when bullied
No individual pens – unless special provision made	Empty individual pens possible – hospital pens
No mixing at end	Mixing at end. More fighting and skin marks
Split sex rearing difficult	Sex splitting easier
Possibly more variation in pen	Less variation in a pen
Activity energy use	Less pig movement – better FCR
Run injuries as pigs can gain speed	Pigs do not run at great speeds
Easier for small pigs	Harder for small pigs
Building effects	
Cheaper per pig space	More expensive per pig space
Easier to clean, quicker and less water	Cleaning small pens takes more time and more water
AIAO easier	AIAO out needs more planning and more discipline
Choice of environment	Environment has to be absolutely correct
Zone behaviour	No zone behaviour
Faeces in one area (initially)	Faeces in each pen – no order
Well defined sleeping area	Sleeping area required for each pen
More drinkers available to an individual – water choice	Needs two drinkers per pig
Water pipeline length can be shorter	Water pipeline to each pen
More feeders available to an individual – feeder choice	Have to use feeder in pen – bully problem
Feed auger distance can be shorter	Feed auger for each pen
Gruel feeding easier	Post-weaning feeding with gruel takes time
More space per pig – floor choice	Needs more space per pig
No loss of production with passageway	Passageway – loss of production space
Less roof	More roof
Temperature variation around room possible	Room has to be at one temperature
Less humidity	More humidity
Less draughts/chilling pigs can move away	Pigs may be chilled in some pens
Good cost utilisation of space	Poor cost utilisation of space
More pigs per cubic space	Less pigs per cubic space
Under floor ventilation (passageways) not possible	Passageway ventilation possible
Easier biosecurity	Internal biosecurity per pen not possible
Rodent biosecurity – less hideaways	Rodent biosecurity more difficult

(Continued)

Table 10.21 *(Continued)* **Production comparison between big and small pens. Red indicates a negative aspect.**

BIG PEN	SMALL PEN
Stockpersons	
No passageway – more difficult to quickly see pigs	Manager able to check up quickly
Dead pigs more difficult to remove	Dead pigs easier to remove
Lameness is more noticeable	Sick pigs easier to remove
Stockperson in with pigs – great if you love pigs	Easier for people who do not love pigs
Splitting of group easy	Pen group uneven or mixed
Variation in pigs	Weighing individuals easier
Autosort gives better sorting	Autosort possible but more difficult
Aggressive behaviour towards stockpersons	Pigs ignore stockpersons
Reduced cost of production	Increased cost of production
Pigs can choose for themselves	Man chooses for the pig
Better for healthy pigs in a group	Better for sick pigs as individuals
Better for stockpersons who really care for pigs	Better for stockpersons who are not that bothered about pigs
Better for buildings	More building space required
Better use of time and labour	Takes more time and labour

Adult space
Females
Breeding area: To optimise oestrus detection a floor space of 2.8 m² per pig is recommended.

Sow pens: The total unobstructed floor area after breeding for each gilt should be at least 1.64 m². The total unobstructed floor area for each sow and gilt in mixed groups should be 2.25 m².

If gilts or sows are kept in a group of less than six, then the space needs to be increased by 10%. If gilts or sows are kept in groups of more than 40, then the space may be decreased by 10%.

The internal area of a pen should not be less than the square of the length of the pig (a sow is 2 m long, therefore the internal area of the pen should be >4 m²). The internal sides of the pen should measure a minimum of 2.8 m in length unless the group is less than six individuals, when the minimum length will be 2.4 m. However, the free access stall, feeding trough or other intrusions must not be included.

If free access stalls have their backs towards a solid wall, the space between back of the stall and the wall needs to be at least the length of a sow (2 m). Free access stalls and back-to-back with a central pen require a minimum distance between them of 3 times the length of pig from the front of the stalls (6 m), with a 1.5 times (3 m) gap between the ends of the stall.

Sow stalls: In general, sows may be kept in stalls until pregnancy checked. In many parts of the world, after pregnancy checking (4 weeks after breeding) the sows will be loose housed in pens.

Sows stalls should be at least 60 cm wide. The back of a breeding sow stall should be designed to allow easy access to the sow's rear by the stockperson. It should not be necessary to open the rear gate to breed the sow.

Farrowing place
Indoors: An environmentally controlled farrowing place and creep area should be 0.5 × 2.02 m with a 3.2 m² piglet escape area. The escape area around a farrowing place should be 30 cm wide. The heat mat should be a minimum of 0.6 m². Eight kg piglets are 60 cm long.

If a farrowing pen is used, the shortest side of the pen should be 1.8 m, and the total area of the pen not less than 5.6 m² per sow. Outdoor farrowing arcs should have a floor area of 4.5 m².

Outdoor production: gestation and farrowing
Farrowing and lactating sows should be kept in groups of 9–14 sows/hectare. Pregnant sows should be kept in groups of 15–25 (UK) or 20–25 (Australia) sows/hectare.

Boars

Individual living accommodation for an adult boar should have a floor area of not less than 6 m². If the boar pen is also used for collection, it is recommended to be 10 m². Within the EU it is not legal to house boars in stalls; however, if local regulations do permit stalls, the boar stall should be 0.7 m wide and 2.4 m long.

Floor type

The floor of a pig barn is a vital part of maintaining pig health. It is essential to properly construct the floor. Making concrete can be very difficult and the floor is intended for possibly decades of wear. Use rolled river stone not aggregate/flint stone with sharp edges.

Solid versus slatted

Within the EU, total slatted areas are banned. There is a minimum requirement for 0.95 m² for gilts and 1.3 m² for sows to be solid. No more than 15% of the solid area should be reserved for drainage openings.

Size of slats

Within the EU there is legislation over the size of slats that may be used in pig production (*Table 10.22*).

Table 10.22 **Slatted floor suggestions. Based on 2001/88/EC.**		
	VOID WIDTH (mm)	CONCRETE SLAT WIDTH (mm)
Sow and litter	8–11	50
Pre-nursery	8–11	50
Nursery	8–14	50
Grow/finish	10–18	80–100
Gestating sows		
Pens	10–20	80–100
Stalls	10–20	80–100
Boars	20	100–130

Wire mesh, metal or plastic slats are preferred in farrowing and nursery areas. The slat edges should be rounded, not sharp or chipped. If the slat is damaged, it should be replaced or repaired.

Bedding

Bedding is being increasingly used to cover and insulate floors. While some of these materials can provide good environmental control, poor use of bedding contaminated with mould spores can be seriously detrimental to health. The improper use of bedding and inadequate cleaning routines can result in pigs being forced to sleep on wet bedding, which has serious consequences for respiratory health. It is very important to ensure that there is adequate rodent control with stored bedding. All straw should be stored on 9 mm of sand to reduce rodent infestation and to assist draining/drying of the straw.

For grow/finish pigs the estimated straw usage is about 3 kg/head/week. For sows, allow 1 tonne of straw per year.

Steps

Where a step cannot be avoided the height should be as small as possible. Recommended maximum step heights would be 100 mm for breeding stock or finishing pigs but only 50 mm for weaners. The edge of the step should be rounded.

Slope

Slopes should not exceed 20 degrees. This can be significant in loading areas and approaches to a truck, especially when placing pigs on the top deck.

Walls and doors

Boars

Boar pen divisions should not be less than 1.5 m high to reduce the likelihood that the boar will escape. In designing an AI collection area, safety bollards to protect humans should be provided. The bollards should be 12 cm wide, 760 cm high and 30 cm apart.

Gates

For weaners, ensure that gaps are not too great otherwise the weaners get stuck. The bottom of gates should be no more than 5 cm from the ground and the gaps between bars be no greater than 5 cm.

Abrasive points ▶ VIDEO 16

Hygiene achieved in buildings is often grossly inadequate. It is not generally appreciated that poor quality and dirty floors can have a significant impact on respiratory diseases. If the floor is rough and causes trauma to the feet, pathogens (in particular streptococci) gain access to the pig (**Figure 10.225**). They are then transported via the blood straight to the lung parenchyma, where they can result in pulmonary abscesses, endocarditis and possibly polyserositis.

Floors wear where there is more traffic, such as near doorways or around feeders and drinkers (**Figure 10.226**). The presence of water from drinkers increases floor wear. If the farm practices liquid feeding, the combination of liquid feeding, pig saliva and feet wears the surrounding floor rapidly (**Figure 10.227**).

Gates and metal will rust and rot quickly on pig farms (**Figure 10.228**). Many pigs can become seriously damaged by contact from these worn systems.

The presence of rust also makes cleaning very difficult.

Loading pigs

It is important to realise that the farm team's responsibility towards their pigs extends all the way to the slaughterhouse. The loading area, passageways around the farm and the driveway to the farm all need to be in good repair to stop injury to the pig.

Loading area

Loading areas need to be carefully constructed to assist with easy and low-stress movement of pigs (**Figure 10.229**). Electric prodders should not be used.

Transportation of pigs

There are legal requirements in many countries for transportation of pigs. To load the pigs, an elevator is preferred. However, if a ramp is used it needs to have a

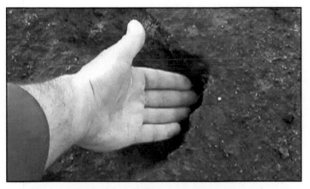

Fig. 10.225 **Hole in the floor resulting in lame pigs.**

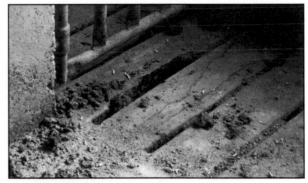

Fig. 10.226 **Slats of variable widths or wear.**

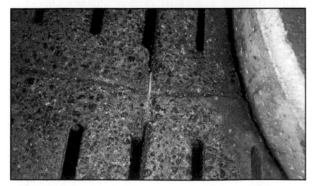

Fig. 10.227 **Worn slats around feeders in a liquid feeding system.**

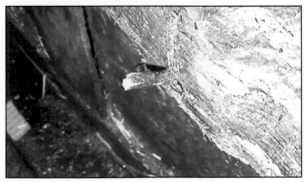

Fig. 10.228 **Abrasive points on rotting gates and walls.**

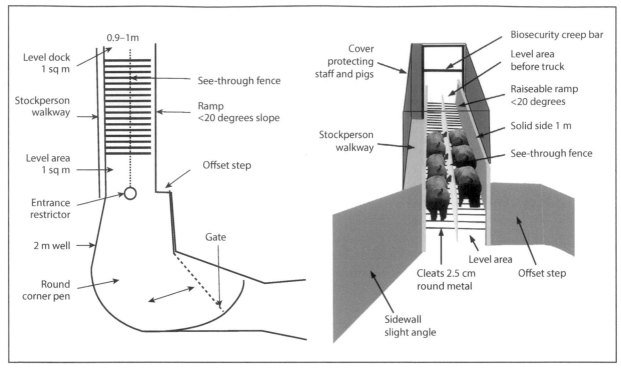

Fig. 10.229 Loading area design.

slope of less than 20 degrees. Once on the truck, pigs of 100 kg should have a minimum space of 235 kg/m². In the summer time, extra space (10–15%) should be provided. Given the cost of transportation, several farms will make this part of their pig flow model to ensure that each truck will be full.

Cleaning protocols

The farm team must understand cleaning protocols. However, most farms do not have adequate cleaning programmes. Batching provides the farm health team with the opportunity to:

- Clean the whole pen including the water, air, feed and the floor areas.
- Repair the pigs' environment and equipment.

Cleaning needs to carefully follow a protocol and should have the following steps:

1 Remove all feed from the house.
2 Remove all pigs from the house.
3 Dampen the building.
4 Apply detergent to the building surfaces.

5 Pressure wash all the building surfaces. Hot water should be used.
6 Disinfect all building surfaces, including the water supply.
7 Allow the building 24 hours to completely dry.

The number one disinfectant is a clean dry surface.

Sow housing options

A potentially controversial area is the housing of sows during gestation and lactation. Sow stalls are being banned, especially post-pregnancy checking, in many parts of the world. Therefore, other options need to be considered. However, all these options, while having some good points that benefit the sows, also have poor points and the farm needs to consider these issues before making a decision regarding housing options (**Figures 10.230–10.241**).

In several countries sows stalls are totally removed. The mixing of unfamiliar sows almost invariably results in aggression. To minimise the adverse effects of aggression on sow fertility, sows should be mixed at weaning by size – parity 1 and 2 sows and the rest of the older sows.

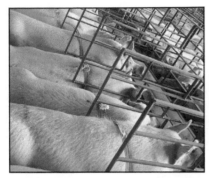

Fig. 10.230 Tethers (illegal in EU).

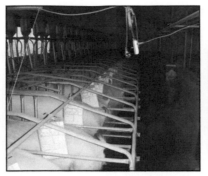

Fig. 10.231 Stalls (illegal after 6 weeks of pregnancy in the EU).

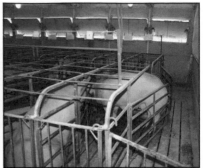

Fig. 10.232 Turn around stalls (illegal after 6 weeks of pregnancy in the EU).

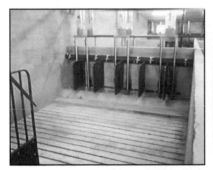

Fig. 10.233 Trickle feeding.

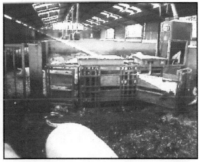

Fig. 10.234 Electronic sow feeding.

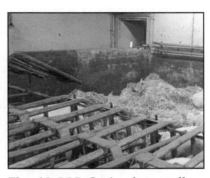

Fig. 10.235 Optional sow stalls.

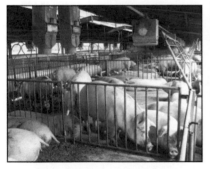

Fig, 10.236 Loose housing – dump feeding.

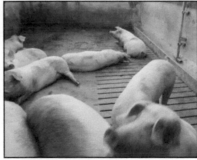

Fig. 10.237 Loose housing – wet feeding.

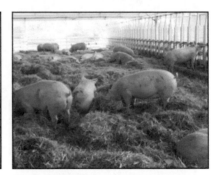

Fig. 10.238 Loose housing – short stall.

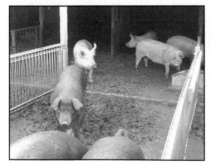

Fig. 10.239 Kennels lots.

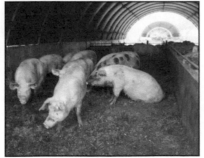

Fig. 10.240 Hoop buildings.

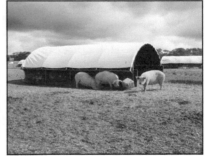

Fig. 10.241 Outdoor.

Examples of poor floor management
See **Figures 10.242–10.267**.

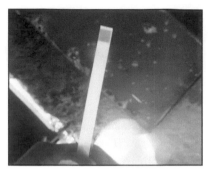

Fig. 10.242 Internal biosecurity is an important aspect of pathogen control. Check the concentration of the disinfectant.

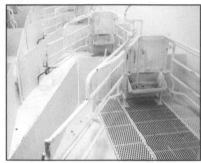

Fig. 10.243 Burnt builder's lime (CaCO₃) washing can provide an inexpensive part of the cleaning programme.

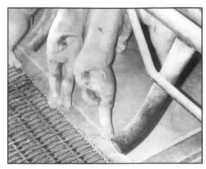

Fig. 10.244 If the burnt builder's lime is not allowed to dry, however, it can scald pigs.

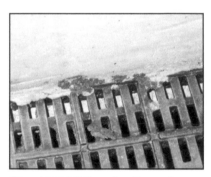

Fig. 10.245 Leaving faeces in corners negates all the cleaning.

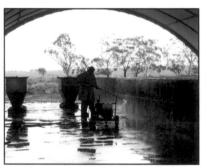

Fig. 10.246 As part of the routine check, ensure that the farm is clean.

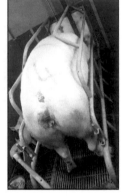

Fig. 10.247 Check that the farrowing place is big enough to accommodate the sow.

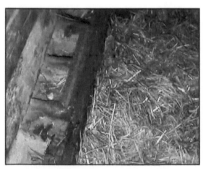

Fig. 10.248 Holes that can damage legs can occur because of unfilled breeze blocks at floor level.

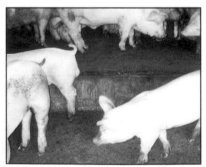

Fig. 10.249 Steps that are too severe can result in leg injury.

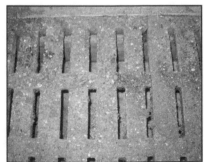

Fig. 10.250 Poorly made concrete causes severe damage to legs and feet.

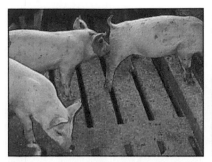

Fig. 10.251 Check the floor gap is not so large that the pigs can damage their feet.

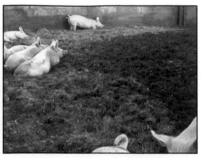

Fig. 10.252 The lying area needs to be looked after; poor bedding leads to encroachment.

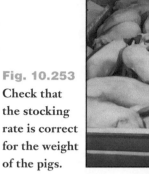

Fig. 10.253 Check that the stocking rate is correct for the weight of the pigs.

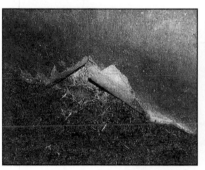

Fig. 10.254 Sharp edges on the bottom of metal work, typically doors.

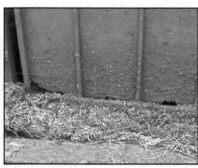

Fig. 10.255 Metal doors that are rotting and corroding at the bottom.

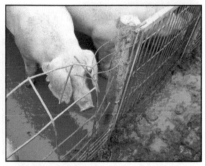

Fig. 10.256 Sharp points sticking out from railing.

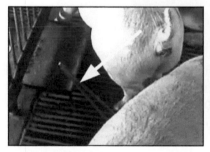

Fig. 10.257 Pieces of the metal floor not repaired (arrow), resulting in extreme risk of injury to the pig.

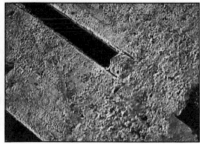

Fig. 10.258 Poorly made and rough new floors can be a major source of lameness in pigs.

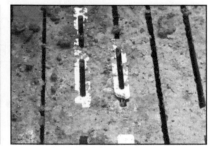

Fig. 10.259 Reducing the void width can unfortunately create sharp edges and make the problem worse.

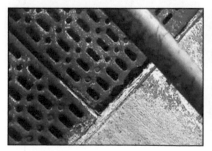

Fig. 10.260 Corrosion of the end of a slat.

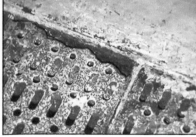

Fig. 10.261 Corrosion continues until pigs can damage their legs and feet.

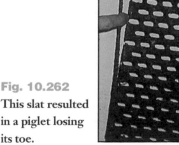

Fig. 10.262 This slat resulted in a piglet losing its toe.

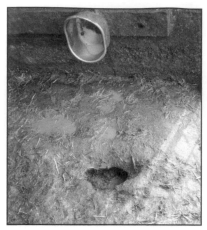

Fig. 10.263 Large hole in the floor.

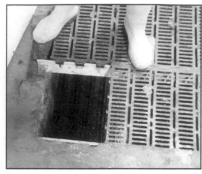

Fig. 10.264 Floors not properly looked after can collapse completely and pigs fall into the pit beneath the floor.

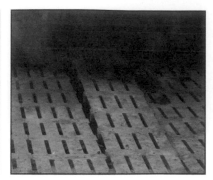

Fig. 10.265 Slats that have become displaced.

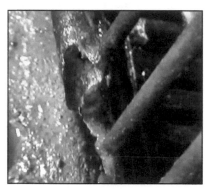

Fig. 10.266 Rusting and corroding metal work can cause problems for the pig.

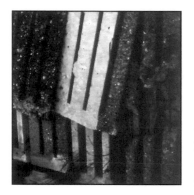

Fig. 10.267 Old slats showing considerable wear. Note the unworn area covered by the feeder.

MANAGEMENT OF STOCKPERSONS

▶ VIDEOS 1–5   ▶ AUDIOS 1–10

Level of stockpersonship

Well trained, dedicated, enthusiastic stockpersons are essential to the efficient running of a pig farm. The good stockperson must have sufficient time to look after the animals and not spend all their time running around maintaining the building (**Figures 10.268–10.271**). Many stockpersons fail to provide sufficient pig care because of a lack of organisation. ▶ VIDEOS 46 and 47

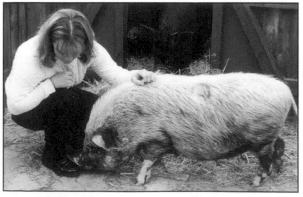

Fig. 10.268 Stockpersons must like pigs.

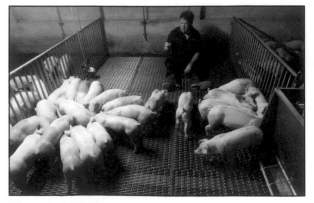

Fig. 10.269 Encourage physical contact between pigs and people; become the pig.
▶ VIDEO 3   ▶ AUDIO 8

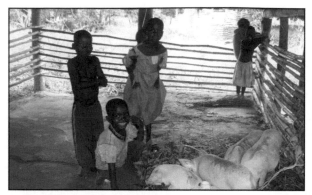

Fig. 10.270 Future stockpersons are an extremely valuable resource.

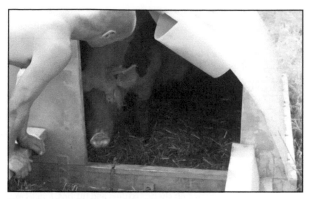

Fig. 10.271 All the components of a successful pig farm: "the other animals looked from man to pig and from pig to man and did not see the difference" (JC Orwell).

Minimum expectation of stockpersons

The stockperson should always be looking out for signs of ill-health in pigs, which include:

- Separation from the group.
- Depressed and quiet behaviour.
- Rapid or irregular breathing.
- Persistent coughing or panting.
- Huddling and shivering.
- Discolouration or blistering of the skin.
- Loss of body condition.
- Sneezing.
- Lameness.
- Lack of coordination.
- Swollen navel, udder or joints.
- Constipation.
- Diarrhoea.
- Vomiting.
- Poor appetite.
- Dead.

Teaching stockpersonship

Stockpersons should be taught the basic signs of ill health (*Table 10.23*).

Training stockpersons

A major role of the veterinarian is to teach good management techniques. The title 'doctor' means 'teacher' in Greek – not healer! The veterinarian and senior farm management team needs to develop a series of training programmes for the whole team (*Table 10.24*).

A chart outlining typical stockperson duties and training levels is shown in **Figure 10.272**.

Table 10.23 **The basic signs of ill health.**

ANIMAL BEHAVIOUR	STAGE OF THE DISEASE	ACTION REQUIRED
Does not get up quickly	Early	Caution
Stomach not full	Early	Look further
Agitated	Early	Look further
Rapid breathing	Fairly early	Look further
Looks gaunt	Fairly early	Intervene
Does not come to eat	Fairly early	Intervene
Remains at back of group	Fairly early	Intervene
Arched back	Fairly early	Intervene
Hair stands on end	Fairly early	Intervene
Pale, long hair	Fairly late	Intervene
Straggler	Late	Intervene
Losing weight	Very late	Improve process
Slow growth	Very late	Improve process
Small in the group	Very late	Improve process

Table 10.24 **Classification of stockpersons.**

Untrained	One week
Level 1	First 3 months
Level 2	3–6 months
Level 3	6 months to 1 year
Level 4	1 year on farm and some off-farm training
Level 5	1–2 years on farm and recognised off-farm training
Level 6	2–3 years on farm and formal farm training
Senior level 7	3 years on farm and capable of all tasks required on the farm

TYPICAL STOCKPERSON DUTIES AND TRAINING LEVELS									
Duties as required by stockpersons		Level of training: numbers indicate level of stockperson							
		UT	1	2	3	4	5	6	7
Bioscurity	effluent removal and disposal								
	clean accommodation pens, fittings and equipment								
	control and maintain protective footware and clothing								
	control procedures can be applied								
	deceased stock disposal								
	clean and maintain buildings and equipment								
	maintain machinary and equipment								
Building	install new or replacement equipment and fittings								
	maintain sheds, fixtures and fittings, fences and surrounds								
	remove faulty or damaged equipment and fittings								
Condition-score pigs									
	be able to perform								
Feed	mix and mill feed								
	feed and water for all stock								
Fire-fighting equipment trained									
Health	recognise signs of bullying								
	administer medicines including injection								
	recognise signs of ill-health								
	care for sick or injured stock								
	recognise heat-distressed pigs								
	recognise lame animals and take appropriate action								
	maintain an adequate environment for the well-being of the stock								
	recognise ill-health and be able to take appropriate remedial action								
	recognise sows that are unsuitable for their accommodation								
	recognise adverse weather from a pig's view								
	medicine usage decisions								
	maintain herd health status at an acceptable level								
	post-mortem examinations of deceased stock								
Husbandy	routines for all stock								
Identification	systems can be administered								
Move, draft and weigh stock									
Order	stores and equipment								
Records	maintain a recording system and interpret data								
Water	check drinkers								
Perform other duties as required									
Specific areas of the farm requiring special skills									
Breeding	artificial insermination								
	able to work with both boars								
	oestrus detection and mate breeding stock								
	pregnancy diagnosis								
	replacement breeding stock selection								
Farrowing	teeth clipping								
	tail docking								
	ear notching								
	castration								
	assist sows and piglets at farrowing								
Health	recognise a piglet that has not eaten within 24 hours of birth								

Y Yes, work unsupervised
S Work but needs supervision
D Direct supervision required
N Must not be carried out without specific training

Note: UT = untrained new employee

Fig. 10.272 Typical stockperson duties and training levels.

Supervision

Staff should work with pigs with various levels of supervision depending on training. Direct supervision implies an employee working with a stockperson level 2 or more within the same room/area. Supervision implies an employee working with a stockperson a level higher than the employee who is present within earshot on the same site.

With this concept, tasks at which the stockperson is expected to be competent can be established.

EXPLANATION OF INFRARED PICTURE INTERPRETATION

When using an infrared camera, the image is colour graded to indicate a scale of temperatures. This means that these cameras can be used as a clinical tool (**Figures 10.273, 10.274**).

Fig. 10.273
Interpretation of the infrared image as a clinical tool.

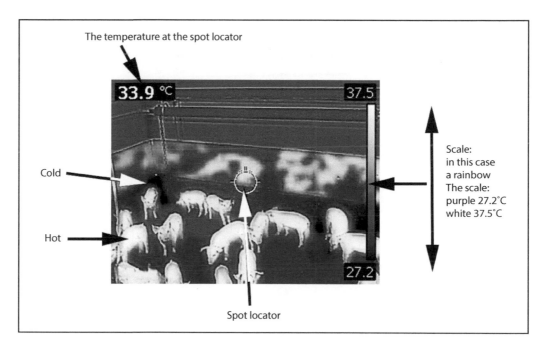

Fig. 10.274 The infrared image illustrating healthy pigs in a nursery. Note the reflected heat images (arrows) of the piglets off the shiny metal walls!

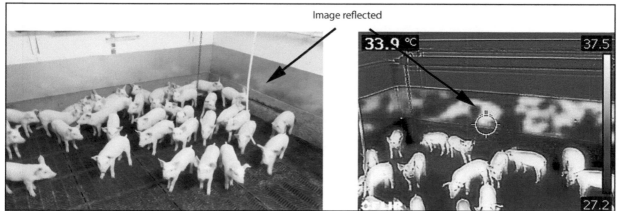

CLINICAL QUIZ

10.1 List some pig behaviours that may indicate inadequate water supply (see **Figure 10.14** [p. 319])?

10.2 How do you read a maximum/minimum thermometer (see **Figure 10.45** [p. 326])?

10.3 What is wrong with the pig in the middle in **Figure 10.61** (p. 329).

10.4 What are the characteristics of sleeping versus defecation areas? Fill in the empty boxes in *Table 10.20* (see p. 368).

The answers to these questions can be found on pages 477–478.

PIG HEALTH MAINTENANCE

INTRODUCTION

Veterinarians aim to maintain or improve the health of the pigs under their care and to reduce treatments. Health maintenance is therefore composed of keeping new pathogens off the farm (i.e. external biosecurity) and containing pathogens within the farm (internal biosecurity). Emerging pathogens will challenge pork producers at an increasing rate because of globalisation. Producers can reduce pathogen loads on a farm by sanitation, all-in/all-out (AIAO) and by reducing age variation within batches. The previous chapter discussed the provision of an adequate environment to house the various ages of pigs. Pathogen load can also be reduced by appropriate use of vaccines and judicial use of therapeutic antibiotics.

In some circumstances, there may be pathogens that are difficult to control or have such an economic impact that they limit the ability of the farm to economically function in the medium term.

In a production environment a veterinarian aims to combine high welfare of the pigs with the farm being economically viable and producing high-quality, safe and wholesome pork.

REDUCING THE RISK OF INTRODUCTION OF NEW PATHOGENS

Farm biosecurity principles

The classical pyramid production system moves desirable genes from a nucleus farm to the production farms. This system also provides a means to move health benefits. If the top of the pyramid is free of a pathogen, it is possible to move this pathogen-free status to the multiplication and ultimately to the production farms, thus maintaining or enhancing the health and wellbeing of the whole production pyramid.

To maintain the system, it is necessary to understand specific pathogen movement. This provides additional stimuli to veterinarians to develop national and international biosecurity standard operating procedures (SOPs) (**Figure 11.1**).

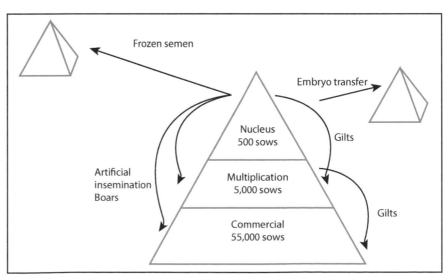

Fig. 11.1 **The pyramid breeding structure. The need to move genes down the pyramid, and between pyramids, lead to the development of biosecurity standard operating procedures.**

Philosophy – diseases or pathogens?

The veterinarian should understand the difference between disease and pathogens.

Disease is a term describing clinical signs and often is associated with economic costs. Farms cannot be 'disease' free. It is only by using the term 'pathogen' that the veterinarian can start writing control and elimination programmes. Organisms continue to evolve, drift, recombine and mutate, triggering a non-economic organism to become a major pathogen. An example is porcine circovirus type 2 (PCV2). This virus was present for many years in global pig populations before it became recognised as a major pathogen in 1996. When historical texts are examined it can be difficult to recognise modern diseases from the clinical signs described.

Pathogens that may or may not be economically eliminated from a commercial farm

See *Table 11.1.*

Understanding how pathogens can enter a farm

Before constructing and writing a biosecurity SOP, the whole farm health team must understand how pathogens can be introduced into the farm (*Table 11.2* and **Figure 11.2**).

Understanding how each of these introduction methods vary with each specific pathogen

Generally, pathogens enter by live animal, transportation or aerosol. Understanding the primary

Table 11.1 **Pathogens that currently may or may not be economically eliminated from a commercial farm.**

PATHOGENS THAT CAN BE ELIMINATED FROM THE FARM	PATHOGENS THAT ARE UNLIKELY TO BE ELIMINATED FROM A FARM
Actinobacillus pleuropneumoniae	*Actinobacillus suis*
African swine fever virus	*Brachyspira pilosicoli*
Aujeszky's disease virus (pseudorabies virus)	*Erysipelothrix rhusiopathiae*
Brachyspira hyodysenteriae	*Escherichia coli*
Brucella suis	Haemagglutinating encephalomyelitis coronovirus virus (vomiting and wasting disease virus)
Classical swine fever virus (hog cholera)	*Haemophilus parasuis*
Foot and mouth disease virus – vesicular diseases	*Lawsonia intracelluaris*
Haematopinus suis	*Leptospira* spp.
Leptospira pomona	*Mycobacterium avium*
Mycobacterium bovis	*Mycoplasma hyorhinis*
Mycoplasma hyopneumoniae	*Mycoplasma hyosynoviae*
Porcine epidemic diarrhoea virus	Parvovirus *Pasteurella multocida*
Porcine delta coronavirus	Porcine circovirus type 2 or 3 Rotavirus
Porcine reproductive and respiratory syndrome virus	*Salmonella* spp.
Salmonella enterica serotype *choleraesuis*	*Staphylococcus hyicus*
Sarcoptes scabiei var *suis*	*Streptococcus suis*
Swine influenza virus*	*Streptococcus* spp.
Toxigenic *Pasteurella multocida*	
Transmissible gastroenteritis virus	

* Swine influenza virus may be introduced into a pig farm by staff, but it can be eliminated again.

Table 11.2 **Potential biosecurity risks to a farm. The relative order of importance of the risk can change depending on many circumstances.**

POTENTIAL THREAT
Other pigs – gilt and boar introductions
Other pigs – AI or embryo transfer
Pork products (ham, salami, sausage, pizza)
Dead disposal - rendering (placement of dead disposal area)
Transportation systems
Locality of neighbouring pig units
Presence of a major road
Purchased second-hand equipment
Clothing from another unit
Birds, rodents, cats, dogs, flies
Feed (ingredients) and water
Modified live vaccines
Bedding (note source of manure used to fertilise straw)
Staff owning their own stock
Staff visiting animal markets, shows and slaughterhouses
Vets and other advisors (clothing)
Visitors (e.g. electricity and gas personnel)
New utensils

transmission routes is key to prevention (*Table 11.3*). However, since the aim is to prevent introduction of multiple pathogens, all risks need to be minimised. The most obvious risk of pathogen transfer is through the movement of pigs themselves. This includes wild/feral members of the Suidae family (not just wild *Sus scrofa*). Movement by faecal spread is particularly important in the spread of enteric pathogens such as porcine epidemic diarrhoea virus (PEDV) and *Brachyspira*.

Veterinarians should realise that they must not play the role of fomite in the spread of faeces from farm to farm. Veterinarians are a particular risk. They must be aware that not only can faeces be spread by their actions, but also other organics, such as blood, which may be even more contagious than faeces.

The veterinarian

Before veterinarians can suggest biosecurity standards, they must determine that their own standards are adequate to ensure that they are not a fomite in pathogen transfer. In general, pathogens are species specific, excluding specific zoonotic pathogens, therefore humans are a low risk to pig units. **Figure 11.3** illustrates how the veterinarian could act as a fomite and/or vector for a number of

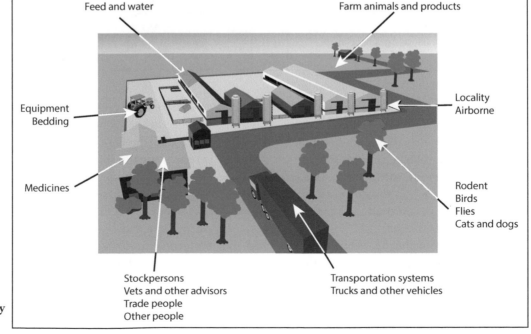

Fig. 11.2

Illustration of the potential threats to a farm. Note the isolation unit further down the road. This would have its own biosecurity SOPs.

Feed and water

Farm animals and products

Equipment Bedding

Locality Airborne

Medicines

Rodent Birds Flies Cats and dogs

Stockpersons Vets and other advisors Trade people Other people

Transportation systems Trucks and other vehicles

Table 11.3 **Major pig pathogens and their potential route of spread. The blocked cells are possible routes of spread. Cells highlighted in red indicate that the risk is highly suspected. Cells highlighted in blue indicate where the risk is predominantly via pig faeces/saliva.**

POTENTIAL RISK	ACTINOBACILLUS PLEUROPNEUMONIAE	AUJESZKY'S DISEASE VIRUS (PSEUDORABIES)	BRACHYSPIRA HYODYSENTERIAE	BRUCELLA SPP.	CLASSICAL AND AFRICAN SWINE FEVER VIRUSES	ESCHERICHIA COLI	FOOT AND MOUTH DISEASE VIRUS	LAWSONIA INTRACELLULARIS	LEPTOSPIRA SPP.	MYCOPLASMA HYOPNEUMONIAE	PASTEURELLA MULTOCIDA	PRRSV	SALMONELLA SPP.	SARCOPTES SCABIEI – MANGE	SWINE INFLUENZA VIRUS	TGEV/PEDV
Other pigs	■	■	■	■	■	■	■	■	■	■	■	■	■	■	■	■
Pork products (ham, salami, sausage, pizza)					■		■						■			
Knackerman (dead pig disposal area)	■	■	■		■	■	■	■	■	■	■	■	■	■	■	■
Transportation systems		■	■		■	■	■	■	■	■	■	■	■	■	■	■
Locality of neighbouring pig units		■			■		■			■		■			■	
Presence of a major road		■			■		■			■		■	■		■	
Purchased second-hand equipment		■	■		■	■	■	■	■	■	■	■	■	■	■	■
Clothing from another unit		■	■		■	■	■	■	■	■	■	■	■	■	■	■
Birds, rodents, cats, dogs, flies		■	■		■	■	■	■	■		■		■			■
Feed and water			■		■	■	■	■	■				■			■
Bedding (note source of manure for straw)			■		■	■	■	■	■				■			■
Staff owing their own pigs	■	■	■		■	■	■	■	■	■	■	■	■	■	■	■
Staff visiting pig markets and slaughterhouses	■	■	■		■	■	■	■	■	■	■	■	■	■	■	■
Vets and other advisors		■	■		■	■	■	■	■	■	■	■	■	■	■	■
Visitors (note electricity and gas people)		■			■		■			■	■	■	■		■	
New utensils																

pathogens by their actions in transferring faeces from farm to farm.

Figure 11.3 also illustrates the number of risk points that the veterinarian must take into consideration before going to the farm. The risk of inviting the veterinarian to the farm can be considerable since veterinarians normally work with sick animals and associated pathogens.

The population health veterinarian has had to learn how to deal with and minimise these risks. The most important risk reduction measure has been to get farms to supply much of their own equipment, so removing the need for veterinarians to take equipment onto the farm. Much of the equipment that

veterinarians use is difficult to clean and sanitise. However, there is no reason why all farms and animal establishments should not provide the visiting veterinarian with boots, overalls, a rectal thermometer, diagnostic supplies and necropsy equipment.

The boot of a farm animal veterinarian's car can be a major biosecurity threat (**Figures 11.4, 11.5**). At any time, day or night, the veterinarian must take biosecurity seriously.

When buying and moving equipment between farms ensure that the equipment can be cleaned and disinfected. For example, the camera or phone can be made waterproof and disinfected between farm visits (**Figure 11.6**).

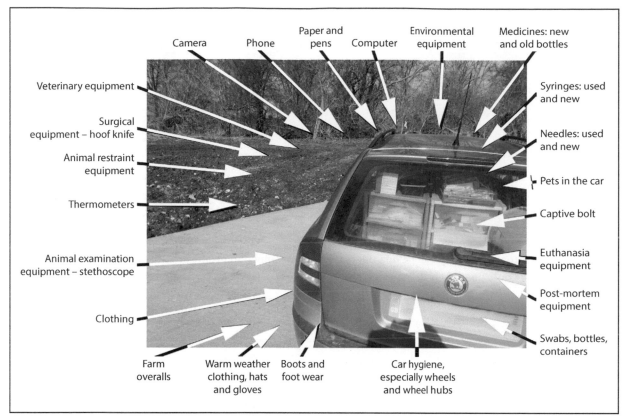

Veterinary equipment

Surgical equipment – hoof knife

Animal restraint equipment

Thermometers

Animal examination equipment – stethoscope

Clothing

Camera Phone Paper and pens Computer Environmental equipment Medicines: new and old bottles

Syringes: used and new

Needles: used and new

Pets in the car

Captive bolt

Euthanasia equipment

Post-mortem equipment

Swabs, bottles, containers

Farm overalls Warm weather clothing, hats and gloves Boots and foot wear Car hygiene, especially wheels and wheel hubs

Fig. 11.3 Potential risk points from the veterinarian and their car.

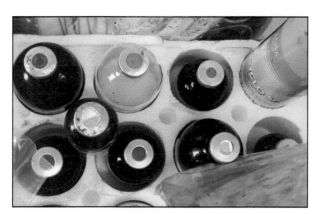

Fig. 11.4 Blood and animal organics on old and adjacent to new medicine bottles in the car boot. There is also a bag of injection needles in direct contact with these contaminated bottles.

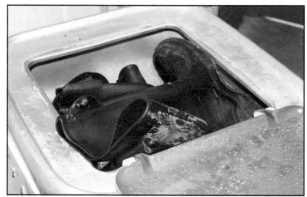

Fig. 11.5 Dirty farm boots going from farm to farm. The plastic container was to keep the car boot clean, not to enhance the client's biosecurity.

Equipment that is difficult to clean should be moved in plastic bags. It can then be quickly cleaned by merely placing the still clean equipment into a new plastic bag and responsibly disposing of the contaminated plastic bag (**Figure 11.7**).

Veterinarians can contaminate their hands just by going into the boot of the car to pick up medicines that have been contaminated from organics from another farm. Viruses (e.g. PEDV) can be transmitted via contaminated plastics.

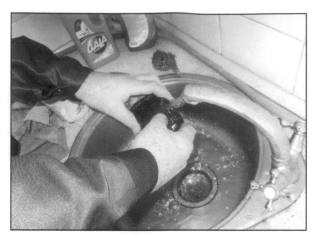

Fig. 11.6 Cameras, phones, data equipment, etc. should only go onto units if they can be disinfected thoroughly; this is only possible if they are waterproof.

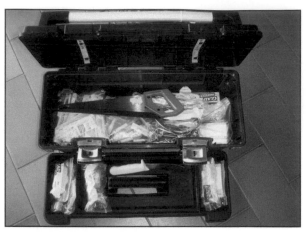

Fig. 11.7 Post-mortem box. All the equipment is wrapped in plastic bags to enhance biosecurity. Ensure the box is easy to clean (see Chapter 1).

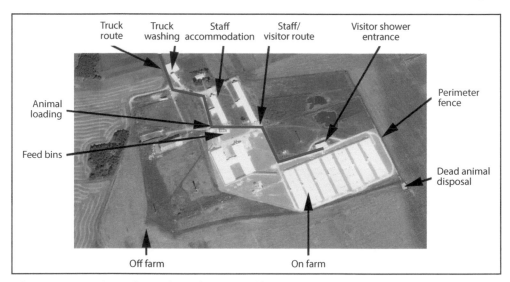

Fig. 11.8 The green zone is on-farm, the red zone is off-farm.

Visit interval

Single farm visits per day allows equipment to be cleaned between visits. Visiting only one farm or pyramid a day has cost implications which, once clients appreciate the importance of maintaining their biosecurity, becomes acceptable.

Reducing the chance of the veterinarian being a zoonotic risk

Influenza viruses are a classical example where the veterinarian can inadvertently carry a new pathogen onto a farm. To reduce this risk, annual vaccination of all members of the practice with the current human influenza strains may help. If veterinarians are sick, they are advised not to visit the farm.

Development of an on-farm and off-farm consciousness

A cornerstone of a farm's biosecurity is to develop the philosophy of off- and on-farm zones (**Figure 11.8**). This needs to be clearly defined and it is vital that the veterinarian does not compromise these zones.

The on-farm zone is all the areas where the pigs, after removal from isolation, have access. This is the specific pathogen-free area and is bound by a clearly defined perimeter fence. Many specific pathogen-free farms, especially those who are porcine reproductive and respiratory syndrome virus (PRRSV) free, may have an intermediate zone where footwear and separate clothing are worn.

Development of biosecurity standard operating procedures

To ensure that the whole farm team understands the requirements to control each risk factor, it is advisable to provide training. The written biosecurity rules then become the farm's SOP. The major areas where SOPs need to be developed are discussed below.

Animal introduction

The introduction of animals/animal products (gilts, boars, semen, embryos, meat and wildlife) are the major method of pathogen spread and have to be given the greatest attention.

An isolation facility is essential on all units. Ideally, it would be a minimum of 50 metres away from the main production facility. This limit of spread may be reduced further if the farm's biosecurity is supported by a workable virus air filtration system.

An introduction programme should be written for all gilts and boars, and it then needs to be strictly implemented (*Table 11.4*).

Table 11.4 **Animal introduction programme SOP.**

ON ARRIVAL

First 2 weeks

1 Ensure animals are separate from native pigs for 2 weeks

2 Ideally separate by 50 metres

3 Attempt to acclimatise the animals to the new environment. Initially attempt to simulate the original environment. Make changes gradually

4 Pay particular attention to:
   • the cooling systems and water supply
   • if possible have bagged feed from original farm or make attempts to match original feed.
   • if pigs come from a straw based system, utilise straw or solid flooring before introducing to slatted systems

5 The animals may require antimicrobial or additional vaccine therapy following introduction. To introduce specific pathogen-negative gilts/boar into a pathogen-positive farm, attempts must be made to introduce the gilts/boar to the circulating farm pathogens. The method changes with pathogen.

2nd to 4th week post introduction

1 Introduce the farm's pathogens to the isolated gilts and boars by feedback programmes. Some farms will use farm animals, but adult animals are very poor shedders of pathogens

2 Change over the environment to match local conditions

3 It may be necessary to medicate the pigs depending on how they respond to the new diseases

4 Start vaccination programmes to pathogens such as parvovirus and *Erysipelothrix rhusiopathiae*. If possible, protect against pathogens before isolation starts. For example, in Asia, classical swine fever and foot and mouth disease vaccines (where applicable) can be administered at 10 weeks of age and will cover the gilt prior to moving into the isolation area.

4th to 8th week post introduction

   If introduced, remove grow/finish animals to allow the new pigs time to recover from any illness

Introduce into the herd

Record all signs of illness over the 8-week period

Table 11.5 **Typical distances a pathogen may move from a farm via airborne spread. The minimum expected spread from an acutely infected farm is highlighted in red.**

POSSIBLE DISTANCE SPREAD FROM AN ACUTELY INFECTED UNIT	ACTINOBACILLUS PLEUROPNEUMONIAE	AUJESZKY'S DISEASE VIRUS (PSEUDORABIES)	BRACHYSPIRA HYODYSENTERIAE	BRUCELLA SPP.	CLASSICAL AND AFRICAN SWINE FEVER VIRUSES	ESCHERICHIA COLI	FOOT AND MOUTH DISEASE VIRUS	LAWSONIA INTRACELLULARIS	LEPTOSPIRA SPP.	MYCOPLASMA HYOPNEUMONIAE	PASTEURELLA MULTOCIDA	PCV2-SD	PRRSV	SALMONELLOSIS	SARCOPTES SCABIEI – MANGE	SWINE INFLUENZA VIRUS	TGEV/PEDV
Less than 10 metres	■	■	■	■	■			■	■	■	■	■	■	■	■		■
10–50 metres		■	■	■	■			■	■	■	■	■	■	■			■
50 metres to 1 km		■			■		■		■	■		■	■	■		■	■
1–10 km					■		■			■			■			■	
More than 10 km					■		■										

Locality of the pig unit

If a pig unit is placed next door to another unit it is likely to share many of the same pathogens and diseases. However, the question is 'how far is safe?'

There is no specific answer as it depends on the pathogen. *Actinobacillus pleuropneumoniae* will be difficult to spread more than a few metres, whereas foot and mouth disease virus (FMDV) may spread 100 km or more. Common sense must prevail in the siting of any new farm and its isolation facility. Even the best placement of the farm can be compromised by the founding of a new farm adjacent to the original farm. *Table 11.5* indicates the distance of likely spread of various pathogens between pig units. The potential movement of smoke from a farm fire is shown in **Figure 11.9**.

Estimating the distance a pathogen may spread is always difficult. Some pathogens, such as *Escherichia coli*

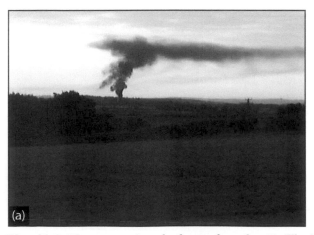
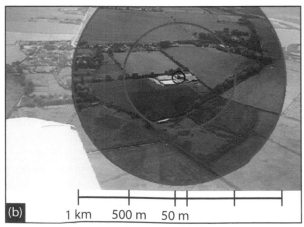

1 km   500 m   50 m

Fig. 11.9 Movement of smoke from a farm fire (a). The likely area of spread of the smoke is demonstrated in (b).

and *Salmonella* spp., are ubiquitous (everywhere). Other pathogens may be spread because they exist in wild animals and movement of the pathogen is dependent on these animals; *Lawsonia intracellularis* and *Brucella* spp. are examples. All the pathogens can be spread by pigs and, therefore, movement of feral pigs will transmit pathogens over their range. In addition, pathogens that are faeces borne and environmentally resistant (which may be seasonal) can be transmitted over vast distances; for example PRRSV: when winter gets below 0°C, the pathogen will survive in frozen faeces carried on boots or vehicles, potentially over hundreds of km. Pathogens such as *A. pleuropneumoniae* do not move far from the pig, and yet are present on almost all pig farms.

The farm may also become compromised by nonporcine species. The best designed isolated boar stud can become compromised by FMDV-positive sheep grazing the road side (**Figure 11.10**).

Mapping programmes and your smart phone are increasingly useful in providing the location of the farm and neighbours, wind directions and other climate conditions together with a GPS location. The American Association of Swine Veterinarians has a useful tool named PADRAP (Production Animal Disease Risk Assessment Program), which is designed to assess pathogen introduction risks. This programme assesses external and internal biosecurity risks.

As part of the on- and off-farm concept, the farm needs to clearly define its perimeter. The perimeter will vary depending on the site and what vehicles have access to the site.

Unit security

A set of rules regarding entry to the unit for animals and people is required. The rules illustrated in *Table 11.6* would be for a high health unit. Your own rules may be more or less than these.

Trucking and transportation rules

There are many trucks that visit a pig farm and an SOP is required for each (**Figure 11.11** and *Table 11.7*). Important trucks can be broken down into three major sections including those that deliver or remove livestock (including semen), those that deliver feed and those that deliver supplies.

Truck cleaning is an important area to monitor. For some pathogen control it may be necessary to heat the truck or use specific disinfectants. The use of bacterial surface test strips may be required to check that the truck is sufficiently clean, but first ensure that all the faecal materials are visibly removed. In very cold climates, antifreeze may have to be added to detergents.

Disposal of dead stock

The collection of dead stock by rendering trucks is potentially a serious risk to a farm (*Table 11.8* and **Figure 11.12**). Ideally, composting of all dead stock should be encouraged. However, composting is not legal in some areas of the world.

Clothing and equipment
Clothing from other units

Outer clothing from another farm is a serious pathogen transfer threat and ideally all off-farm clothing should be removed prior to entering the farm. Ensure that footwear is removed before entering the showering facilities. Showering facilities ensure that off-farm clothing is removed prior to entry to the farm. Disposable underwear for visitors greatly helps the practical implementation of these rules.

Needles, syringes and medicines

It is essential that equipment, needles, syringes and medicines are not shared between units.

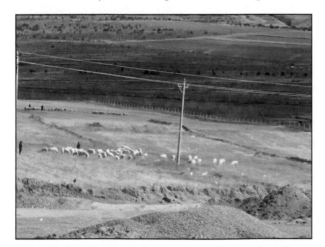

Fig. 11.10 Sheep grazing next to an isolated nucleus farm may pose a biosecurity risk for FMD.

Table 11.6 **Unit security.**

BASIC DESIGN

1	The unit must be surrounded by a complete fence
2	The fence should be 2.5 metres high and 0.5 metres deep to stop pigs and other mammals entering and leaving the unit
3	A car park should be sited away from the unit and appropriately marked
4	All entrances through the fence must be locked
5	All personal items including personal clothing, watches, cigarette lighters, cell phones etc. must remain outside the entrance area
6	Spectacles, cameras and other visitor equipment must be washed or enter through a UV chamber or be disposable and be inspected by a member of staff before being allowed onto the unit
7	All meters (electrical, gas and water) must be situated off-farm and placed in a locked area
8	The farm manager's office should be situated near the entrance
9	A horn switch should be placed by the car park to attract staff attention to visitors
10	None of the staff should own or come into contact with other pigs
11	No staff should visit animal markets, pig shows or slaughterhouses
12	No unauthorised pigs, pig products or pig faecal material must be allowed onto the farm
13	Unit rules regarding last pig contact must be strictly adhered too
14	All entry and exit points should be well lit, ideally with proximity sensors

THE FOLLOWING ENTRANCES/EXITS ARE PERMITTED

1	Entrance via a locked door into staff shower facility
2	Entrance via a locked door into a visitor shower facility
3	Connector to the feed bins allowing the feed bins to be filled from off-farm
4	Exit via a raised ramp for livestock
5	Exit for dead animal disposal through a locked gate
6	The straw barn has an entrance from off-farm and an entrance on-farm. Both should be kept locked. Staff are not allowed to leave the farm through the straw barn
7	Slurry disposal through underground pipe to slurry store off-farm

Table 11.7 **Loading ramp rules for animal movement.**

1	Trucks must have no pigs on board, must be clean, disinfected and dry
2	The off-farm disinfectant/washing area (see **Figure 11.11**) must be prepared prior to each loading by the unit staff (wearing off-unit clothing) and then they must re-enter the farm
3	The truck driver must inform a member of staff upon arrival
4	Truck drivers must wash their hands and wear over-boots (and possibly clothing) and dip their boots in the disinfectant provided
5	The truck driver's name and vehicle number should be logged in the animal movement book
6	Farm staff must not cross the security line or the loading ramp line of separation between vehicle and ramp
7	The loading ramp area must be thoroughly cleaned after loading each batch of pigs
8	The truck driver must not enter the the on-farm ramp to assist the loading
9	All entry and exit points should be well lit, ideally with proximity sensors
10	The sorting area and on-farm loading area must be thoroughly cleaned and disinfected once the pigs have arrived or left

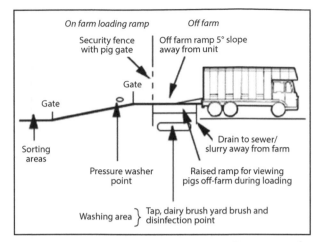

Fig. 11.11 Unit animal entry or exit loading protocol.

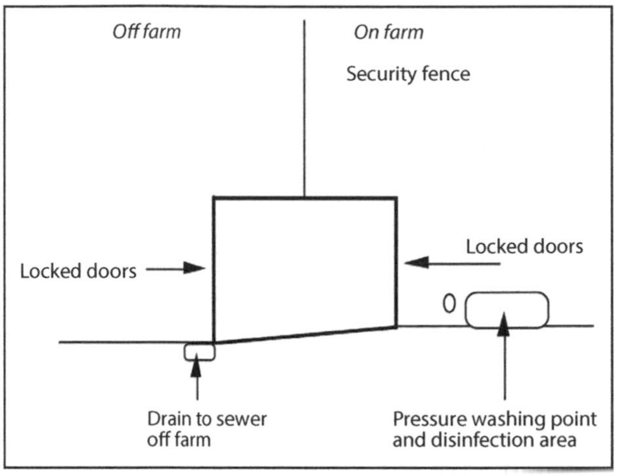

Fig. 11.12 Design of a dead pig area.

Table 11.8 **Disposal of a dead pig SOP.**
1	When a dead animal is identified it should be recorded
2	The farm manager should decide if a post-mortem examination is required
3	The animal should be removed from the house as soon as possible
4	The animal should be moved to the perimeter fence dead area
5	The dead pig area should be designed as shown in **Figure 11.12**
6	Once the dead pigs are removed by the rendering company the dead box should be pressure washed and disinfected
7	The dead box should be emptied at least once a week, twice in the summer months
8	Cover cuts and abrasions when handling sick or dead pigs
9	Always wash your hands after handling sick or dead pigs
10	The rendering truck must not have any other dead pigs on board prior to arrival. Only reputable rendering companies with properly constructed trucks should be utilised

Equipment purchase

All equipment that is going to come into contact with the animals must be purchased new and with no previous contact with animals. All equipment must look new on arrival and be clean otherwise entry to the farm must be refused. On no account must equipment be shared between farms.

Other animals

Birds, rodents, cats, dogs, flies

Control programmes must be written and implemented to reduce and ideally prevent the introduction and maintenance of other animals on a pig farm (*Table 11.9*).

Production of an SOP does not by itself reduce the rodent population. The veterinarian has to work continually by checking that the rules are understood and implemented by the whole farm team (**Figure 11.14**). For example, at each visit check the bait points and that they actually contain bait (**Figure 11.15**).

Feed and water

Feed and all feed ingredients must come from known sources and effective control of food-borne diseases such as salmonellosis implemented. Drinking water quality is important and the source should be routinely checked for possible contamination, or mains water should be used. In areas where surface water is used, it should be treated with chlorine dioxide, hydrogen peroxide or ultraviolet light. Routine analysis should be conducted to insure pathogen inactivation is being achieved.

Table 11.9 Protocol required to provide rodent control.

1	Rodents do not like exposed situations. Remove all rubbish and overgrown vegetation from outside the buildings. All buildings should be surrounded by a 1 metre wide concrete walkway or crushed rock. Remove all weeds and grass
2	Ensure all bagged feed is stacked tidily on pallets off the floor and at least 0.35 metres from the walls
3	Food must be stored in closed containers
4	All spilt food under feed bins must be swept up and discarded in designated area
5	All rubbish must be placed in rodent proof containers
6	Block all holes wherever possible. Wire mesh on windows must be 6 mm to keep out mice. Seal junctions between walls, floors and ceilings with metal sheeting
7	Seal water cisterns and header tanks
8	Cats and dogs are not to be used as rodent control as they are a health risk to the pigs (e.g. Aujeszky's disease and toxoplasmosis)
9	Prepare a map of the farm and examine for evidence of rats. Examine at least 100 metres around the farm
10	On the map mark out the position of the permanent baits and where clearance baits are to be placed (**Figure 11.13**). Bait stations should be located every 15 metres externally and internally of the facility
11	Clearance baits Check baits every week and continue baiting for one week after baits have stopped being taken
12	Permanent baits Check baits every 2 weeks. If signs of feeding are found replenish the bait and re-survey the premises. Place baits in drainpipes placed at the base of straw
13	Burn all dead rodents found and all unused clearance bait boxes
14	Prevent access to the bait by children and other animals
15	Wear impervious gloves when handling dead rodents and baits
16	Wash your hands thoroughly after handling baits or rodents
17	Operator must be familiar with the safety rules for the rodenticide/baits being used
18	Empty rodenticide/bait containers must not be reused for any purpose
19	In buildings that can be sealed, fumigation may be effective to reduce a serious infestation to controllable levels

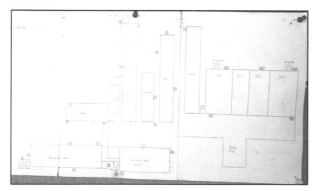

Fig. 11.13 Farm map with the various rodent control bait points marked as blue dots.

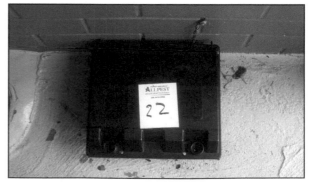

Fig. 11.14 Numbering rodent bait points and having a farm map is an essential component of compliance.

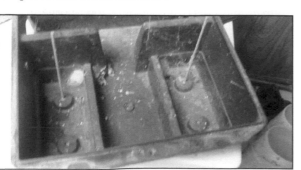

Fig. 11.15 Rodent bait points need to have bait to attract rodents.

Bedding

Bedding represents a critical risk to the farm's biosecurity from potential contamination from applied animal wastes, wildlife contamination, transport contamination and impracticality of disinfection. Any bedding used on the farm must come from approved sources. A system of storage in a vermin-free shed maintained at ambient temperatures may be most practical.

Staff and other people

Humans are often considered to be the biggest risk, but there are very few zoonotic pathogens from humans to pigs and thus humans actually are of very low risk to a pig farm. Humans can act as a vector if they do not practice reasonable hygiene.

Staff should not have access to other pigs and no uncooked pig products, including pizza, ham or salami sandwiches for instance, should ever come onto the unit. Farms should supply clothing and boots for all visitors. Showering is an excellent tool to minimise risks as it requires total disrobing, washing of body and hair and using clothes that are part of the farm.

Showering and clothing

For facilities that do not have showers, farm-supplied clothing is an absolute requirement. A designated area where personal clothing is removed and farm clothing and boots are provided should be created. This can be made easier by the use of different coloured boots and overalls (**Figures 11.16–11.19**). Veterinarians should not move clothing and boots between farms, irrespective of how well they are cleaned.

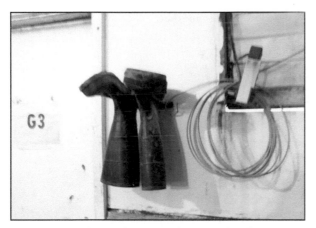

Fig. 11.16 **Change foot wear between batches.**

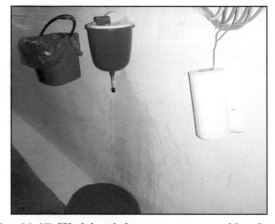

Fig. 11.17 **Wash hands between rooms and batches. Use gloves if pigs are sick, especially diarrhoea.**

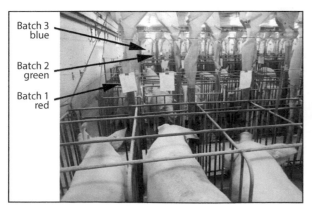

Fig. 11.18 **Some farms colour code the records to ensure dirty records are not moved between batches.**

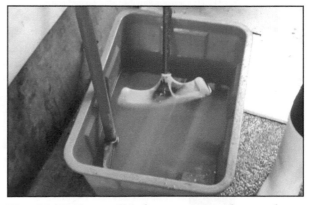

Fig. 11.19 **Ensure disinfectants are used properly.**

DEVELOPMENT OF INTERNAL FARM BIOSECURITY

Once on the farm the veterinarian can play a vital role in enhancing internal farm biosecurity. Three areas where the veterinarian can train and instruct the farm team are described below.

Multi-site production – development of all-in/all-out

Multi-site pig production systems are now well established. They utilise breaks in the production from the gilt development, breeding/gestation/farrowing to weaning, then the wean to finish (sometimes split into wean to grower and then grower to finish facilities). This development from family farm to corporate is illustrated in **Figure 11.20**. However, AIAO is only achieved by batch farrowing, which strictly and accurately controls the size of each batch, thus pig flow.

This model has now evolved into parity segregation models (**Figure 11.21**). A parity segregated system offers the best biosecurity options. In addition, because the offspring of gilts have a poorer immune status than those of multiparity sows, they should also be housed separately.

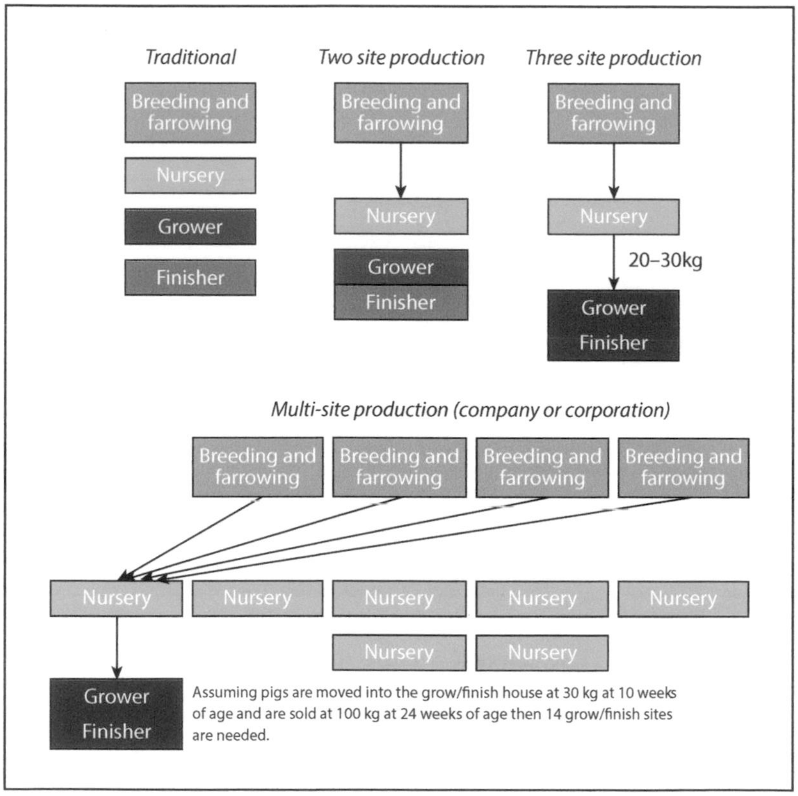

Fig. 11.20 The traditional farm has evolved into separated production sites to facilitate AIAO batches. The arrows indicate where pigs leave one site and move to another.

Fig. 11.21 Parity segregation models.

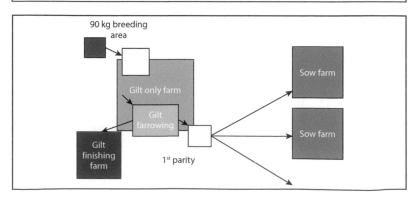

Intra-farm batch equipment

The farm's batches can be further separated from the rest of the farm by using colour coding (**Figures 11.22–11.25**). Then each area, for example the pig farrowing area, has a specific brush and shovel. This has significantly reduced the prevalence of neonatal diarrhoea problems.

Wearing different boots in each area also reduces the risk of pathogen transfer by reduction of faecal transmission via the boots. Having different coloured boots reduces the risk of human error. Boots are important because the first thing pigs will do when the stockperson enters their pen is lick the boots and overalls and they are particularly attracted to organic materials such as faeces (**Figures 11.26, 11.27**).

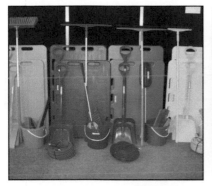

Fig. 11.22 Different coloured equipment can be used to further separate batches and age groups.

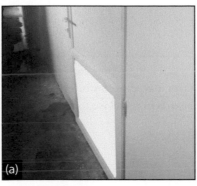

Fig. 11.23 (a, b) The yellow equipment is only used in the yellow room. All equipment is numbered.

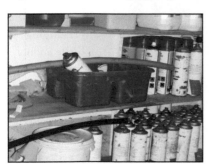

Fig. 11.24 Medicines and equipment can be moved around; the blue tray is for the farrowing area only.

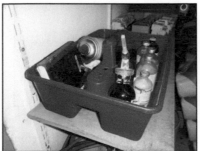

Fig. 11.25 Medicines in a red tray are for the nursery area only. Other colours indicate other departments.

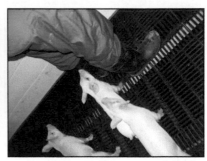

Fig. 11.26 Pigs pay particular interest to the boots.

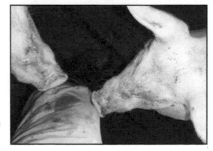

Fig. 11.27 Pigs love licking organic material off overalls.

Examples of biosecurity problems on pig farms

Location of the farm
See **Figures 11.28–11.30**.

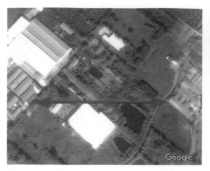

Fig. 11.28 Farms are too close, but this also depends on which pathogens require control.

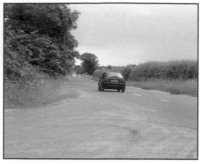

Fig. 11.29 Major road next to the farm may allow for infected pigs to be driven too close to the unit.

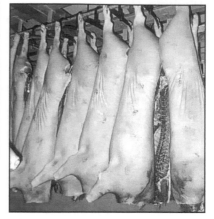

Fig. 11.30 Farms near a slaughterhouse will have an increased number of off-farm pigs driving past the farm.

Perimeter of the farm
See **Figures 11.31–11.35**.

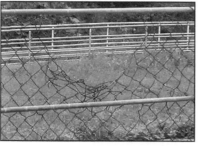

Fig. 11.31 Damaged fencing caused by children gaining access to the farm.

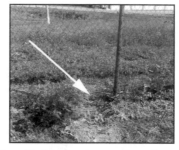

Fig. 11.32 Fencing not into the ground. Pigs will burrow, therefore fencing needs to be buried (arrow) otherwise wild pigs can gain access.

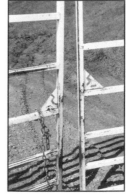

Fig. 11.33 Gates unlocked. Hanging the chains around the gate does not lock the gate or restrict access.

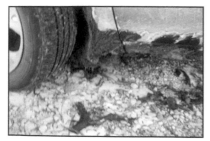

Fig. 11.34 Vehicles transporting snow, especially in the wheel hub area. PRRSV and *Brachyspira hyodysenteriae* can be easily transported in snow and ice.

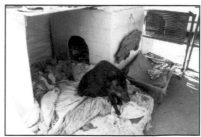

Fig. 11.35 Feral pig adopted as a pet making itself at home. There was a commercial pig farm within 1 km.

Visitor security
See **Figures 11.36–11.38**.

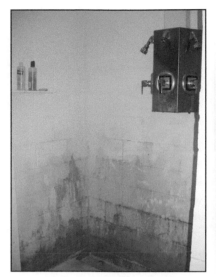

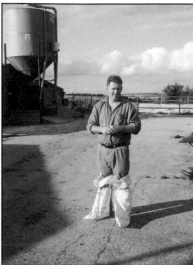

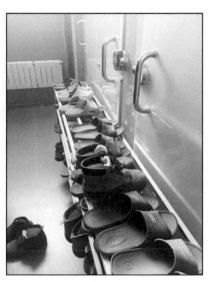

Fig. 11.36 The shower has to have running hot and cold water with soap. If the shower is cold, dirty and unattractive, visitors will be reluctant to shower adequately.

Fig. 11.37 No unit clothing. If the unit does not provide unit clothing, whatever pathogens are alive on your outer clothing will gain access to the pigs.

Fig. 11.38 Different styles and colours of boots can assist the AIAO programme.

Equipment
See **Figure 11.39**.

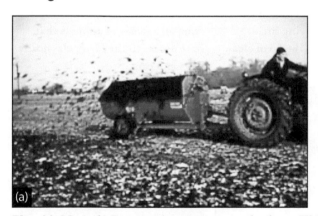

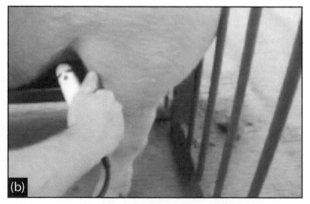

Fig. 11.39 (a, b) Borrowed equipment on the farm. This can be a very neighbourly thing to do. Slurry dispersal systems are classic examples. In the event of major pathogens being involved, such as FMDV, the government should consider both farms as one unit.

Internal biosecurity
See **Figures 11.40–11.53**.

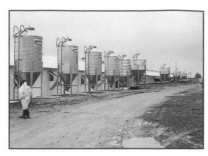

Fig. 11.40 No feed security. To fill the feed bins, the truck has to drive right up to the feeders. Movement of pigs into the buildings utilises the same roadway.

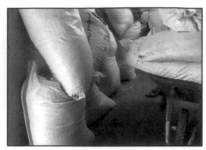

Fig. 11.41 Food stored on floor. This is a major rodent risk as well as the food becoming damp and increasing the risk of moulds. Feed bags themselves are high risk and mechanical handling of feed or transfer from bags should occur.

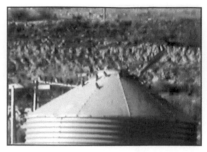

Fig. 11.42 Poor food bin management. The feed bin lids were left open and birds were able to gain access to the food storage, resulting in an outbreak of salmonellosis on the unit.

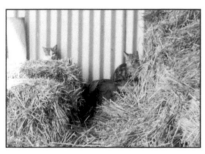

Fig. 11.43 Poor bedding storage with poor understanding of vermin control.

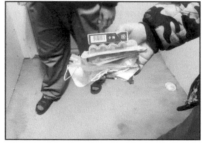

Fig. 11.44 Poor personal hygiene by the farm staff having little respect for keeping the farm clean and tidy.

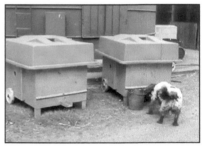

Fig. 11.45 Be aware of the risk from all species of animals that have access to the farm, classically dogs and cats.

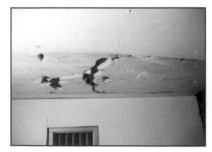

Fig. 11.46 Rodent damage clearly evident. The insulation has been eaten away by rodents.

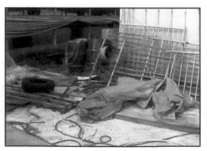

Fig. 11.47 Rodent control poor. It is impossible to have rodent control on farms with poor litter control.

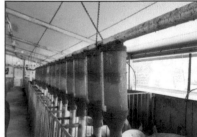

Fig. 11.48 Bird control poor. Birds were entering the building, eating feed and potentially bringing pathogens into the building.

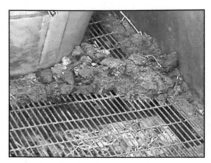

Fig. 11.49 Poor cleaning between batches. This outside weaner arc was supposed to be cleaned and ready for the next batch of pigs.

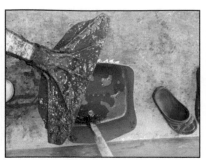

Fig. 11.50 No inter-room bio-security. When attempting to ensure biosecurity between rooms, make sure that scrapers and brushes are individually marked. The equipment must be clean before it is disinfected. You cannot disinfect faeces.

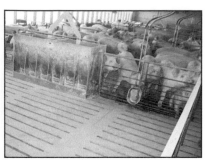

Fig. 11.51 No AIAO. The nursery shown did not practice AIAO and the farm has empty pens, a serious loss of revenue.

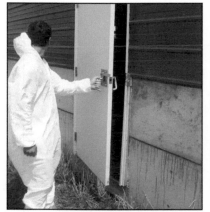

Fig. 11.52 Poor door security, especially any door that leads to off-farm.

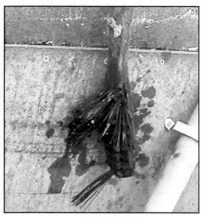

Fig. 11.53 Poor boot cleaning facilities. You cannot clean boots with a brush with no bristles.

Fallen stock management
See **Figures 11.54–11.58**.

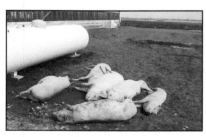

Fig. 11.54 Dead animals around the farm. It is not acceptable to just throw out the dead. This would encourage dogs and cats to the unit – an Aujeszky's disease risk.

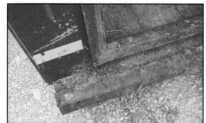

Fig. 11.55 Poor vehicle biosecurity. Vehicles are a major biosecurity risk and need their own security protocols.

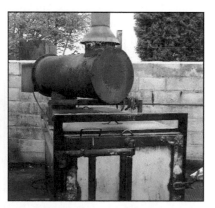

Fig. 11.56 Poor incinerator management. There are rules covering the use and handling of incinerators and these need to be carefully followed.

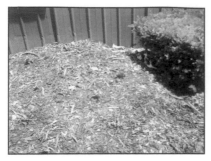

Fig. 11.57 Poor placement of a composting pile. Composting is a useful method of animal control. However, do not place too close to buildings or fly control can be poor.

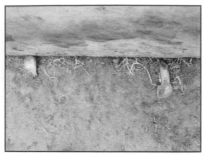

Fig. 11.58 Poor composting management. If the compost pile is not correctly managed to achieve animal decomposition, animal remains may attract dogs and cats, who can carry materials from the farm.

Other livestock on the farm
See **Figures 11.59–11.62**.

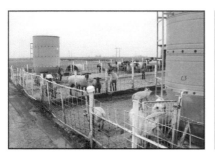

Fig. 11.59 The presence of other animals poses their own specific risks. Foot and mouth disease would be one obvious risk. Sheep running loose to keep the grass short around pig buildings may die from eating rodent bait.

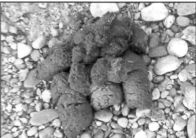

Fig. 11.60 Look for clear evidence of other animal's access to the farm. These stool samples come from raccoons that can carry rabies.

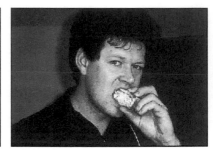

Fig. 11.61 Human food, in particular pork products, should not be present on farms as they pose a risk for classical and African swine fever as well as foot and mouth disease.

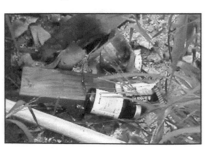

Fig. 11.62 Medicines disposal systems should be reviewed. This image demonstrates a lack of care and concern by the farm staff.

Isolation facilities
See **Figure 11.63–11.65**.

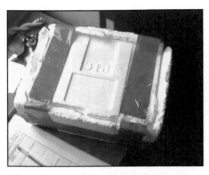

Fig. 11.63 AI box – broken and dirty. If an AI box arrives at the farm broken, there has been a biosecurity breach as well as possible semen storage problems.

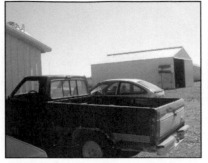

Fig. 11.64 Isolation too close. An isolation area should be at least 50 metres away from the main unit. This isolation area was only 10 metres away – *Mycoplasma hyopneumoniae* and PRRSV could not be controlled.

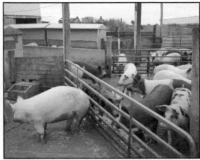

Fig. 11.65 No isolation available. Many commercial farms have no isolation facility available. The farmer simply hopes that the source farm is safe.

Transport systems (see also specific figures in previous sections)
See **Figures 11.66–11.68**.

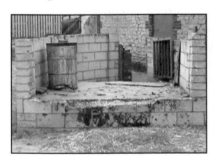

Fig. 11.66 There is no specific loading area. The area shown is not secure and is dirty. Entry and exit areas need to be clean.

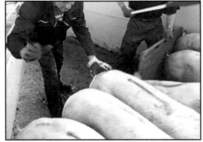

Fig. 11.67 On some farms there is no loading area, they just take their chance. Note that the driver and stockperson are loading the pigs, which provides direct contamination between the slaughterhouse and the farm.

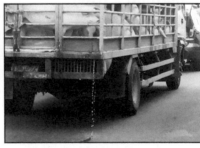

Fig. 11.68 Trucks should avoid getting too close to other trucks. Be aware of cafés and other truck stops. Note the slurry pouring off the back of the truck and thus contaminating the tailgating truck's wheels.

Staff issues
See **Figures 11.69–11.71**.

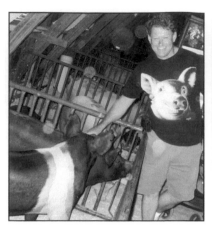

Fig. 11.69 If you visit a market, you have to adhere to the normal 'visitor' biosecurity rules.

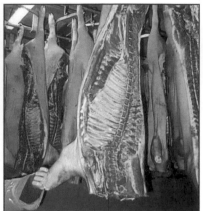

Fig. 11.70 When visiting a slaughterhouse, it is essential to practice advanced entry precautions on your return to the farm.

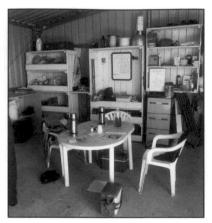

Fig. 11.71 Poor staff room. Practice tidy home rules in the staff room. There are zoonotic diseases of pigs that could infect staff.

REDUCING THE PATHOGEN LOAD ON A PIG FARM

Cleaning a room

It is often forgotten that the key to reducing the pathogen load in a building is simply being able to clean the room properly. *Table 11.10* illustrates an SOP used to teach and ensure that the cleaning protocols are properly followed by the farm health team. Cleaning has seven components:

- Preparation – removing animals and feed.
- Soaking.
- Detergent (often missed).
- High-pressure washing. Hot water wash.
- Partial drying.
- Disinfection.
- Terminal drying.

All-in/all-out programmes ⏵ VIDEO 46

AIAO needs good pig flow and must have even pig numbers between each batch. AIAO is not only about pigs and floors, but also includes air, feed, water and veterinary supplies.

Achieving AIAO is the key to current farming programmes. AIAO can be simply defined as 'pigs do not enter a building before the building is totally emptied of pigs and cleaned and prepared'.

The principles appear simple, but in practice farms seem unable to achieve AIAO. The first requirement is to understand the animal flow on a pig farm. Farms often grow either by increasing sow inventory or improving output, and unfortunately the growth is generally not coordinated. This results in production in one department (nursery for example) being greater than can be legally accommodated in the next phase (finishing in this example). As the production flow increases it becomes more challenging to compensate for the normal growth decline that occurs in hot summer months, making it difficult to allow adequate time for cleaning and drying.

While the industry considers AIAO to be about animals and properly cleaned buildings, in reality it is about the whole area (i.e. buildings, equipment and medicines) (**Figure 11.72**).

AIAO must start in the farrowing area; you cannot do it in only one part of the farm. AIAO cannot be achieved without a well-constructed batching pig

Table 11.10 **Room cleaning SOP suggestion.**

PREPARATION

1	Remove all the animals from the building
2	Ideally all feed should have been eaten by the previous occupants. Remove all remaining feed from the room
3	Dismantle as many movable objects as possible and remove from the room
4	Isolate all electrics. Ideally, all electrics should be encased in a box within the room. Comply with current Health and Safety Recommendations

PRE-CLEANING

1	Turn off the water supply that goes into the room or the header tank
2	Remove end drinker and drain water supply
3	Remove accumulations of dirt from the water supply, especially header tanks, if used
4	Re-fit the end drinker. Restore the water supply to the room and add disinfectant
5	The dung channels should be drained and emptied. This should include all large faecal accumulations, tanks and gullies
6	All old or blistered paint work on animal housing should be smoothed down with a wire brush
7	Remove cobwebs by brushing and all other material either by brushing it into the slats or picking it up using a shovel
8	Repair any broken pieces of equipment/housing
9	Place a water sprinkler in the room attached to an external water supply, close doors and soak room for at least 1 hour or even overnight. Note any problem with the electrics etc. that may arise. If soaking is not possible, move to the next section

CLEANING OF ALL REMOVABLE OBJECTS

1	All removed drinkers and feed troughs should be cleaned out thoroughly so that all food and faecal material is removed
2	All removed items should be soaked in water for 5 minutes
3	Spray detergent using low-pressure washing (2 mPa) or the foam gun application at a concentration of 2%
4	Allow detergent contact time of 30 minutes; do not allow surfaces to dry
5	Thoroughly wash down with hot water using a pressure washer set at 3.5 mPa
6	All creep light fittings should be thoroughly cleaned. Beware that bulbs may blow if they are hot and water is splashed on them
7	Disinfect all utensils by soaking in disinfectant for 1 hour if possible; otherwise apply disinfectant using a knapsack sprayer or pressure washer set at 2 mPa
8	Allow all utensils time to thoroughly dry

CLEANING THE ROOM

1	When the room is ready, spray with detergent using a low-pressure washer (2 mPa) or the foam gun application
2	Allow detergent contact time of 30 minutes; do not allow surfaces to dry
3	Pressure wash the house using hot water and a pressure washer set at 3.5–10.3 mPa with a 45-degree angle jet. Pressure washing is a very labour intensive job and particular effort must be made on all surfaces below pig height. However, surfaces above pig height must also be washed. Using hot or steam washing can reduce the time of the operation compared with cold water washing
4	Prior to entering the room with a pressure washer, ensure that the operator is properly trained and clothed. Wear waterproofs, goggles and gloves and any additional equipment as required by Health and Safety. Electrically operated pressure washers should not be connected in the room to be washed.
5	Start at the apex of the room and work down the walls to the floor, paying particular attention to corners and other areas where dirt accumulates. Caked soiling should be brushed if necessary to aid removal
6	If the slats can be easily raised, wash the undersurface of the slats to ensure that faecal material does not remain underneath slats within reach of pigs' tongues
7	Store pressure washer and equipment clean. Ensure that the washer is stored so that it is protected from frost during the winter months

(Continued)

Table 11.10 *(Continued)* **Room cleaning SOP suggestion.**

RE-BUILDING THE ROOM

1	Remove end drinker and drain disinfectant/water
2	Re-fit the end drinker. Restore the water supply and check that all the drinkers work
3	Allow the house to dry for 2 hours, then disinfect using a knapsack sprayer or a pressure washer set at 2 mPa with a 45-degree spray head
4	Spray into the apex of the roof and work down the walls to the floors
5	Open up all the ventilation systems and maximise air flow through the building for at least 2 hours to completely change the air in the building
6	Allow the room to dry completely, using additional heaters if necessary before pigs are placed in the room
7	Make sure that there are no residues of disinfectant around before rehousing pigs
8	Ensure room environment is satisfactory for the pigs before they enter the room
9	Place a foot bath filled with disinfectant outside the room. Practice colour coding batch room biosecurity

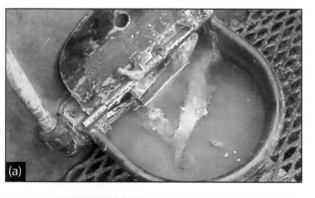
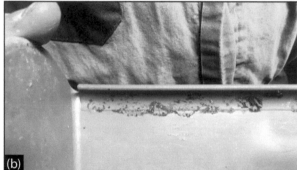
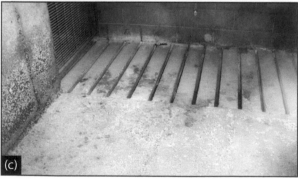
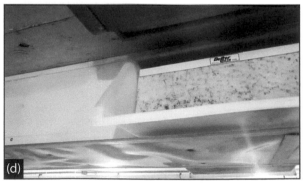

Fig. 11.72 Poor AIAO. (a) Water; (b) food; (c) floor; (d) air.

flow model. The farrowing stage is challenging as the normal gestation length is 112–120 days unless intervention occurs by inducing sows to farrow or stockpersons moving sows between rooms before they farrow to keep the room times tight.

Normal gestation lengths

One issue with gestation length is that it starts with a human intervention (mating) and not reality, which is ovulation. Therefore, gestation lengths are farm specific (**Figure 11.73**).

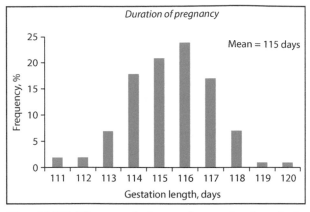

Fig. 11.73 **The spread of normal gestation lengths in the pig.**

The rationale behind AIAO is that when a problem occurs during one batch it does not spread to the next batch. However, this depends on the pathogens involved. AIAO is not:

- In over a time period.
- Almost all out before in.
- All in, plus a few more later.
- All-in, but variable numbers per batch.
- Some this week, some the next week and some the week after, but then AIAO.
- Continuous flow farrowing, but AIAO nursery and then continuous flow finishing (or any variant of the above).

Designing and implementing a batching pig flow model

The easiest pig flow model to design is when the farm is still on the drawing board. The aim of pig farming is to achieve production at the best cost, given the opportunities. Maintaining health contributes significantly to reducing the cost of production and the only way to resolve and maintain health is to achieve AIAO.

Pig farming is about perfecting the art of repetition. Unfortunately, the pig industry will cheat on AIAO (from time to time) and then hopes to 'get away' without issues. However, nature has a way of making the farm pay. The more cheating that occurs, the more desperate cleaning protocols become, rooms are not rested and the pigs are overstocked or understocked; continuous flow or the equally ludicrous all-out only programme starts. Health issues then occur,

resulting in failure of growth and ventilation systems. The farm is on a negative health spiral.

Farms generally need to take a long hard look at their layout and design a layout that will:

- Allow for buildings to have at least a 24-hour rest between groups/batches, repeatable 52 weeks of the year
- Produce repeatable outputs in meat supply (52 weeks of the year). To allow for possible summer infertility issues the sow herd size should change over the year, being bigger in summer and smaller in winter. Therefore, farm assessments using 'pigs/sow/year' have no significance in real cost control measures.
- Predict gilt requirements and thus allow batch breeding targets to be set and easily reached (52 weeks of the year), making allowances for summer infertility issues.
- Minimise cost of production.
- Create discipline and understanding of the needs of the farm by the stockpersons.
- Produce a farm that is socially acceptable in terms of stockpersons' time and holidays.
- Produce a farm that is legal within the area the farm is located and the requirements of the slaughterhouse.

Of course new farms are a novelty. Farms grow and perhaps the farm was built with an ideal pig flow. With time new buildings are added, generally without pig flow being a consideration. The chaos then builds up.

All-in/all-out – the only magic in the medicine box

To run a pig farm by AIAO ideals allows:

- For the pathogens of the previous batch to be reduced in number before the next batch of pigs enter the room.
- For the rooms to be maintained and fixed.

All farms batch

Many producers think that batching is just a term used by small farms. However, to achieve AIAO farms must batch; it is just the batch time interval that varies. Although many batch intervals are possible, the most common intervals are weekly, or at 2, 3, 4 or 5 week intervals.

Which weaning age should I pick?

Within the European Union, there is little real choice as it is not legal to wean before 28 days of age unless specialised accommodation for pigs older than 21 days can be provided. Weaning age is a balance between regulations, reproductive output, wean to finish performance and facility costs. The goal is to maintain a balanced system that optimises value throughout the systems. Research suggests that a 0.5 kg heavier pig at weaning will result in a 2 kg heavier pig at slaughter in the same number of growing days post weaning. The weaning age should be determined by the quality of the nursery and available feeds. Genetic lines vary but in general a lactation shorter than 19 days reduces parity 1 sow production, lactations shorter than 17 days reduce parity 2 sow production; if parity 1 and 2 sows are added up this is half the females in a normal parity structure herd. Sows older than parity 3 do not generally suffer a production reduction with short lactations. Outside of the EU, restrictions on weaning age are not mandatory, but the veterinarian should confirm any local government requirements.

One way to assess if a farm weaning weekly is adopting a formal AIAO programme is to examine the average weaning age. Many textbooks and papers discuss increasing weaning age by a day or two and the advantages this will invoke in your herd, but with weekly weaning the weaning age can only move by 7 whole days, unless you change the day of the week you wean, which farms generally do not do.

Designing a pig flow model

Where should you start? What about using a 100 sow or 1,000 sow farm and then you can scale up or down by size?

The slaughter weight and thus the finishing floor area should be the starting point. Unfortunately, many farms adopt a variety of finishing systems with different sizes and pen layouts. In addition, many farms have no idea of the size of the unobstructed floor area available for their pigs. Therefore, in practice, the farrowing area is a good start and allows the farm to at least achieve AIAO to the point of weaning. If you do not practice AIAO by weaning, you do not practice AIAO anywhere.

What matters in the farrowing area?

To adopt an AIAO programme the farm needs to create equal batches of sows within a recognised time period ('the batch'). The farm therefore needs to know:

- How many farrowing places are present on the farm?
- How many farrowing rooms/air spaces are present on the farm?
- How the farrowing places are distributed within these rooms/air spaces?

Should I wean twice a week or every 5 weeks?

The answer to this question should be determined by the flow, which allows for the maximum AIAO programme (*Table 11.11*).

With the 0.5 week system it is possible to reduce the room number; however, this does compromise the sow pre-farrowing by reducing cleaning time, but reduces cost.

A 'room' is defined as the space taken by all the air spaces required for one batch. For example, one batch may farrow in two air spaces of 10 farrowing places, whereas the next batch is one air space of 20 farrowing places. This can be illustrated graphically (**Figure 11.74**). In all the Tables the following colour codes apply:

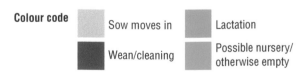

Colour code — Sow moves in | Lactation | Wean/cleaning | Possible nursery/otherwise empty

Table 11.11 **Number of rooms required to allow for all-in/all-out.**

BATCH TIME	0.5	1 WEEK	10 DAYS	2 WEEKS	3 WEEKS	4 WEEKS	5 WEEKS
Weaning age							
20 days	8 (7)	4		2		1	
27 days	10 (9)	5	2		3		1

Note: Several models will not work over the 52 calendar weeks or groups do not align. For example, biology cannot be cheated; a mated sow will farrow 115 days later and needs a farrowing place to be available. With the 0.5 week batch, if sows are moved into the room at the point of farrow, a room/time can be saved.

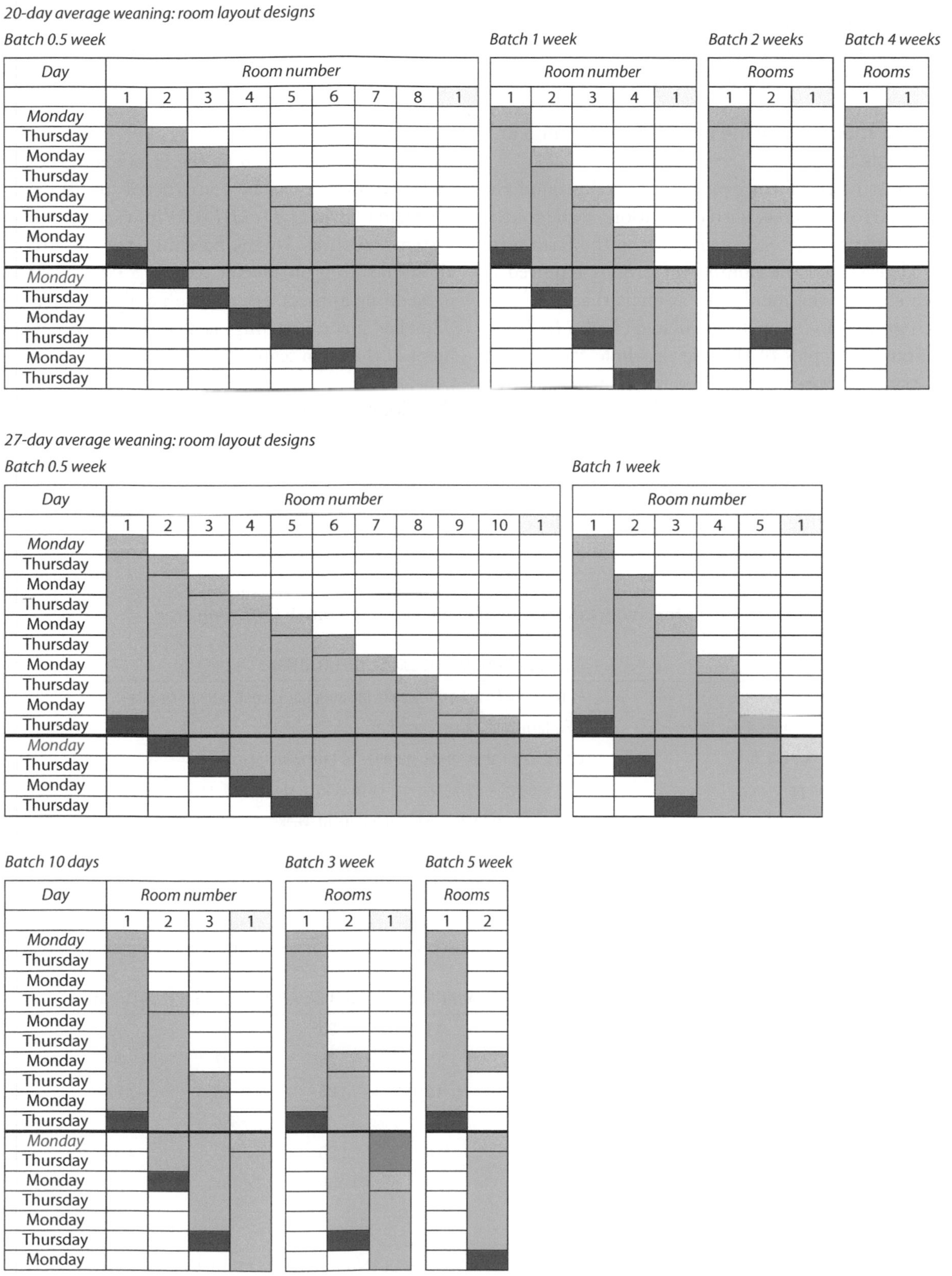

20-day average weaning: room layout designs

Batch 0.5 week

Day	Room number								
	1	2	3	4	5	6	7	8	1
Monday									
Thursday									
Monday									
Thursday									
Monday									
Thursday									
Monday									
Thursday									
Monday									
Thursday									
Monday									
Thursday									
Monday									
Thursday									

Batch 1 week

Room number				
1	2	3	4	1

Batch 2 weeks

Rooms		
1	2	1

Batch 4 weeks

Rooms	
1	1

27-day average weaning: room layout designs

Batch 0.5 week

Day	Room number										
	1	2	3	4	5	6	7	8	9	10	1
Monday											
Thursday											
Monday											
Thursday											
Monday											
Thursday											
Monday											
Thursday											
Monday											
Thursday											
Monday											
Thursday											
Monday											
Thursday											

Batch 1 week

Room number					
1	2	3	4	5	1

Batch 10 days

Day	Room number			
	1	2	3	1
Monday				
Thursday				
Monday				
Thursday				
Monday				
Thursday				
Monday				
Thursday				
Monday				
Thursday				
Monday				
Thursday				
Monday				
Thursday				
Monday				
Thursday				
Monday				

Batch 3 week

Rooms		
1	2	1

Batch 5 week

Rooms	
1	2

Fig. 11.74 **Different weaning room layout designs for different batch options. Note: 20-day average weaning is illegal within the European Union.**

The plans are designed around Monday and Thursday weaning for the 0.5 week batch and Thursday weaning for the other batch models.

Pig flow models from the batch farrowing area to the whole farm

The rest of the farm can be designed around the batch farrowing area, with estimations made for the space required for each group. Once the farm team has determined the number of groups required in each section, the number of animals that will be in each group can be easily calculated (*Table 11.12*).

Some examples of the use of whole farm model predications based on the batch farrowing area are shown in *Table 11.13*. The calculations are based on the following assumptions:

- 12 weaned per batch farrowing place;
- 82% farrowing rate;

- 95% finishing rate[*];
- 9-week gilt introduction programme using a one week batch programme.

Pig flow calendars

Once a model is agreed by the farm team, then calendars of events can be constructed for all parts of the farm (*Tables 11.14, 11.15*). With various batching systems, such as 3-week batching, this programme allows farming on specific days (e.g. Christmas Day or wedding anniversaries) to be a quiet day each year. This has made batching part of the social development of the farm team (*Table 11.16*).

Developing a farm model

To explain the pig flow around the farm, visual farm models can be devised. Google Earth produces great farm maps, which can then be used to illustrate pig flow (**Figure 11.75**).

Table 11.12 **Minimum targets for whole farm production based on the batch farrowing area.**

ANIMAL GROUP	CALCULATION (USING EXCEL NOTATIONS)
Gilts pool requirement	= (BF/10) × (number of weeks introduction)/batch time in weeks
Breeding females required per batch	= FS/farrowing rate (round up)
Farrowing sows per batch	Visual calculation of the number of farrowing places
Numbers weaned per batch	= FS × numbers weaned per farrowing place (round down)
Numbers sold per batch	= WB/finishing rate × 52/batch time in weeks (round down)

BF, breeding females required per batch; FS, farrowing sows per batch; WB, numbers weaned per batch.

Table 11.13 **Examples of the use of the whole farm model predications based on the batch farrowing area.**

	MINIMUM NUMBER OF ANIMALS IN EACH CATEGORY					
Gilts pool requirement	6	11	20	30	40	49
Breeding females required per batch	7	13	25	37	49	61
Farrowing sows per batch	**5**	**10**	**20**	**30**	**40**	**50**
Numbers weaned per batch	60	120	240	360	480	600
Numbers sold per batch	57	114	228	342	456	570
Numbers sold annually	2,964	5,928	11,856	17,784	23,712	29,640

---

[*] The 'finishing rate' is the percentage of weaned pigs that have a saleable value (**Note:** Farming 10-batch farrowing places every week is approximately a 250 sow unit.)

Table 11.14 **Calendar of daily events in the adult herd. The example herd used a 3-week batch, 27-day weaning programme. The group identification (number) starts with the breeding/service group and ends with the finished pigs at market.**

2017		BATCH TIME 3 weeks			WEANING AGE 27 days					
MONTH		MONDAY	TUESDAY		WEDNESDAY	THURSDAY		FRIDAY		SATURDAY	SUNDAY
EVENT	W	D	D	SERVICE G	D	D	WEAN G	D	FARROW G	D	D
January	1	2	3	S1	4	5		6		7	8
	2	9	10		11				F3	14	15
	3	16	17		18	19	W2	20		21	22
	4	23	24	S2	25	26		27		28	29
	5	30	31		1	2		3	F4	4	5
February	6	6	7		8	9	W3	10		11	12
	7	13	14	S3	15	16		17		18	19
	8	20	21		22	23		24	F5	25	26
	9	27	28		1	2	W4	3		4	5

W, week; D, day; G, group number.

Table 11.15 **Weekly events in the grow/finish herd in the same herd as in Table 11.14. The numbers in the Table indicate which group of pigs are at which weight; group identification starts with the breeding sows and gilts at mating.**

2017					BATCH TIME 3 weeks	WEAN 4 weeks	
MONTH		10 week	12 week	15 week	20 week	24 week	
EVENT	W	30 kg	45 kg	60 kg	95 kg	110 kg	
January	1	G6					
	2				G3		
	3		G6	G5		G1	
	4	G7					
	5				G4		
February	6		G7	G6		G2	
	7	G1					
	8				G5		
	9		G1	G7		G3	

W, week; G, group number.

Changing the weaning day

Some farms have changed to weaning on a Monday to allow for the most attention to be given to the newly weaned pig's growth and socialisation, accommodating the larger weaning numbers per batch farrowing place (*Table 11.17*). This also allows farrowing to occur without inducing during the working week.

Table 11.16 **Calendar of events for stockperson routines around a pig flow model. The Table indicates which group of pigs require a specific task. This work sheet is designed for weaning once every 3 weeks at 27 days of age.**

TASK\WEEK	1	2	3	4	5	6	7	8	9	10	11	12	13	14	15	16	17	18	19	20	21	22	23	24	25	26
Move wean sows		2			3			4			5			6			7			1			2			
Breed	1			2			3			4			5			6			7			1			2	
Heat check 1	7			1			2			3			4			5			6			7			1	
Heat check 2		7			1			2			3			4			5			6			7			1
Condition score sows		+		+		+		+		+		+		+		+		+		+		+		+		
Vaccinate 1 (6 weeks)	5			6			7			1			2			3			4			5			6	
Vaccinate 2 (3 weeks)	4			5			6			7			1			2			3			4			5
Move into farrow	3			4			5			6			7			1			2			3			4	
Boars to vaccinate	+																									
Completed initials																										

Note: The numbers in the Table refer to the identity of each group of sows, with the numbers starting at the point of breeding.

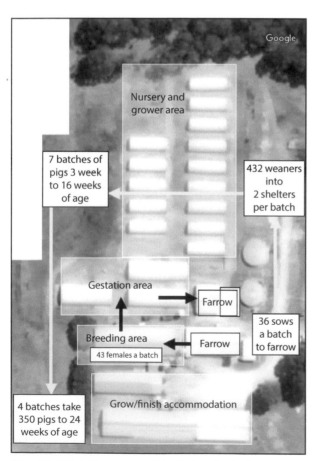

Fig. 11.75 A farm map with the batch pig flow illustrated for the whole farm team.

Table 11.17 **Production events dependent on the day of weaning.**

WEANING DAY	MAIN BREEDING DAY (5 DAYS LATER)	FARROWING DAY (115 DAYS LATER)
Thursday	Tuesday	Friday
Wednesday	Monday	Thursday
Monday	Saturday	Tuesday

Can pig flow assist with cash flow analysis?

This is probably one of the greatest advantages in running a pig farm around its flow. Once the farm is run based on production output targets, the whole cost of production can be assessed.

Analysis of cost of production: See *Table 11.18.*

Achieving an all-in/all-out pig flow batch (example)

This is demonstrated using a real life example farm (*Table 11.19*). Farrow to finish farm with 101 farrowing crates. Three rooms - [40] [40] [21]. The farm weans at 4 weeks of age, but admits this is a little chaotic. It produces 981 tonnes of pork per year (85 kg deadweight) but fails to achieve AIAO.

Solution: Split the two rooms of 40 into 4 rooms of 20 to produce 5 rooms of 20. The extra farrowing

Table 11.18 **Costings for a farm of 10 batch farrowing places. The breakdown costs are arbitrary in order to give examples.**

BATCH TIME		1	1	2	3	4	Weeks
TOTAL COSTS (£ STERLING)		1,178,012	589,006	294,503	196,335	147,252	annual
Feed costs %	66	777,488	388,744	194,372	129,581	97,186	annual
Labour costs %	14	164,922	82,461	41,230	27,487	20,615	annual
Genetic costs %	6	70,681	35,340	17,670	11,780	8,835	annual
Health costs %	4	47,120	23,560	11,780	7,853	5,890	annual

Assumptions: A £1/kilogram deadweight cost (pound sterling has been used as the price unit, local currencies can easily be inserted); 12 weaned per batch farrowing place; 95% finishing rate (the post-weaning pigs that have a saleable value); deadweight 82 kg. Different countries use different carcase calculations, ranging from liveweight to dressed carcase weight.

Table 11.19 **Real example of a pig flow model.**

BATCH TIME	WEEKLY
Weaning age	27 days
Farrowing house layout	20 20 20 20 20
Gilts pool requirement	22
Minimum breeding females per batch	25
Weaned sows per batch	20
Minimum number weaned per batch	240
Number sold per batch	228
Number sold annually	11,856
Weight sold annually	1,007 tonnes

Note: This pig flow model provides a more disciplined approach. The farm can produce an extra 26 tonnes of pig meat, reducing the cost of production.

place is not required. The division of the room of 40 was easy to achieve without affecting the ventilation system.

Monitoring the batching system

A series of production boards can be introduced to the farm team (**Figure 11.76**). These boards record events in real time batch on batch. Three production boards are particularly useful:

- Breeding to weaning board.
- Nursery board.
- Grow/finish board.

Using colours for changes and failure to reach targets allows the board to be easily read and analysed.

Production boards have proven to be extremely useful in team building.

Records based on pig flow

The whole farm revolves around the batch farrowing place plan. A plan of action is then determined around this single number, based on some assumptions. For example:

- The batch farrowing place. This is the minimum number of sows that need to farrow each batch (e.g. 20 batch farrowing places).
- From this, the minimum number of females to breed would be 20/farrowing rate (e.g. 20/0.82 = 25 females per batch [round up]).
- The minimum number of weaners per batch; 20 × numbers weaned per batch farrowing place (e.g. 20 × 12 = 240 weaners per batch [round up]).
- The minimum number of finishers per batch = 240 × finishing rate (i.e. minus the number of pigs that die/are culled between weaning and finish) (e.g. 240 × 0.95 = 228 pigs to finish each batch [round up]).
- The minimum weight of pigs paid for each batch = 228 × dressed weight (e.g. 228 × 85 kg = 19,380 kg per batch paid for).

Production records

The farm records need to be compared with the required output. The target output is placed at 100%; the rest of the production results are then related to the 100% for each parameter. This data can be illustrated graphically to demonstrate past, current and future production trends (**Figure 11.77**).

Batch number	12 (13) SRG	Heat check weeks 3–6 / Week of gestation — 1	2	3	4	5	6	7 (cull week)	8	9	10	11	Order new gilts weeks 10 to 14 — 12	13	14	15	16	17	Farrowing house weeks — 1	2	3	4	Batch week	W
1	10+1+1	12	12	11	11	11	11	11	11	11	11	11	11	11	11	11	11	11	10	10	10	10	22	125
2	9+1+2	12	12	11	10	10	11	11	11	10	10	10	11	10	10	10	10	10	10	10	10	10	23	118
3	10+1+1	12	12	12	11	11	12	11	11	11	11	11	11	11	11	11	10	11	10	10	10	10	24	122
4	8+0+2	10	10	9	8	8	8	8	8	9	8	8	8	8	8	8	8	8	8	8	8	8	25	104
5	9+1+2	12	12	12	11	11	11	11	11	9	9	9	9	9	9	9	9	9	9	9	9	9	26	110
6	8+0+4	12	12	11	10	11	10	10	10	10	10	10	10	10	10	10	10	10	10	10	10		27	
7	10+1+2	13	13	13	12	12	11	11	11	11	11	11	11	11	11	11	11	11	11	11			28	
8	10+1+2	12	12	12	12	11	11	11	11	11	11	11	11	11	11	11	11	11	11				29	
9	9+1+2	12	13	13	12	11	11	11	11	11	11	9	10	10	10	11	10	11					30	
10	9+2+1	12	12	11	10	10	10	10	10	10	9	10	10	10	9	10	10						31	
11	10+1+2	12	13	12	11	11	11	10	11	11	11	10	10	10	11	11							32	
12	10+1+1	12	12	12	12	12	10	10	10	10	10	11	10	10	10								33	
13	10+2+2	14¹	14	14	13	12	11	10	10	10	10	10	10	10									34	
14	10+1+1	12	12	11	10	10	11	10	10	10	10	10	11										35	
15	9+1+2	12	12	11	10	10	11	10	10	10	10	10											36	
16	8+1+3	12	12	12	11	11	11	11	11	11	11												37	
17	9+1+1	12	12	12	11	11	11	12	11	11													38	
18	8+0+4	12	12	10	9	9	9	9	9														39	
19	10+1+1	12	12	11	11	11	11	11															40	
20	10+1+1	12	12	11	10	11	10																41	
21	10+0+2	12	12	10	10	10																	42	
22	10+1+1	12	12	11	11																		43	
23	9+2+1	12	12	10																			44	
24	9+1+2	12	12																				45	
25	10+0+2	12																					46	
26																							47	
27																							48	

Fig. 11.76 The breeding board completing the cycle from breeding back to breeding again. Red denotes when there has been a change in output; blue is a failure to reach targets. Green denotes deliberate culling to reduce variation. SRG = sows, returns, gilts; W = number of pigs weaned.

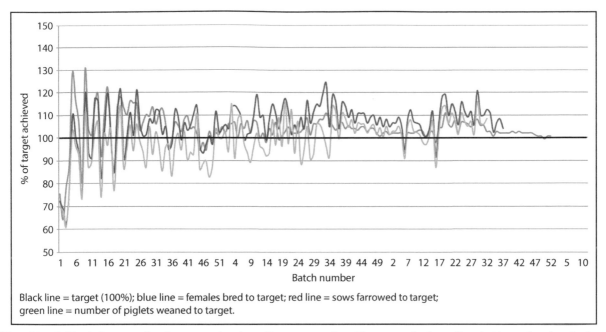

Black line = target (100%); blue line = females bred to target; red line = sows farrowed to target; green line = number of piglets weaned to target.

Fig. 11.77 Real time production records – breeding to weaning. For example, breeding is 17 weeks ahead of farrowing, which is 4 weeks ahead of weaning and 26 weeks ahead of finishing (not shown to make the graphics cleaner). The graph is, therefore, able to predict likely future production trends.

Analysis power of these production graphs

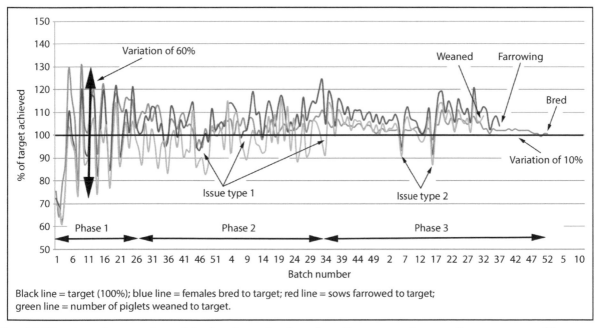

Black line = target (100%); blue line = females bred to target; red line = sows farrowed to target; green line = number of piglets weaned to target.

Fig. 11.78a At a glance review of the farm's production – breeding to weaning over 3 years on a weekly batching farm. Using a 100% target means that the actual size of the farm is not relevant, only how well it performs to its target expectations.

Production change over time: There are three phases to the farm's production (**Figure 11.78a**).

Phase 1. Batch 1 to batch 28 year 1: The farm before the implementation of a batch production system concept. The farm bred whatever females were in oestrus during the breeding week. The various production departments did not talk to each other and had no concern over the problems they created downstream. On normal farms, the variation batch on batch is around 40%, and on this farm was closer to 60%. Note how the number of females bred is directly related to the number that will farrow and, therefore, the number of piglets to be weaned. The farm has repeated over- and understocking of the nursery. This results in movement of pigs between rooms and batches and a failure in AIAO.

Phase 2. Batch 28 year 1 to batch 34 year 2: The farm agrees to a batching pig flow AIAO system. The breeding team needs to stabilise the number of females bred each batch by changing the culling programme and the judicious introduction of gilts. The variation in the system was progressively reduced as the farm's production was brought under control.

Phase 3. Batch 35 year 2 to batch 52 year 3: The farm adopts the batch production system. The farm production is modified to ensure that the batch farrowing places will be filled in each batch by adapting overbreeding by 5%.

Examination of the performance by batch (illustrated in detail in **Figure 11.78b**): Interpretation if the actual result of one point is above or below another:

- above – target overachieved;
- under – target underachieved.

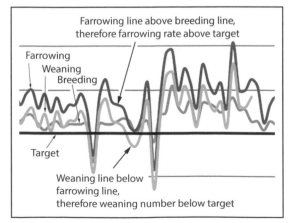

Fig. 11.78b Detail of batch analysis. Batch 49 year 2 to batch 37 year 3.

Farm production issues

The production record graph (**Figure 11.77**) can also be used to predict problems on the farm.

Issue 1: At three points, around batch 43 to 50 year 1, batch 6 to 8 year 2 and batch 33 year 2, there was a major reduction in the number of pigs weaned per batch. This was associated with an increase in the number of gilts in the breeding batch. With the increased number of gilts, this precipitated a diarrhoea outbreak in the farrowing area and a decrease in the numbers weaned per batch farrowing place. However, the farm team quickly realised the issues created by too many gilts in the breeding pool and changed their management of the farrowing house accordingly to minimise the impact.

Issue 2: At two points in year 3, the breeding team failed to reach batch breeding target. This was associated with a failure in gilts to cycle on time and an increase in wean-to-service interval in the sows. This failure to reach the batch breeding target resulted in a failure to farrow sufficient number of sows and subsequent failure to wean sufficient weaners and, ultimately, failure to produce sufficient pork from the farm.

Summary of the use of these production graphics

- The production veterinarian is able to demonstrate the effect of strategic advice quickly.
- The advantages of using this system of recording is that neither farm size nor batch interval is irrelevant, allowing different farms to be easily compared.
- The records are very predictive and allow for future problems to be visualised by the whole team.
- The system encourages a reduction in variations on the pig production.
- The system enforces honesty as any cheating is rapidly identified by all members of the farm team.

All points help bring about the whole farm working together.

Examples of poor pig flow
See **Figures 11.79–11.89**.

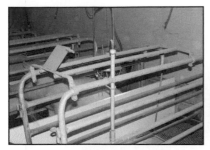

Fig. 11.79 Empty farrowing place. If breeding targets are not met it is likely that there will be empty farrowing places. This is an extremely expensive mistake.

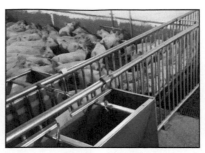

Fig. 11.80 Empty nursery pen. Empty farrowing places generally result in too few weaners and thus empty pens.

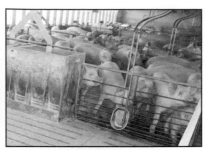

Fig. 11.81 Empty growing and finishing pen. If the nursery area has insufficient pigs this permeates throughout the farm into the finishing area.

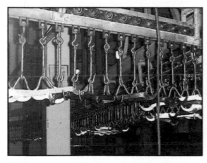

Fig. 11.82 Empty shackle space.

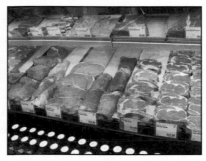

Fig. 11.83 Lack of pork sales. This is the final aspect of pig flow where meat is not sold.

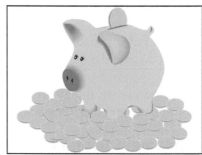

Fig. 11.84 Increase in cost of production. Where there is a lack of pigs in the system the remaining pigs must shoulder the cost over feed, thus the cost of production increases.

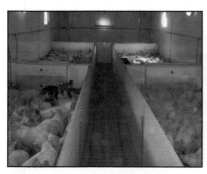

Fig. 11.85 Overstocked pens. If breeding targets are overreached there will be more pigs in the system, resulting in overstocking and generally more respiratory problems.

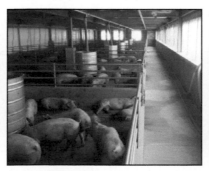

Fig. 11.86 Understocked pens. If breeding targets are underrreached there will be insufficient pigs into the system, resulting in chilling and generally more intestinal problems.

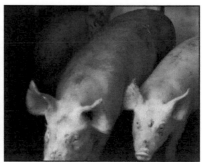

Fig. 11.87 Uneven growth. Especially with overstocking, there is not only a lack of space, the water and feeding spaces also become limiting, increasing the variation within the batch.

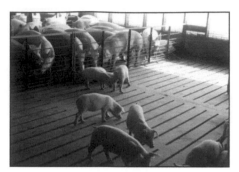

Fig. 11.88 Failure in AIAO. If there are uneven numbers of pigs in each group there is a tendency for the farm team to cheat and move pigs from batch to batch (i.e. a failure in AIAO).

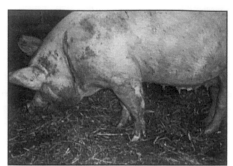

Fig. 11.89 Decreased health: increased medicine use. With increased variation in pig flow, the cumulative effects of over- and understocking results in decreased health and thus increased medicine use.

MANAGEMENT OF MEDICINES ON PIG FARMS

Medicine storage and administration is the cornerstone of any preventive medicine programme.

Equipment useful for monitoring medicine management
See **Figures 11.90, 11.91**.

Medicines use
The use of medicines in animals is required to ensure that food supplies are healthy, which is a major reason why human health has improved over centuries. However, the veterinary profession must ensure that medications are used appropriately.

There are five stages that can be recommended to our clients to assist in medicine management:

1 Only use medications when prescribed or administered by a veterinarian.
2 Follow the recommended dosage and length of treatment even if the pig appears to have recovered.
3 Exclusively obtain medications from authorised sources.
4 Vaccinate and institute good hygiene and husbandry practices to prevent infections.
5 Keep adequate written records of all medications used as well as the laboratory results.

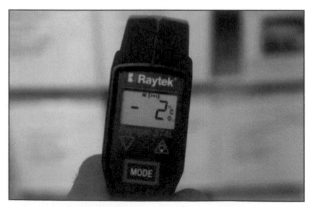

Fig. 11.90 Infrared thermometer allows instant review of the fridge temperature.

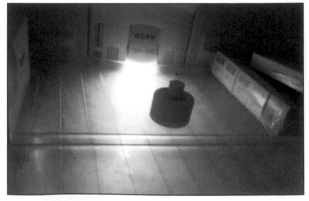

Fig. 11.91 For long-term permanent temperature records use a temperature logger.

Medicine storage

A proper medicine storage area, which is temperature controlled, lockable and safely away from children and animals, should be available on every farm. It is essential that all medicines are stored clean and dust free. The car is an unsuitable place to store medicines as the boot/trunk can be too hot or too cold depending on the season.

Medicine storage examination can be divided into two main sections, cold and warm.

Cold medicine storage

Read the data sheets carefully. These medicines generally need to be kept in a refrigerator between 2° and 8°C.

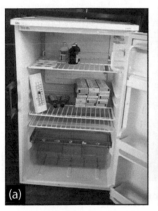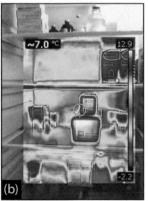

Fig. 11.92 (a) A well managed cold medicine store. (b) The infrared temperature map of a well managed cold medicine store. Details on how to read an infrared temperature map can be found at the end of Chapter 10.

Freezing most vaccines will render them useless, and the entire preventive medicine programme is negated. Refrigerators that have a freeze thaw cycle must therefore be avoided. Do not rely on the refrigerator temperature control dial to monitor the temperature. Place a maximum and minimum thermometer in the body of the fridge and monitor the temperature fluctuations at least weekly. It is important that the farm team is able to read a max/min thermometer. Ideally, a temperature logger should be placed in the fridge and the temperature print out can be included in the quarterly veterinary report (**Figures 11.92, 11.93**).

Check that the door seals to ensure the fridge at least attempts to maintain a steady temperature. Know the temperature distribution of your fridge. Ensure that medicines are placed in the body of the fridge. The door and the vegetable tray are generally above 8°C and are therefore unsuitable areas for cold medicine storage. The fridge should be kept clean at all times.

A major problem found on farms is the presence of human food in the medicine fridge, including soft drinks. Aside from the obvious health and safety issues of storing human food stuffs in a chemical store, there is a potential risk of the spread of some of the most significant pig pathogens. FMDV and classical swine fever virus are examples where the pig's ingestion of human food containing pork products has resulted in the loss of millions of animal's lives and crippling costs to the local swine industry. Both PRRSV and PCV2 have been isolated in fresh pork. If human food is to be brought onto the

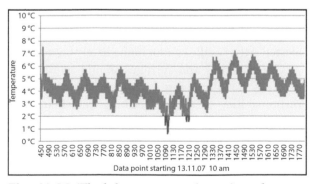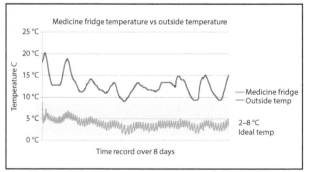

Fig. 11.93 The left temperature logger's readout records one incident where the fridge nearly froze. The green band is acceptable temperature. The right records indicate that the outside temperature had no impact on the fridge temperature.

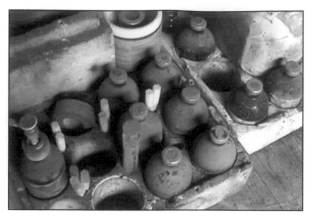

Fig. 11.94 This warm medicine storage is appalling and yet never even created a comment by the local veterinarian.

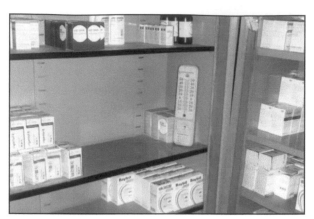

Fig. 11.95 Proper warm medicine store on a large commercial pig farm.

farm, a) it should not include any pork products and b) it should be stored in a separate area.

Warm medicine storage

Some pharmaceuticals used on farms (e.g. antimicrobials) should be stored at temperatures generally not exceeding 25°C and this includes in-feed medications. A max/min thermometer should also be in the warm medicine storage area. The temperature of 25°C may seem like room temperature, but in many parts of the world this temperature will be easily exceeded in the summer months. Therefore, it may not be adequate to store medicines in an office (**Figures 11.94, 11.95**).

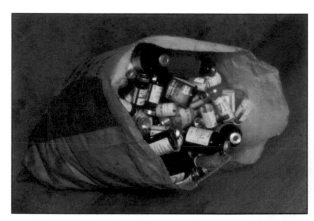

Fig. 11.96 Inadequate empty medicine bottle disposal.

Medicine bottle disposal

A formal protocol should be drawn up detailing the procedures for disposal of used medicine bottles (**Figure 11.96**). Local regulations will direct your options but just dumping them into the local trash collection is not appropriate. Pharmaceutical bottles should be returned to the prescribing veterinary practice or pharmacy, but note the risk of pathogen transfer. It is the responsibility of the prescribing veterinarian to dispose of used pharmaceutical products.

Needles and syringes   VIDEO 35

Protocols on cleaning and sanitising syringes, needles, scalpels, etc. should be available. These protocols must ensure that their use will allow adequate

injection techniques without risk of abscessation. A broken needle policy should be in place. On many farms, needles now have to be counted out and returned or accounted for. Any pig that has a needle break should be tagged and the slaughter plant alerted if the needle cannot immediately be removed.

Used needles and syringes should be disposed of safely, ideally using a sharps container. It is a responsibility of the prescribing veterinarian to ensure safe disposal of used needles and syringes (**Figures 11.97, 11.98**).

Needleless technology should be explored if available. It is realised that there is still a lot of work needed to perfect the system for general use. Needleless technology administers the product intra- or subdermally.

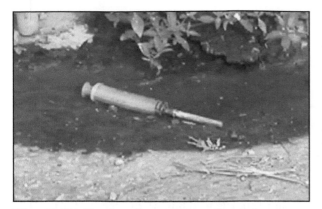

Fig. 11.97 Careless disposal of needles and syringes can result in serious health and safety issues.

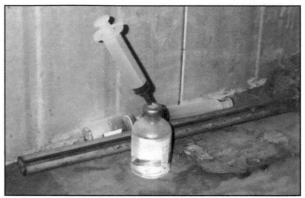

Fig. 11.98 Dirty needle and bottle use. Such practices should be stopped.

Injection site and needle use

At this time, most antimicrobials and vaccines continue to be administered by injection (*Table 11.20*). Injections should be administered into the neck behind the ear to minimise carcase blemish issues, but this is an important cut in many parts of the world and it should be remembered that the pig is a global commodity. Injections are most commonly given subcutaneously or intramuscularly depending on manufacturer and product.

Accidental injection or medication ingestion by farm staff protocols

In the case of accidental needle stick injury or medication ingestion, the protocols listed below should be followed:

1 Inform manager (or assistant manager) immediately.
2 Obtain relevant data sheet.
3 Telephone local medical centre for advice.
4 Be taken to the medical centre. Do not drive yourself.
5 Go to local medical centre with data sheet and name, telephone and email address of the farm veterinarian
6 Fill in the accident book and date and sign it.

Water supply medication

The water supply can be an ideal route for medication of pigs. For it to work it must be checked to be sure that all the drinkers are working within specifications. This should include:

- Height.
- Angle.
- Flow.
- Pressure of the water.
- Absence of leaks in the water system.

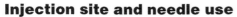

Table 11.20 **Needle length and size.**

INTRAMUSCULAR INJECTIONS			kg	SUBCUTANEOUS INJECTIONS		
Piglet	16 mm	0.8 mm	1–7	Piglet	16 mm	0.8 mm
Weaner	25 mm	1.1 mm	8–25	Weaner	16 mm	0.8 mm
Grower	35 mm	1.1 mm	26–60	Grower	16 mm	1.1 mm
Finisher	35 mm	1.3 mm	61–100	Finisher	16 mm	1.1 mm
Adult	40 mm	1.3 mm		Adult	25 mm	1.1 mm

Note: Adult pigs require a needle of 40 mm in length to enter the muscular tissues. Vaccinating into subcutaneous fat will significantly reduce the effectiveness of the vaccine.

When medications go into the water supply ensure that they are mixed properly, otherwise medicine residues may occur. Many medications and vaccines require that specific chemicals, such as chlorine, are removed from the water supply prior to their administration. Some water medications are actually difficult to dissolve; for example, amoxicillin can be very difficult to dissolve unless the pH of the water is changed. Some water medications may contain sugars and this may stimulate biofilm production, resulting in blocked drinkers.

Many waterers waste a lot of water, possibly 20–50% of the volume actually drunk. Therefore, there can be considerable environmental contamination through wasted antimicrobials.

The water supply is becoming a very useful method of supplying vaccines to large numbers of pigs without the stress of restraint and injection.

Feed medications

The use of medication via the feed supply is a normal route of administration in pig production. Many pathogens affect whole groups of pigs (even subclinically) and then the whole group need to receive antimicrobial medication. However, there are issues with in-feed medication:

- **Time**. To treat clinically sick animals, the time delay in getting the feed to the farm means

that the pigs can suffer mortality and reduced welfare.

- **Appetite**. With several diseases, such as *Actinobacillus pleuropneumoniae* infection, the pig is clinically sick and does not eat. Therefore, sick pigs will not get the intended medication.
- **Feed bin management**. Good management of the feed bin is essential to ensure that the correct pigs are medicated. Have all feed bins numbered (**Figure 11.99**). Understand how feed moves in the feed bin. Medicated feed placed on top of unmedicated feed in a feed bin will not result in the medication being delivered at the required concentration. The new feed will move though the centre of the older feed, reducing the medication dose (**Figure 11.100**).
- **Medication residues**. Once the period of medication has finished it is essential to ensure that the feed system is thoroughly cleaned, including the feed trough in the pens, otherwise medicine residues may inadvertently occur in the pig meat.

Pig identification and medication systems

A properly run medication programme relies on accurate pig and pen identification (**Figures 11.101, 11.102**). A review of the medication records is an essential component of the health audit.

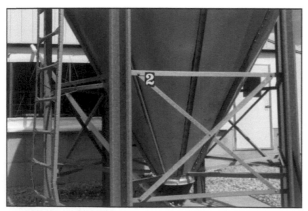

Fig. 11.99 Feed bins must be numbered.

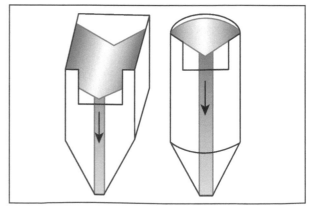

Fig. 11.100 Feed movement within a feed bin is through the centre of the bin.

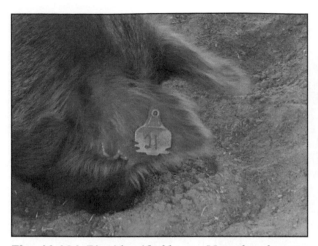

Fig. 11.101 Pigs identified by tag. Note that the tag is notched, making it easier to read.

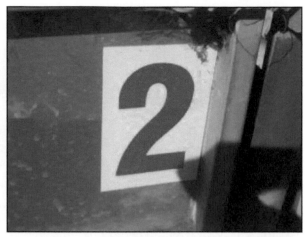

Fig. 11.102 Identify each pen – an ear tag can work well on a wall.

Examples of poor medicine management
Refrigerator management – frozen vaccines will not work
The farms in these examples generally had no preventive medicine programme (**Figures 11.103–11.114**).

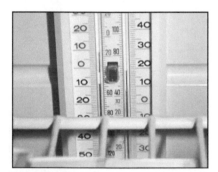

Fig. 11.103 Ensure the fridge has a working max/min thermometer to record the extremes.

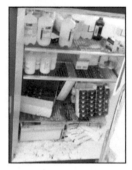

Fig. 11.104 Fridge very dirty. Note there is no ice box cover. Overstocked with medicines.

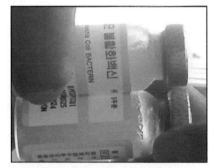

Fig. 11.105 Fridge too cold resulting in products that have frozen. Storage that is too hot will inactivate medications.

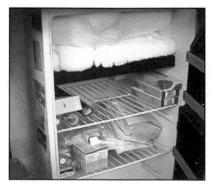

Fig. 11.106 Fridge requires defrosting. The products are at a serious risk of freezing.

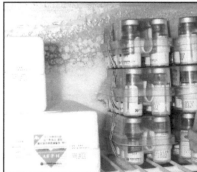

Fig. 11.107 The rear of the fridge is frozen and medicines are in contact with the back plate.

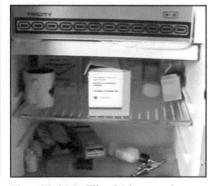

Fig. 11.108 The fridge needs to be defrosted before the medicines become frozen.

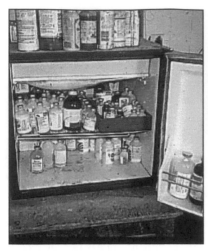

Fig. 11.109 Fridge overstocked. This was only a 150 sow unit. Also requires defrosting.

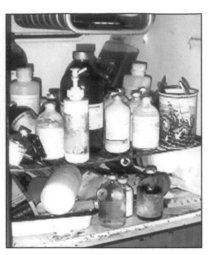

Fig. 11.110 The fridge has no management – medicines just thrown in.

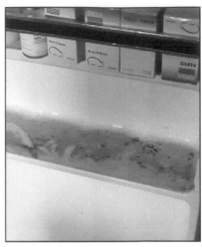

Fig. 11.111 Vaccines in door of fridge and therefore too warm. Note fridge is not very clean.

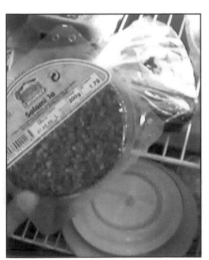

Fig. 11.112 Food in fridge, especially pork products. This is a serious biosecurity risk.

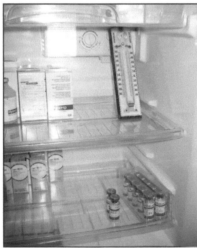

Fig. 11.113 A well managed fridge; minimal medicines and temperature storage check possible.

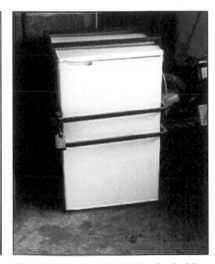

Fig. 11.114 Is the fridge lockable and secure? Is it away from children?

General bottle management
See **Figures 11.115–11.122**.

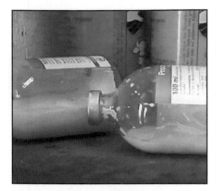

Fig. 11.115 Multiple bottles of the same medicine open at the same time.

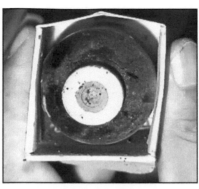

Fig. 11.116 Bottles stored dirty. This is a serious abscess risk.

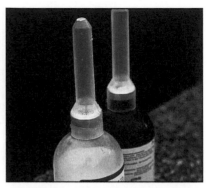

Fig. 11.117 Keep the tops of bottles clean by covering them or placing them under cover.

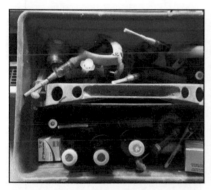

Fig. 11.118 This degree of bottle contamination is unacceptable.

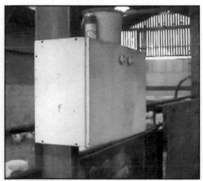

Fig. 11.119 A finishing yard's simple lockable cupboard.

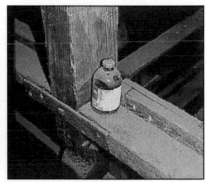

Fig. 11.120 Medicines cannot be 'stored' on convenient walls.

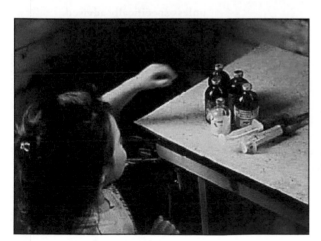

Fig. 11.121 Keep all medicines out of the reach of children.

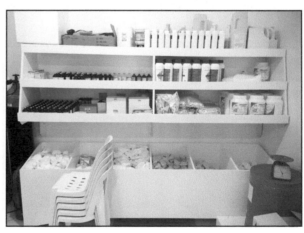

Fig. 11.122 Too many medicines. This was only a 200 sow unit.

Needle and syringe management
See **Figures 11.123–11.130**.

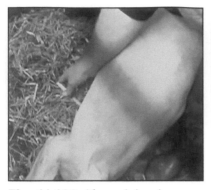

Fig. 11.123 Always inject into the neck of pigs. Review the use of needleless technology.

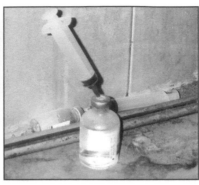

Fig. 11.124 Do not leave bottles and syringes lying around.

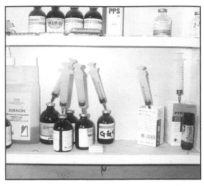

Fig. 11.125 Do not store needles and syringes in the bottles.

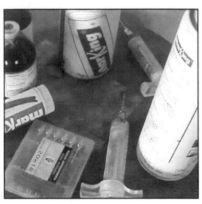

Fig. 11.126 Do not leave syringes and needles 'ready' on tops.

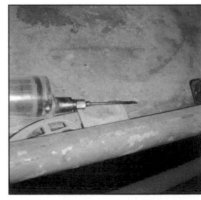

Fig. 11.127 This syringe is very dirty and unusable.

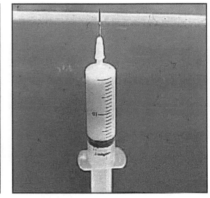

Fig. 11.128 Do not mix medicines unless specifically advised.

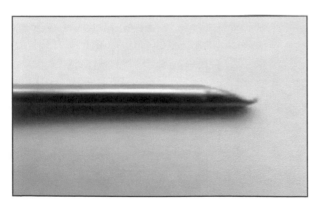

Fig. 11.129 Blunt needles cause a lot of trauma when used.

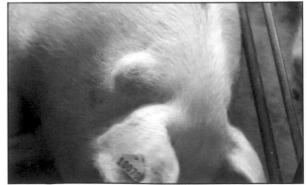

Fig. 11.130 Shoulder/neck abscess from dirty injection technique.

Disposal of used medicines, needles and syringes – review local requirements
See **Figures 11.131–11.134**.

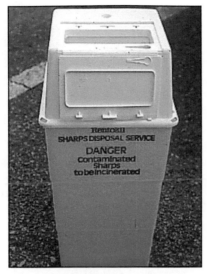

Fig. 11.131 Use a sharps tin to dispose of all needles, blades etc.

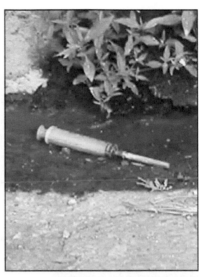

Fig. 11.132 Do not carelessly dispose of syringes and needles.

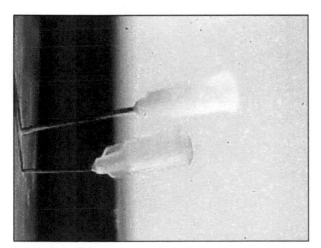

Fig. 11.133 Doorways or building supports are not for disposal of needles.

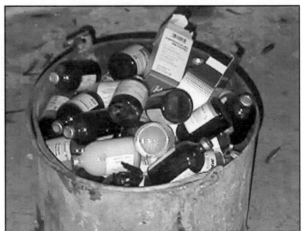

Fig. 11.134 Poor medicine bottle disposal.

Records and preventing medicine residues
See **Figures 11.135–11.138**.

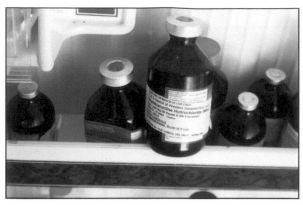

Fig. 11.135 Always read and understand the label on the bottle.

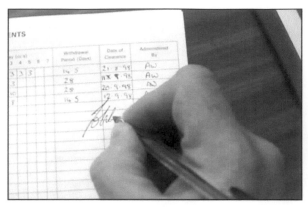

Fig. 11.136 Complete medicine records as soon as possible.

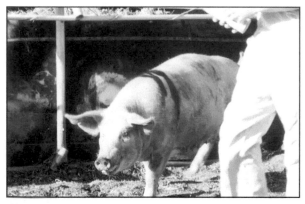

Fig. 11.137 Mark medicated pigs or pens adequately.

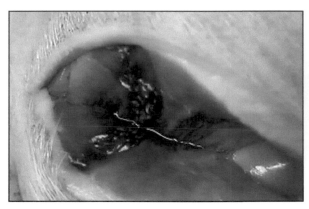

Fig. 11.138 Residues are not that hard to find in the slaughterhouse.

Other medicine administration methods
See **Figures 11.139–11.142**.

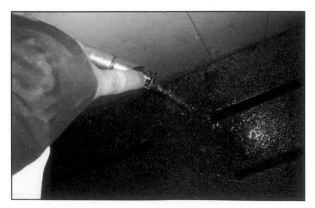

Fig. 11.139 Medication through the water supply – ensure that the supply is adequate. Check for leaks.

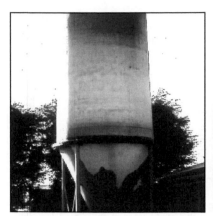

Fig. 11.140 Medicating through feed bin management.

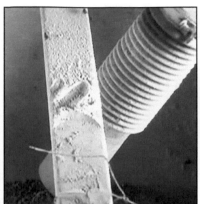

Fig. 11.141 When top dressing ensure that the medicine is mixed with the feed. Carelessness leads to residues.

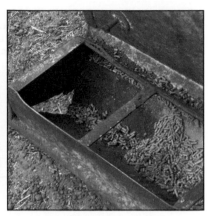

Fig. 11.142 Ensure that the feeding system is adequate for the pigs and no wastage occurs.

TREATMENT GUIDELINES

The following sections discuss the variety of chemicals and treatments that can be used on pig farms (*Table 11.21*). When dealing with pet pigs it is important to remember that certain products and chemicals may be banned from use within pigs without exception. It is vital to check your local regulations.

Pain relief in pigs

There are a few products that can be used to provide pain relief in pigs. Many treatment regimes will be enhanced if appropriate pain relief is offered. The medication can be injected or, preferably, administered via the water supply. It can also be given in tablet form offered in a 'treat' such as a grape or banana. These are generally the options when treating pet pigs. In many countries, procedures such as castrating, notching or tail docking require medication to reduce post-procedural pain. Sows may be in pain with full mammary glands or during parturition.

Suggestions for pain relief medication include:

- **Meloxicam** at 0.4 mg/kg body weight orally or intramuscular injection.
- **Ketoprofen** at 3 mg/kg body weight once daily
- **Sodium salicylate** at 35 mg/kg body weight is commonly used in water and in feed. This can

be useful in mass medication and in outbreaks of PRRSV or swine influenza virus (SIV). It may also be useful in compromised pigs.
- **Phenylbutazone.** This medicine is very useful in treating painful conditions such as acute lameness and torn muscles, bush foot infections or acute mastitis. It can be given by injection or orally. In many countries phenylbutazone cannot be used in food producing animals.

Use of vaccines in pigs

Pathogens for which vaccines are commercially available in pigs are listed in *Table 11.22*. A decision tree for vaccine selection is shown in **Figure 11.143**.

Care of the compromised pig ▶ VIDEO 18

Unfortunately, pigs do get sick. It is essential to have a programme in place to care for these compromised pigs. Are they treated in their pen, will they be able to manage in the presence of their pen mates or do they need to be removed and placed in the passageway or specialised accommodation (*Table 11.23*, **Figures 11.144–11.146**)? One major problem governing the treatment of pigs is that pigs are bullies and will bully a sick animal, restricting its access to feed and water. Once removed from a group, replacing the pig can be difficult as the whole group will turn on the 'new' pig.

Table 11.21 **Pathogen antimicrobial therapy possibilities. Green: 70% or more isolates sensitive. Red: up to 50% of isolates resistant. Where the row is white, antimicrobials are generally not available for therapy. They may still be useful to control secondary pathogens. Tiamulin may be beneficial in PRRSV as the antibiotic modulates the macrophage function (pink box). Antimicrobials are not generally antiparasitic.**

ANTIMICROBIAL AGENT / PATHOGEN	AMINOCYCLITOLS — SPECTINOMYCIN	AMINOGLYCOSIDES — GENTAMICIN	AMINOGLYCOSIDES — NEOMYCIN	CEPHALOSPORINS — CEFTIOFUR	DITERPINES — TIAMULIN	FLUROQUINOLONE — ENROFLOXACIN	LINCOSAMIDES — LINCOMYCIN	MACROLIDES — TILMICOSIN	MACROLIDES — TULATHROMYCIN	MACROLIDES — TYLOSIN TARTRATE	MACROLIDES — VALNEMULIN	PENICILLINS — AMPICILLIN	PENICILLINS — PENICILLIN	SULPHONAMIDES — SULPHONAMIDES	SULPHONAMIDES — TRIMETHOPRIM/SULFAMETHOXAZOLE	TETRACYCLINES — FLORFENICOL	TETRACYCLINES — TETRACYCLINE
Actinobaculum suis																	
Actinobacillus suis																	
Actinobacillus pleuropneumoniae																	
African swine fever virus																	
Ascaris suum																	
Aujeszky's disease virus (pseudorabies)																	
Bordetella bronchiseptica																	
Borrelia spiralis																	
Brachyspira hyodysenteriae																	
Brachyspira pilosicoli																	
Brucella suis																	
Classical swine fever virus																	
Circovirus types 1 and 2																	
Clostridium difficile																	
Clostridium perfringens																	
Congenital tremor virus																	
Cystoisospora suis *																	
Cytomegalovirus																	
Escherichia coli																	
Erysipelothrix rhusiopathiae																	
Foot and mouth disease virus and other vesicular viruses																	
Haemophilus parasuis																	
Haematopinus suis																	
Hyostrongylus rubidis																	
Lawsonia intracellularis																	
Leptospira spp.																	
Metastrongylus apri																	

(Continued)

Table 11.21 *(Continued)* **Pathogen antimicrobial therapy possibilities. Green: 70% or more isolates sensitive. Red: up to 50% of isolates resistant. Where the row is white, antimicrobials are generally not available for therapy. They may still be useful to control secondary pathogens. Tiamulin may be beneficial in PRRSV as the antibiotic modulates the macrophage function (pink box). Antimicrobials are not generally antiparasitic.**

ANTIMICROBIAL AGENT / PATHOGEN	AMINOCYCLITOLS — SPECTINOMYCIN	AMINOGLYCOSIDES — GENTAMICIN	AMINOGLYCOSIDES — NEOMYCIN	CEPHALOSPORINS — CEFTIOFUR	DITERPINES — TIAMULIN	FLUROQUINOLONE — ENROFLOXACIN	LINCOSAMIDES — LINCOMYCIN	MACROLIDES — TILMICOSIN	MACROLIDES — TULATHROMYCIN	MACROLIDES — TYLOSIN TARTRATE	MACROLIDES — VALNEMULIN	PENICILLINS — AMPICILLIN	PENICILLINS — PENICILLIN	SULPHONAMIDES — SULPHONAMIDES	SULPHONAMIDES — TRIMETHOPRIM/SULFAMETHOXAZOLE	TETRACYCLINES — FLORFENICOL	TETRACYCLINES — TETRACYCLINE
Mycoplasma hyopneumoniae																	
Mycoplasma hyosynoviae																	
Mycoplasma suis																	
Oesophagostonum dentatum																	
Parvovirus																	
Pasteurella multocida																	
PEDV																	
PRRSV																	
Ringworm (*Trichophyton mentagrophytes*)																	
Rotavirus																	
Salmonella spp.																	
Sarcoptes scabiei																	
Spirochaetal colitis																	
Staphylococcus hycius																	
Stephanurus dentatus																	
Streptococcus spp.																	
Strongyloides ransomi																	
Swine influenza virus																	
Swine pox virus																	
Teschovirus																	
TGEV																	
Toxoplasma gondii																	
Trichonella spiralis																	
Trichuris suis																	
Trueperella pyogenes																	

* *Cystoisospora suis* – use toltrazuril.

Table 11.22 **Pathogens and toxins for which vaccines are available in pig production.**

PATHOGEN/TOXIN	COMMENTS ABOUT USE
Actinobaccilus pleuropneumoniae	To growing pigs
Aujeszky's disease virus (pseudorabies)	Whole herd twice or more yearly. Vaccine gene deleted to allow identification
Classical swine fever	To pigs over 10 weeks of age. Vaccine gene deleted to allow identification
Clostridial infections	
Clostridium perfringens	To gilts and sows pre-farrowing for piglets via colostrum
Clostridium novyi	Twice a year to adults
E. coli	
F4 and F5	To gilts and sows pre-farrowing for piglets via colostrum, or at weaning
F18	To weaners via water supply
Erysipelas	Available via injection or water
Gilt	At selection, two injections 2–4 weeks apart
Sows	Sows at weaning and for piglets via colostrum at the next lactation
Boars	Twice a year
Growing pigs	After 30 kg
Foot and mouth disease	To pigs over 10 weeks of age
Haemophilus parasuis	To piglets or weaned pigs. To gilts and sows pre-breeding for piglets via colostrum
Lawsonia intracellularis	To weaner to growing pigs via water or injection
Japanese encephalitis	Once or twice a year to adult breeding stock
Leptospirosis	To gilts during acclimatisation To gilts and sows pre-farrowing
Mycoplasma hyopneumoniae	To piglets or weaned pigs
Parvovirus	To gilts during acclimatisation
Porcine coronavirus type 2	To sows pre-farrowing for weaners via colostrum To piglets at weaning
Porcine epidemic diarrhoea	To sows pre-farrowing for piglets via colostrum
Porcine reproductive and respiratory syndrome	To weaned pigs To gilts during acclimatisation To gilts and sows pre-farrowing for piglets via colostrum
Rotavirus	To gilts and sows pre-farrowing
Salmonellosis	Via water supply to growing pigs
Swine influenza	To sows twice a year
Toxins from *Pasteurella multocida* and *Bordetella bronchiseptica*	To gilts and sows pre-farrowing for piglets via colostrum
Transmissible gastroenteritis	To gilts during acclimatisation To gilts and sows pre-farrowing for piglets via colostrum

Note: Not all of these vaccines are available in all countries. Timing and requirements may change between different countries. It is essential to be aware of the local legal situation. In addition, there may be a number of autogenous vaccines to specific pathogens available.

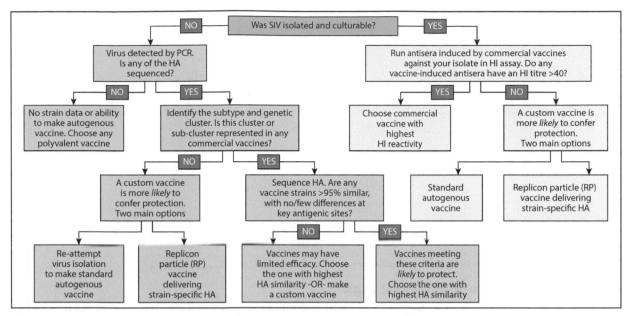

Fig. 11.143 Decision tree for vaccine selection strategy using swine influenza virus (SIV) as an example. HA, haemagglutinin gene of SIV; HI, haemagglutination inhibition test.

Table 11.23 **Design of a hospital pen for compromised pigs.**

1	Deep dry straw bedding covering a non-slip, insulated concrete floor
2	Good draught free ventilation. A kennelled area should be available
3	Provide an individual feeder, which is hand filled twice daily. There should never be a lot of food in the feeders so that in-feed medication is possible
4	Provide a bowl drinker that is set at 30 cm above the ground for pigs 20 kg or more. This drinker should be fed from a separate header tank to enable easy medication if necessary
5	Easy entry and exit points that do not necessitate lifting the animal over steps
6	Pigs in this pen should be examined a minimum of twice daily and the hospital pen records should be completed
7	All hospital pen pigs should be tagged and treated as individuals on entry
8	Pigs in the sick pen may need a companion
9	Each hospital pen should be of adequate size to hold up to ten pigs

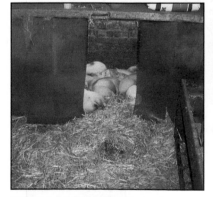

Fig. 11.144 Hospital pen for nursery and growing pigs.

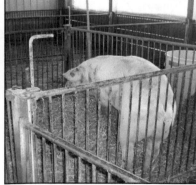

Fig. 11.145 Hospital pen for adults.

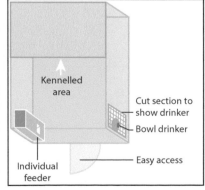

Fig. 11.146 Drawing of a simple hospital pen.

Hospital pen records

An example of a hospital pen record sheet is shown in the chart below.

DATE STARTED	ANIMAL NUMBER	DISEASE CONDITION	TREATMENT	RESPONSE DAYS AFTER START X = STILL SICK √ = RECOVERED													
				1	2	3	4	5	6	7	8	9	10	11	12	13	14

What to do with compromised pigs

A decision tree that will help plan the care and management of compromised pigs is shown in **Figure 11.147**.

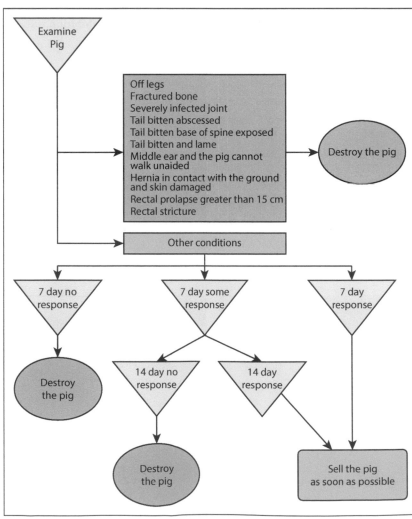

Fig. 11.147 Decision tree for planning the care and management of compromised pigs.

Grow/finish pigs (*Table 11.24*)

- To send to slaughter, all grow/finish pigs must be over 60 kg in weight and have a body condition score of 3 or greater.
- If less than condition score 3, treat or destroy.
- All pigs hospitalised must be identified with a numbered ear tag. All medication withdrawal periods must be complied with.

Table 11.24 **Actions to be taken for certain conditions (grow/finish pigs).**

CONDITION	EXTENT	IMMEDIATE ACTION	ACTION AFTER X DAYS
Lameness (**Figures 11.148–11.150**)	Unable to use back legs	Euthanase	
	Infected joints with soft pus filled abscess	Treat or euthanase	Euthanase if 7 days with no improvement
	Multiple joints infected	Euthanase	
	Single infected joint with non-discharging abscess less than golf ball size and able to walk unassisted	Treat as necessary	Send to slaughter as soon as possible
	Cannot walk with all four feet on ground	Treat or euthanase in hospital pen	Euthanase if 7 days with no improvement
	Fractured bone	Euthanase	
Hock sores (**Figure 11.151**)	Less than 3 cm and walking without lameness	Keep on deep straw in hospital pen	If healed in <14 days send to slaughter as soon as possible. Euthanase if no improvement
Bush foot but not lame (**Figure 11.152**)	One joint only. No discharge and no swelling up leg	Treat as necessary	When the pig goes to slaughter send in separate pen
Tail bitten (**Figures 11.153–11.155**)	Abscessed	Euthanase	
	Base of spine exposed	Euthanase	
	Tail bitten and lame	Euthanase	
	Infected with no abscesses	Treat in hospital pen	If healed within 14 days, retain separate until slaughter
	Fresh with no infection	Treat in hospital pen	Send to slaughter as soon as possible
Open wounds (**Figure 11.156**)	Cuts (damage through the whole skin) of any type	Treat in hospital pen	When healed send to slaughter as soon as possible
	Grazes (surface skin damage only) less than 6 cm	Treat if necessary	Send to slaughter as soon as possible
Flank bites (**Figure 11.157**)	Greater than 6 cm or infected	Treat in hospital pen	Once healed send to slaughter as soon as possible
	Fresh. No infection, less than 6 cm and superficial	Treat if necessary	Send to slaughter as soon as possible
Beaten up pigs (**Figure 11.158**)	Numerous fight marks	Treat in hospital pen individually	Euthanase if sick for more than 3 days
Aural haematoma (**Figure 11.159**)	Large with infection and swelling	Treat in hospital pen	Leave a week, then if necessary lance and when healed send to slaughter as soon as possible
Crumpled ear (**Figure 11.160**)	Healed and no infection	No treatment necessary	Send on normal load
Middle ear infection (**Figure 11.161**)	Can walk unaided	Treat as necessary	Send to slaughter as soon as possible
	Cannot walk unaided	Euthanase	

(Continued)

Table 11.24 *(Continued)* **Actions to be taken for certain conditions (grow/finish pigs).**

CONDITION	EXTENT	IMMEDIATE ACTION	ACTION AFTER X DAYS
Hernia **(Figure 11.162)**	Belly, scrotal or groin hernia and 9 cm clear of ground with no damage or infection	No effective treatment possible	Send to slaughter as soon as possible
	Pedunculated hernia with no damage or infection	No effective treatment possible	Send to slaughter as soon as possible, separate on the truck
	Hernia in contact with ground, with skin damage or infected	Euthanase	
	Any pig with a hernia that is bigger than 30 cm should be euthanased. Send pigs with large hernias to the cutter market at 70 kg rather than trying to get them to bacon weights		
Rectal prolapse **(Figure 11.163)**	Fresh, no smell, no bigger than 15 cm	Send to slaughter as soon as possible	Or stitch in and send to slaughter as soon as possible
	Larger than 15 cm	Euthanase	
Rectal stricture **(Figure 11.164)**	Any type	Euthanase	
Pneumonia **(Figure 11.165)**	Walking but off food	Treat in pen	If no improvement in 24 hours, move to hospital pen. Euthanase if no response to treatment for 7 days
Thin pig **(Figure 11.166)**	With or without scour	Treat in hospital pen	Euthanase if no response clinically within 7 days and no visible improvement within 14 days
PCV2-SD		Treat in hospital pen	Euthanase if no response clinically within 7 days and no visible improvement within 14 days
Porcine dermatitis and nephropathy syndrome **(Figure 11.167)**		Treat in hospital pen	Euthanase if no response within 7 days
Kinky back or other abnormality **(Figure 11.168)**	Visibly deformed and affects ability to slaughter pig	Mark in the pen	

All pigs that present with a condition that makes them unlikely to be slaughtered for human consumption should be euthanased as soon as this decision is reached

It is essential that the appropriate therapy is used for each condition and that all pigs are slaughtered after the relevant withdrawal period has elapsed

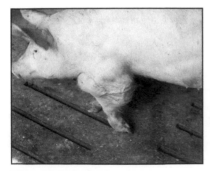

Fig. 11.148 Broken leg.

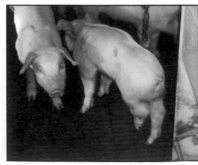

Fig. 11.149 Swollen joint.

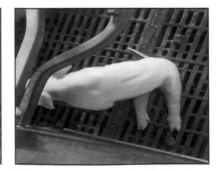

Fig. 11.150 Broken back.

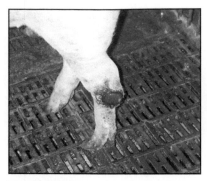

Fig. 11.151 Hock sores.

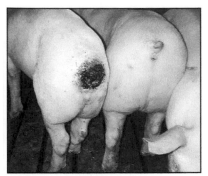

Fig. 11.152 Bush foot.

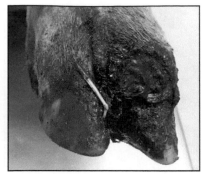

Fig. 11.153 Tail bitten: severe.

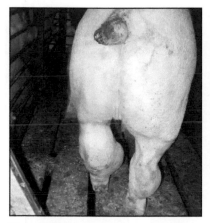

Fig. 11.154 Tail bitten and lame.

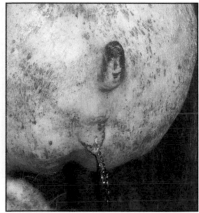

Fig. 11.155 Tail bitten: fresh and no infection.

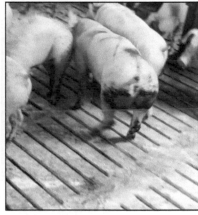

Fig. 11.156 Open wounds. In this pig from a lime burn wound.

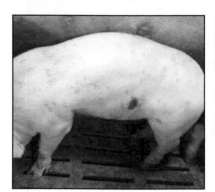

Fig. 11.157 Flank biting.

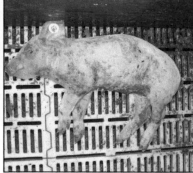

Fig. 11.158 Beaten up pig.

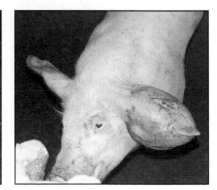

Fig. 11.159 Aural haematoma.

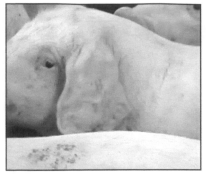

Fig. 11.160 Crumpled ear.

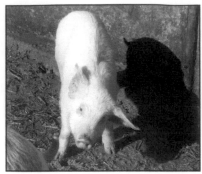

Fig. 11.161 Middle ear infection.

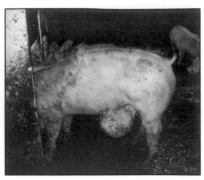

Fig. 11.162 Pig with a large hernia.

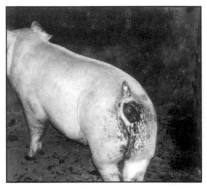

Fig. 11.163 Rectal prolapse.

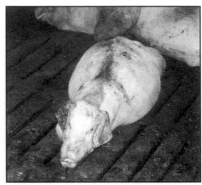

Fig. 11.164 Rectal stricture.

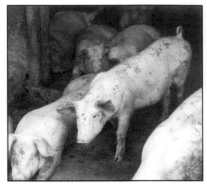

Fig. 11.165 Pig with pneumonia.

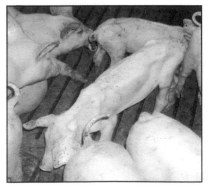

Fig. 11.166 Thin pig.

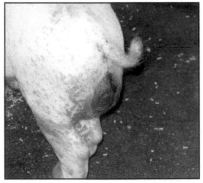

Fig. 11.167 Porcine dermatitis and nephropathy syndrome.

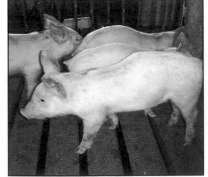

Fig. 11.168 Kinky back.

Compromised adults (*Table 11.25*)

- To send to slaughter, all adults must have a body condition score of 2 or greater.
- If less than condition score 2, treat or euthanase.
- All hospitalised adults must be identified with a numbered ear tag

Is the problem real? The use of statistical process control

One of the issues that the clinician faces is determining if there is an outbreak on the farm. A rise in mortality may be part of the normal pattern of events or it may be an indicator of a major problem starting.

Table 11.25 **Actions to be taken for certain conditions (adults).**

CONDITION	EXTENT	IMMEDIATE ACTION	ACTION AFTER X DAYS
Prolapses (**Figures 11.169, 11.170**)	Uterine	Immediate treatment or euthanase	
	Vagina	Immediate casualty slaughter	
		Treat if found fresh	Sell as soon as possible. Euthanase if re-prolapses
	Rectum	Immediate casualty slaughter if not excessive	
		Treat if found fresh and undamaged	Sell as soon as possible. Immediate culling if re-prolapses
Open wounds (**Figures 11.171–11.173**)	Traumatic injuries, cuts and wounds	Severe – euthanase	
		Not severe – treat	Sell when healed
	Shoulder sores and ulcerated hocks	Treat and move to bedded area.	Sell when healed
Lameness (**Figures 11.174–11.176**)	Off back legs	Euthanase	
	Acutely lame	Severe – euthanase	
		Not severe – treat	Euthanase if still lame after 7 days
	Lame with no obvious cause	Severe – euthanase or treat	Euthanase if still lame after 7 days
		Not severe – treat in bedded area	Euthanase if still lame after 7 days
		Casualty slaughter as long as pig can bear weight on all four legs and is willing to walk unaided and without being forced	
Emaciated (**Figure 11.177**)	Score 1, ribs visible	Euthanase	
		Treat	Review after 7 and 14 days
Dystocia (**Figure 11.178**)		Treat	Review when farrowing finished
		If live pigs are present	Use a Doppler pregnancy tester; consider euthanasia and immediate hysterectomy
		Euthanase	Note: Do not send a sow with retained piglets for slaughter as it will be condemned
All pigs that present with a condition that makes them unlikely to be slaughtered for human consumption should be euthanased as soon as this decision is reached			
It is essential that the appropriate therapy is used for each condition and that all pigs are slaughtered after the relevant withdrawal period has elapsed			

Using statistical process control allows the veterinarian to assist the farm in determining the normal expected pattern of mortality or morbidity and to make treatment decisions. However, the clinician must understand the concept of a normal population in biology.

What is a normal population?

A normal population is defined as a group of animals that are 2 standard deviations (SDs) either side of the mean (average), and will include 95% of the whole population (**Figure 11.179**). The animals in the 2.5% above and 2.5% below are outside the normal population.

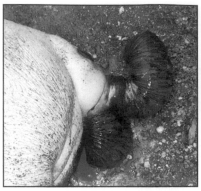

Fig. 11.169 Uterine prolapse.

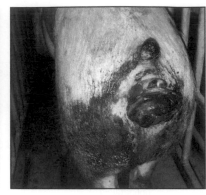

Fig. 11.170 Rectal prolapse.

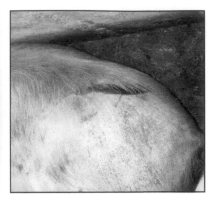

Fig. 11.171 Traumatic injuries.

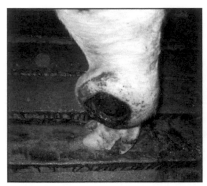

Fig. 11.172 Ulcerated granuloma.

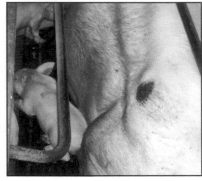

Fig. 11.173 Shoulder sore.

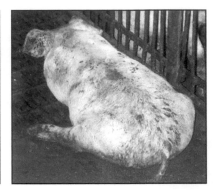

Fig. 11.174 Off back legs.

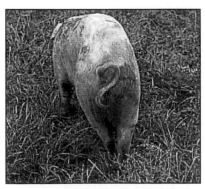

Fig. 11.175 Acutely lame.

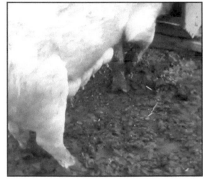

Fig. 11.176 Lame sow.

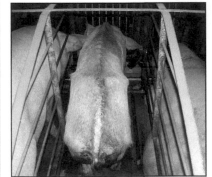

Fig. 11.177 Very thin sow.

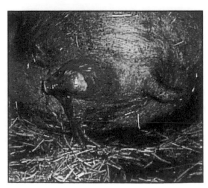

Fig. 11.178 Sow with dystocia.

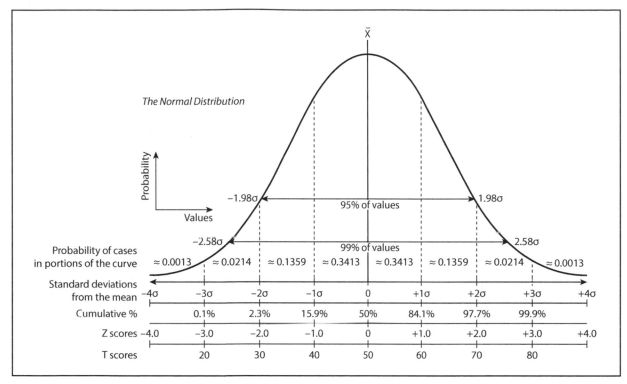

Fig. 11.179 Graph of a normal population.

If this is applied over time using the parameter of mortality, a pattern of expected results can be built up. To make an assessment of events on a farm, it is possible to use statistical process control. For example, statistical process control can be applied to post-weaning mortality. This method allows for outbreaks to be recognised, analysed and treated. This results in treatment being targeted to problems rather than be wasted on 'normal' variation.

To determine if the system is in control, maximum and minimum control limits are set. These are often set at 6 sigma points – this would be 3 SDs above and below the mean. If the results are within the two control limits, the system is said to be 'in statistical control'. If the system is 'in statistical control' then we can predict that the process will continue with approximately the same average.

How do I collate and analyse the data?
Method
1 Collect at least 20 data points to establish your control lines.
2 Determine the mean (centre line).

3 Determine control limits – 3 SDs from the mean – upper and lower.
4 Determine midline between mean and upper control limit – this is 1.5 SDs.

Example
A farm with a weekly batch production. Collecting 2 years of data on post-weaning mortality we can graph out the data as shown (**Figure 11.180**). The mortality varied from 1% to 7% from batch to batch.

Analysing the example
Mean calculated to be 3.0%, indicated by the green line

The SD is 1.3%

Therefore, the upper control limit is $3 + (3 \times 1.3) = 6.9$, indicated by the red line

Lower control limit is $3 - (3 \times 1.3) = -0.9$, not indicated as we are looking at mortality

The midline between upper control limit and mean is $([6.9 - 3]/2) + 3 = 4.95$, indicated by the black line

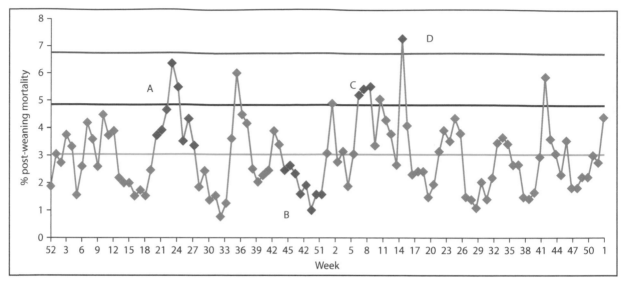

Fig. 11.180 Statistical process control review of post-weaning mortality. Mean – green line; upper control limit – red line; midline – black.

When is the post-weaning performance 'out of control'?

There are three rules to determine if the system process is out of control:

1. A single point outside control limits.
2. Three out of four consecutive points closer to the control limit than to the centre line.
3. Eight or more successive points on one side of the centre line.

Therefore, from a veterinarian's view, using the example above, the system was out of control at four incidences:

A In batches 19 to 22 in year 1 the mortality progressively increased and medication/management enhancement was required to bring the system under control, which happened in weeks 23 to 26.

B In batches 44 to 52 in year 1 there was a consistent low post-weaning mortality. There was no particular explanation to this reduction and after this period the system returned to a higher normal. Occasionally, the reduction can be maintained (e.g. following a new vaccination programme), and the farm then enters a new system control model.

C In batches 5, 6 and 7 in year 2, mortality was rising slowly, management enhancement was implemented and the system returned to within control.

D In batch 14 year 2 the mortality was suddenly out of control. This was probably a mechanical failure rather than a pathogen incursion and therefore no need to mass medicate.

The other batch fluctuations are within 'normal' variation and do not warrant any change in the health maintenance programme.

Explanation of the pattern

Normal variation is explained by 'Common causes', associated with inherent random variation. Variation outside the control limits is associated with 'Special causes', which are sporadic, unstable and unpredictable (e.g. a power failure or absence of personnel).

Use of early weaning to enhance health

It is possible to reduce the number of pathogens and even eliminate some pathogens by the use of early weaning. This programme utilises the colostral antibodies that are transferred from the mother to her offspring within 6–12 hours of birth. This method, however, is fraught with potential risks:

Table 11.26 **Persistence of specific colostral IgG antibodies in the piglet.**

WEEK WHEN MOST ANTIBODY LOST	AGENT
Week 1	*Escherichia coli*
Week 2	Transmissible gastroenteritis virus
	Porcine epidemic diarrhoea virus
Week 3	*Actinobacillus pleuropneumoniae*
	Brachyspira hyodysenteriae
	Haemophilus parasuis
	Porcine reproductive and respiratory syndrome virus
Week 4	*Pasteurella multocida*
	Bordotella bronchiseptica
Weeks 6–9	Aujeszky's disease virus (pseudorabies)
	Teschovirus
	Mycoplasma hyopneumoniae
	Porcine circovirus
	Porcine respiratory coronavirus
	Respiratory syncytial virus
	Swine influenza virus
Week 10	Classical swine fever virus
	Foot and mouth disease virus
Week 12	*Erysipelothrix rhysiopathiae*
Week 24	Parvovirus

- The piglet may not consume sufficient colostrum.
- The colostrum may not contain sufficient antibodies to the desired pathogen.
- Colostral antibodies may decline to a level that will not protect the piglet.
- The sow may be sick and not produce sufficient colostrum.

If the groups of piglets do consume sufficient antibodies from the colostrum, *Table 11.26* provides a guide to the weaning age required to 'ensure' that the piglets can be weaned free of the pathogen. Note that rigorous testing and isolation procedures are also required to ensure that the whole programme is successful. Also, the pigs need to be weaned before maternal antibodies have waned too much.

As a guide, 14 days should be the oldest age to wean pigs to achieve a segregated weaning programme.

Partial depopulation

The effect of disease can become crippling. In some cases, a partial depopulation with thorough cleaning and refurbishment of the post-weaning accommodation can help restore the farm's health, thus greatly improving the pig's welfare (*Table 11.27*). Reducing

Table 11.27 **Typical protocols required in a partial depopulation.**

DAY	EVENT
Pre-	Organise alternative accommodation for the finishers
	Purchase or make nursery kennels
	Calculate pig flow requirements
0	Weaning day. Wean all pigs older than 21 days into off-site weaner accommodation
	Stockpersons working with adults and farrowing house must not enter finishing accommodation
	All stockpersons working with adult and farrowing houses must wear clean overalls and boots
0–4	Empty grow/finish accommodation
1	Clean fridge and all tops of bottles. Dispose of all used needles and syringes
4–24	Clean out buildings, starting with weaner accommodation
7	Wean piglets into off-site weaner accommodation
	Move next week's farrowing sows into cleaned farrowing room
7–28	Repair buildings, starting with weaner accommodation
10	Veterinary check of cleaning programme
24	Wash all overalls and boots used by all personnel
	Start re-populating weaner accommodation
	Stockpersons cleaning finishing accommodation are not allowed into farrowing, adult sow or weaner accommodation
28	All buildings should be functional and ready to accept the pigs

the food conversion rate and enhancing the growth rate may also restore the farm's profitability.

Elimination of specific pathogens from farms

Pathogens can become so destructive to the farm that the welfare of the pigs is unacceptably compromised and the farm becomes economically non-viable. It will then be necessary to completely remove the pathogen. For some pathogens this is almost impossible (e.g. PCV2, *Bordetella bronchiseptica* or *Lawsonia intracellularis*). These pathogens exist in other common animals and, therefore, when eliminated the farm rapidly becomes reinfected.

However, some of the most serious pathogens in pigs can be eliminated from farms (e.g. African swine fever virus, classical swine fever virus [hog cholera], FMDV, transmissible gastroenteritis virus/porcine epidemic diarrhoea virus and Aujeszky's disease virus [pseudorabies]). This section discusses some techniques that may be used to eliminate various pathogens. The key to pathogen elimination is a thorough understanding of the epidemiology, physical characteristics and diagnostic capabilities of the specific pathogen. In addition, a pathogen is not necessarily eliminated from a farm just because it cannot be detected in the laboratory.

Also, you cannot eliminate 'disease' – only specific pathogens. This is why a term like 'high health' is meaningless. All elimination programmes hinge on the availability of negative pigs to purchase or that internal replacements will be negative (*Tables 11.28–11.31*).

Table 11.28 Elimination programmes.

1 Depopulation and repopulation

All pigs, pig products and faecal contaminants must be removed from the farm, followed by fumigation and resting of the farm. The farm is then repopulated with animals negative to the pathogen

2 Hysterectomy and move piglets to a new farm

A sow at the point of farrowing is euthanased and her uterus removed and placed in disinfectant and carried 50 metres from the euthanasia point. Here the piglets are removed from the uterus and immediately placed in a warm box and taken from the area. None of the reproductive or systemic diseases can be eliminated. Hysterectomy can be used to eliminate pathogens such as *Actinobacillus pleuropneumoniae*, *Mycoplasma hyopneumoniae* and *Sarcoptes scabiei*

3 Direct pathogen exposure

All susceptible animals are exposed to the pathogen and infected animals develop immunity. If the pathogen has no long-term carrier status it will die out on the farm. New animals are negative to the pathogen. Enteric viruses (e.g. TGEV and PEDV) are classic pathogens that may be controlled. PRRSV has also been controlled by this method combined with herd closure

4 Vaccination

All susceptible animals are vaccinated. The pathogen then dies out on the farm. Generally, it is important to identify vaccinated from wild/field pathogen infected animals. Aujeszky's disease (pseudorabies) is controlled by vaccination, combined with test and remove

5 Segregated early weaning

Segregated early weaning utilising maternal colostrum antibodies, possibly combined with medication, has proved effective at eliminating several pathogens (e.g. *Mycoplasma hyopneumoniae*). Toxigenic *Pasteurella multocida* may be eliminated but will need vaccination control and very early removal of the piglets. *Actinobacillus pleuropneumoniae* has been eliminated but requires pre-day 8 weaning of the piglets

6 Partial depopulation

Partial depopulation is where the susceptible population is removed and the pathogen is removed from the remaining adult stock. *Mycoplasma hyopneumoniae* and PRRSV are examples

7 Test and remove

All infected animals are identified and removed before they spread the pathogen to remaining susceptible animals. This can be very difficult to achieve. Combined with vaccination, Aujeszky's disease (pseudorabies) has been successfully eliminated by this method

(Continued)

Table 11.28 *(Continued)* **Elimination programmes.**

8 Herd closure

The pathogen dies out of the farm over time. Combined with vaccination and direct pathogen exposure, PRRSV and SIV have been eliminated by this method

9 Medication programmes

The pathogen has to be susceptible to medication; viruses, for example, cannot be eliminated. *Sarcoptes scabiei* (mange) and *Haematopinus suis* (lice) can be eliminated by avermectins. Tilmicosin or tulathromycin has eliminated *Mycoplasma hyopneumoniae*, especially when combined with segregated weaning and partial depopulation. Tiamulin may be effective in eliminating *Brachyspira hyodysenteriae* when combined with cleaning and partial depopulation

Table 11.29 **Possible elimination methods for the major pathogens of pigs. A hatched block indicates it is only sometimes possible.**

PATHOGEN	DEPOPULATION AND REPOPULATION	HYSTERECTOMY AND MOVE PIGLETS TO A NEW FARM	DIRECT PATHOGEN EXPOSURE	VACCINATION	SEGREGATED EARLY WEANING	PARTIAL DEPOPULATION	TEST AND REMOVE	HERD CLOSURE	MEDICATION PROGRAMMES
Actinobacillus pleuropneumoniae	■				■				
African swine fever virus	■								
Ascaris suum	▨	■							
Aujeszky's disease virus (pseudorabies)	■	▨		■			■		
Brachyspira hyodysenteriae	■								■
Brucella suis	■								
Classical swine fever virus	■								
Foot and mouth disease virus	■								
Haematopinus suis	■	■							■
Hyostrongylus rubidis	■	■							
Leptospira pomona	■								
Metastrongylus apri	▨	■							
Mycoplasma hyopneumoniae	■	■			■	■			■
Oesophagostonum dentatum	▨	■							
Pasteurella multocida (toxigenic)	■	■				▨			
Porcine epidemic diarrhoea virus	■	■	■	■					
Porcine reproductive and respiratory syndrome virus	■	■			■			■	
Sarcoptes scabiei	■	■					■		▨
Transmissible gastroenteritis virus	■	■	■						

Table 11.30 Depopulation/repopulation as a means of eliminating pathogens.

SCIENTIFIC POINTS

	Negative stock is commercially available
	The pathogen does not exist naturally in the environment or locally in common wild animals
	The pathogen can be eliminated from the contaminated building easily/quickly by routine cleaning

STANDARD DOWNTIMES

	This depends on the pathogen to be eliminated. For instance, with *Brachyspira hyodysenteriae* it should be a minimum of 8 weeks
	For routine restock, 6 weeks would be the suggested minimum

Depopulation

	Depopulation means removal of all pigs and their products from the farm for the downtime period

DEPOPULATION PROCEDURES

1	Rodent control should start and be vigorous. Place baits near water to encourage intake
2	As animals are sold, buildings become empty and should then be cleaned and repaired
3	Run down all stocks of medicines, feed and disposables
4	It will probably be necessary to arrange personnel schedules to ensure that 'dirty' stockpersons do not enter cleaned buildings

CLEANING PROTOCOLS

1	Ensure pressure washing is carried out thoroughly
2	In addition: pay particular attention to the removal of all faecal material. The building should be brushed down thoroughly and then dry cleaned using a knife and scraper to remove all visible faeces. The small amounts should be removed with a dustpan and brush. This has to be very thorough and on your hands and knees
3	Remove dust by vacuuming where possible
4	Areas of particular note – pigs have long tongues
	Under and around gate posts and gates
	Corners at the back of pens
	Around fittings (i.e. farrowing places)
	Under drinkers and troughs
	Where cracks and holes exit in the concrete
5	Repair all large cracks and holes in concrete by: cleaning out where possible; pouring in a suitable disinfectant; once dry, repair by screeding over with concrete
6	All wooden partitions should be removed and replaced with new cleanable partitions. Place outside in sunlight to dry
7	Drain and clean the slurry channels and pits. Remove all available faeces. Sometimes this is impractical but it is essential to clean to 30 cm below the removable slats
8	Ideally, lime wash all surfaces, especially up to 2 metres in height. Spray with a disinfectant using a knap sack sprayer into the ceiling and loft areas
9	Ensure that the water supplies are adequately disinfected
10	Repair all equipment to the necessary standards

(Continued)

Table 11.30 (Continued) Depopulation/repopulation as a means of eliminating pathogens.

Water	Ensure adequate flow is obtainable from all drinkers. This may necessitate replacement of all pipelines. Ensure water pressure is adequate around the system
Air	Ensure all ventilation systems are thoroughly cleaned. All fans must be checked to ensure that they perform as required. Repaint all blades. Check fan speeds with a tachometer and volt meter
Floor	All floors must be non-abrasive. All sharp points should be removed or covered. Note worn doorways, concrete under water points and around feeders, in particular wet feeding systems. All holes and cracks should be repaired. Worn rough slats must be repaired or replaced
Feed	Ensure all feeders work as required. All old food needs to be removed and sharp edges smoothed. Any holes repaired and if feeder's leak and cannot be repaired, they must be thrown away. Feed is the major cost and any waste should be minimised
Vermin	Bird proof all buildings where possible

CLEANING PROTOCOLS WHEN FARM EMPTY

	Ensure unit perimeter secure
	Finish cleaning the last building
	Dispose of all medicines, needles and syringes
	Remove all disposables from the farm, including all feed. Empty all feed hoppers and feed bins. Ideally all feed should have been eaten
Surfaces	Ensure all surfaces are cleaned. This must include the fridge, chemical store, feed stores, changing rooms and staff room
Midden area	Spread all the midden material, lagoons and slurry store
	The soil within the proximity of the midden area will have faeces still remaining from the old unit. Skim off this area to a depth of 80 cm. Spray the soil with a suitable disinfectant and then rescree over the 80 cm of soil
Straw and other bedding	Old straw should be disposed of as part of the cleaning as it can harbour mice/rats from the pre-cleaned unit
Dogs and cats	Discuss dog and cat protocols. Treatment may be required depending on the pathogens to be eradicated
Tractors	Ensure all tractors and equipment, in particular muck spreading and bob cats, are thoroughly cleaned and disinfected
	Burn all straw and used bedding
	Dispose of all brushes, shovels and scrapers
	Dispose of all overalls, boots and protective clothing
	Purchase clothing for the new clean unit

FARM CLEANING PROTOCOLS

1	Pressure wash all buildings
2	Lime wash all buildings
3	Fumigate all buildings
4	Seal all buildings as each building becomes clean
5	Dispose of all clothing, boots and purchase new when whole farm finished

ONCE WHOLE FARM FUMIGATED

1	Restore water supplies and check all drinkers work. Note that when water supplies are cleaned, the loosened deposits can block the drinkers
2	Ensure rodent controls are maintained, particularly at the perimeter of the farm

NEW STOCK INTRODUCTION AND BIOSECURITY PROTOCOLS

1	The new stock require isolation procedures
2	Note biosecurity requirements; these vary depending on the health of the incoming stock

Table 11.31 Depopulation and repopulation Calendar of Events – Week (7 day) batch

36	35	34	33	32	31	30	29	28	27	26	25	24	23	22	21	20	19	18	17	16	15	14	13	12	11	10	9	8	7	6	5	4	3	2	1	1	2	3	4

Breeding replacement farm

- Gilts arrive (week 2)
- Farrow (week 1)
- 1st Gilt breeding (weeks 14–17)
- Gilt preparation 9 weeks (weeks 21–27)
- Clean replacement

Depopulation and repopulation farm

- Breed last sows (week 34)
- Farrow last group of sows (week 28)
- Sell sows at weaning from now on (weeks 30 onwards)
- To sell 30 kg weaners (week 16)
- Last 30 kg born (week 17)
- Sell 7 kg (week 10)
- Clean farm / Fumigate (weeks 6–9)

Or if a weaner market

- Breed last sows (week 25)
- Farrow last sows (week 24)
- Sell sows at weaning from now on (week 24)
- Last finishers born (week 30)
- Last finishers enter grow finish (week 17)
- Sell all 30 kg pigs (week 20)
- Sell weaners (week 12)

Farm emptied of all stock

Start rodent control programme and prepare for the refurbishment and cleaning of the farm

■ = gilts are bred only over a 7-day period (Friday to Thursday, for example). It is essential to get the batches together. The batches of gilts mated in the hatched weeks are mated on the clean farm. Organise gilts using altrenogest and possibly also use PG600.

□ = the week of an event.

The slaughter weight is assumed to be reached at 22 weeks of age.

Weaners are at maximum 28 days of age.

Depopulation and repopulation problems

Some examples of how repopulations have encountered problems are shown in the following sections.

Inadequate planning
See **Figures 11.181–11.186**.

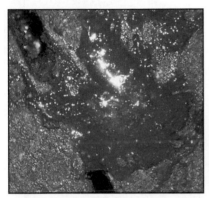

Fig. 11.181 Pathogens not recognised – *Brachyspira hyodysenteriae* is one example where failure to recognise its presence will result in too short a downtime.

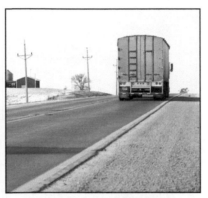

Fig. 11.182 Unrealistic pathogen removal associated with pathogens in the same district too close to the farm. Note the location of the "isolation" unit.

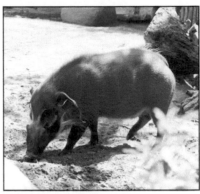

Fig. 11.183 The presence of wild pigs, even from different species, in the vicinity and poor fencing.

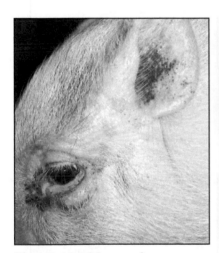

Fig. 11.184 New stock are infected with pathogens; *Sarcoptes scabiei* is an example.

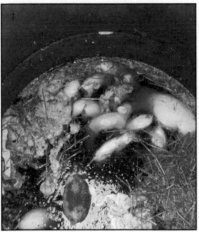

Fig. 11.185 Inadequate removal of previous dead animals.

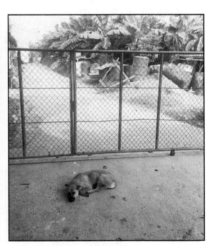

Fig. 11.186 Inadequate review of surrounding wildlife

Inadequate preparation
See **Figures 11.187–11.192**.

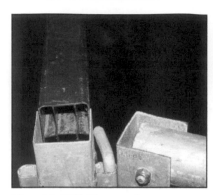

Fig. 11.187 Pipes and gates may contain faeces on the inside.

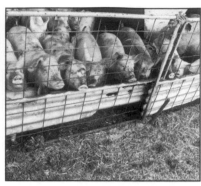

Fig. 11.188 Gates require to be fixed before cleaning. Note particularly under the gate.

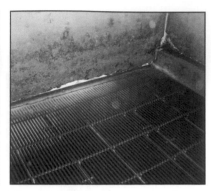

Fig. 11.189 Inadequate repair of buildings. Note the holes in the walls and the large cracks.

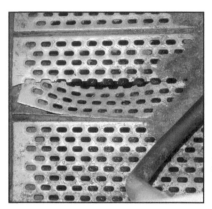

Fig. 11.190 Destroy and remove all broken equipment.

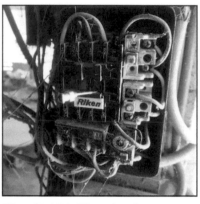

Fig. 11.191 Electrics that are not cleaned.

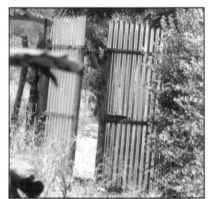

Fig. 11.192 Poor farm security during and after cleaning.

Greed
See **Figures 11.193–11.198**.

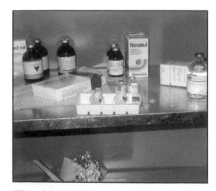

Fig. 11.193 Keeping 'old' medicines on the farm. Even unopened packages should be suspected.

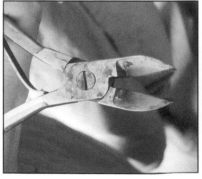

Fig. 11.194 Keeping old equipment such as piglet processing equipment.

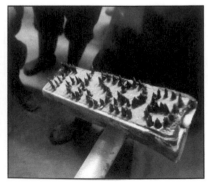

Fig. 11.195 Slap markers are a classic to remain on the farm.

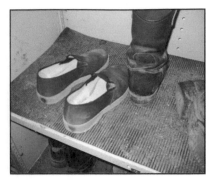

Fig. 11.196 Keeping boots (e.g. the favourite slippers).

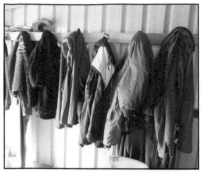

Fig. 11.197 Attempting to clean overalls, especially pressure washing protective clothing.

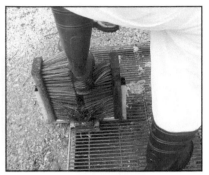

Fig. 11.198 Keeping other equipment that has been in direct contact with the previous pigs.

Inadequate cleaning
See **Figures 11.199–11.207**.

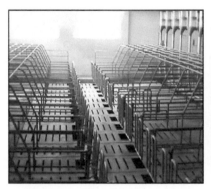

Fig. 11.199 Examine cleaned area extremely carefully.

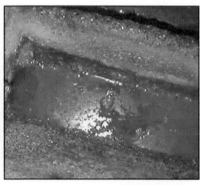

Fig. 11.200 Water unclean with faeces from previous groups.

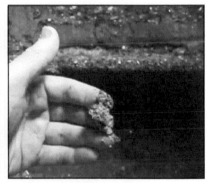

Fig. 11.201 Examine floor for faeces. The building should be checked by the veterinarian.

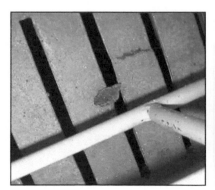

Fig. 11.202 Even small pieces of faeces need to be manually removed.

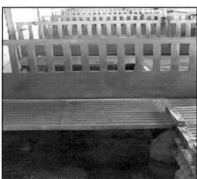

Fig. 11.203 Under the slatted floor can be extremely difficult to clean.

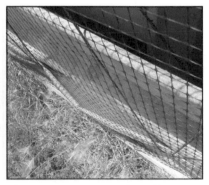

Fig. 11.204 Remember all areas where dirt can hide (e.g. inside curtains).

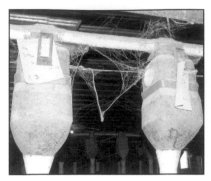

Fig. 11.205 Cobwebs should be manually removed, especially around electrics.

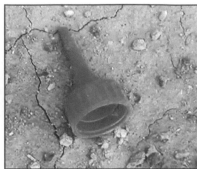

Fig. 11.206 Evidence of the previous pig farm may be clear, such as this AI top.

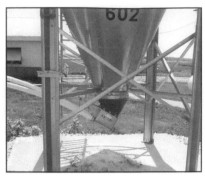

Fig. 11.207 Old feed on a farm in bags and in feed bins and pipelines.

Poor repair of farm facilities
See **Figures 11.208–11.213**.

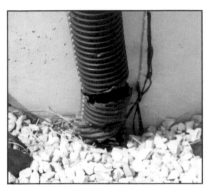

Fig. 11.208 Downpipes left unfixed are a rodent risk.

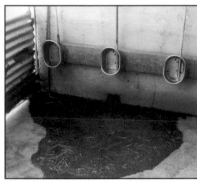

Fig. 11.209 Waterers that are leaking.

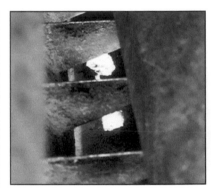

Fig. 11.210 Feeders with holes.

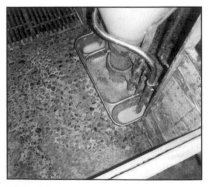

Fig. 11.211 Floors that are worn, especially under waterer and feeders.

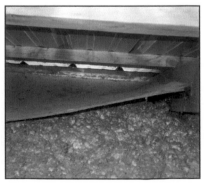

Fig. 11.212 Ventilation systems broken (e.g. blocked attic inlets).

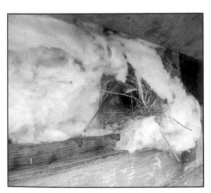

Fig. 11.213 Insulation that requires replacing.

Post-repopulation problems
See **Figures 11.214–11.228**.

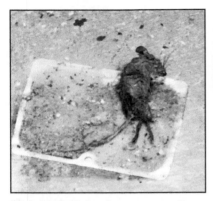

Fig. 11.214 Inadequate vermin control programmes.

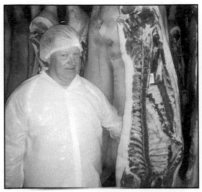

Fig. 11.215 Biosecurity rules broken by stockpersons (e.g. slaughterhouse visits).

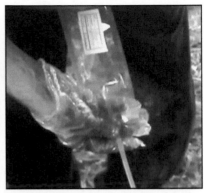

Fig. 11.216 Introduction of pathogens. Remember pigs are the number one risk.

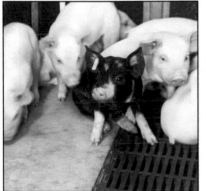

Fig. 11.217 Congenital tremor. Can be a particular problem in start-up herds and a risk to new gilts

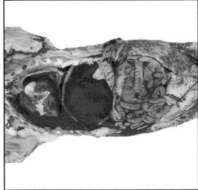

Fig. 11.218 Mulberry heart. With increased growth rate, increase vitamin E supplementation to the weaners. Figure shows classic liver rupture and abdomen full of blood.

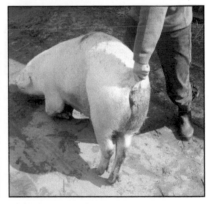

Fig. 11.219 Slippery floors associated with extremely good cleaning. Can result in damage to the hips of gilts or weaned sows.

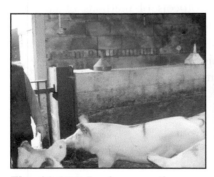

Fig. 11.220 Inadequate gilt numbers provided or selected and batch breeding targets missed.

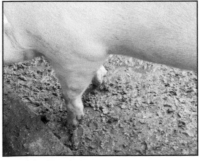

Fig. 11.221 Poor selection of gilts associated with pressure of the 'sale'; in particular, check backs, legs and teats.

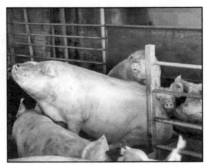

Fig. 11.222 Poor feeding control resulting in breeding of overweight pigs or too young gilts being mated.

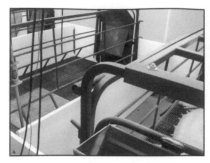

Fig. 11.223 Over optimistic gilt reproduction resulting in empty farrowing places.

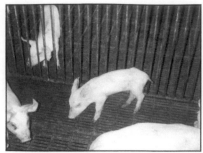

Fig. 11.224 Too many gilts bred, again resulting in poor pig flow and poor weaners.

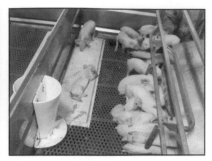

Fig. 11.225 Pre-weaning diarrhoea due to poor parity 1 immune status

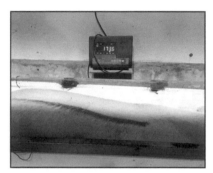

Fig. 11.226 Overweight/fat finishing pigs as growth rates are unexpectedly high.

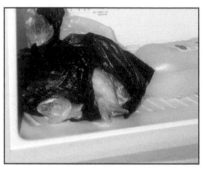

Fig. 11.227 Careless breach of biosecurity, bringing pork products onto the farm.

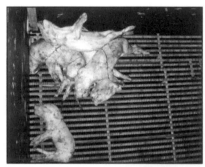

Fig. 11.228 In the long term, if poor parity control occurs, the herd ages and stillbirth rates increase.

Depopulation and subsequent repopulation can be a great success if the process is fully planned, orchestrated and then implemented. The major reasons for problems are failing to set formal goals and then setting out to complete these goals. Remember that the repopulation is about gilts and if they are rushed the consequences are far reaching. Coordinate the gilt growth, introduction, flow and future care with all members of the health team.

Finally, remember that not all 'pathogens' can be eliminated (e.g. *Erysipelothrix rhusiopathiae*). Some are brought rapidly back onto the farm (e.g. *Bordetella bronchiseptica*) and some are present in other animals (e.g. *Lawsonia intracellularis*).

In some cases, perhaps, the organism should not be eliminated as its absence makes new stock introduction impossible and movement of the produced stock difficult (e.g. *Haemophilus parasuis*).

Examples of pathogen elimination methods

Some example protocols of methods of eliminating pathogens are shown in *Tables 11.32–38*. In these examples, specific antibiotics are discussed. However, as science progresses, other antibiotics may be more suitable.

Table 11.32 **Hysterectomy and moving pigs to a new farm to help eliminate *Actinobacillus pleuropneumoniae* infection.**

SCIENTIFIC ASSUMPTIONS

The organism is not normally present on the skin

The organism not normally present in the blood

The organism is not passed through the placenta to the fetus

SOW PREPARATION PROTOCOLS

The sow should be presented at 112–114 days of gestation.
The day before the hysterectomy, the sow should be washed without causing stress

DAY BEFORE HYSTERECTOMY

1 It is better to not try to delay the farrowing but sometimes it will necessary. Three compounds may be considered. Check that these compounds are legal: (1) Progesterone: 300 mg intramuscularly day before, and (2) clenbuterol: 10 mL (300 mg) intramuscular dose every 12 hours. (3) Altrenogest may assist in delaying parturition

2 Ensure that a foster mother is going to be available on the new farm

PREPARATION PROTOCOL

1 The sow must not be in labour and giving birth. If any piglets have been born or there is placenta showing, the sow must not be moved off the unit

2 The sow should be gently driven to the site of hysterectomy

3 The truck, driver and support staff must stay at least 50 metres away from the piglet end of the hysterectomy

4 The driver and support staff must wear clean outer clothing on the day of the hysterectomy. Particular areas of concern are the wearing of clean boots and washed hands

5 The truck used to transport the sow should be cleaned and disinfected and not used to move pigs for 12 hours after cleaning and disinfection

6 The breeding company must ensure all parties know that the hysterectomy is to be carried out the next morning

HYSTERECTOMY SITE

1 The hysterectomy site must be secure and discreet

2 The site should be arranged so that the piglet area and dam area are clearly separated by a minimum of 50 metres

3 No staff should move between the two sites at any time except briefly when moving the uterus

4 After the hysterectomy has been completed all material must be removed and the site disinfected

5 If the carcase remains at the hysterectomy site, it must be placed in a covered and/or purpose built dog proof building. The carcase must be removed within 24 hours of slaughter. The carcase must have been removed prior to another hysterectomy being carried out

PREPARATION FOR HYSTERECTOMY

Day prior to hysterectomy

Stockpersons responsibilities

1 Prepare the bath, ensure that it is thoroughly cleaned and disinfected

2 Ensure the hysterectomy table is thoroughly clean

WITHIN 15 MINUTES OF THE START OF THE HYSTERECTOMY

1 The bath is to be filled to a water depth of 30 cm with hot tap water

2 Add suitable mild disinfectant to the water

(Continued)

Table 11.32 *(Continued)* **Hysterectomy and moving pigs to a new farm to help eliminate *Actinobacillus pleuropneumoniae* infection.**

3	Move the bath to the clean site of the hysterectomy
4	Have one additional bucket of warm clean water ready to clean post slaughter
5	If the hysterectomy is not carried out within 25 minutes of filling the bath, then the bath should be refilled with water at the required temperature

SLAUGHTER PROCEDURE

Three people are required: stockpersons 1 and 2 and one veterinarian

1	The piglet area must be ready
2	The sow must be securely snared and restrained by stockperson 1
3	The veterinarian gives stockperson 2 the pithing rod and the knife
4	Both stockpersons must stand behind the veterinarian. The veterinarian shoots the sow using a captive bolt
5	Immediately the veterinarian passes the discharged gun to stockperson 2 by the handle, keeping the gun pointing at the floor at all times
6	Then stockperson 2 passes the pithing rod to the veterinarian
7	The veterinarian attempts to insert the pithing rod into the cranial hole. A certain degree of force may be required to fully penetrate the cranium
8	Stockperson 1 must stay behind the veterinarian and continue to restrain the sow on the snare
9	The pithing rod is passed down the spinal cord of the sow and slowly moved in and out until all excessive movement stops
10	Leave the pithing rod in place until after the hysterectomy

HYSTERECTOMY PROCEDURE

1	The sow is rolled on to her back with stockperson 1 holding one hind leg
2	Stockperson 2 passes the knife to the veterinarian then places the gun back in its gun box
3	Stockperson 2 prepares to bring the hot water bath to the side of the sow
4	Starting at the xyphoid process, the veterinarian cuts through the skin and fat, down to between the hind legs. Do not penetrate the abdomen. Cut only through skin and fat
5	Penetrate the abdominal cavity at the xyphoid process. Make a sufficiently large hole to allow the hand to be inserted into the abdominal cavity. Reverse the cutting method and raising the abdominal wall with the hand, cut along the *linea alba*. Take particular care not to penetrate any internal organs
6	Place the knife blade into the muscles of the fore leg
7	Bring the hot water bath to the side of the sow
8	Pull the uterus into the bath. Pull and tear the ovarian end. In some cases the cervical end can even be torn, but in most cases the cervical end will need to be severed by the knife
9	Once the whole uterus is in the water bath, both stockpersons must briskly walk with the bath to the piglet area

POSSIBLE PROBLEMS DURING HYSTERECTOMY

A	A small hole has been made in the uterus but no piglets are released. Ignore and continue
B	A larger hole has been made in the uterus and a piglet is released. Keep pulling the uterus into the water bath and proceed with the hysterectomy. The released piglet must not be moved to the piglet processing area but is dried and returned, whenever possible, to the sow source farm

(Continued)

Table 11.32 *(Continued)* **Hysterectomy and moving pigs to a new farm to help eliminate *Actinobacillus pleuropneumoniae* infection.**

THE PIGLET SITE

Day before hysterectomy

1 Processing table. Ensure the table is cleaned and disinfected thoroughly at least 12 hours before the hysterectomy. The table is designed to have a grill to allow water though but not the uterus and piglets

2 Piglet transportation box. Make sure the box is cleaned and disinfected thoroughly at least 12 hours before the hysterectomy. Ensure the box can be warmed effectively, that there is an adequate number of boxes and that they are big enough to take the maximum number of piglets

3 The truck to transport the piglets to the new farm. Make sure it is cleaned and disinfected thoroughly at least 12 hours before the hysterectomy

DAY OF HYSTERECTOMY

1 The piglet area should be discretely sited

2 The veterinarian, nurse and stockperson from the destination farm should have clean outer clothing and boots. Plastic outer protectors should be worn

3 Hands should be cleaned prior to arrival and washed with surgical scrub disinfectant. Gloves can be worn by the operators. However, gloves can interfere with the processing time as it can make it more difficult to remove the piglets from the uterus

4 Tools required are: 24 pairs of naval clamps, sterilised curved blunt ended scissors, dry towels and revival solutions

PIGLET PROCESSING

1 The two stockpersons approach the processing table and pour the water and disinfectant onto and through the processing table

2 The two stockpersons then walk back to the hysterectomy site

3 All three operators (one vet, nurse and stockperson) open the uterus and remove the piglets. Do not cut into the piglets

4 The veterinarian then moves the blood up the cord towards each pig and places a navel clamp approximately 5 cm from the umbilicus. The umbilical cord is then cut from the placenta from each piglet

5 During all this time the nurse and stockperson use dry towels to massage and dry the piglets. The nurse and stockperson must talk to the piglets and encourage the piglets to breath

6 Piglets should squeal and move vigorously before being moved into the transportation box

7 If piglets are having problems with breathing, attempt to recover using a suitable revival solution dripped on the tongue. Despite the temptation, mouth to mouth resuscitation is not to be attempted as pathogen transmission may occur

8 Once all the piglets are in the transportation box the stockperson, transportation box and transport truck must leave for the new farm

9 Any piglets with any deformity likely to affect production must not enter the piglet transportation box. For example, deformed legs or cleft palate (if noticed)

10 The piglet processing area is now thoroughly cleaned down and all disposable equipment disposed of hygienically (plastic overcoat, gloves etc.)

AT THE NEW FARM

New farm has no sow available

The farm facilities must be extremely clean

Note the new piglets will have received no colostrum and, therefore, will have no natural immunity

Provide artificial colostrum supplements. Cow colostrum may be a good substitute. Provide 50 mL per piglet at 10 mL per dose by stomach tube.

Inject each piglet with 3 mg ceftiofur or 5 mg tulathromycin

(Continued)

Table 11.32 *(Continued)* **Hysterectomy and moving pigs to a new farm to help eliminate *Actinobacillus pleuropneumoniae* infection.**

New stock being moved to an established farm

Induce sows to farrow on the day of the hysterectomy

Foster pigs of sows as they farrow. If short of sows, box up sow's natural piglets and give them artificial colostrum and once all pigs are born, give them one suckle of the sow

Hysterectomy piglets must be given priority. When hysterectomy piglets arrive, do not fuss over them. Put shredded paper in the pen and extra lights. Ensure foster sow has not suckled in the last hour, and then just leave the hysterectomy piglets to get on with it

Inject each piglet with 3 mg ceftiofur or 5 mg tulathromycin

Table 11.33 **Segregated early weaning to eliminate *Mycoplasma hyopneumoniae*.**

SCIENTIFIC ASSUMPTIONS

Sows remain infected all their lives

M. hyopneumoniae colostrum antibodies remain for 14 days post consumption

M. hyopneumoniae can be killed with tilmicosin, tiamulin, tulathromycin or chlortetracycline

M. hyopneumoniae can be eliminated by cleaning of an off-site nursery

The absence of *M. hyopneumoniae* antibodies and that PCR is an effective diagnostic tool at 10 weeks of age

Source of *M. hyopneumoniae*-negative pigs is available.

M. hyopneumoniae only spreads 3 km between farms

SOW PREPARATION PROGRAMME

8 weeks pre-farrowing

Vaccinate the sows. The success of the programme relies on colostrum antibodies and the key to this is vaccination. Ensure vaccines are stored properly and administered using a 40 mm 1.3 mm needle

Possible vaccinations are: *Actinobacillus pleuropneumoniae*, atrophic rhinitis (toxin), clostridia, *E. coli*, erysipelas, *Haemophilus parasuis*, *Lawsonia intracellularis*, *Mycoplasma hyopneumoniae*, porcine reproductive and respiratory syndrome (dead), swine influenza and rotaviruses

Provide the sows with feedback using nursery faeces and diarrhoea from the farrowing house.

4 weeks pre-farrowing

Repeat the vaccine and feedback programme

2 weeks pre-farrowing

Provide in-feed medication of tilmicosin (400 g/tonne) and chlortetracycline (800 g/tonne) to the sows until the piglets are weaned at 10 days of age

7–5 days pre-farrowing

All sows must be healthy; move into farrowing house

| General bacteria | Tetracycline long acting | 30 mg/kg IM into the neck using a 40 mm 1.3 mm needle |

(Continued)

Table 11.33 *(Continued)* **Segregated early weaning to eliminate *Mycoplasma hyopneumoniae.***

WEANER PROGRAMME

Day of life

1	Iron	200 mg IM into the neck using a 16 mm 0.8 mm needle
	Colostrum	
2	Avermectin	300 µg/kg SC into the neck using a 16 mm 0.8 mm needle
	Tulathromycin	2.5 mg/kg IM into the neck using a 16 mm 0.8 mm needle
	Enrofloxacin	Oral medicator – 10 mg (not legal in any country)
4	Toltrazuril	7 mg/kg oral dose – to control coccidiosis
5	Ceftiofur	5 mg/kg IM into the neck using a 16 mm 0.8 mm needle
9	Ceftiofur	5 mg/kg IM into the neck using a 16 mm 0.8 mm needle
10	Weaned; move to the off-site nursery – note biosecurity of truck and site	

POST WEANING AT THE CLEAN OFF-SITE NURSERY

	Tiamutin 12.5% solution	180 ppm through the water supply supplied for the first 7 days post weaning
	Chlortetracycline	800 g per tonne of creep feed, to be fed for 21 days post weaning
	Tilmicosin	400 g per tonne of creep feed, to be fed for 21 days post weaning
	Avermectin	300 µg/kg SC into the neck using a 16 mm 0.8 mm needle
	Tulathromycin	2.5 mg/kg IM into the neck using a 16 mm 0.8 mm needle

TESTING THE PIGS

Deaths	All deaths should be subject to post-mortem examination
Diarrhoea	Investigate all cases of diarrhoea
Coughing	Investigate all cases of coughing and sneezing. Note that post-weaning sneezing may occur
10 weeks of age	Pigs should be tested to ensure that they are negative. Ensure that the testing does not detect maternal colostrum antibodies
Sentinel	Place known negative gilts into contact with grow/finish pigs and blood test after 1 month. Note any coughing experienced by these gilts

MOVE THE PIGS TO THE CLEAN SECOND SITE GROW/FINISH FARM

| | Assuming all the pigs are negative, move the pigs to the new grow/finish operation. If there is any question over the health of the pigs, they must not be moved to the new farm |

Table 11.34 **Partial depopulation as a method of eliminating *Mycoplasma hyopneumoniae.***

SCIENTIFIC ASSUMPTIONS

Sows remain infected all their lives

M. hyopneumoniae colostrum antibodies remain for 14 days post consumption

M. hyopneumoniae can be killed with tilmicosin, tiamulin, tulathromycin or chlortetracycline

M. hyopneumoniae survives in the environment for only a couple of days

The absence of *M. hyopneumoniae* antibodies, PCR and/or immunohistochemistry are effective diagnostic tools at 12 weeks of age

Source of *M. hyopneumoniae*-negative pigs is available.

M. hyopneumoniae only spreads 3 km between farms

(Continued)

Table 11.34 *(Continued)* **Partial depopulation as a method of eliminating *Mycoplasma hyopneumoniae.***

PREPARATION OF THE PROGRAMME

All animals older than 10 days of age and less than 10 months of age will be removed from the farm

Farrow to finish farm – review protocols of partial depopulation with the inclusion of the need to care for piglets from 10 days of age

Review the pig flow programme to ensure that sufficient young sows will be available to compensate for the shortfall of gilts that will occur for a 3 month period

Cull all sows/boars where necessary to reduce the herd size if appropriate, with considerations for maintaining pig flow

Cull all unhealthy sows and boars

The eradication should be programmed for the summer months, which will aid environmental removal of the mycoplasma

As buildings become empty ensure that a full cleaning, repair and refurbishment programme is instigated

8 weeks before start of the programme

Vaccinate the sows and boars against *M. hyopneumoniae*. It is essential to ensure that all piglets get colostrum and sows are not shedding *M. hyopneumoniae* while in the farrowing house. The success of the programme relies on colostrum antibodies and the key to this is vaccination. Ensure vaccines are stored properly and administered using a 40 mm 1.3 mm gauge needle

Provide the sows and boars with feedback, using nursery faeces and diarrhoea from the farrowing house. All the adults must be immune to *M. hyopneumoniae*

4 weeks before start of the programme

Repeat the vaccine and feedback programme

Start of the 6 week eradication programme

Ensure that all sows and boars will be provided with 3 kg a day of medicated feed. Boars may require more to ensure adequate medication for their weight or use in combination with injection

Boar alternative medication is via injection – consider using tulathromycin (2.5 mg/kg) once every 7 days. Weigh boars as necessary

Provide in-feed medication of tilmicosin (400 g/tonne) and chlortetracycline (800 g/tonne) to the sows. This should be provided for a period of 6 weeks. Tilmicosin may be very bitter, therefore provide sugar in the feed to assist palatability of feed

In the farrowing house provide 3 kg of medicated feed in the morning and unmedicated feed in the evening

Inject any sick or inappetent sow (in oestrus, for example) with tulathromycin (2.5 mg/kg). If a sow is sick for 3 days, it should be euthanased. *M. hyopneumoniae* must not be allowed to remain in weakened adults

MANAGEMENT OF PIGLETS IN THE FARROWING HOUSE TO ASSIST SURVIVAL OF 10-DAY WEANED PIGLETS

Day of life

1	Iron	200 mg IM into the neck using a 16 mm 0.8 mm needle
	Colostrum	All piglets must receive colostrum from sows. If there is any suspicion that a piglet has failed to receive adequate colostrum, it should be euthanased.
2	Ceftiofur	5 mg/kg IM into the neck using a 16 mm 0.8 mm needle
	Enrofloxacin or tulathromycin	Oral medicator – 10 mg (not legal in any country). Tulathromycin by injection – 2.5 mg/kg
4	Toltrazuril	7 mg/kg oral dose – to control coccidiosis
5	Ceftiofur	5 mg/kg IM into the neck using a 16 mm 0.8 mm needle
9	Ceftiofur	5 mg/kg IM into the neck using a 16 mm 0.8 mm needle
10	Weaned piglets moved to the off-site nursery – note biosecurity of truck and site	

(Continued)

Table 11.34 *(Continued)* **Partial depopulation as a method of eliminating *Mycoplasma hyopneumoniae*.**

MANAGEMENT OF THE EARLY WEANED SOW

Place the early weaned sow onto altrenogest 1 day before weaning. Maintain altrenogest until normal expected weaning day. This is essential to maintain pig flow. It is possible to provide altrenogest via toasted bread or train the pig to take from a drench using apple juice or canola oil for 3 days prior to dosing regime

CONFIRMING ERADICATION OF *MYCOPLASMA HYOPNEUMONIAE*

Deaths	All deaths should be subject to post-mortem examination
Coughing	Investigate all cases of coughing and sneezing. Note post-weaning sneezing may occur
12 weeks of age	The pigs should be tested to ensure that they are negative. Ensure that the testing does not detect maternal colostrum antibodies.
Sentinel	Place known negative gilts into contact with grow/finish pigs and blood test after 1 month. Note any coughing experienced by these gilts
Time	The farm should be examined serially over a period of at least 1 year, utilising clinical examination, blood serology and slaughterhouse tests. Perform immunohistochemistry on any suspect lesions

Table 11.35 **Vaccination and test and remove. Aujeszky's disease virus (pseudorabies) eradication programme from a low infected farm.**

SCIENTIFIC ASSUMPTIONS

Aujeszky's disease virus is a stable DNA virus

There is an effective vaccine

A diagnostic test differentiates between vaccinated and field infected animals

VACCINATION

1	All pigs over 10 weeks of age should be vaccinated with a gene deleted vaccine. Continue vaccination for 6 months. This will keep the virus at bay while the herd is cleaned up. Stringent biosecurity measures need to be in operation.

TEST AND REMOVE

2	Blood test all the boars, sows and gilts and examine by serology. Blood test 30–50 pigs in the following groups: 30–45 kg, 45–70 kg and 70+ kg range
	If less than 10% of the animals are positive, remove any positive boars, sows and gilts immediately. Then move to point 3. If more than 10% are positive, either depopulate or set up an off-site weaning programme. This would need its own programme
3	30 days later, blood test all the boar, sows and gilts and examine by serology. Repeat serological profile
	Any positive boars/sows or gilts should be removed from the herd immediately. If some of the finishers are positive, ear tag/notch negative pigs at 30 kg, place them around the grower facility and specifically retest these animals every 6 weeks. These will act as sentinels
	If all animals are negative, go to point 4
4	A minimum of 120 sows should be tested and retested 90 days later. Repeat serological profile
	Any positive boars/sows or gilts should be removed from the herd immediately and go back to point 3
	If all animals are negative, go to point 5
5	Retest 6 months later. Any positive boars/sows or gilts should be removed from the herd immediately and go back to point 3
6	If all animals are negative, it is highly likely you now have a negative herd. The vaccination programme can be dismantled over the next 18 months
7	Declare the farm free of Aujeszky's disease virus (pseudorabies)

Table 11.36 **Herd closure and pathogen exposure. Example: porcine reproductive and respiratory syndrome virus (PRRSV).**

SCIENTIFIC ASSUMPTIONS

No long-term (over a specified time) carrier status for PRRSV in sows or boars
PRRSV particles are excreted for less than 100 days following infection (see note at bottom)
Piglets less than 14 days of age are protected by maternal colostrum-deprived antibodies
Spread of PRRSV is difficult/unlikely over 1,000 metres
It is not significantly present in other animal species

DIFFICULTIES

PRRSV is not excreted in many body fluids consistently
Reproductive problems of PRRSV may be accentuated by the treatment advised

TECHNIQUE

Purchase sufficient young gilts to provide breeding animals for 100 days
Close the farm to all inputs, except for PRRSV-free semen

INFECT ALL ANIMALS ON THE FARM – PATHOGEN EXPOSURE

	Vaccinate all sows, gilts and boars with a suitable PRRSV vaccine; a live vaccine is acceptable if no previous exposure
	Create a 'vaccination model' from the native pigs. For example, obtain tonsillar scrapes from all animals with acute signs. This is made up to vaccinate all sows, gilts, boars and young future breeding stock
	Practice feedback of of rope chewed by acutely ill pigs from the nursery that has become covered in saliva and nasaoral fluids and therefore will contain farm PRRSV, and also aborted materials; aborted materials; macerate piglets that die with clinical signs. Feed this material for 14 days
	At the end of the infection period, throw away all used needles and syringes
2 weeks later	Vaccinate all sows, gilts and boars with a dead PRRSV vaccine to reduce viral shedding
	At the end of the infection period, throw away all used needles and syringes

HERD CLOSURE

The farm must be totally closed (except for PRRSV-free semen) for 100 days minimum
All piglets over 14 days of age are weaned off the farm for 100 days
Enhance biosecurity measures

CLEAN FARM

At 90 days post infection, disinfect the entire farm with a suitable disinfectant. Disinfect the walls and ventilation system, and also the water supply. Wash all clothing and boots. Throw out all used needles and syringes. Note that the pigs are present

CHECK THE EFFECT OF THE ERADICATION

1	Purchase 20 PRRSV-free gilts
2	Introduce gilts into the farm and place the animals all around the farm
3	After 21 days, bleed the 20 gilts
4	After 35 days, re-bleed the 20 gilts
5	If the gilts are negative, declare the farm free of PRRSV and allow the weaning age to increase
6	If any of the gilts are positive, all the gilts should be removed. The farm remains closed for another 30 days and the test repeated

POST CONTROL

All gilts and boars introduced into the farm through an adequate isolation area are PRRSV negative
Ideally, practice on-farm semen collection
Do not use a live vaccine on the introduced animals
Continue enhanced biosecurity measures

Table 11.37 Porcine reproductive and respiratory syndrome virus elimination. Calendar of events.

Week 1	Infect all sows and boars – live vaccine and own material from farm Ensure all staff are well aware of biosecurity measures Isolation animals – infect all with dead vaccine and own materials Move materials from the isolation area? Purchase new stock for 100 days and ensure all animals are exposed Close the herd
Week 2	Stop live vaccines Continue feedback (rope and feedback) for 14 days
Week 3	Throw away all used needles and syringes Start 100-day countdown All piglets older than 14 days weaned off farm Limit or cease cross-fostering
Weeks 4–14	All piglets older than 14 days weaned off farm Limit or cease cross-fostering
Week 14	Disinfect walls, floors, air and water, vehicles and utensils Throw away all clothing, boots etc., needles and syringes Order 20 PRRSV-negative gilts
Week 18	Introduce the 20 gilts into the isolation. Order 20 PRRSV-negative gilts.
Week 21	Bleed gilts. If negative, go to next week. Move additional 20 PRRSV-free gilts onto main farm If gilts are positive, immediately remove from the isolation area Close farm for 30 days and re-start checking programme
Week 24	Bleed gilts in isolation and main farm. If negative, go to next week If any gilt is positive, immediately remove from the isolation area Close farm for 30 days and re-start checking programme
Week 25	Start weaning as normal
Week 27	Bleed all 40 gilts again. If negative: re-start gilt introduction programme; declare the farm free of PRRSV

Note: This programme has successfully eliminated PRRSV from a number of farms. As science progresses, PCR technology has revealed PRRSV virus in tissues for 200 days post exposure. Therefore, in designing the herd closure programme the health team must consider the relative risks. In certain circumstances a 200-day closure programme may be adopted rather than the 100-day programme discussed.

Table 11.38 Medication as a means of eliminating pathogens. Example: *Sarcoptes scabiei* var *suis* from a farrow to wean unit.

SCIENTIFIC POINTS	
	Avermectin remains active in the pig for 7 days post treatment
	Sarcoptic eggs are resistant to avermectins
	Sarcoptic eggs hatch in 5 days
	Sarcoptic mites may live off the host for 21 days, but in the summer months this is reduced to 5 days
	It is difficult to estimate the weight of boars so they are often underdosed – a major reason for the programme failure
Animal	Programme
Suckling pigs	Inject in the neck with an avermectin (300 µg/kg) using a 16 mm 0.8 mm needle and an insulin syringe
Gilt pool	In-feed medication for 7 days with an inclusion of avermectin (100 µg/kg). Ensure all animals eat 2.75 kg per day

(Continued)

Table 11.38 *(Continued)* **Medication as a means of eliminating pathogens. Example:** *Sarcoptes scabiei* var *suis* from a farrow to wean unit.

SCIENTIFIC POINTS	
Breeding and pregnant sows	In-feed medication for 7 days with an inclusion of averectin (100 µg/kg). Ensure all animals are fed 2.7 kg of feed per day. Ignore condition score
Lactating sows	Feed 2.7 kg of the dry sow ration, with an inclusion of avermectin (100 µg/kg) in the morning for 7 days. Feed lactator in the evening
Boars	Feed dry sow ration with an inclusion of avermectin (100 µg/kg). For large boars increase quantity of feed. For instance, for a 200 kg boar feed 2.7 kg per day for 7 days; 250 kg boar feed 3.3 kg per day for 7 days; and for a 300 kg boar feed 4 kg per day. Alternatively, inject with an avermectin (300 µg/kg)
Hospital pens	Inject all pigs in the neck with an avermectin (300 µg/kg)
All adults off feed for more than 24 hours	Inject in the neck with an averectin (300 µg/kg). Note sows in oestrus
Buildings	At the end of the 7-day animal treatment period spray all houses with amitraz 0.1% (40 mL per 10 L of water) using a knapsack sprayer
Clothing	Stockpersons attending to the grow/finish herd should not wear the same overalls when attending to the breeding herd
	At the end of the 7-day animal treatment period all overalls and boots should be washed thoroughly, disinfected and re-washed in amitraz 0.1%
Repeat injection programme 14 days after initial treatment started and repeat medicated feed 7 days after previous treatment ended	
Feed bin management	All feed lines should be flushed with normal food after the 7-day period to remove any treated feed material

Note: If this programme is combined with a partial depopulation or a clean pen break system, mange can be eliminated from a farrow to finish farm.

ANTIBIOTIC-FREE FARMING

Farming without antibiotic medications (raised without antibiotics [RWA]) is not difficult, but does take determination by the whole health team to want to make it happen. Farming the pigs (even most of them) without antibiotics has to be the aim of health maintenance; however, sick pigs still require treatment. The aim of antibiotic-free farming is to enhance the health of most of the pigs and to manage any pig that becomes compromised into a streamed programme.

Note: All meat sold today is free of unacceptable antimicrobial residues provided withdrawal times on medications are followed by the whole farm health team. Pork is 'antibiotic free'.

Before embarking on an antibiotic-free farm regime, a health team needs to be constructed. This should involve owners, manager, stockpersons and the veterinarian, and it also needs the understanding of the genetic and nutrition suppliers. A degree of openness is required, which is alien to many farms who are more used to a degree of silence about actual farm events. This takes trust and honesty. Each member of the farm health team has specific roles; the veterinarian plays the vital role of the 'pig' speaking up for the animal's biology and is the 'honest broker' with robust checking systems.

Antibiotic-free farming is about getting the management right:

- Management of pathogens.
- Management of pig flow.
- Management of immunity.
- Management of the environment.
- Management of any compromised pigs.
- Management of people.

All the sections need to be understood. In this section the minimum requirements to be followed are discussed. Antibiotic-free farming is the combination of all the previous sections and chapters, and as such is an interesting summary of pig health.

Management of pathogens requirements for an antibiotic-free system

Location

The farm should be at least 1 km away from the nearest pig farm. An isolation area is essential. Each of the isolation areas then runs as a strict AIAO programme. Each isolation area needs to be at least 50 metres from the main farm and obviously each more than 1 km from adjacent farms. The prevailing wind should be from the main farm towards the isolation areas. This can prove impossible in many areas (**Figure 11.229**).

There must be good lines of communication between the genetic supplier's veterinarian and the farm veterinarian. The genetic company should prepare a health declaration and be willing to prioritise the antibiotic-free farm with regard to health information. Consistent and quality gilt supply is an essential component to pig flow.

Vermin control has to be proactive. Buildings should be bird proofed wherever possible.

Cleaning of batch areas. The antibiotic-free farm needs to minimise contact with pathogens. Pathogen reduction is achieved by removing all faeces and allowing the room to dry.

Reducing internal spread of pathogens:

- From weaning to 30 kg (10 weeks of age) the stockpersons should wear a different specific coloured set of boots for each batch of pigs.

- In the farrowing area, each batch should have its own brush and scrapers, ideally colour and number coded.
- Do not move oral medicators, needles and syringes between batches of pigs.
- Footbaths can assist by improving stockperson attitude and can disinfect clean utensils. Brush clean all boots before using the disinfectant footbath.

Always examine healthy pigs before any sick pigs and move from the youngest to the oldest pigs.

Pathogen review

Before embarking on an antibiotic-free regime, elimination of certain pathogens would make the enterprise more likely to succeed. The major pathogens that should be removed from a commercial farm include: *Brachyspira hyodysenteriae* (swine dysentery), *Sarcoptes scabiei* var *suis* (mange), *Mycoplasma hyopneumoniae* (enzootic or mycoplasma pneumonia), PRRSV and Aujeszky's disease virus. It is assumed that the farm is free of major World Organisation for Animal Health (OIE) pathogens or active vaccine programmes are in place to control the pathogens.

Certain pathogens may be difficult to remove but acute clinical signs of the disease should be absent from the farm. These include *Streptococcus suis* II *et al.*, (meningitis), *Haemophilus parasuis* (*Glässer's disease*)/*Mycoplasma hyorhinis/Streptococcus* spp./ *Actinobacillus suis* (polyserositis), *Escherichia coli* F18

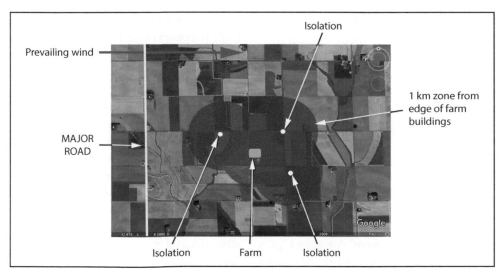

Fig. 11.229 Review of the farms position in terms of potential pathogen spread.

(oedema disease) and *Actinobacillus pleuropneumoniae* (porcine pleuropneumonia).

Management of pig flow

Adopting the batch concept

Any farm attempting to have an AIAO programme must run a batch system.

Correct stocking densities facilitate good health

The purpose of instigating a pig flow model is to eliminate over- and understocking of the farrowing house, nursery and finishing area. It is only when a room is empty of pigs that it can be cleaned and, as importantly, maintained. The farm must resist the temptation to 'make up' losses by over producing later on. This particularly involves post-summer heat issues that have resulted in a reduced farrowing rate and slower finishing growth. When farming without antibiotics it is imperative that the pigs are not overstocked and that stocking rates are adhered to in practice.

The second inevitable event the health team must accept is that if the farm is described in terms of sows, for example a 1,000 sow unit, the production of pork/bacon must vary as farrowing rates will fall over the summer months. This variation in output can be 15% over the year. To stabilise the pork/bacon output the herd size must vary (i.e. being bigger at the beginning of summer and smaller at the beginning of winter).

Management of immunity

Innate immunity

The best immunity is achieved by using animals that have no receptor sites for the 'pathogen'. The selection of pigs and the use of DNA mapping will enhance our knowledge of the pig's natural resistance to pathogens. Lines of pigs are already commercially available that are 'resistant' to *Escherichia coli* F18 (oedema disease) and F4 (K88) (pre- and post-weaning diarrhoea) or PRRSV. Several breeding companies are already recording resistance to diseases/pathogens and disorders within their selection pressures; for example, not selecting future gilts and boars from sows and gilts whose piglet's demonstrate pre-weaning diarrhoea (**Figure 11.230**).

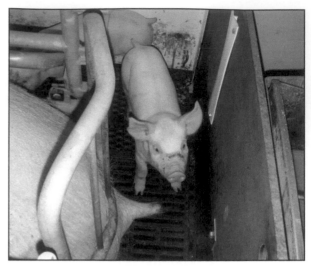

Fig. 11.230 These piglets should not be selected for future breeding as they have demonstrated a tendency towards having pre-weaning diarrhoea.

Acquired immunity

Preventive medicine programmes rely on a healthy immune system being stimulated via effective vaccines or endemic pathogens using protocols such as feedback programmes or direct exposure.

Immune suppression

Any agent or factor that can impair the pig's immune system should be avoided. For example, mycotoxins can be introduced into the herd through feed, poor feed storage or bedding. A careful review of these items is required by the health team. It may be better to use old rotten straw for composting rather than bedding, especially if it results in either an abortion storm or a PRRS breakthrough affecting the gilt's immune system.

Pathogens can affect the immune system; SIV is a prime example. If the herd undergoes a SIV break, this may affect the gilt's immune response to the preventive vaccination programme. This may result in the need to extend the isolation and acclimatisation time or revaccination. The batch must still be achieved.

In the piglet and weaner, iron anaemia can result in ill-health, particularly post-weaning diarrhoea. Proper administration of iron at 3–5 days of age by injection is advised. Note that iron should not be administered to piglets that have diarrhoea. Iron supplementation is not required if the pigs are pasture reared.

Adult herd

Healthy adult herd and introduction of new genetics: A major risk to the herd's health is the introduction of live animals into the herd. The farm has two major options to obtain new breeding gilts: (1) breed their own gilts, or (2) purchase breeding gilts from a genetic supplier.

If the farm is large enough, parity segregation should be considered as a better option to reduce the risk of pathogen introduction and spread around the farm.

Teaser boars should be sourced from on-farm stock. Male genes should be obtained through AI. In general terms AI is a highly efficient and biosecurity safe method of moving male genes. On-farm AI stations should be considered.

Parity profile: A herd's natural immunity can be disturbed by the introduction of large numbers of gilts. The pig flow model will predict the number of gilts required, allowing for careful planning of isolation.

Herd immunity: To reduce the necessity for antibiotics, the health of the adult herd needs to be enhanced by the use of vaccines. However, if vaccines are not stored properly, they will be inactivated. Feedback programmes can be used to cover pathogens not available in vaccines.

Piglets

The runt pig: Piglets born less than 800 g weight should be euthanased at birth before they have consumed any colostrum. Colostrum is limited and must be used wisely. Do not waste colostrum on piglets that have a 90% chance of dying before 115+ kg liveweight.

Gilt litters: Ideally, all gilt litters should also receive some colostrum from an adjacent sow by spilt suckling.

Infectious load: Reduce the infectious load on the piglet by excellent cleaning and drying of the farrowing accommodation. Washing the sow pre-entry into the farrowing area reduces faecal contamination of the udder and reduces the number of parasite eggs (e.g. *Ascaris suum*). In non-pasture reared sows remove the faeces from behind the sows daily for 3 days pre- and post farrowing.

Coccidiosis: *Cystoisospora suis* is an insidious pathogen of piglets and results in chronic, often subclinical, injury to the small intestine.

Iron deficiency anaemia: Sow's milk is deficient in iron. The piglet naturally would acquire the necessary iron from eating soil from the farrowing nest environment.

Blood-borne pathogens: Do not unnecessarily spread blood-borne pathogens between litters (e.g. *Mycoplasma suis* and PRRSV). Take care with castration blades between litters. At most, use one needle per litter.

Avoid piglet growth limitations: All measures that may reduce or interfere with the piglet's growth should be avoided, including most piglet processing: teeth clipping, tail docking, castration and ear notching. Fostering should be practiced only minimally and only to even up litters and not after day 3, unless absolutely necessary.

Birth to weaning: Evening up of litters by day 3 post farrowing has enormous benefits. However, this must be managed to maximise the colostrum intake of each piglet. After day 3, fostering should be avoided whenever possible.

The weaned pig

Weaning the pig: Weaning the pig is extremely stressful. The weaned piglet has little idea where to eat, drink, sleep or defecate, especially in a new foreign environment. If the building has been adequately cleaned, the natural landmarks have disappeared. It is essential that you create these environmental signals. A big pen environment is the easiest to assist this:

- Create a sleeping area away from any draught (less than 0.2 m/s) and water supplies.
- Create a defecation area that is cold, damp, possibly draughty (about 0.3 m/s) and dark/dim.
- Teach the new weaner when and how to eat; on the day of weaning they were being fed every hour by their mother, who told them when to eat. They are not hunger driven.
- Provide copious amounts of freely accessible water, but not from a nipple that has low flow rates and is out of reach (because it is still set for the previous 30 kg pigs).

Vaccines at weaning: Administer vaccines to the pig where applicable. Ileitis (porcine intestinal adenopathy, *Lawsonia intracellularis*) occurs on most farms. Vaccines are available, which can be administered at or even before weaning.

Streaming – not all pigs are born equal: The smallest 10% of pigs at weaning should be removed from the main group and given special attention and time to adapt to their circumstances. On many antibiotic-free farms, these are actually removed from the system altogether and farmed along traditional lines with the use of conventional prophylactic treatment methods. This also allows for any fall-out pigs from the antibiotic-free group/room/batch to be treated humanely.

Grow/finish

It is essential that the pigs remain in their own cohort. Neither pigs nor materials from other batches should enter their environment. Ideally, on batch antibiotic-free farms, a wean to finish system should be employed as this reduces the pig's exposure to novel pathogens.

Management of the environment

Set parameters for the environment and ideally have them posted in a prominent position; for example, on the entry door. The health team should be provided with suitable equipment to measure and adjust the environment of the pigs. The building, prior to the pig's entering, must be suitable for the animals to move into. It must be capable of maintaining a suitable environment for the entire duration of the animal's occupancy. Animals are not there to warm and dry the building.

Management of compromised pigs

The compromised pig is a major health threat to the farm as well as creating enormous welfare problems. Farm staff must realise that euthanasia is a good welfare option and keeping severely compromised pigs alive is cruel. Production figures should be about realities rather than just numbers. Killing pigs on the first of the month in order to reduce last month's figures is not acceptable.

Management of people

The success of an antibiotic-free programme depends on the stockpersons. Training, encouragement and provision of confidence in the system is essential. Stockpersons need to realise that they cannot cheat the system. Antibiotics are easily revealed in the slaughterhouse and food processing laboratories.

Production targets only matter once the farm is profitable

Moving from a traditional farm towards an antiobiotic-free farm. The programme below takes about 2 years to complete.

Current farm	Antibiotics to 70 kg liveweight in the finishing herd
1st phase	Remove antibiotics from adult herd
	Remove antibiotics from growing pigs heavier than 30 kg
2nd phase	Remove antibiotics from weaned pigs heavier than 18 kg
3rd phase	Remove prophylactic antibiotics from all healthy pigs Use only injectable or oral medication for the compromised pigs
4th phase	Separate all medicated compromised pigs from the main farm unit

CLINICAL QUIZ

11.1 What species is shown in **Figure 11.183** (see p. 449)?

11.2 What breeds are shown in **Figure 11.217** (see p. 452)?

The answers to these questions can be found on page 478.

CONVERSION FACTORS

To convert from SI units to old/conventional units, divide by the conversion factor.

	SI UNITS	CONVERSION FACTOR	OLD/ CONVENTIONAL UNITS
Haematology			
PCV	l/l	0.01	%
RBCs	$\times 10^{12}$/l	1	$\times 10^6$/µl
Erythrocytes	$\times 10^9$/l	1	$\times 10^3$/µl
Nucleated cell count	$\times 10^9$/l	1	$\times 10^3$/µl
Eosinophils	$\times 10^9$/l	1	$\times 10^3$/µl
Fibrinogen	g/l	100	mg/dl
MCV	fl	n/a	fl
MCH	pg	n/a	pg
MCHC	g/l	10	g/dl
Biochemistry			
ALP	U/l	1	IU/l
ALT	U/l	1	U/l
ACTH	pmol/ml	0.22	pg/ml
Albumin	g/l	10	g/dl
Ammonia (NH_4)	µmol/l	0.587	µg/dl
Amylase	U/l	1	U/l
AST	U/l	1	U/l
Bilirubin	µmol/l	17.1	mg/dl
Calcium	mmol/l	0.2495	mg/dl
Carbon dioxide	mmol/l	1	mEq/l
Chloride	mmol/l	1	mEq/l
Cholesterol	mmol/l	0.0259	mg/dl
Copper	µmmol/l	0.157	µg/dl

	SI UNITS	CONVERSION FACTOR	OLD/ CONVENTIONAL UNITS
Cortisol	nmol/l	27.59	µg/dl
Creatine kinase (CK)	U/l	1	IU/l
Creatinine	µmol/l	88.4	mg/dl
GGT	U/l	1	U/l
GLDH	U/l	1	U/l
Globulin	g/l	10	g/dl
Glucose	mmol/l	0.0555	mg/dl
Iron, binding	µmol/l	0.179	µg/dl
Iron, total	µmol/l	0.179	µg/dl
Lipase	U/l	1	IU/l
	U/l		Cherry-Crandall U
Magnesium	mmol/l	0.4114	U/l
Osmolality	mmol/l	1	Osm/kg
Phosphorus	mmol/l	0.323	mg/dl
Potassium	mmol/l	1	mEq/l
Protein, total	g/l	10	g/dl
SDH	U/l	1	IU/l
Selenium	µmol/l	0.1266	µg/dl
Sodium	mmol/l	1	mEq/l
Triglycerides	mmol/l	0.0113	mg/dl
Triiodothyronine (T3)	nmol/l	0.0154	µg/dl
Thyroxine (T4)	nmol/l	12.5	µg/dl
Urea nitrogen	mmol/l	0.357	mg/dl
Uric acid	mmol/l	59.48	mg/dl
Vitamin E	µmol/l	2.322	mg/ml

(Continued)

Needle size conversions

LENGTH		GAUGE	
MM	IN	MM	G
16	5/8	0.8	21
25	1	1.1	19
35	1 3/8	1.3	18
40	1 5/8		

CLINICAL QUIZ: ANSWERS

CHAPTER 1

1.1 *Look at the clinical signs shown in* **Figures 1.21–1.105**. *Can you identify what condition or conditions, where applicable, are illustrated.* Note that the clinical signs are only part of the differential diagnosis. The diagnoses provided here are what was found in these cases; after investigation other diagnoses could have been possible.

1.21	Porcine pleuropneumonia	1.51	Rectal stricture	1.78	Porcine epidemic diarrhoea
1.22	Normal	1.52	Congenital oedema and double muscling	1.79	*Ascaris suum*
1.23	Pneumonia	1.53	Congenital deformity of the foot	1.80	Normal
1.24	Glässer's disease			1.81	Colitis
1.25	Leukaemia	1.54	Ear biting	1.82	Ileitis
1.26	Pneumonia	1.55	Vulva biting	1.83	Constipation water issues
1.27	Iron anaemia	1.56	Tail biting	1.84	Ileitis
1.28	Erysipelas	1.57	Prolapsed uterus	1.85	Swine dysentery
1.29	Staphylococcal infection from poor teeth clipping	1.58	Rectal prolapse	1.86	Swine dysentery
		1.59	Perineal prolapse	1.87	Liver failure
1.30	Hock trauma	1.60	Pneumonia/Glässer's disease	1.88	*E. coli* post-weaning scour
1.31	Mange			1.89	Normal
1.32	*Salmonella enterica* serotype *choleraesuis*	1.61	Porcine pleuropneumonia	1.90	Cystitis
		1.62	Streptococcal meningitis	1.91	Pyelonephritis
1.33	Fat blind			1.92	Mycotoxicosis
1.34	Greasy pig disease	1.63	Stroke	1.93	Normal
1.35	Foot and mouth disease	1.64	Mange	1.94	Normal
1.36	Bush foot	1.65	Split hips	1.95	Monorchid
1.37	Joint ill	1.66	Broken leg	1.96	Normal; the pig has drawn his left testicle closer to his body, making it look as though there is atrophy
1.38	Ulcerative granuloma	1.67	Infected foot		
1.39	Abscess	1.68	Normal		
1.40	Aural haematoma	1.69	Normal		
1.41	Melanoma	1.70	Shortage of feed	1.97	Streptococcal orchitis
1.42	Oedema disease	1.71	Chemical burn eye	1.98	T2 toxin
1.43	Overgrown toes	1.72	Progressive atrophic rhinitis	1.99	Normal
1.44	Chronic mastitis			1.100	PRRS
1.45	Scrotal hernia	1.73	Mange	1.101	Mycotoxicosis
1.46	Umbilical hernia	1.74	Atrophic rhinitis	1.102	PRRS
1.47	Acquired hernia trauma	1.75	Salmonellosis	1.103	Normal
1.48	Cyclops	1.76	Vulval discharge	1.104	Leg abscess
1.49	Kyphosis	1.77	Gastric ulcer	1.105	PCV2-SD
1.50	Atrophic rhinitis				

1.2 *Figures 1.231–1.283 illustrate what might be seen when undertaking a post-mortem examination. Can you identify the different conditions that may be associated with these findings?*

1.231	Porcine pleuropneumonia	1.248	Cystic ovaries	1.265	Scrotal haemangioma
1.232	Erysipelas	1.249	Infarct in kidney	1.266	Chronic mastitis
1.233	Rectal stricture	1.250	Lymphosarcoma in the rib cage	1.267	Purulent dermatitis
1.234	Renal hyoplasia			1.268	Embryonic folding – kidney
1.235	Greasy pig disease	1.251	Stomach with oedema disease		
1.236	Melanoma of the skin			1.269	Skin tumour
1.237	PDNS	1.252	Ileitis	1.270	Pericarditis
1.238	Mange along the dorsum	1.253	Necrotic ileitis	1.271	Enzootic (mycoplasma) pneumonia
		1.254	Carpal erosions in a piglet		
1.239	Flank biting	1.255	*Borrelia* granuloma	1.272	Skull of peccary – note teeth pointing forward
1.240	1, normal; 2, normal; 3, red – cystitis; 4, blood – pyelonephritis	1.256	End-stage kidney	1.273	Normal faecal pellet
		1.257	Chronic mastitis	1.274	Colitis faeces
1.241	Endocardiosis	1.258	Leiomyoma of the uterus	1.275	Streptococcal abscess
1.242	Ringworm	1.259	Mulberry heart disease	1.276	Fluid-filled abscess
1.243	Pityriasis rosea	1.260	Gastric ulceration	1.277	Clostridial hepatopathy
1.244	Tearing of the uretero-vesical junction	1.261	Oesophageal stricture	1.278	Urinary calculi
		1.262	Nasal tumour	1.279	Chronic mange
1.245	Congenital swine pox lesions	1.263	*Salmonella enterica* serotype *choleraesuis* in the lung	1.280	Normal nose
				1.281	PRRSV in lungs
1.246	Skin tumour			1.282	Udder oedema
1.247	Pyelopnephritis	1.264	Thymic tumour	1.283	Shoulder abscess

CHAPTER 2

2.1 *In the middle of oestrus how long does a sow stand for mating?* (E) 15 minutes

2.2 *In the middle of oestrus, after being in standing heat, how long will it take for an average sow to respond to a boar by standing again?* (D) 45 minutes

2.3 *Some reproductive viruses are classified as SMEDI viruses. What is the meaning of this acronym? Give two examples of porcine viruses that may create these clinical signs.* SMEDI viruses refer to viruses that can result in stillborn, mummified, embryonic death and infertility as combined clinical signs. Two examples of porcine viruses could include:

- Porcine circovirus 2
- Japanese encephalomyelitis virus
- Porcine parvovirus
- Porcine teschovirus

- Porcine reproductive and respiratory syndrome virus
- Aujeszky's disease virus (pseudorabies)
- Classical swine fever virus

2.4 *Which mycotoxin is a phytoestrogen?* The mycotoxin zearalenone is a phytoestrogen and can mimic maternal recognition signals.

CHAPTER 3

3.1 *Identify the other lesion/s in the lung in* **Figure 3.58** *that are not associated with the Ascaris migration.* There is cranioventral consolidation – enzootic (mycoplasma) pneumonia. Note that the lesion extends further caudal than would be the case with uncomplicated EP.

3.2 *Why do ceftiofur, penicillin and amoxicillin have no effect on Mycoplasma hyorhinis?* The 'penicillin' family destroys the bacterial cell wall. As mycoplasma organisms do not have a cell wall, this family of antibiotics cannot have any action on *M. hyorhinis*.

3.3 *The pig's anatomy affects the pathogenesis of enzootic (mycoplasma) pneumonia. Explain. Mycoplasma hyopneumoniae* is a descending infection of pigs; the cranial part of the lung is affected first. Thus the lesion is cranioventral rather than caudal. The fact that the pig has a tracheal bronchus on the right-hand side (see **Figure 3.7**) results in the right apical lobe being the first lung lobe to be affected with enzootic (mycoplasma) pneumonia, therefore this lobe will tend to have more consolidation than other lobes.

CHAPTER 4

4.1 *Look at the clinical signs illustrated in* **Figures 4.16a–4.16j**. *What conditions may be associated with the different colours of the faeces?*

4.16a   *E. coli*, coccidiosis, 'milk scour', salmonellosis.

4.16b   *E. coli* post weaning, colitis (*Brachyspira*), ileitis, PED, nutritional scours.

4.16c   Swine dysentery, ileitis.

4.16d   Ileitis, swine dysentery.

4.16e   Rectal blood associated with constipation.

4.16f   Gastric ulcer, ileitis (haemorrhagic).

4.16g   *E. coli*, rotavirus, coronavirus diarrhoea (PED/TGE).

4.16h   *Salmonella enterica* serotype *choleraesuis*.

4.16i   Possible liver issues or old faeces.

4.16j   *Ascaris suum*.

4.2 *Look at the gross pathology illustrated in* **Figures 4.17–4.26**. *What are the classic conditions for each of the pathology states described? Do not just look at the figure.*

4.17   Rectal stricture, *E. coli*, PED, starvation.

4.18   Coccidiosis, ileitis, salmonellosis, clostridial enteritis, spirochaetal colitis.

4.19   Ileitis, swine dysentery, haemorrhagic bowel syndrome, clostridial enteritis, torsion, intussusception.

4.20   Salmonellosis, classical swine fever, gastric ulcer.

4.21   Colitis, swine dysentery.

4.22   *Clostridium difficile*, PCV2-SD.

4.23   Regional ileitis.

4.24   Clostridial enteritis, post-mortem emphysema.

4.25   Rectal stricture, oesophageal stricture.

4.26   Mesenteric ossification: gross and radiographic image.

4.3 *What do you see in* **Figure 4.59** *that could affect pre-weaning diarrhoea control measures?* The farrowing house room looks clean and well managed. However, there is a significant pre-weaning diarrhoea problem affecting 7 to 12-day-old piglets from multiple parities. Looking at the photograph you will see that there is a lot of air movement in the house, as indicated by the sow cards (arrows). At piglet level this air movement was 0.4 m/s cold air (i.e. a draught). Once this was controlled the pre-weaning diarrhoea problem resolved.

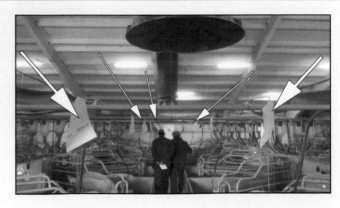

CHAPTER 5

5.1 *Identify the anatomical structures in* ***Figure 5.4***.

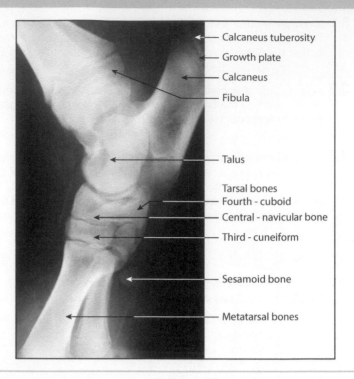

Calcaneus tuberosity
Growth plate
Calcaneus
Fibula
Talus
Tarsal bones
Fourth - cuboid
Central - navicular bone
Third - cuneiform
Sesamoid bone
Metatarsal bones

5.2 *Why does auscultation at one end and tapping the other end of the bone not work for diagnosing epiphysiolysis?* The greater trochanter of the femur and the lateral condyle of the femur are available for auscultation and percussion. However, in epiphysiolysis these components of the femur are still connected. The epiphysiolysis lesion is in the femoral neck.

CHAPTER 6

6.1 *Identify the structures in* ***Figure 6.1***.

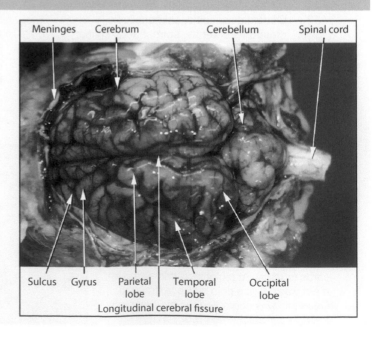

Meninges   Cerebrum   Cerebellum   Spinal cord

Sulcus   Gyrus   Parietal   Temporal   Occipital
lobe   lobe   lobe
Longitudinal cerebral fissure

CHAPTER 7

7.1 *Identify the major organs and the tumour shown in* **Figure 7.25**.

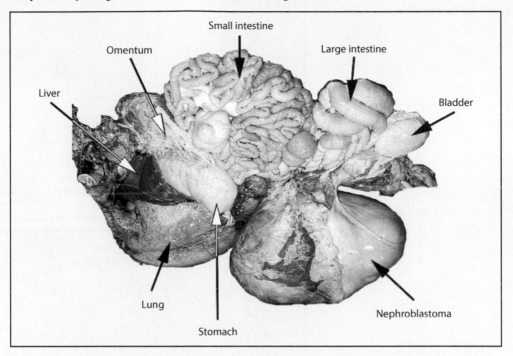

7.2 *Identify the major structures shown in* **Figure 7.27**.

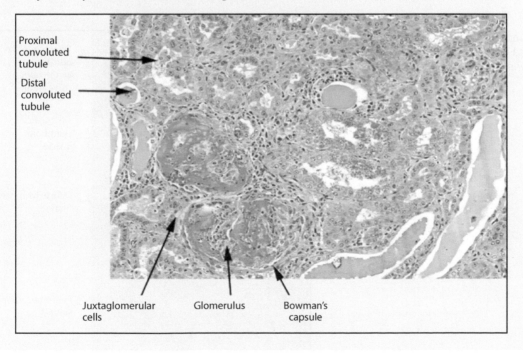

CHAPTER 8

8.1 *Identify the superficial lymph nodes arrowed in **Figures 8.1a, b**.*

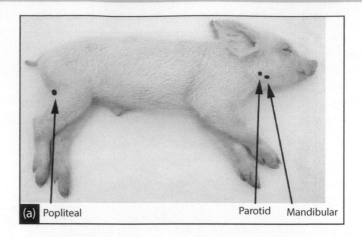

(a) Popliteal   Parotid   Mandibular

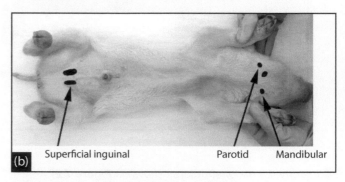

(b) Superficial inguinal   Parotid   Mandibular

8.2 *Identify the structures shown in the histological section of a porcine lymph node in **Figure 8.3**.*

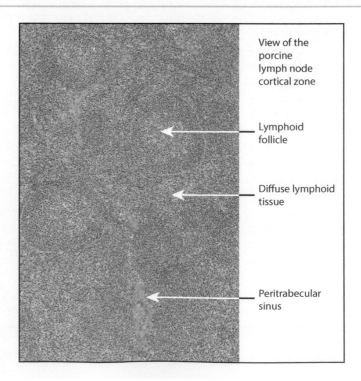

View of the porcine lymph node cortical zone

Lymphoid follicle

Diffuse lymphoid tissue

Peritrabecular sinus

CHAPTER 9

9.1 *Label the other structures shown in Figure 9.21.*

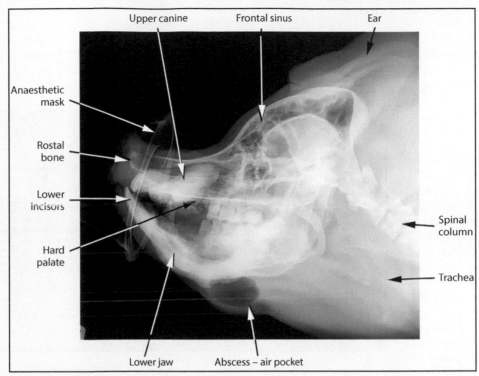

Upper canine

Frontal sinus

Ear

Anaesthetic mask

Rostal bone

Lower incisors

Hard palate

Spinal column

Trachea

Lower jaw

Abscess – air pocket

CHAPTER 10

10.1 *List some pig behaviours that may indicate inadequate water supply (Figure 10.14).*

- Crowding around drinkers.
- Increased time spent drinking
- Increased aggression.
- Bizarre behaviour patterns.

- Off feed.
- Changes in anatomy.
- Reduction in growth rates.
- Variable performance within the same group.

10.2 *How do you read a maximum/minimum thermometer?*

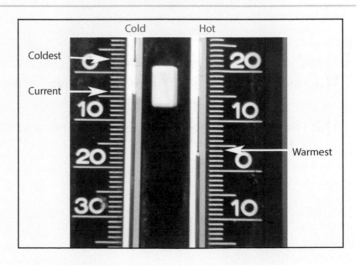

Cold

Hot

Coldest

Current

Warmest

10.3 *What is wrong with the pig in the middle in* **Figure 10.61.** The pigs in general are dirty and this is generally an indication that their general environment is too hot. The pig in the middle (arrow) has two clinical problems:

1. He has a very large umbilical hernia (arrowhead).
2. He is not eating properly and is in poor body condition – compare this pig with the pigs on either side of him.

The pig on the left, however, was very talkative and looks happy!

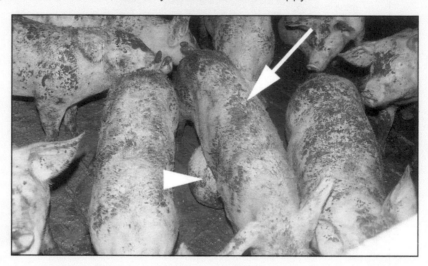

10.4 *What are the characteristics of sleeping versus defecation areas? Fill in the empty boxes in Table 10.20.*

SLEEPING	DEFECATION
Dry	Wet
Warm/hot	Cold
No draughts	Draughty
Light	Dark
Open	Private
Comfortable	Uncomfortable

CHAPTER 11

11.1 *What species is shown in* **Figure 11.183**? A red river hog (*Potamochoerus porcus*).

11.2 *What breeds are shown in* **Figure 11.217**? The centre black and white piglet is a Berkshire, the others are Large White/Yorkshire pigs.

You can access the resources that are referenced in the text and listed in *Tables A* and *B* below via the companion website by using the following link:

https://www.crcpress.com/9781498704724

It will take you to a webpage where you can click on Downloads/Updates to access the resources themselves.

VIDEO CLIPS

The videos do not describe the ideal environment for raising pigs as such ideals do not exist. In each video, there are areas where the veterinary surgeon could recommend improvement to benefit the welfare and wellbeing of the pigs. The video clips of groups of pigs can be used to compare the clinical cases.

- Review the videos and history and describe what you see.
- Prepare a differential diagnosis list.
- What tests would you perform to confirm/reduce the differential list?
- Review each of the differentials you have listed and review the treatment options.
- Make a diagnosis!
- Also review the video clips on normal pigs at various stages of production and the audio files.
- Enjoy.

Table A gives the numbers of the video clips, the page numbers of the text they are associated with, and commentaries that summarise the video content and clinical cases.

Table A **Video clips**		
VIDEO NUMBER	**PAGE NUMBER**	**COMMENTARY**
1	1, 54, 55, 378	Breeding area – a breeding group demonstrating artificial insemination in a teaching environment where sows are both in oestrus and not in oestrus
2A, B, C	1, 62, 89, 262, 378	Farrowing area. Note the disparity in size and climate requirements of piglets and lactating sows. Three videos: (A) demonstrating the farrowing process; (B) suckling process in piglets a few days old; (C) piglets at 3 weeks of age.
3A, B	1, 378	Nursery. Two videos demonstrating the nursery behaviour on a farm: (A) where stockpersons talked and interacted with their weaners and farm; (B) where the weaners were well looked after, but the stockpersons had little interaction with them, but did their job.
4	1, 357, 378	Interaction at feeding time between pigs.

(Continued)

Table A *(Continued)* **Video clips**

VIDEO NUMBER	PAGE NUMBER	COMMENTARY
5A, B, C, D	1, 311, 378	Finishing pigs: (A) on straw; (B) in a tunnel-ventilated evaporative cool cell finishing house; (C) outside with a large wallow; (D) finishing pigs with a toy.
6	3	*Obvious clinical signs:* A Vietnamese Pot Belly pig presents with skin inflammation in the skin folds of the groin. The pig is reluctant to freely move. The pig is grossly overweight. The other three pigs are also overweight. The cross-bred white pig also has a lachrymal discharge on its face and may be 'fat blind'. *History indicates:* That these are pet pigs in a sanctuary. *Diagnosis:* Overweight pigs are liable to serious joint issues in later life. Fat blindness may also be a problem in later life.
7	54, 55	*Obvious clinical signs:* While walking the farm you notice a group of sows pushing, fighting and being vocal to each other. *History indicates:* That these sows were weaned 5 days previously. *Diagnosis:* Oestrous behaviour. The sow in the background is almost in oestrus and may stand. The sow in the foreground is coming into oestrus.
8	75	*Obvious clinical signs:* A female 110 kg Large White gilt in a gilt development pen presents with a protrusion from the vulva. Examination revealed this was an enlarge clitoris. The building is a little dark. This makes checking the gilts more difficult and lighting patterns may influence reproductive performance. The tails on these selected gilts are too short, especially for breeding stock. Despite this being a pen of future gilts, there is also a castrated boar. *History indicates:* That there was some confusion over gilt selection protocols. These two pigs were missed. *Diagnosis:* Hermaphrodite.
9	85	*Obvious clinical signs:* A large Vietnamese Pot Belly-cross female pig, 14 years of age. The pig has a very large abdomen, which is distended, especially ventrally. She is walking slowly but is not lame. Her toes are a little long, both the main digits and the supernumerary digits. *History indicates:* That the enlarged abdomen has been under observation for 6 months. The sow eats, drinks, defecates and urinates every day. She is happy to walk around and look for food. She lives with two other pigs and has good accommodation. *Diagnosis:* Leiomyoma.
10	85	*Obvious clinical signs:* A sow presents with a white purulent discharge from her vulva about 3 weeks after breeding. *History indicates:* That the pig was seen yesterday at 18 days' post breeding. No other pigs are presenting with the same clinical sign. However, the farrowing rate is 78% and this is not an uncommon occurrence. *Diagnosis:* 14–21-day post-service vulval discharge.
11	87, 266	*Obvious clinical signs:* A cross-bred gilt of about 50 kg bodyweight presents with an enlarged vulva. There appears to be blood on her flank. Another pig is sitting hunched on its own. *History indicates:* That there were a number of other young gilts also with enlarged vulvas. Examination also revealed enlarged nipples in both female and male growing pigs. *Diagnosis:* Zearaleonone mycotoxicosis.

(Continued)

Table A *(Continued)* **Video clips**

VIDEO NUMBER	PAGE NUMBER	COMMENTARY
12	90	*Obvious clinical signs:* A sow presents with a large ventral mass. There appear to be two healing ulcerated areas associated with the mass. The other mammary tissue has receded.
		History indicates: That the sow farrowed 60 days ago and was weaned 32 days ago. She has just been scanned pregnant and the stockperson has requested a clinical examination to determine her future on the farm.
		Diagnosis: Chronic mastitis.
13A, B, C, D	105, 123, 129, 148, 172, 295	*Obvious clinical signs:* A, B and C are clinical cases where the presenting sign is coughing; D shows a group of pigs who are not coughing:
		(A) Finishing Large White pigs around 80 kg liveweight with a cough. Multiple pigs are affected. (The problem had occurred for several years on the farm).
		(B) Finishing Large White pigs around 50 kg liveweight with a cough. Multiple pigs are affected. Note the overflowing feeder resulting in wasted feed.
		(C) Growing outdoor Berkshire pigs about 40 kg liveweight with a cough. One pig has a large lump ventrally.
		(D) Growing pigs on a *Mycoplasma hyopneumoniae*-negative unit without an audible cough.
		History indicates:
		(A) That this problem was very common on the farm and in each batch; some pigs would start to cough at around 60–80 kg.
		(B) That it was unusual and the cough occurred suddenly and spread rapidly around the farm and affected all age groups.
		Diagnosis:
		(A) Enzootic (mycoplasma) pneumonia.
		(B) Swine influenza.
		(C) *Ascaris suum*, umbilical hernia.
		(D) Healthy pigs.
		Comment: Pigs on pasture are more likely to have parasites, although *Ascaris suum* is also common on indoor farms. In all the different videos note and recognise the different breeds illustrated: Large White (Yorkshire), Landrace, Duroc, Berkshires, Gloucestershire Old Spot pig and various cross-bred pigs.
14A, B, C	118	*Obvious clinical signs:* The farm has experienced a sudden increase in mortality in finishing pigs. Three videos:
		(A) There is a finishing pig, 45 kg bodyweight, in lateral recumbency and dying in the pen. The pig is mouth breathing. There are a large number of flies. Other pigs appear normal. The pigs are wet fed. The house is very quiet;
		(B) In another pen in the same house, there is a dead pig under the feeder. The other pigs appear cold and huddled together. A few are lying correctly. The pigs look in good body condition. The house is very quiet.
		(C) In another house with 60 kg bodyweight pigs there are a large number of pigs not eating. There was a low degree of coughing. The breathing pattern of several pigs was more visual that normal.
		History indicates: That the farm is specific pathogen free of *Mycoplasma hyopneumoniae* and porcine reproductive and respiratory syndrome. There is no history of swine influenza on the farm. Normal finishing rate is 96%, but 100 finishing pigs have died in the last 6 days. The farm weans 3,000 pigs a week. Post-mortem examination of the two dead pigs indicated a pleuropneumonia in the diaphragmatic lobe of both pigs.
		Diagnosis: Actinobacillus porcine pleuropneumonia.
		Laboratory: *Actinobacillus pleuropenumoniae* cultured and antimicrobiogram prepared.

(Continued)

Table A *(Continued)* **Video clips**

VIDEO NUMBER	PAGE NUMBER	COMMENTARY
15	123, 284, 359	*Obvious clinical signs:* Post-weaning/young growing pigs presenting with a foreshortened snout. The pigs are in good body condition. The foreshortened snout is present in a number of pigs. Note the short sneezing bouts. One pig presents with epistasis in the left nostril. One pig presents with an aural haematoma, possibly because the pigs are sneezing and shaking their heads. With cases of epistasis it is likely to be acute rather than long-standing.
		History indicates: That this was the first outbreak on an otherwise negative farm.
		The problem was only in the weaners and early growers.
		Diagnosis: Progressive atrophic rhinitis associated with toxigenic *Pasteurella multocida* D. Aural haematoma. Note the good feeder management.
16	134, 217, 367, 373	*Obvious clinical signs:* A male cross-bred finishing pig in good body condition, which is lame on both front legs. Both front legs are unnaturally bent at the carpal joint. The pig has been noticed by the stockperson, as indicated by the mark on its back.
		History indicates: That this is not an uncommon occurrence in the finishing herd. There is also a high incidence of pleurisy in the slaughterhouse.
		Diagnosis: Poor floors and overstocking resulting in polyarthritis associated with a range of bacterial organisms. The farm has a background of problems with Glässer's disease.
17A, B	134	*Obvious clinical signs:* Two pigs isolated in a recovery pen. One pig, a 30 kg Large White growing pig, has dyspnoea and is in poor body condition. The ribs are showing and the pig is having serious problems breathing. Neither pig is up and talking to the other pigs outside their recovery pen. The pigs look cold and there is no obvious coughing or sneezing.
		Post-mortem findings: Severe septic pericarditis.
		History indicates: That this was not an unusual occurrence on the farm. The farm has a finishing rate of 93%.
		Diagnosis: Glässer's disease.
		Laboratory: Haemophilus parasuis and *Streptococcus suis* were isolated.
18	134, 139, 429	*Obvious clinical signs:* A cross-bred growing pig about 35 kg bodyweight. The pig is losing weight and is hairy and gaunt. The pig has been noticed by the stockperson and may be receiving treatment. Other pigs also have treatment marks on their back, so this might be a recovery pen. There is no obvious diarrhoea or lameness.
		History indicates: That this was a hospital pen. The finishing rate for this farm is 94%.
		Diagnosis: Mixed respiratory distress with Glässer's disease and pasteurellosis. *Laboratory: Haemophilus parasuis* and *Pasteurella multocida* isolated.
19A, B	143, 274	*Obvious clinical signs:* During a routine visit you notice 3–4 week old pigs in the farrowing area that are lethargic and reluctant to move. The piglets have dyspnoea and cyanosis of the ears. You continue your visit to the nursery and notice that the hospital pen in the nursery is full of pigs that are sick and poor doing. The weaners are 1-week post-weaning. They are lethargic and some have lost weight, with their spine and ribs visible. Some have become hairy. The weaners are being supported with additional heat and gruel feed in a long trough. Mortality has doubled. All the pigs in the hospital pen have been given tulathromycin (25 mg/kg bodyweight) by injection.
		History indicates: That the farm is positive for porcine reproductive and respiratory syndrome (PRRS), classical swine fever, porcine circovirus type 2 and *Mycoplasma hyopneumoniae*. There are vaccination programmes against all of these pathogens. Five sows have aborted and the sows have not eaten properly over the last 2 weeks. Whole farm PRRS vaccination occurred a month ago.
		Post-mortem exmination: Post-mortem of the piglets revealed few gross findings; the lungs appeared not to collapse properly. Post-mortem of the nursery pigs revealed many cases of polyserositis – Glässer's disease. Some euthanased pigs had no gross changes.

(Continued)

Table A *(Continued)* **Video clips**

VIDEO NUMBER	PAGE NUMBER	COMMENTARY
		Diagnosis: PRRS.
		Laboratory: Introduction of a novel strain on an already positive farm. Confirmed by sequence analysis of the RNA of the novel strain.
20	188	*Obvious clinical signs:* Examination of a grower pen on a specific pathogen free nucleus farm reveals a dysenteric faecal mass. The majority of the pigs in the pen look normal and healthy albeit variable in size. One pig, however, looks gaunt and underweight. Examination of this individual pig demonstrates that the dysentery is being passed from this pig.
		History indicates: That the farm has not had a problem with dysentery, although there has been a low-grade diarrhoea present in the growing pigs, which is believed to be nutritionally based. The farm is free of a range of pathogens including *Brachyspira hyodysenteriae* and classical swine fever.
		Post-mortem examination: Reveals a haemorrhagic distal ileitis with bloody faeces also present in the caecum and colon. *Lawsonia intracellularis* is known to be present on the farm.
		Diagnosis: L. intracellularis infection.
		Laboratory: L. intracellularis identified on immunohistochemistry.
21	188	*Obvious clinical signs:* Two cross-bred growing pigs around 40 kg bodyweight present with profuse diarrhoea. The diarrhoea is very liquid and is a light grey colour. There is no blood, mucus or frothing. There is an older puddle of diarrhoea. Other piles of faeces appear normal.
		History indicates: That the farm has a history of low-grade diarrhoea in grower and finishing pigs. The farm is specific pathogen free of *Brachyspira hyodysenteriae*, *Mycoplasma hyopneumoniae* and porcine reproductive and respiratory syndrome.
		Diagnosis: Lawsonia intracellularis ileitis. Note this could be a swine dysentery breakdown.
		Laboratory: No *Brachyspria hyodysenteriae* isolated or identified by PCR.
22A, B	190	*Obvious clinical signs:* Two videos: (A) On entry to the farrowing area it is apparent there is a major problem with the young suckling piglets. Nearly all the litters appear to have severe diarrhoea. The piglets appear very cold. There is very watery diarrhoea evident on the floor and on the pigs. There are numerous areas of vomit. The litter size is very small. The stockpersons have placed charcoal in the pens for the piglets to eat. The sows are very quiet and not eating properly. Walk around the rest of the farm. (B) The adult sows are very unresponsive and not talking. There are puddles of diarrhoea, which is greenish in colour, evident on the floor, together with more normal looking faeces.
		History indicates: That the clinical problems started 2 days ago. Previously the farm was consistently weaning 100 kg of piglet per sow at 27 days with minimal problems. The sows were healthy with an 87% farrowing rate.
		Diagnosis: Porcine epidemic diarrhoea (PED).
		Laboratory: PED 2a infection confirmed.
23	195, 196	*Obvious clinical signs:* Growing Large White pigs about 35 kg bodyweight. One pig with red stockperson marks presents with a large abdomen. The pig does not move away from the veterinarian quickly. The pig is thin and the spinal vertebrae, ribs and shoulder blades can be visualised. Other pigs look normal.
		History indicates: That this was an individual pig on the farm.
		Diagnosis: Rectal stricture as a sequela of a rectal prolapse.
24A, B	198, 200	*Obvious clinical signs:* (A) Cross-bred weaned pigs. The weaner presents with yellow diarrhoea on the perianal region and tail. The weaner has lost a lot of condition and is very emaciated. Other pigs in the group are in much better body condition. (B) A view of the hospital pen from the same farm. There are a number of other emaciated pigs.

(Continued)

Table A *(Continued)* **Video clips**

VIDEO NUMBER	PAGE NUMBER	COMMENTARY
		History indicates: That 2 weeks ago the farm started with a serious diarrhoea problem in the nursery. The diarrhoea lasts around 10 days. The mortality in the nursery has escalated.
		Post-mortem examination: Revealed a diphtheritic typhlitis and colitis.
		Diagnosis: Salmonella enterica serotype *typhimurium.*
		Laboratory: Confirmation of the presence of *Salmonella enterica* serotype *typhimurium* and an antimicrobiogram prepared.
25	216	*Obvious clinical signs:* Kune kune pig with a horizontal crack on the medial side of the left front foot running parallel to the coronary band. The crack also runs forward along the base of the toe. The pig is reluctant to place full weight on the left front foot. He is eating.
		History indicates: That the crack appeared 2 days ago. The pig was very lame initially but following administration of pain relief its stance has improved and he has started to eat again.
		Diagnosis: Split hoof requiring remedial care.
26	218, 345	*Obvious clinical signs:* Duroc and Large White gilts – four in the pen. One of the Duroc gilt is lame on her right hind leg. The pig is able to place her foot on the ground but is reluctant to place all her weight on the foot. The solid part of the pen, intended for sleeping, is covered in faecal material, which has not been cleared away. There is a hanging drinker at the interface of the solid and slatted part of the pen. There is a light flashing to the right of the pen.
		History indicates: That these pre-mating gilts were sound when they were moved from the isolation area and placed in the pen 10 days ago. This shifting lameness is seen frequently affecting the mainly the hind legs and responds to a course of tiamulin treatment.
		Diagnosis: Mycoplasma hyosynoviae arthritis.
27	220	*Obvious clinical signs:* A Duroc sow post-weaning presents with a large swelling on its right fore foot. The lesion is large with surface cracks. The pig is placing weight on the foot. The pig is also lame on the right hind leg and is only just weight bearing on this foot. There is a horizontal crack at the coronary band. When moving the right hind foot is not placed properly, and from time is placed under the body of the sow. The left fore leg also has a lump over the elbow joint.
		History indicates: That the pig was seen to develop an injection in the right fore foot 1 week before farrowing. The farm team treated the sow and decided to allow her to farrow and suckle her piglets. At weaning the sow has been placed in the cull sow pen and the veterinarian has been called to determine if she needs on-farm euthanasia or can be sent to the slaughterhouse. She is outside all medicine withdrawal periods.
		Diagnosis: Bush foot.
28	220	*Obvious clinical signs:* Cross-bred piglets about 3 days post-farrowing. One stockperson marked piglet is 10/10 lame on it right front leg. The right elbow appears swollen. An additional piglet is slightly hairy and has a stockperson mark but appears lively. The litter on the right are a couple of days older and have been tail docked.
		History indicates: That the lame pig was noticed this morning and treated. The other piglet yesterday had a mild diarrhoea and treatment with electrolytes was initiated.
		Diagnosis: Streptococcus suis I synovitis.
29	222	*Obvious clinical signs:* The Landrace gilt is lame on the left hind leg. When the pig moves the left hind leg swings in underneath the body.
		History indicates: That the gilt was normal in oestrus yesterday and was walking normally. She ate and drank normally yesterday. The stockperson found her this morning reluctant to rise. When the stockperson managed to get the pig onto her feet she was reluctant to walk.
		Diagnosis: Epiphysiolysis.

(Continued)

Table A *(Continued)* **Video clips**

VIDEO NUMBER	PAGE NUMBER	COMMENTARY
30	223, 231	*Obvious clinical signs:* Piglets in the farrowing house. Large White piglets presenting with neurological problems. This is called dancing piglets. Occurs in a number of the piglets. Piglets are vigorous and trying to suckle. Splay leg in day-old piglets on the left and the piglet on its own. No obvious signs on diarrhoea. Other litters are unaffected.
		History indicates: That the dancing occurs predominately in the party 1 litters.
		Diagnosis: Congenital tremor II and splay leg.
31	223	*Obvious clinical signs:* Cross-bred piglets 1 day of age. One pig is unable to rise. The pig is ridge backed. The pig's hind legs are splayed and the pig cannot get them under his body. Other walking piglets are slipping on the heat pad. The ears have been notched.
		History indicates: That such pigs are common on the farm.
		Diagnosis: Splay leg.
32	233	*Obvious clinical signs:* Cross-bred weaned pigs about 6 kg bodyweight. One pig is in lateral recumbency and is paddling. Note the paddling marks in the bedding. The pig is aware of its surroundings but unable to rise. There is a small degree of ophthalmos.
		History indicates: That the pig was weaned 4 days previously and was not noticed to be sick at the morning check.
		Diagnosis: Meningitis.
		Laboratory: Bacteriology revealed *Streptococcus suis* II from the meninges and post-mortem examination a meningitis associated with gram-positive cocci.
33	236	*Obvious clinical signs:* Young cross-bred weaner about 6 kg liveweight in a group of 10 kg weaners presents with a head tilt. The pig's head is tilted to the right and the pig circles to the right. The pig has been noted by the stockperson as indicated by the mark on its head. The pig is underweight, has noticeable breathing and is hairy. The pig is tail docked and other pigs are not tail docked.
		History indicates: That the farm has no history of similar cases.
		Diagnosis: Middle ear disease.
34A, B	269	Two different farms present with identical clinical signs: A is a North American farm; B is a Eastern European farm.
		Obvious clinical signs:
		(A) A few smaller cross-bred finishing pigs in a group of larger pigs. Average weight of the bigger pigs is 90 kg; the smaller pigs range from 35 to 60 kg. The small 35 kg pig is also thin and is breathing more heavily than normal.
		(B) A pen of growing pigs, about 30 kg, that contains a number of variable weight smaller pigs (five at least). One pig has a cough. Another pig defecates with normal faeces.
		History indicates: That in farm A the finishing rate had fallen to 80% over the last 3 batches (15 weeks) – the farm utilised 5-week batching and the problem was getting worse, with a particular problem with full hospital pens. Antibiotics did not improve the situation and the poor pigs were very slow recovering. In farm B the finishing rate again had fallen to 85%. The problem has only been seen in the last 6 weeks, with a sudden change in otherwise great performance. Antimicrobial medication appears to have minimal effect. The farm has attempted to change the feeding routines, again with no change in performance.
		Both farms are positive for porcine circovirus type 2 and do not vaccinate.
		Post-mortem examination: On the wasting pigs revealed few gross signs but a loss of body fat. Bronchial lymph nodes were enlarged.
		Diagnosis: PCV2-SD.

(Continued)

Table A *(Continued)* **Video clips**

VIDEO NUMBER	PAGE NUMBER	COMMENTARY
35	282, 420	*Obvious clinical signs:* Large White sow in the farrowing house with piglets about 10 days of age. The sow presents with a large 4 cm diameter lump behind her left ear at the normal site of injection. The lump is red and inflamed. There is no heat mat for the piglets; additional head is provided by a heat lamp. *History indicates:* That the last injection for this sow was 3 weeks prior to farrowing when the sow was vaccinated using an *Escherichia coli* vaccine. The stockperson claims there was no lump at this time. *Diagnosis:* Abscess.
36	134, 284, 310	*Obvious clinical signs:* Grower cross-bred pigs about 35 kg in an autosort feeding system present with ear biting in a majority of the pigs. One pig presents with a bitten tail. Several pigs present with an aural haematoma. One thin hairy pig with stockperson marks appears behind the feeders. *History indicates:* That the ear biting started in the nursery. However, tail biting is also common at 60 kg. *Diagnosis:* Vice ear biting, aural haematoma, Glässer's disease.
37	287	*Obvious clinical signs:* Large White female 60 kg finishing pig in good body condition. The pig's skin has red diamond-shaped lesions on the skin. Other pigs look all right. Pig would normally be pyrexic, off its food and lethargic. *History indicates:* That this was an acute case. No other pigs were affected on the farm. *Diagnosis:* Erysipelas.
38	293	*Obvious clinical signs:* Nursery cross-bred female weaner about 6 kg bodyweight. The pig's skin is dark and greasy. The ears and neck appear particularly affected with crusty material in/on the skin. The lesions appear circular is shape but are often coalesced into plaque areas. The pig is subdued. The weaners are against the rear wall and are not approaching the stockperson. Other pigs are biting the tails of pen mates. One male pig has numerous marks on the face and neck. Some of the pigs are licking the far wall. *History indicates:* That this problem is common in pigs but generally resolves at about 3 weeks post-weaning. There are some cases also seen in the farrowing house. Affected pigs may be pyretic. *Diagnosis:* Greasy pig disease. *Laboratory:* Isolation of *Staphylococcus hyicus* provided a suitable antimicrobiogram.
39	297	*Obvious clinical signs:* During routine examination of a group of weaner pigs about 25 kg in bodyweight, small black marks are noted adherent to the pigs. Examination reveals that they are numerous and some are moving around. *History indicates:* That this is a well-established small family farm with 20 sows. *Diagnosis:* Pig lice (*Haematopinus suis*).
40	297	*Obvious clinical signs:* Adult Large White sows and a Duroc in a breeding row. Several of the sows are pruritic (itchy). No other obvious clinical abnormalities. *History indicates:* That this has been an ongoing problem on the farm for several years. Affects all age groups, especially in the late growers seasonally. *Diagnosis:* Mange. *Laboratory:* *Sarcoptes scabiei* var *suis* demonstrated.

(Continued)

Table A *(Continued)* **Video clips**

VIDEO NUMBER	PAGE NUMBER	COMMENTARY
41	301	*Obvious clinical signs:* A 30 kg growing pig presents with skin lesions that have spread over the surface of the skin. The lesions are circular and many are merged. The lesions are rough with a crusty centre and a raised edge, which is blanched. The pig is otherwise healthy with a 38°C rectal temperature and eating and drinking normally.
		History indicates: That this is the only pig with this condition on the farm. Similar pigs have been seen over the last couple of years and the lesions gradually resolved over 1 month.
		Diagnosis: Pityriasis rosea.
42	301	*Obvious clinical signs:* Landrace castrated male pig, about 80 kg bodyweight and in good body condition, presents with purple blotches over its body, concentrated towards the rear of the pig and high contact places – shoulders. The lesions appear circular with a darker centre and outer ring. The pig is walking freely and appears curious regarding its surroundings.
		History indicates: That the farm has serious problems with wasting and ill thrift in the growing phase. The are a couple of cases with skin issues a month. The farm is porcine circovirus I and II positive. The farm does not vaccinate sows or nursery pigs with PCV2 vaccine.
		Diagnosis: Porcine dermatitis and nephropathy syndrome.
43	310	*Obvious clinical signs:* Large White finishing pigs around 80 kg bodyweight present with blood and ulceration of the tail tip. The tail is black. The tail of the pig in the foreground is swollen. The affected pigs are eating. A third pig appears where the tail appears to have been lost altogether. A fourth pig has blood clearly evident at the tip of the tail. Unaffected pigs have variable tail lengths post-docking. Other pigs that also have damage to their tails are seen in the pen.
		History indicates: That there has been a problem with a variety of vices over the last month. It is winter time and the weather is very cold outside.
		Diagnosis: Vice and stress problems in the pigs, which is revealed by the tail biting.
44A, B, C	321	(A) Water flow poor for growing pigs who require 1 litre per minute. The flow was 0.5 litres per minute. (B) Removal of the drinker in A revealed blocked filters. Once cleaned the drinker worked adequately. (C) Water flow too much for nursery pigs – requirement would be 0.7 ml per minute. This flow was over 4 litres per minute and at a high pressure.
45	326	Air pattern around house as demonstrated by smoke at the inlet.
46	188, 356, 378, 404	*Obvious clinical signs:* Variable finishing pigs between 35 and 50 kg. A large pig is dominating a feeder. The feeder has too much food and food has been spilt. The large pig is stopping the smaller pig from having access to the feeder.
		Action: Feeder management should be reviewed. Examine the role of ileitis on the farm. Examine the pig flow management of all-in-all-out.
47	378	*Obvious clinical signs:* A Duroc sow in a farrowing place. There are no piglets and the behaviour of the sow indicates that it is trying to adopt nesting behaviour. There is a small amount of feed in the feeder.
		History indicates: That the sow should farrow tomorrow.
		Action: Training opportunity in stockpersonship in providing for the expression of normal behaviour. Lack of toys and nesting material.

AUDIO FILES

Clinicians need to learn to 'talk to their clients'; this includes the pigs under their care. It is important that clinicians learn to use all their senses when making a clinical diagnosis. In this exercise, we strengthen the sense of sound. It should be possible to recognise normal pig talking around the farm and then distinguish sounds of distress and clinical problems.

The audio files are presented twice: once with a black screen so that you can only listen, and then with the video active so you can confirm what you thought your ears were telling you.

Table B **Audio files**

AUDIO NUMBER	PAGE NUMBER	
S1	1, 378	Lactating sow calling piglets to suckling.
S2	1, 378	Finishing pig's general talking.
S3	1, 378	Piglets talking general.
S4	1, 378	Pig general greeting.
S5	1, 378	Piglets trying to encourage sow to lie down and suckle.
S6	1, 378	Finishing pigs asleep.
S7	378	Finishing pig's active.
S8	378	Weaners just moved distressed.
S9	141, 378	Mild sneezing in nursery pigs.
S10	129, 139, 378	Coughing with enzootic (mycoplasma) pneumonia.

INDEX

T - #0554 - 071024 - C512 - 261/194/23 - PB - 9780367893408 - Gloss Lamination